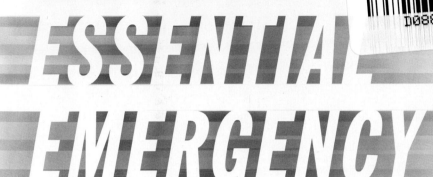

ESSENTIAL EMERGENCY IMAGING

ESSENTIAL EMERGENCY IMAGING

Editors

Resa E. Lewiss, MD
St. Luke's-Roosevelt Hospital Center
Assistant Professor of Clinical Medicine
Columbia University College of Physicians and Surgeons
New York, New York

Turandot Saul, MD
St. Luke's-Roosevelt Hospital Center
Assistant Professor of Clinical Medicine
Columbia University College of Physicians and Surgeons
New York, New York

Kaushal H. Shah, MD
Associate Professor
Mt. Sinai School of Medicine
New York, New York

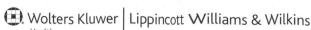

. Wolters Kluwer | Lippincott Williams & Wilkins
Health

Philadelphia · Baltimore · New York · London
Buenos Aires · Hong Kong · Sydney · Tokyo

Senior Acquisitions Editor: Frances DeStefano
Product Director: Julia Seto
Production Manager: Alicia Jackson
Senior Manufacturing Manager: Benjamin Rivera
Senior Marketing Manager: Angela Panetta
Design Coordinator: Holly McLaughlin
Production Service: Aptara, Inc.

© 2012 by **LIPPINCOTT WILLIAMS & WILKINS, a WOLTERS KLUWER business**
2001 Market Street
Philadelphia, PA 19103 USA
LWW.com

Printed in China

Library of Congress Cataloging-in-Publication Data

Essential emergency imaging / editors, Resa E. Lewiss, Turandot Saul,
Kaushal H. Shah.
   p. ; cm. – (Essential emergency medicine series)
 Includes bibliographical references and index.
 ISBN 978-1-60831-893-3 (pbk. : alk. paper)
 1. Diagnostic imaging. 2. Medical emergencies. I. Lewiss, Resa E.
II. Saul, Turandot. III. Shah, Kaushal. IV. Series: Essential emergency
medicine series.
 [DNLM: 1. Diagnostic Imaging. 2. Emergencies. WN 180]
 RC78.7.D53E866 2012
 616.07'57–dc23

                                        2011022701

To purchase additional copies of this book, call our customer service department at (800) 638-3030 or fax orders to (301) 223-2320. International customers should call (301) 223-2300.

Visit Lippincott Williams & Wilkins on the Internet: at LWW.com. Lippincott Williams & Wilkins customer service representatives are available from 8:30 am to 6 pm, EST.

10 9 8 7 6 5 4 3 2 1

RRS1106

Dedication

Resa E. Lewiss

People grow through experience if they meet life honestly and courageously. This is how character is built (E. Roosevelt). To those individuals who have inspired me to live honestly and courageously.

Turandot Saul

I dedicate this book to my mother Ruth, my husband Josh and my twin boys, Zachary and Asher.

Kaushal H. Shah

I would like to dedicate this book to all the medical providers who stand with me in awe of the amazing medical technology available to us and yet think really hard before ordering that next imaging test despite the medico-legal environment and other external pressures.

And I would also like to dedicate this book to my wife, Vanisha, and our new daughter, Naya, without whom life would not be complete.

Contributors

Mara S. Aloi, MD
Assistant Professor
Department of Emergency Medicine
Drexel University School of Medicine
Philadelphia, Pennsylvania;
Program Director
Emergency Medicine Residency
Allegheny General Hospital
Pittsburgh, Pennsylvania

Phillip Andrus, MD, FACEP
Assistant Professor
Department of Emergency Medicine
The Mount Sinai School of Medicine
New York, New York

Brecken J. Armstrong-Kelsey, MD, MSt
Emergency Physician
Department of Emergency Medicine
Harbor-UCLA Medical Center
Torrance, California

Faizan H. Arshad, MD
Resident Physician
Department of Emergency Medicine
Yale New Haven Hospital
New Haven, Connecticut

Richard G. Bachur, MD
Associate Professor
Department of Pediatrics
Harvard Medical School;
Chief, Division of Emergency Medicine
Department of Medicine
Children's Hospital Boston
Boston, Massachusetts

Michael J. Barra, MD
Chief Resident
Division of Emergency Medicine
Washington University School of Medicine
St. Louis, Missouri

Marc N. Baskin, MD
Assistant Professor
Pediatrics
Harvard Medical School;
Senior Associate Physician
Division of Emergency Medicine
Children's Hospital
Boston, Massachusetts

Sarah M. Battistich, MD
Fellow and Clinical Instructor
Department of Emergency Medicine
Yale University School of Medicine
New Haven, Connecticut

Theresa M. Becker, DO
Instructor
Department of Pediatrics
Harvard Medical School;
Attending Physician
Division of Emergency Medicine
Children's Hospital Boston
Boston, Massachusetts

Suzanne K. Bentley, MD
Chief Resident
Department of Emergency Medicine
The Mount Sinai Medical School;
Chief Resident Physician
Department of Emergency Medicine
The Mount Sinai Medical Center
New York, New York

Kriti Bhatia, MD
Associate Residency Director,
Harvard Affiliated Emergency Medicine
Residency
Brigham and Women's/Massachusetts
General Hospitals
Staff Physician,
Department of Emergency Medicine
Brigham and Women's Hospital
Clinical Instructor,
Harvard Medical School

William D. Binder, MD
Assistant Professor
Division of Emergency Medicine
Harvard Medical School
Attending Physician
Department of Emergency Medicine
Massachusetts General Hospital

Glen D. Blomstrom, MD
Yale-New Haven Hospital Resident Physician
Department of Emergency Medicine
Yale University School of Medicine
New Haven, Connecticut

Laura J. Bontempo, MD, FACEP
Assistant Professor
Department of Emergency Medicine
Yale University;
EM Program Director
Department of Emergency Medicine
Yale-New Haven Hospital
New Haven, Connecticut

Pierre Borczuk, MD
Assistant Professor
Department of Medicine
Harvard Medical School;
Attending Physician
Emergency Services
Massachusetts General Hospital
Boston, Massachusetts

Mark F. Brady, MD, MPH
Resident
Department of Emergency Medicine
Yale-New Haven Hospital
New Haven, Connecticut

David F.M. Brown, MD
Vice Chair
Department of Emergency Medicine
Massachusetts General Hospital
Associate Professor
Division of Emergency Medicine
Harvard Medical School

Lara L. Bryan-Rest, MD
Clinical Fellow
Department of Radiology
Yale University School of Medicine
New Haven, Connecticut

Greg Buehler, MD
Assistant Professor
Section of Emergency Medicine
Department of Medicine
Baylor College of Medicine
Houston, Texas

Casey Buitenhuys, MD
Clinical Instructor
Department of Emergency Medicine
Harbor-UCLA Medical Center
Torrance, California

David Burbulys, MD
Associate Professor of Clinical Medicine
Department of Medicine
David Geffen School of Medicine at UCLA
Los Angeles, California;
Residency Program Director
Department of Emergency Medicine
Harbor-UCLA Medical Center
Torrance, California

Marc A. Camacho, MD, MS
Instructor
Department of Radiology
Harvard Medical School;
Section Chief, Emergency Radiology
Department of Radiology
Beth Israel Deaconess Medical Center
Boston, Massachusetts

Crystal Cassidy, MD
Assistant Professor
Section of Emergency Medicine
Department of Medicine
Baylor College of Medicine
Houston, Texas

Douglas Mark Char, MD, MA, FACEP, FAAEM
Associate Professor
Emergency Medicine
Washington University in St Louis;
Attending Physician
Emergency Medicine
Barnes-Jewish & St Louis Children's Hospitals
St Louis, Missouri

Betty Chen, MD
Resident
Division of Emergency Medicine
Washington University School of Medicine
St. Louis, Missouri

Samuel Clarke, MD
Medical Education Fellow
Emergency Medicine
Harbor-UCLA Medical Center
Los Angeles, California

Mieka Close, MD
Attending Physician
Jersey City Medical Center

Brian Cohn, MD
Clinical Instructor
Division of Emergency Medicine
Washington University School of Medicine
St. Louis, Missouri

Matthew Constantine, MD
Clinical Assistant Professor
Department of Emergency Medicine
Downstate/Kings County Hospital
Brooklyn, New York

Moira Davenport, MD
Assistant Professor
Department of Emergency Medicine
Allegheny General Hospital/Drexel University
College of Medicine;
Attending Physician
Department of Orthopaedic Surgery
Allegheny General Hospital/Drexel University
College of Medicine
Pittsburgh, Pennsylvania

Mark Deaver, MD, MBA
Resident
Department of Emergency Medicine
Harbor-UCLA
Torrance, California

Jason DeBonis, MD
Attending Physician
Los Angeles, California

Stephanie Donald, MD
Resident Physician
Department of Emergency Medicine
Harbor-UCLA Medical Center
Torrance, California

Nicholas Drakos, MD
Resident Physician
Emergency Medicine
Harbor-UCLA Medical Center
Torrance, California

Andrea Dugas, MD
Attending Physician
John Hopkins University
Baltimore, Maryland

Jonathan A. Edlow, MD
Associate Professor of Medicine
Department of Medicine
Harvard Medical School;
Vice Chair of Emergency Medicine
Department of Emergency Medicine
Beth Israel Deaconess Medical Center
Boston, Massachusetts

Daniel J. Egan, MD
Associate Residency Director
Department of Emergency Medicine
St. Luke's-Roosevelt Hospital Center
New York, New York

Robert R. Ehrman, MD
Chief Resident
Department of Emergency Medicine
Yale University School of Medicine
New Haven, Connecticut

Joy English, MD
Physician
Department of Emergency Medicine
Washington University School of Medicine
Saint Louis, Missouri

Chuck Feronti, DO
Resident Physician
Department of Emergency Medicine
Allegheny General Hospital
Pittsburgh, Pennsylvania

Jason W.J. Fischer, MD, MSc
Assistant Professor of Pediatrics
Department of Pediatrics
University of Toronto;
Staff Physician
Division of Emergency Medicine
Hospital for Sick Children
Toronto, Ontario

Jonathan I. Fischer, MD
Chief Resident
Department of Emergency Medicine
Yale School of Medicine
New Haven, Connecticut

Megan Fix, MD
Assistant Professor
Division of Emergency Medicine
University of Utah School of Medicine;
Associate Residency Director
Division of Emergency Medicine
University of Utah
Salt Lake City, Utah

Emily Fontane, MD, FACEP, FAAP
Associate Professor
Department of Emergency Medicine
University of Central Florida
Orlando, Florida

Samantha Foy, MD
Resident Physician
Department of Emergency Medicine
Beth Israel Deaconess Medical Center
Boston, Massachusetts

Christopher Freeman, MD
Assistant Professor
University of Texas Health Science Center
Attending Physician
Department of Emergency Medicine
Memorial Hermann Healthcare System
Houston, Texas

Joseph M. Fuentes, MD
Emergency Medicine
Washington University School of Medicine
St. Louis, Missouri;
Attending Physician
Department of Emergency Medicine
Kaiser Permanente San Jose
San Jose, California

Jennifer Galjour, MD, MPH
Department of Emergency Medicine
The Mt. Sinai Hospital
New York, New York

Michael Ganetsky, MD, FACEP
Clinical Instructor, Harvard Medical School
Department of Emergency Medicine
Beth Israel Deaconess Medical Center
Boston, Massachusetts

Joshua N. Goldstein, MD, PhD, FACEP
Assistant Professor
Department of Surgery
Harvard Medical School;
Attending Physician
Department of Emergency Medicine
Massachusetts General Hospital
Boston, Massachusetts

Moses B. Graubard, MD
Attending Physician
Department of Emergency Medicine
Kaiser Oakland Medical Center
Oakland, California

Richard T. Griffey, MD, MPH
Assistant Professor
Division of Emergency Medicine
Washington University School of Medicine;
Associate Chief
Division of Emergency Medicine
Barnes-Jewish Hospital
St. Louis, Missouri

Samuel Gross, MA, MD
Resident
Department of Emergency Medicine
Beth Israel Deaconess Medical Center
Boston, Massachusetts

Lisa Freeman Grossheim, MD, FACEP
Assistant Professor
Department of Emergency Medicine
University of Texas Medical School at Houston
Houston, Texas

Shamai A. Grossman, MD, MS
Assistant Professor
Medicine
Harvard Medical School;
Director, The Cardiac Emergency Center and
Clinical Decision Unit
Division of Emergency Medicine
Beth Israel Deaconess Medical center
Boston, Massachusetts

Iman Hassan, MD
Clinical Assistant Professor
Division of Pulmonary & Critical Care Medicine
University of Texas Health Science Center at
Houston
Houston, Texas

Nathan Hemmer, MD
Resident
Department of Emergency Medicine
Allegheny General Hospital
Pittsburgh, Pennsylvania

Daniel Henning, MD
Resident
Department of Emergency Medicine
Beth Israel Deaconess Medical Center
Boston, Massachusetts

Leah Honigman, MD
Resident Physician
Department of Emergency Medicine
Beth Israel Deaconess Medical Center
Harvard University School of Medicine
Boston, Massachusetts

Timothy Horeczko, MD
Clinical Instructor of Medicine
Emergency Medicine
David Geffen School of Medicine at UCLA
Los Angeles, California;
Attending Physician
Department of Emergency Medicine
Harbor-UCLA Medical Center
Torrance, California

Erin Roxanne Horn, MD
Chief Resident
Department of Emergency Medicine
Harvard Affiliated Emergency Medicine
Residency
Beth Israel Deaconess Medical Center
Boston, Massachusetts

Zoe D. Howard, MD
Resident Physician
Department of Emergency Medicine
Massachusetts General Hospital
Boston, Massachusetts

Randall A. Howell, DO, FAAEM, FACOEP, FACEP
Assistant Professor
Department of Emergency Medicine
Washington University School of Medicine
Saint Louis, Missouri

Jonie J. Hsiao, MD
Assistant Clinical Professor
Department of Medicine
David Geffen School of Medicine at UCLA
Los Angeles, California

Jonathan S. Ilgen, MD, MCR
Acting Assistant Professor
Division of Emergency Medicine
University of Washington School of Medicine
Seattle, Washington

Jason Imperato, MD, MBA, FACEP
Assistant Professor
Department of Medicine
Harvard Medical School
Boston, Massachusetts;
Attending Physician
Department of Emergency Medicine
Mount Auburn Hospital
Cambridge, Massachusetts

John E. Jesus, MD
Chief Resident
Department of Emergency Medicine
Beth Israel Deaconess Medical Center
Boston, Massachusetts

Christopher Kabrhel, MD MPH
Assistant Professor
Department of Surgery
Harvard Medical School;
Attending Physician
Department of Emergency Medicine
Massachusetts General Hospital
Boston, Massachusetts

Amy H. Kaji, MD, PhD
Assistant Professor
Emergency Medicine
Harbor-UCLA Medical Center
Torrance, California

Jacob B. Keeperman, MD
Fellow, Emergency Medical Services
Department of Emergency Medicine
Washington University in Saint Louis School of
Medicine;
Fellow, Critical Care Medicine
Department of Anesthesia
Washington University in Saint Louis School of
Medicine
Saint Louis, Missouri

Patrick R. Kennedy, MD
Resident
Division of Emergency Medicine
Washington University in St. Louis School of
Medicine
St. Louis, Missouri

Atif N. Khan, MD
Research Fellow
Department of Radiology
Beth Israel Deaconess Medical Center
Boston, Massachusetts

Jonathan Kirschner, MD
Assistant Professor
Attending Physician
Department of Emergency Medicine
Indiana University School of Medicine

Jessica H. Klausmeier, MD, MPH
Resident Physician
Department of Emergency Medicine
Beth Israel Deaconess Medical Center
Boston, Massachusetts

Jean E. Klig, MD, FAAP
Assistant Professor of Pediatrics
Harvard Medical School;
Associate Chief, Division of Pediatric
Emergency Medicine
Department of Emergency Medicine
Massachusetts General Hospital
Boston, Massachusetts

Jasmine A. Koita, MD
Resident Physician
Department of Emergency Medicine
Mount Sinai School of Medicine
New York, New York

Daniel A. Kopp, MD
St. Joseph's Hospital
St. Charles, Missouri

Katherine E. Kroll, MD
Resident
Department of Emergency Medicine
Beth Israel Deaconess Medical Center
Boston, Massachusetts

Khoshal Latifzai, MD
Resident Physician
Department of Emergency Medicine
Yale School of Medicine
New Haven, Connecticut

Christopher H. Lee, MD
Clinical Instructor
EMS and Disaster Medicine
Department of Emergency Medicine
Yale University School of Medicine
New Haven, Connecticut

Jarone Lee, MD, MPH
Attending Physician
Department of Emergency Medicine
St Luke's Roosevelt Hospital Center of
Columbia University
New York, New York

Lois K. Lee, MD, MPH
Assistant Professor
Department of Pediatrics
Harvard Medical School;
Attending Physician
Division of Emergency Medicine
Children's Hospital Boston
Boston, Massachusetts

Jill F. Lehrmann, MD, MPH
Assistant Professor
Department of Emergency Medicine
Northwestern University Feinberg School of
Medicine
Chicago, Illinois

Robin B. Levenson, MD
Instructor of Radiology
Division of Emergency Radiology
Department of Radiology
Beth Israel Deaconess Medical Center
Harvard Medical School
Boston, Massachusetts

Mark D. Levine, MD, FACEP
Assistant Professor
Division of Emergency Medicine
Washington University School of Medicine;
Attending Physician
Emergency Department
Barnes-Jewish Hospital
St. Louis, Missouri

Daniel Lindberg, MD
Instructor
Department of Emergency Medicine
Harvard Medical School;
Attending Physician
Department of Emergency Medicine
Brigham & Women's Hospital
Boston, Massachusetts

Ari M. Lipsky, MD, PhD, FACEP
Attending Physician
Department of Emergency Medicine
Santa Monica-UCLA Hospital Center
Santa Monica, California

Michael Lohmeier, MD
EMS Fellow
Emergency Medicine
Washington University School of Medicine at
Saint Louis
Saint Louis, Missouri

Keith A. Marill, MD
Assistant Professor
Department of Medicine (Emergency Medicine)
Harvard Medical School;
Attending Physician
Department of Emergency Medicine
Massachusetts General Hospital
Boston, Massachusetts

Daniel McGillicuddy, MD
Associate Director of ED Clinical Operations
Emergency Medicine
Beth Israel Deaconess Medical Center
Harvard Medical School
Boston, Massachusetts

Julie McManemy, MD, MPH
Assistant Professor
Department of Pediatrics
Washington University School of Medicine
St. Louis, Missouri

William P. Meehan III, MD
Instructor
Emergency Medicine
Children's Hospital Boston;
Instructor
Sports Medicine
Children's Hospital Boston
Boston, Massachusetts

Delwin Merchant, MD
Resident Physician
Department of Emergency Medicine
Washington University in St Louis School of
Medicine
St. Louis, Missouri

Sara Miller, MD
Assistant Professor
Department of Emergency Medicine
University of Texas Health Science Center at
Houston
Houston, Texas

Kyle Minor, MD
Chief Resident
Department of Internal Medicine
Division of Emergency Medicine
University of Wisconsin
Madison, Wisconsin

Christopher L. Moore, MD
Assistant Professor
Department of Emergency Medicine
Yale University School of Medicine
New Haven, Connecticut

Ravi Morchi, MD
Assistant Professor
Department of Emergency Medicine
Harbor UCLA Medical Center
Torrance, California

Hawnwan Moy, MD
Physician
Emergency Medicine
Washington University Barnes Jewish Hospital
Saint Louis, Missouri

Joshua Nagler, MD
Assistant Professor
Department of Pediatrics
Harvard Medical School;
Attending Physician
Division of Emergency Medicine
Children's Hospital Boston
Boston, Massachusetts

Jolene Nakao, MD, MPH
Resident
Department of Emergency Medicine
St. Luke's-Roosevelt Hospital Center
Columbia University College of Physicians and
Surgeons
New York, New York

Sreeja Natesan, MD
Resident Physician
Department of Emergency Medicine
Barnes Jewish Hospital/St. Louis Children's
Hospital
St. Louis, Missouri

Bret P. Nelson, MD, RDMS, FACEP
Associate Professor
Department of Emergency Medicine
Mount Sinai School of Medicine
New York, New York

David D. Nguyen, MD, FACEP
Assistant Professor
Department of Medicine/Division of Emergency
Medicine
Baylor College of Medicine
Houston, Texas;
Assistant Professor
Department of Surgery/Division of Emergency
Medicine
The University of Texas Medical Branch
Galveston, Texas

Vicki E. Noble, MD
Director, Division of Emergency Ultrasound
Department of Emergency Medicine
Massachusetts General Hospital
Assistant Professor, Harvard Medical School
Boston, Massachusetts

Kevin Nuttall, MD
Resident
Emergency Medicine
Beth Israel Deaconess Medical Center
Boston, Massachusetts

Joanne L. Oakes, MD, FACEP
Associate Professor
Department of Emergency Medicine
The University of Texas Health Science Center
at Houston
Houston, Texas

Ryan O'Neill, DO
Resident
Department of Emergency Medicine
Allegheny General Hospital
Pittsburgh, Pennsylvania

Ngozi Onyenekwu, MD
Resident
Emergency Medicine/Internal Medicine
Allegheny General Hospital
Pittsburgh, Pennsylvania

Joshua A. Ort, MD
Department of Emergency Medicine
Allegheny General Hospital
Pittsburgh, Pennsylvania

Michael R. Osborne, MD, FACEP, RDMS, RDCS
Associate Professor
Department of Emergency Medicine
University of Kentucky College of Medicine
Lexington, Kentucky

Caroline Pace, MD
Assistant Professor
Department of Emergency Medicine
Medical College of Wisconsin
Milwaukee, Wisconsin

Peter D. Panagos, MD, FACEP, FAHA
Associate Professor
Department of Emergency Medicine
Washington University;
Associate Professor
Department of Neurology
Washington University
St Louis, Missouri

Ram A. Parekh, MD
Assistant Professor
Emergency Department
Mount Sinai School of Medicine
New York, New York;
Attending Physician
Emergency Department
Elmhurst Hospital Center
Queens, New York

Ashley K. Peko, MD, MS
Resident Physician
Department of Emergency Medicine
McGaw Medical Center of Northwestern University
Chicago, Illinois

Joshua Penn, MD
Resident
Division of Emergency Medicine
Harvard Affiliated Emergency Medicine Residency
Harvard Medical School
Boston, Massachusetts

Catherine E. Perron, MD
Assistant Professor
Department of Pediatrics
Harvard University Medical School;
Attending Physician
Division of Emergency Medicine
Children's Hospital Boston
Boston, Massachusetts

M. Tyson Pillow, MD
Assistant Professor
Department of Medicine
Baylor College of Medicine;
Assistant Residency Program Director
Section of Emergency Medicine
Ben Taub General Hospital
Houston, Texas

Cori McClure Poffenberger, MD
Assistant Professor
Clinical Medicine
David Geffen School of Medicine at UCLA
Los Angeles, California;
Director, Adult Emergency Department
Department of Emergency Medicine
Harbor-UCLA Medical Center
Torrance, California

Brian Popko, MD, FACEP
Attending Physician
Department of Emergency Medicine
Allegheny General Hospital
Pittsburgh, Pennsylvania

Stacey L. Poznanski, DO
Clinical Instructor
Department of Emergency Medicine
Boonshoft School of Medicine
Wright State University
Kettering, Ohio

Bridget J. Quinn, MD
Attending Physician
Department of Orthopedics Division of Sports Medicine
Children's Hospital Boston;
Attending Physician
Department of Orthopedics Division of Sports Medicine
Beth Israel Deaconess Medical Center
Boston, Massachusetts

Nicholas Rathert, MD
Resident
Emergency Medicine
Washington University School of Medicine
St. Louis, Missouri

Gregory S. Rebella, MD
Assistant Professor
Pediatrics and Medicine
University of Wisconsin School of Medicine and
Public Health
Madison, Wisconsin

Michael J. Rest, MD
Assistant Professor
Department of Emergency Medicine
Yale University
New Haven, Connecticut

Hector Rivera, MD
Resident
Department of Emergency Medicine
Yale University School of Medicine
New Haven, Connecticut

Thomas E. Robey, MD, PhD
Department of Emergency Medicine
Yale-New Haven Hospital
New Haven, Connecticut

Carlo L. Rosen, MD
Associate Professor
Department of Medicine
Harvard Medical School;
Program Director and Vice Chair for Education
Harvard Affiliated Emergency Medicine
Residency
Beth Israel Deaconess Medical Center
Boston, Massachusetts

Gregory E. Rumph, MD
Assistant Professor
Section of Emergency Medicine
Department of Medicine
Baylor College of Medicine
Houston, Texas

Amina Saghir, MBBS, MD
Department of Internal Medicine
Saint Vincent Hospital
Worcester, Massachusetts

Christopher S. Sampson, MD, FACEP
Assistant Professor
Emergency Medicine
Washington University in Saint Louis
Saint Louis, Missouri

Leon D. Sanchez, MD, MPH
Assistant Professor
Department of Medicine
Harvard Medical School;
Attending Physician
Department of Emergency Medicine
Beth Israel Deaconess Medical Center
Boston, Massachusetts

Turandot Saul, MD
Assistant Professor
Department of Emergency Medicine
Columbia University School of Medicine;
Attending Physician
Department of Emergency Medicine
St. Luke's Roosevelt Hospital
New York, New York

Sara A. Schutzman, MD
Assistant Professor
Department of Pediatrics
Harvard Medical School;
Attending Physician
Division of Emergency Medicine
Children's Hospital Boston
Boston, Massachusetts

Sonya Seccurro, MD, MS
Chief Resident
Department of Emergency Medicine
St. Luke's-Roosevelt Hospital Center/Columbia
University
New York, New York

Todd A. Seigel, MD
Assistant Professor (Clinical)
Department of Emergency Medicine
Warren Alpert School of Medicine
Brown University;
Attending Physician
Department of Emergency Medicine
Rhode Island Hospital
Providence, Rhode Island

Magdy H. Selim, MD, PhD
Associate Professor
Department of Neurology
Beth Israel Deaconess Medical Center
Harvard Medical School;
Co-Director, Stroke Center
Beth Israel Deaconess Medical Center
Boston, Massachusetts

David Seltzer, MD
Assistant Professor
Division of Emergency Medicine
Washington University in St Louis School of
Medicine
St. Louis, Missouri

Emily L. Senecal, MD
Clerkship Director
Department of Emergency Medicine
Harvard Medical School;
Attending Physician
Department of Emergency Medicine
Massachusetts General Hospital
Boston, Massachusetts

Karen D. Serrano, MD
Chief Resident
Division of Emergency Medicine
University of Wisconsin School of Medicine &
Public Health
Madison, Wisconsin

Sachita P. Shah, MD
Assistant Professor
Department of Emergency Medicine
Warren Alpert Medical School of Brown
University;
Attending Physician
Department of Emergency Medicine
Rhode Island Hospital
Providence Rhode Island

Sejal Shah, MD, MS
Instructor
Department of Radiology
Beth Israel Deaconess Medical Center
Boston, Massachusetts

Kaushal H. Shah, MD, FACEP
Associate Professor
Emergency Department
Mount Sinai School of Medicine
New York, New York;
Associate Residency Director
Emergency Department
Elmhurst Hospital
Elmhurst, New York

Pranav P. Shetty, MD
Resident Physician
Department of Emergency Medicine
Harbor-UCLA Medical Center
Torrance, California

Sanjay Shewakramani, MD
Assistant Professor
Department of Emergency Medicine
Georgetown University Hospital
Washington, District of Columbia

Sandy S. Sineff, MD
Assistant Professor
Department of Emergency Medicine
Washington University School of Medicine;
Attending Physician
Department of Emergency Medicine
Barnes-Jewish Hospital
St. Louis, Missouri

Craig A. Sisson, MD, FACEP
Assistant Clinical Professor
Department of Emergency Medicine
East Carolina University, Brody School of
Medicine
Greenville, North Carolina

Peter B. Smulowitz, MD, MPH, FACEP
Instructor
Department of Medicine
Harvard Medical School;
Attending Physician
Department of Emergency Medicine
Beth Israel Deaconess Medical Center
Boston, Massachusetts

Aaron Sodickson, MD, PhD
Assistant Professor
Radiology
Harvard Medical School;
Assistant Director of Emergency Radiology
Department of Radiology
Brigham and Women's Hospital
Boston, Massachusetts

Jeffrey Peter Spear, MD
Resident
Emergency
Beth Israel Deaconess Medical Center
Boston, Massachusetts

Jeffrey W. Spencer, MD
Resident Physician
Emergency Medicine
Washington University School of Medicine
St. Louis, Missouri

Adarsh K. Srivastava, MD
Resident
Department of Emergency Medicine
Allegheny General Hospital
Pittsburgh, Pennsylvania

Anne M. Stack, MD
Assistant Professor
Department of Pediatrics
Harvard Medical School;
Senior Associate Physician
Department of Medicine
Children's Hospital Boston
Boston, Massachusetts

Dana A. Stearns, MD
Assistant Professor
Department of Emergency Medicine
Massachusetts General Hospital;
Assistant Professor
Department of Surgery
Harvard Medical School
Boston, Massachusetts

Sean P. Stickles, MD
Resident Physician
Division of Emergency Medicine
Washington University in St. Louis School of
Medicine
St. Louis, Missouri

Shannon Straszewski, MD
Resident
Emergency Medicine
Beth Israel Deaconess Medical Center
Boston, Massachusetts

Keith J. Strauss, MSc, FAAPM, FACR
Clinical Instructor
Department of Diagnostic Radiology
Harvard Medical School;
Director Radiology Physics and Engineering
Department of Radiology
Children's Hospital Boston
Boston, Massachusetts

Darrell Sutijono, MD
Clinical Instructor
Department of Emergency Medicine
Yale University School of Medicine;
Attending Physician
Department of Emergency Medicine
Yale-New Haven Hospital
New Haven, Connecticut

James E. Svenson, MD, MS
Associate Professor
Division of Emergency Medicine
University of Wisconsin
Madison, Wisconsin

Christopher R. Tainter, MD
Resident Physician
Department of Emergency Medicine
The Mount Sinai Hospital
New York, New York

Katrin Takenaka, MD, MEd, FACEP
Assistant Professor
Department of Emergency Medicine
University of Texas Medical School at Houston
Houston, Texas

Marsha L. Tallman, MD
Resident
Department of Emergency Medicine
Allegheny General Hospital
Pittsburgh, Pennsylvania

Nathan Teismann, MD
Assistant Professor
Department of Emergency Medicine
University of California—San Francisco School
of Medicine
San Francisco, California

Lisa E. Thomas, MD
Chief Resident
Emergency Medicine
Harvard Affiliated Emergency Medicine
Residency
Massachusetts General Hospital & Brigham &
Women's Hospital
Boston, Massachusetts

Elga Tinger, MD
Attending Physician
Department of Emergency Medicine
White Memorial Medical Center
Los Angeles, California

Susan B. Torrey, MD
Associate Clinical Professor
Department of Pediatrics
Baylor College of Medicine;
Attending Physician
Pediatric Emergency Medicine
Texas Children's Hospital
Houston, Texas

Caleb J. Trent, MD
Resident
Division of Emergency Medicine
Barnes-Jewish Hospital
Washington University School of Medicine
St. Louis, Missouri

Shefali Trivedi, MD
Department of Emergency Medicine
Mount Sinai School of Medicine
New York, New York

Janis P. Tupesis, MD, FACEP, FAAEM
Associate Professor, Residency Director
Division of Emergency Medicine
University of Wisconsin
Madison, Wisconsin

David Paul Turley, MD
Assistant Professor
Department of Emergency Medicine
University of Kentucky
Lexington, Kentucky

Reinier Van Tonder, MBChB
Clinical Instructor
Department of Emergency Medicine
Yale University School of Medicine
New Haven, Connecticut

Rebecca L. Vieira, MD
Instructor
Department of Pediatrics
Harvard Medical School;
Staff Physician
Emergency Medicine
Children's Hospital Boston
Boston, Massachusetts

Irena V. Vitkovitsky, MD
Resident Physician
Department of Emergency Medicine
Washington University School of Medicine
Saint Louis, Missouri

Kathryn A. Volz, MD
Resident
Department of Emergency Medicine
Beth Israel Deaconess Medical Center
Boston, Massachusetts

Lauren R. Wade, MD
Resident Physician
Division of Emergency Medicine
University of Wisconsin School of Medicine and
Public Health
Madison, Wisconsin

Sarah N. Weihmiller, MD
Pediatric Emergency Medicine
AI duPont/Nemours Hospital for Children
Wilmington, Delaware

Scott G. Weiner, MD, MPH
Assistant Professor
Department of Emergency Medicine
Tufts University School of Medicine;
Attending Physician
Department of Emergency Medicine
Tufts Medical Center
Boston, Massachusetts

Brian Wessman, MD
Fellow, EM/Critical Care
Department of Anesthesiology
Washington University in Saint Louis
St. Louis, Missouri

Kathleen A. Wittels, MD
Clinical Instructor
Department of Medicine
Emergency Medicine
Harvard Medical School;
Associate Director of Student Programs
Department of Emergency Medicine
Brigham and Women's Hospital
Boston, Massachusetts

Lalena M. Yarris, MD, MCR
Assistant Professor
Department of Emergency Medicine
Oregon Health & Science University
Portland, Oregon

Michael Yeh, MD, MS
Resident
Department of Emergency Medicine
Allegheny General Hospital
Pittsburgh, Pennsylvania

Christian C. Zuver, MD, FACEP
Assistant Professor—CHS
Division of Emergency Medicine
University of Wisconsin School of Medicine and
Public Health
Madison, Wisconsin

Preface

Emergency physicians are responsible for ordering, interpreting, and sometimes performing imaging specific to the presentation and diagnosis of the emergency department patient. This handbook is designed for the reader to have a bedside image-focused manual with pathognomonic images readily available. Emergency physicians, primarily residents and medical students but even the seasoned attending, will appreciate the focus on classic images and guide to image evaluation and interpretation. We have presented classic images of common complaints in an attempt to serve as an easy to access and understand guide for physicians.

We have created a user-friendly text after many rounds of editing by section editors as well as senior editors. It was particularly challenging to distill each topic to the most relevant information and to create tables of estimates of radiation exposure and advantages and disadvantages of each modality.

The text contains 14 sections organized generally by organ system and 132 chapters authored by emergency physicians, pediatric emergency physicians, and radiologists from medical centers all over the country. The first section, Pediatrics, falls outside of this organ system organization. Two unique chapters "Introduction to Emergency Radiation" and "Radiation Considerations in Children" are particularly timely and relevant to physicians making decisions and recommendations that will affect a patient's cumulative lifetime radiation exposure. Most chapters follow a similar format divided into subsections: Background with a focus on the epidemiology of the diagnosis, a table listing classic history and physical examination findings, helpful laboratory values if relevant, and classic images organized by the modality beginning with radiographs.

We provide the reader with our best *estimate* of the radiation exposure (as an approximate effective dose) if the modality utilizes radiation. The reality is that the true dose varies a great deal depending on multiple factors such as age, weight, gender, machine settings, and institutional protocols. We believe that the specific number is not as important or useful as the relative comparison and should be used as such.

In addition to identifying whether the study is best performed with IV and/or PO contrast, in most cases we provide pearls on how to read and interpret the images. Each chapter concludes with basic management bullet points and a final chart of advantages versus disadvantages of each imaging modality. In some instances, we included modalities that may not be readily available in the reader's practice center or in a timely fashion. If we included these images, it was for illustration and education purposes for the reader to appreciate the full scope of the disease process.

The practice of medicine is extremely complex and the purpose of this text is not to present a standard of care or an authoritative resource but rather a clinical guide. The information provided in this text should not be a substitute for institutional protocols or replace a real-time discussion with your radiology colleagues or any other specialists.

We hope you find *Essential Emergency Imaging* clinically valuable and useful in providing excellent patient care.

Acknowledgments

We would like to acknowledge Frances DeStefano, Senior Acquisitions Editor and Julia Seto, Product Director at Lippincott Williams & Wilkins as well as Sarah Granlund, freelance editor, for their dedication to this book and their flexibility with creating it as close to our vision as possible.

Contents

1

CT Radiation Risks

Aaron Sodickson

Introduction

As anyone reading this chapter knows, CT has tremendously advanced our diagnostic capabilities in the emergency department and broadly throughout medicine. These diagnostic benefits have combined with widespread availability and rapidity of scanning to produce tremendous increases in CT utilization, currently estimated at approximately 70 million CT scans per year in the United States. However, the rapidly increasing utilization has heightened concerns about the collective radiation exposure to the population as a whole and about the high levels of cumulative exposure that may occur in patients undergoing recurrent imaging for chronic conditions or persistent complaints.

Radiation risks have been alternately downplayed and exaggerated in the literature and lay media, resulting in great confusion about the magnitude of these risks. While conventional x-ray, fluoroscopy, and nuclear medicine studies also expose patients to ionizing radiation, CT has appropriately received the greatest scrutiny because of the relatively high radiation dose per examination—although it comprises about 15% of all medical imaging procedures, it produces approximately half of the population's medical radiation exposure. The basic anatomy of a CT machine is a gantry rotating around the patient, which contains on one side a source of x-rays (the x-ray tube) and on the opposite size a detector array that captures the x-rays passing through the patient. CT scanners gather x-ray attenuation data from a large number of angles around the patient and use advanced reconstruction techniques to create cross-sectional images.

The objective of this chapter is to convey some understanding about the approximate levels of risk imparted by CT, and the factors influencing these risks, to encourage a more rational decision-making process by enabling risk estimates to be weighed against the perceived benefits of imaging.

Radiation Terminology

- *Absorbed dose*: This is the energy absorbed by tissue, divided by the mass of the tissue. It is measured in gray or rad (1 rad = 0.01 Gy).
- *Equivalent dose*: This reflects the biological effect of ionizations in tissue, and depends on the type of radiation. For x-rays and gamma rays used in diagnostic imaging, equivalent dose numerically equals absorbed dose, but units change to sievert or rem (1 rem = 0.01 Sv).
- *Effective dose*: This multiplies each organ's equivalent dose times its relative risk of radiation-induced carcinogenesis to infer the whole-body equivalent dose that would be expected to produce the same overall cancer risk as the partial-body exposure received. It is often used as a single number to compare exposures to different body parts, rather than cataloging individual organ doses and risks.

Approximate Doses from Different CT Examinations

Table 1.1 gives the approximate effective dose values for many of the common CT examinations performed in the ED. These are only approximate numbers, as the dose that a patient truly receives from a CT scan may vary widely depending on several technical and patient factors.

TABLE 1.1: Approximate effective doses for various anatomic regions

Scanned anatomy	Approximate effective dose per CT (mSv)
Head, face	2
C-spine, neck	2
Chest, PE, T-spine	8
Abdomen/pelvis, L-spine	15
Abdomen or pelvis alone	7.5

The available CT technology, enabled dose-reduction tools, and selected CT parameters all greatly influence dose to the patient. Dose-reduction tools are commonly available, with more being developed by the CT manufacturers. These tools and growing scrutiny of CT doses will likely lead to a continued downward trend in dose per examination.

Patient size is a crucial variable as well: For fixed CT technique, smaller patients receive a higher dose, as there is less intrinsic shielding of their radiosensitive internal organs. However, to maintain diagnostic quality scans, large patients require substantially more x-ray tube output. In combination, these two competing effects result in larger doses to larger patients for appropriately performed examinations where technique has been correctly adjusted to patient size. As an approximate rule of thumb, extremely large or small adult patients may be expected to receive doses varying by up to a factor of 2 from the "typical" values of Table 1.1.

Radiation Risk

Much of what we know about radiation biology comes from long-term follow-up of atomic bomb survivors and relatively small studies of medical or occupational exposure. These studies have demonstrated increases in cancer incidence for exposures on the order of 50–100 mSv, but controversy persists about the shape of the dose-response curve from smaller exposures or from fractionated or prolonged exposures. Until more data become available that directly explores risk models in these lower-dose regimes, radiation risk estimation will typically be performed using a linear-no-threshold (LNT) model in which cancer risk is assumed to rise linearly as a function of exposure.

Figure 1.1 shows results from the widely used BEIR-VII (Biological Effects of Ionizing Radiation) report that uses an LNT model. For a given exposure, female patients are at a higher risk than male patients and risk per dose increases at younger ages due both to the increased radiation sensitivity of younger tissues and the longer remaining life expectancy in which a radiation-induced cancer may develop. The lifetime attributable risk (LAR) represents an additive risk above baseline cancer rates (42% in the US population).

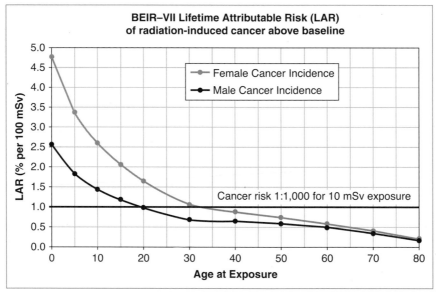

FIGURE 1.1: Expected lifetime attributable risk of radiation-induced cancer. For a 10-mSv exposure, approximate cancer risk is 1 in 1,000 for a 33-year-old woman or a 19-year-old man (solid horizontal line). (Data from National Research Council (U.S.). Committee to Assess Health Risks from Exposure to Low Level of Ionizing Radiation. Health risks from exposure to low levels of ionizing radiation: BEIR VII, Phase 2. Washington, DC: National Academies Press, 2006.)

These curves may be used for rough estimates of risk levels based on the patient's age, gender, and level of exposure. However, it is important to realize that these models assume standardized US life expectancies. Radiation-induced cancers typically have a 10- to -20-year latency (depending on the organ), and so patients with short remaining life expectancy have very little associated risk from radiation exposure.

Cumulative Risk

The risk from most individual CT scans is small, but many patients undergo large amounts of imaging over time. As radiation risks are generally believed to accumulate additively, recurrent imaging can lead to large cumulative risks over time. In addition, it is often the case that patients who have been frequently imaged in the past are likely to be frequently imaged in the future. These high-risk patients warrant particular attention and special consideration during decision making about diagnostic imaging using ionizing radiation.

Estimating cumulative risk is challenging, and ultimately will best be extracted from the electronic medical record by using embedded informatics tools. Until that is widely available, one can make a reasonable ballpark estimate of a patient's cumulative risk by following these steps:

Approach for rough estimation of cumulative risk

1. Count all prior chest and abdomen/pelvis CT scans.

2. Divide the count by 10. The result is the approximate LAR in percent above baseline.

To incrementally improve these estimates

3. Adjust for scan type: The simplified approach above assumes that each CT scan imparted a 10 mSv effective dose. If all the scans were abdomen/pelvis, increase by 50% (see Table 1.1). If there are many head CTs, these can be included by adding 1/5 of them to the "scan count" of step 1.

4. Adjust for patient size: Assuming appropriate dose modulation techniques, increase by a factor of 2 for extremely obese patients and decrease by a factor of 2 for very small patients.

5. Adjust for age and gender: Multiply by the appropriate y-axis value from Figure 1.1.

6. Understand that these estimates are high for patients with life expectancy substantially shorter than age and sex-matched peers.

As an example, assume a moderately obese 60-year-old man has had 40 CT scans (step 1) of the abdomen/pelvis, giving a crude LAR estimate of 4% above baseline (step 2). As all of these scans are relatively higher-dose abdomen/pelvis scans, adjust to 6% (step 3) and then adjust to 9% for moderate obesity (step 4). Finally, multiply by 0.5 (y-axis value from Figure 1.1) to adjust for his gender and age (step 5). The result is an LAR estimate of 4.5% above baseline, increasing his expected lifetime cancer risk from 42% to 46.5%. If the patient is unlikely to survive this hospital admission, radiation risk estimation is irrelevant (step 6).

Note that there are many approximations involved in this type of risk estimation, and further methodology development is needed at each stage to make these estimates more accurate. These types of calculations will ultimately be performed with appropriate extraction of relevant information from the electronic medical record.

Methods to Reduce Radiation Risk

There is substantial ongoing effort to standardize and reduce the radiation dose for each CT scan performed through collaborative efforts of radiologists, CT manufacturers, CT technologists, and medical physicists.

But the primary lever available to nonradiologist providers is control over the frequency of scanning for any given patient. This requires a thoughtful risk/benefit assessment of the role of imaging in the particular patient's care, and is especially important in patients likely to undergo large amounts of cumulative imaging. Some important considerations in this process are:

- Order scans only if they will impact management.
- Review the patient's prior imaging history as thoroughly as possible, not just the last one or two studies.
- Move beyond the incremental risks of the single scan being considered at present, and balance the benefits of recurrent imaging against cumulative radiation risks.
- Take a longitudinal view of the patient. If numerous prior scans for the same complaint have been unrevealing, a new approach may well be warranted.
- Consider other imaging or diagnostic alternatives for focused questions if the desired information is available by other means.
- Increase spacing between scans when possible.

2 Abusive Injuries

Daniel Lindberg

Background

Child abuse is common, with approximately 3 million cases of abuse and neglect involving almost 5.5 million children reported annually. In a 10-year review, abuse accounted for 10% of children younger than 5 years admitted for blunt trauma. Although abused children may be critically injured, many present with relatively minor injuries. Common abusive injuries include fractures, intracranial injuries, and intra-abdominal injuries. Head injury is the most important cause of death in abused children with the vast majority of abusive head trauma occurring in children younger than 3 years. Abdominal trauma is second only to brain injury as a cause of death from abuse.

TABLE 2.1: Concerning history and physical

History
Serious brain injury with a short fall
Serious injury inflicted by a young sibling
Unexplained delay in seeking care
History changes over time or between caregivers
No history of trauma offered for serious injury
History inconsistent with developmental abilities of the child

Physical
Bruising in children who cannot yet "cruise"
Bruising to the pinna, abdomen, or neck
Patterned bruises or burns
Retinal hemorrhages
Oral (labial, sublingual) frenulum tears
Abdominal bruising

TABLE 2.2: Potentially helpful laboratory tests

LFTs (AST/ALT, lipase)	Screening for occult abdominal injury
CBC	Can be useful in excluding mimics of abuse, especially if injuries
PT/PTT	are restricted to bleeding and/or bruising*
Urine	RBCs due to renal injury

ALT, alanine aminotransferase; AST, aspartate aminotransferase; CBC, complete blood count; LFTs, liver function tests; PT, prothrombin time; PTT, partial thromboplastin time; RBCs, red blood cells.
*The full list of tests that might be obtained to exclude mimics of abuse is extensive, and beyond the scope of this chapter.

Skeletal Survey
- Most useful screening study for physical abuse
- Twenty percent yield for occult injury in infants with concern for abuse
- Lower yield, but still significant for ages 1–2 years
- American Academy of Pediatrics recommendation: skeletal survey is mandatory for all children younger than 2 years with concern for physical abuse
- Consider in children between the ages of 2 and 5 years and especially in children with illnesses that limit mobility or communication or predispose to bone fragility
- Requires high-resolution technique and interpretation by a skeletal survey experienced radiologist
- Avoid imaging the whole infant in one, or a handful of films
- **Classic images:** corner or bucket handle fractures, rib fractures, and multiple fractures in various stages of healing
- Look for periosteal reactions and radiopaque calcifications signifying healing fractures

TABLE 2.3: Skeletal survey–required views

Arms (AP)
Forearms (AP)
Hands (PA)
Thighs (AP)
Legs (AP)
Feet (AP)
Thorax (AP; lateral)
Abdomen, pelvis, L-spine (AP)
L-spine (lateral)
C-spine (AP; lateral)
Skull (frontal and lateral)

Adapted from Kleinman et al. Diagnostic imaging of child abuse. *Pediatrics* 123: 2009; 1430–1435.

TABLE 2.4: Skeletal survey x-ray

IV contrast	No
PO contrast	No
Amount of radiation	3–4 mSv*

*Approximate dose.

Classic Images

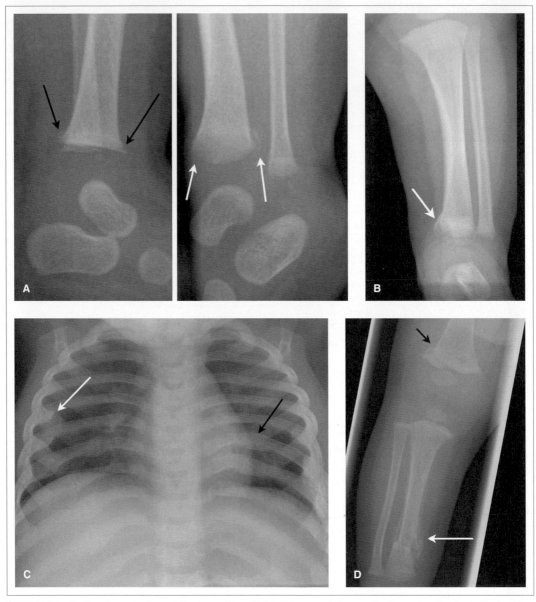

FIGURE 2.1: A: Classic metaphyseal fracture of the distal tibia seen in two projections showing "chip-fracture" (*black arrows*) and "bucket-handle" (*white arrows*) appearances. **B:** Classic metaphyseal lesion with more developed periosteal calcification. **C:** AP chest x-ray from skeletal survey showing more than a dozen rib fractures with evidence of healing. One representative posterior (*black arrow*) and anterior (*white arrow*) have been labeled. **D:** Child with multiple fractures at different stages of healing. While the fracture of the distal femur (*dark arrow*) shows very minor, if any, periosteal reaction or calcification, the fracture of the distal tibia (*bright arrow*) shows robust calcification and periosteal reaction. (*Courtesy of Cincinnati Children's Hospital Medical Center, Cincinnati, OH.*)

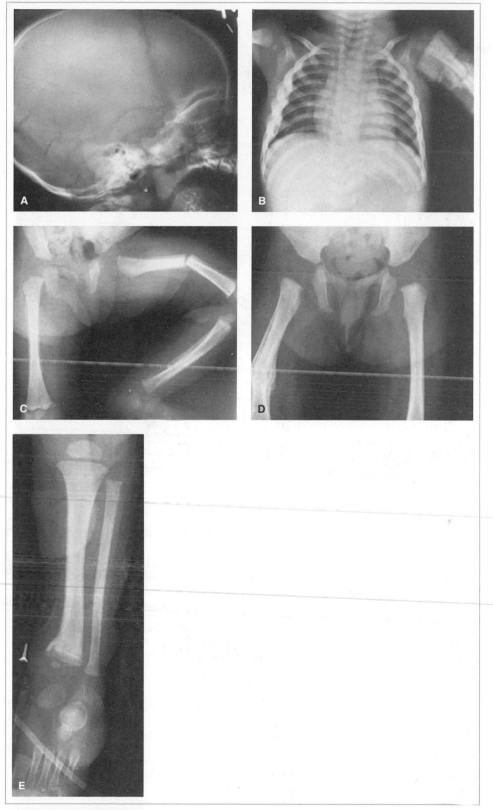

FIGURE 2.2: Radiographic findings of child abuse. **A:** Multiple skull fractures in an infant. **B:** Left humeral fracture and multiple old healing rib fractures. **C:** Left femoral fracture and metaphyseal chip avulsion fractures of the right distal femur. **D:** Healing fracture of the right femur with callus formation and new periosteal bone formation. **E:** "Bucket-handle" deformity of healing distal tibial epiphyseal fracture. (From Fleisher GR, Ludwig S, and Baskin MN. Atlas of Pediatric Emergency Medicine. Philadelphia: Lippincott Williams & Wilkins, 2004.)

Radionuclide Bone Scintigraphy

- Not a first-line study
- Complement to skeletal survey when radiographs are inconclusive or where follow-up skeletal survey is not practical

TABLE 2.5: Skeletal survey bone scan

IV contrast	No
PO contrast	No
Amount of radiation	6 mSv

Classic Images

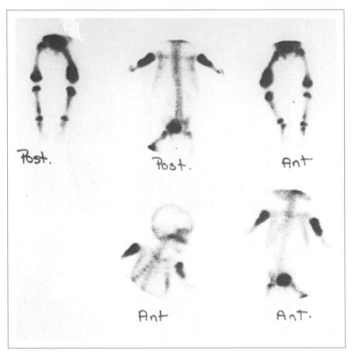

FIGURE 2.3: Bone scan showing multiple areas of skeletal trauma. Despite artifactual uptake in metaphyses and bladder, asymmetry suggests an injury to the right distal femur. (From Fleisher GR, Ludwig S, and Baskin MN. Atlas of Pediatric Emergency Medicine. Philadelphia: Lippincott Williams & Wilkins, 2004.)

Head CT

- Order in patients younger than 6 months in whom any inflicted injury is suspected
- Order in patients with facial bruising, rib fractures, or multiple fractures
- May detect skull fractures missed by skeletal survey and soft tissue swelling missed on physical examination
- May miss fractures oriented in the same plane as the CT cuts
- Subdural hematomas, hypoxic-ischemic injury, cerebral contusions, fractures (especially if multiple or complex), soft tissue swelling, and traumatic subarachnoid hemorrhages
- Intraparenchymal hemorrhages, simple skull fractures, and epidural hemorrhages are less specific for abuse
- Look for interruption or break in the cortex of the bony skull on bone windows
- Look for collections of blood in the epidural, subdural, or subarachnoid spaces along the falx cerebri or the tentorium
- Look for loss of differentiation between grey and white matter, effacement of sulci, and midline shift

TABLE 2.6: CT scan: abusive head trauma

IV contrast	No
PO contrast	No
Amount of radiation	2 mSv*

*Approximate dose.

Classic Images

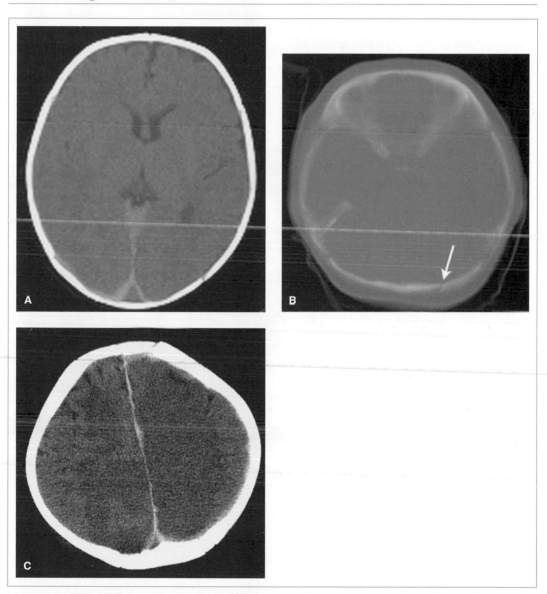

FIGURE 2.4: A: Head CT showing posterior, parafalcine subdural hematoma with extension into the bilateral occipital regions. **B:** Head CT showing occipital bone fracture. **C:** Head CT showing hypoxic/ischemic injury. Note the loss of the grey/white border seen here predominantly on the left hemisphere. This CT also demonstrates the parafalcine subdural hemorrhage commonly seen in abusive head trauma. (*Images courtesy of Children's Hospital Boston and Cincinnatl Children's Hospital Medical Center, Cincinnati, OH.*)

Abdominal CT

- While abusive head trauma is predominantly found in young children (ages 1–3 years), abdominal injuries are found in relatively older children as well.
- Abdominal bruising, tenderness, or distention are concerning, although the physical examination may be normal in as many as 50% of cases with traumatic injury
- While several thresholds have been proposed for the levels of AST/ALT that should imply the need for further imaging, no threshold has been shown to be 100% sensitive.

TABLE 2.7: CT scan: abusive abdominal injury

IV contrast	Yes
PO contrast	No
Amount of radiation	6 mSv*

*Approximate dose.

Classic Images

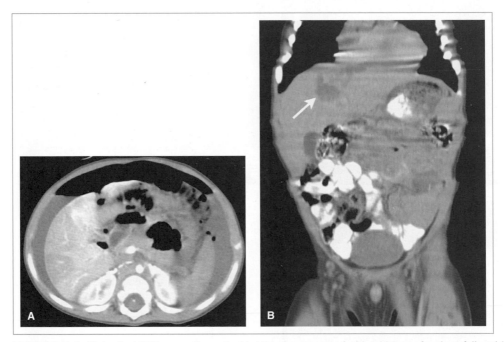

FIGURE 2.5: A: Abdominal CT from an 8-month-old child who presented with a history of a short fall and "funny breathing." The image demonstrates free air, a large amount of free fluid, and hypoperfusion of bowel and solid organs. The child was found on laparotomy to have duodenal perforations. Multiple healing fractures were demonstrated on skeletal survey. **B:** Coronal reformat of a CT demonstrating a large liver laceration that was clinically occult. (*Images courtesy of Cincinnati Children's Hospital Medical Center, Cincinnati, OH and University of Massachusetts Medical Center, Worcester, MA.*)

Brain MRI

- Can demonstrate subdural blood missed on initial CT
- Often a second-line study, but may be first line in stable infants in order to decrease radiation exposure.

Classic Images

Ultrasound

- Not considered a first-line test to screen for abusive injuries
- Sensitivity not sufficient to demonstrate many traumatic injuries
- Positive findings should be confirmed using another modality

Basic Management

- Resuscitation and stabilization with emphasis on airway, breathing, and circulation
- Perform and document a complete neurological examination
- Keep the child in a safe environment
- All reasonable concerns for abuse must be reported to appropriate public agencies and/or to a hospital-based child protection team
- Transfer or admit a stable patient if necessary in order to obtain a useful skeletal
- A follow-up skeletal survey (omitting skull films that do not show normal signs of healing) may be useful 7–14 days after the initial survey
- A postmortem skeletal survey as a component of the postmortem examination may be indicated
- Hospital admission may be necessary pending safe environment availability
- Avoid definitive statements about the etiology of an injury in favor of more neutral statements such as "I'm concerned that someone may have hurt your child"
- Consider whether other children in the household may be at risk or may require evaluation and screening
- Consider injury-specific consultative services, e.g., trauma surgery, general surgery, neurosurgery, or orthopaedic surgery

Summary

TABLE 2.8: Advantages and disadvantages of imaging modalities in child abuse

Imaging modality	Advantage	Disadvantage
X-ray (skeletal survey)	Better resolution of metaphyses Fast Low cost Minimal radiation	May miss early injuries May not delineate fracture or extent of fracture
Bone scan	May be more sensitive for subtle rib or long-bone fractures	Sedation required Time intensive More radiation More expensive Misses skull injuries Misses metaphyseal fractures Cannot estimate age of fracture
CT	Fast Available Identifies injuries needing acute intervention	Radiation exposure Expensive
MRI	More sensitive for some injuries No radiation	Sedation required May be less sensitive for acute blood

3

Foreign Body Aspiration

Joshua Nagler

Background

Foreign body aspiration (FBA) can lead to significant morbidity and mortality in children. Acutely, aspirated material can result in respiratory compromise due to airway obstruction. When aspiration goes unrecognized and the diagnosis is delayed, material in the tracheobronchial tree can lead to chronic pulmonary infections and bronchiectasis. More than 75% of FBA cases occur in children between 1 and 3 years of age. Peanuts as well as other organic materials such as seeds and popcorn are most common causes of FBA, particularly in infants who are not able chew adequately prior to the development of molars. Inorganic material including plastic, wood, and metal objects are more likely to be aspirated by older, ambulatory children who have a tendency to put such objects in their mouths. Aspirated material lodges in the right more commonly then the left mainstem bronchus. Obstruction of the trachea or larynx is less common, occurring in less than 10% of cases.

TABLE 3.1: Classic history and physical

Presenting signs and symptoms	
Constellation of (1) choking or gagging; (2) acute onset of coughing; (3) unilateral wheezing or decreased aeration is highly suggestive of FBA	Triad seen in minority of cases
Choking or gagging episode	75–90% cases
Coughing	Most common symptom
Respiratory distress	Variable
Stridor	
Unilateral wheezing	
Unilateral decreased or absent aeration	
Fever, recurrent or persistent pneumonia, or lung abscess	Delayed diagnoses
Normal physical examination	Does not rule out FBA

FBA, foreign body aspiration.

TABLE 3.2: Potentially helpful laboratory tests

Laboratory tests are not routinely indicated	
Blood gas analysis	May confirm inadequate oxygenation
	No advantage above clinical assessment
WBC	Elevated in retained FBA with postobstructive pneumonia

FBA, foreign body aspiration; WBC, white blood cells.

Chest X-ray

- Order anteroposterior and lateral views
- Primary visible foreign body (10–15% of cases)
- Secondary findings:
  - Air trapping/hyperinflation aka obstructive emphysema
  - Postobstructive atelectasis and pneumonia (delayed presentations)
- Normal (10–50% cases)
  - Typically laryngeal or tracheal foreign bodies
  - Presentation soon after aspiration event
- Inspiratory/expiratory views may accentuate asymmetric hyperinflation seen with foreign bodies lateralizing to the right or left hemithorax
- Lateral decubitus (alternative)
  - Assesses local air trapping with persistent hyperinflation in the dependent hemithorax
  - Useful in young children unable to cooperate with inspiratory/expiratory

TABLE 3.3: Radiographic findings in foreign body aspiration

Radiopaque foreign body	10–15% cases
Air trapping/obstructive emphysema	Asymmetric
	Check valve mechanism
Contraction (absorptive) atelectasis	Delayed presentation
Pneumonia/consolidation	Delayed presentation
Mediastinal shift	
Lobar collapse	
Pneumothorax	
Normal	10–50% cases
	Laryngeal or tracheal FBA
	Early presentations

FBA, foreign body aspiration.

TABLE 3.4: Chest x-ray: foreign body aspiration

IV contrast	No
PO contrast	No
Amount of radiation	0.2 mSv per view*

*Approximate does; 0.1 mSv (2 views).

TABLE 3.5: Diagnostic modality

	Sensitivity	Specificity
History	81–97%	33–76%
Physical examination	24–86%	12–64%
Radiography	49–88%	9–71%

Classic Images

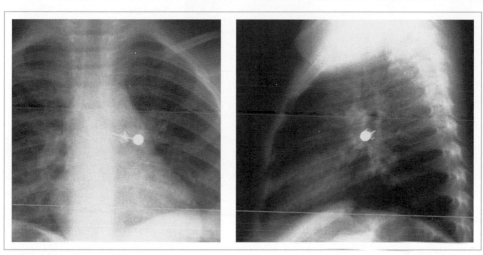

FIGURE 3.1: Aspirated radiopaque foreign body (an earring) located in the left bronchus. (From Fleisher GR, Ludwig S, and Baskin MN. Atlas of Pediatric Emergency Medicine. Philadelphia: Lippincott Williams & Wilkins, 2004.)

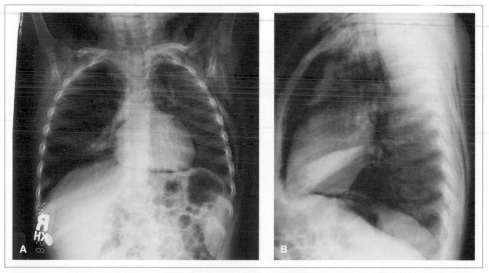

FIGURE 3.2: A 19-month-old child with wheezing since choking on walnut toast. **A:** The posteroanterior view shows subcutaneous air, pneumomediastinum, and right middle lobe (RML) collapse. **B:** The lateral view shows marked hyperinflation with flat diaphragms and increased retrosternal space and RML collapse. (*Courtesy of Dr. Mark Waltzman.*) From Fleisher GR, Ludwig S, and Baskin MN. Atlas of Pediatric Emergency Medicine. Philadelphia: Lippincott Williams & Wilkins, 2004.

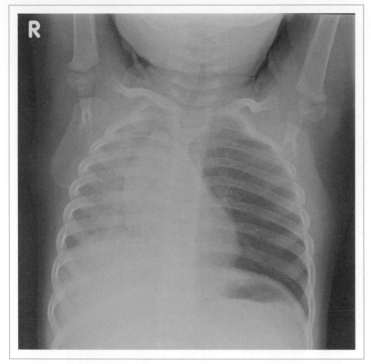

FIGURE 3.3: Air trapping in the left hemithorax from a left mainstem radiolucent foreign body. (*Courtesy of Children's Hospital Boston, Boston, MA.*)

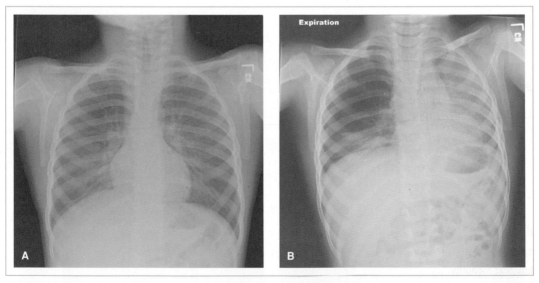

FIGURE 3.4: A: Inspiratory film without radiographic evidence of foreign body aspiration. **B:** Expiratory film of the same patient highlights right-sided air trapping. (*Courtesy of Children's Hospital Boston, Boston, MA.*)

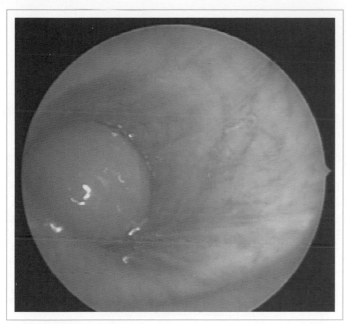

FIGURE 3.5: Bronchoscopic image showing popcorn kernel in left mainstem bronchus. (*Courtesy of Children's Hospital Boston, Boston, MA.*)

Fluoroscopy
- Provides additional information. Findings include:
  - paradoxical movement of the hemidiaphragms
  - "swinging mediastinum" shift away from the affected side with inspiration/expiration
- Data regarding diagnostic accuracy varies

TABLE 3.6: Fluoroscopy: FBA

IV contrast	No
PO contrast	No
Amount of radiation	0.10–5.0 mSv

Basic Management
- Immediate evaluation and treatment of complete airway obstruction
- Obtain radiographs—portable are preferable in the setting of a potentially unstable airway
- Consultation for bronchoscopy
- Rigid bronchoscopy is the gold standard for diagnosis and treatment
- Postprocedural radiographs and observation for suggestion of residual fragments or secondary foreign bodies
- Low suspicion: observe closely for signs and symptoms and consider repeat radiographs in 24–48 hours
- Antibiotics recommended in cases of delayed diagnosis

Summary

TABLE 3.7: Advantages and disadvantages of imaging modalities in FBA

Imaging modality	Advantages	Disadvantages
X-ray	Confirms or supports diagnosis Guides removal Low radiation dose	Negative study does not definitively rule out FBA
Additional views (inspiratory/expiratory or lateral decubitus, fluoroscopy)	May better identify asymmetric air trapping	Additional radiation exposure
Bronchoscopy	Diagnostic and therapeutic Low complication rate	Invasive, requires anesthesia, potential for airway injury

FBA, foreign body aspiration.

4 Bronchiolitis

Marc N. Baskin

Background

Bronchiolitis is the most common lower respiratory tract infection among children 1 month to 2 years of age. Pathologically it is characterized by inflammation, edema, and necrosis of the epithelial cells of the small airways. Many research studies of bronchiolitis limit the diagnosis to infants younger than one or two years of age with their first or second episode of wheezing.

The clinical syndrome of bronchiolitis has been described in the earliest textbooks of pediatrics, and in the past has been called infectious asthma or wheezy bronchitis. Respiratory syncytial virus (RSV) was described in the 1950's and its association with bronchiolitis noted in the 1970s. RSV currently causes about 70% of bronchilitis. Other associated viruses include human metapneumovirus, rhinovirus, influenza, parainfluenza, and adenovirus. In the United States approximately one third of children are diagnosed with bronchiolitis in the first 2 years of life and about 3% of all infants are hospitalized. Younger infants, premature infants, and infants with congenital heart and lung disease are at increased risk for more severe clinical courses.

TABLE 4.1: Classic history and physical

Less than 12–24 mo
Late fall to early spring
Nasal congestion, cough, rhinitis, low grade fever, decreased oral intake
Tachypnea, chest wall retractions, wheezing, and/or crackles

TABLE 4.2: Potentially helpful laboratory tests*

Rapid viral antigen testing	▪ Sensitivity 0.8–0.90, specificity 0.90 ▪ Since many other viruses cause similar clinical findings with similar clinical courses, identifying RSV should not change management ▪ Some hospitals use RSV testing to cohort admitted patients
Blood gas analysis	As needed to assess for respiratory failure

RSV, respiratory syncytial virus.
*None routinely indicated according to American Academy of Pediatrics.

Chest X-ray

- American Academy of Pediatrics guidelines do not recommend routine imaging
- May be useful if another diagnosis is suspected, for example, heart murmur, severe symptoms, or atypical clinical presentation
- In the largest prospective study of patients with clinical bronchiolitis seen in a pediatric emergency department, only 2 of 265 patients (0.7%) had radiographs that were not consistent with bronchiolitis
- Range of image findings:
  - Normal
  - Peribronchial thickening
  - Hyperinflation
  - Atelectasis
  - Consolidation (rarely seen except in severe bronchiolitis and is more consistent with bacterial pneumonia)

TABLE 4.3: Chest x-ray: bronchiolitis

IV contrast	No
PO contrast	No
Amount of radiation	0.1 mSv per view*

*Approximate dose; 0.1 mSv (2 views).

Classic Images

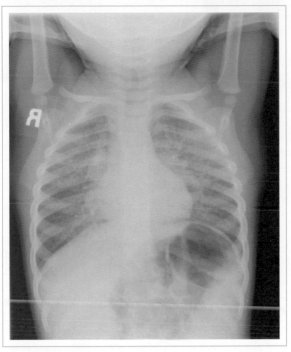

FIGURE 4.1: Twenty-month-old child with respiratory syncytial virus bronchiolitis. Hyperinflated lungs with peribronchial wall thickening in the hilar regions bilaterally. Streaky opacity in the right lung base is consistent with atelectasis. (*Courtesy of Children's Hospital Boston, Boston, MA.*)

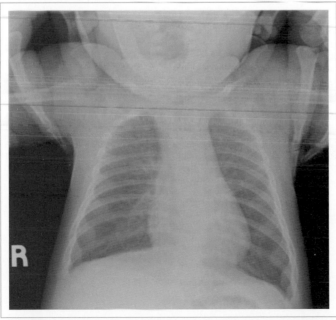

FIGURE 4.2: Three-month-old child with bronchiolitis. Hyperinflated lungs with mild peribronchial wall thickening and minimal bibasilar atelectasis. (*Courtesy of Children's Hospital Boston, Boston, MA.*)

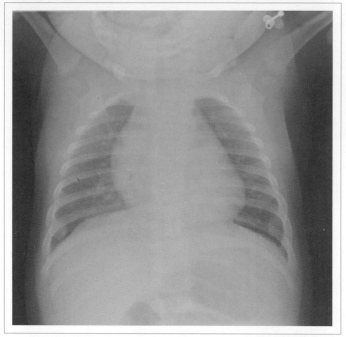

FIGURE 4.3: Three-month-old child with bronchiolitis. This patient's cardiothymic silhouette, especially the superior aspect, appears enlarged but is within normal limits. This is due to the thymus being relatively large compared to the heart in the first few months of life. The patient has mild peribronchial wall thickening and mild hyperinflation. (*Courtesy of Children's Hospital Boston, Boston, MA.*)

Basic Management
- Supportive measures
- Monitor vital signs including pulse oximetry
- Supplemental oxygen and antipyretics as needed
- Assess hydration and ability to take fluids orally
- Consider trial of inhaled bronchodilator with continuation only if there is an objective clinical response
- Antibiotics are not routinely indicated

Summary

TABLE 4.4: Advantages and disadvantages of x-ray in bronchiolitis

Advantages	Disadvantages
Low cost	Often normal
Availability	Nonspecific findings
Minimal radiation exposure	

Retropharyngeal Abscess

Anne M. Stack

Background

Deep tissue infection of the neck is an uncommon but severe disease among children. It can cause serious complications including airway obstruction. Retropharyngeal abscesses (RPA) occur most commonly in infants and children 6 months to 6 years (mean age 1–4 years) of age, although one case series reports children as young as 3 months and as old as 14 years infected with RPA. Finding purulence at surgery is the gold standard for diagnosis.

Anatomically, there are two chains of lymph nodes, in the retropharyngeal space, that are prominent in young children but tend to atrophy before puberty. These nodes are active in the lymphatic drainage of the head and neck. Infections in these areas may lead to suppurative adenitis within the nodes of the deep tissues. Generally, the infections remain contained within the capsule of the node and show progressive changes from cellulitis to phlegmon to suppuration. Very rarely, these infections can spread beyond the capsule to contiguous areas in the deep tissue of the neck. Further complications include carotid sheath involvement leading to septic vascular events, airway obstruction, or mediastinitis if there is nodal rupture. Most infants and children respond very well to appropriate treatment and the infection resolves without sequelae.

TABLE 5.1: Classic history and physical

1- to 2-year-old child with fever, preceding URI
Decreased oral intake, fussiness, limited neck movement, change in voice quality
Tender cervical adenopathy, +/− stridor, possible asymmetry of the posterior wall of the oropharynx
+/− Torticollis, may be worsening stridor when supine

TABLE 5.2: Potentially helpful laboratory test results

CBC	WBC usually >12,000 Neutrophil predominance
Blood culture	Rarely positive

Plain Radiographs: Lateral and Anteroposterior Soft Tissue Neck

- Screening examination for RPA, although not the gold standard
- Obtain a true lateral and AP study in inspiration with neck at neutral to extended position; this avoids the high incidence of false positive widening of the retropharyngeal space
- A soft tissue retropharyngeal space wider than the width of the adjacent vertebral body is highly suggestive of infection
- A soft tissue retropharyngeal space >7 mm at C2 or >14 mm at C6 (22 mm in adults) is highly suggestive of infection
- Associated loss or reversal of normal cervical lordosis may suggest infection
- The lateral neck radiograph may be normal if the RPA is laterally placed
- Sensitivity and specificity of plain radiographs for diagnosis of RPA is not well studied

Classic Images

TABLE 5.3: Soft tissue neck x-ray: retropharyngeal abscesses

IV contrast	No
PO contrast	No
Amount of radiation	0.2 mSv per view*

*Approximate dose.

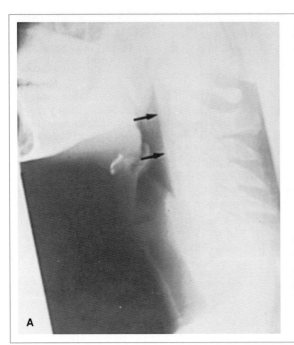
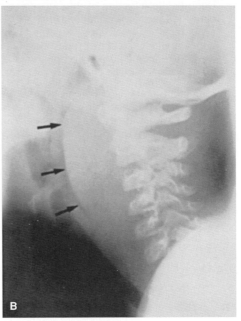

FIGURE 5.1: A: Normal lateral cervical view. **B:** Expansion of prevertebral soft tissues by retropharyngeal abscess. (*Courtesy of Dr. A. Weber, Massachusetts Eye and Ear Infirmary, Boston, MA.*) From Gorbach SL, Bartlett JG, and Blacklow NR. Infectious Diseases, 3rd ed. Philadelphia: Lippincott Williams & Wilkins, 2003.

CT Scan
- IV contrast CT is an excellent way to image deep tissue infections of the neck
- CT demonstrates the extent of the primary infection as well as presence of complications, such as airway compression or spread to adjacent vascular structures
- The sensitivity (64–100%) and specificity (45–82%) of CT in predicting abscess at surgery varies
- Sedation for imaging young children with suspected deeps space neck infections requires extreme care and providers skilled in pediatric advanced airway management

Classic Images

TABLE 5.4: CT scan: retropharyngeal abscesses

IV contrast	Yes
PO contrast	No
Amount of radiation	6.0 mSv*

*Approximate dose.

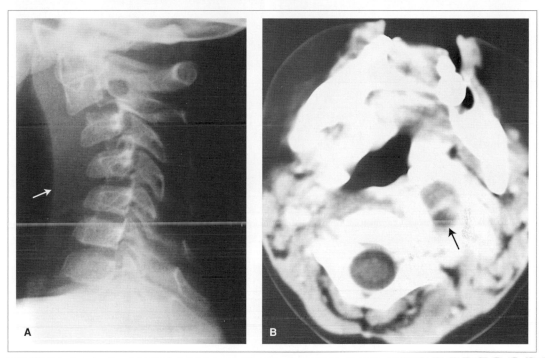

FIGURE 5.2: A: Lateral cervical spine. Observe the increase in the retropharyngeal soft tissues at C2–C4 (*arrow*). **B:** Computed tomography (axial neck). Note the localized area of low density in the left retropharyngeal space, representing an abscess (*arrow*). (From Yochum TR and Rowe LJ. Yochum and Rowe's Essentials of Skeletal Radiology, 3rd ed. Philadelphia: Lippincott Williams & Wilkins, 2004.)

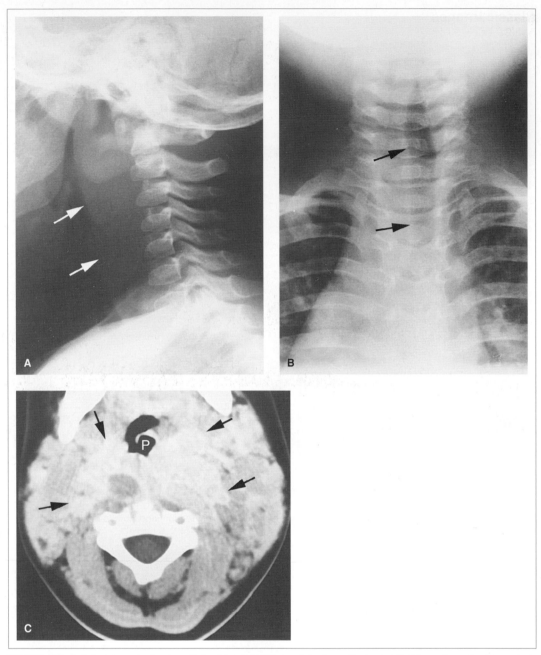

FIGURE 5.3: A: Lateral cervical spine. Note the marked prevertebral swelling extending from the retropharyngeal to retrolaryngeal interspaces (*arrows*). There is no spinal involvement. **B:** Frontal cervical spine. Observe the lateral shift of the trachea (*arrows*). **C:** Computed tomography (axial cervical spine). Note the pharynx (*arrows*). (*Courtesy of David Neal, MD, Columbus, OH.*) From Yochum TR and Rowe LJ. Yochum and Rowe's Essentials of Skeletal Radiology, 3rd ed. Philadelphia: Lippincott Williams & Wilkins, 2004.)

Magnetic Resonance Imaging

Magnetic resonance imaging is not typically performed because of long test time, prolonged sedation, and concern for airway integrity.

Basic Management
- Careful attention to airway patency
- NPO with IV hydration
- IV antibiotics for polymicrobial infection of the neck (e.g., clindamycin, ampicillin/sulbactam [Unasyn])
- Otolaryngology consultation
- Anesthesia consultation if airway emergency
- Admission for IV antibiotics and surgical drainage

Summary

TABLE 5.5: Advantages and disadvantages of imaging modalities in retropharyngeal abscess

Imaging modality	Advantages	Disadvantages
Plain radiographs	Low cost Minimal patient discomfort Minimal radiation Readily available Obtained quickly Can rule out epiglottitis	May be poorly sensitive for small or lateral abscesses Must have true lateral image with patient's neck in extension and during inspiration or prevertebral soft tissues may appear falsely widened
CT scan	Availability Can diagnose complications of RPA and other etiologies	IV contrast Sedation usually required Possible airway compromise Radiation exposure

RPA, retropharyngeal abscesses.

Pyloric Stenosis

Susan B. Torrey

Background

Pyloric stenosis (PS) is an acquired cause of gastric outlet obstruction among infants which develops as the result of hypertrophy of the pylorus muscle. The incidence ranges from approximately 2 to 5 per 1,000 live births (higher numbers among Caucasian population, lower among African American and Asian populations). It occurs more commonly in males than in females (>4:1) and among children with affected mothers. Symptoms usually occur at 3–5 weeks of age and rarely occur after 8 weeks. Approximately 30% of cases occur in firstborn children. The etiology is likely multifactorial, involving genetic and environmental factors. Multiple abnormalities have been identified in hypertrophied muscle (including abnormal innervations, peptide-containing fibers, nitric oxide synthetase activity, and messenger RNA production), many of which return to normal within months of surgical correction. In addition, the development of PS has been associated with the use of macrolide antibiotics, particularly among infants who receive erythromycin within the first 2 weeks of life. The pyloric spasm and PS distinction may be challenging to diagnose, particularly for small infants. Infants with apparent pyloric spasm should receive careful clinical follow-up and may require additional ultrasound evaluations.

TABLE 6.1: Classic history and physical

Male infant 3–5 weeks of age
Nonbilious, often projectile vomiting immediately postprandial; will eat immediately postvomiting
Weight loss
Signs/symptoms of dehydration
"Olive" mass may be palpable in the right upper quadrant
Peristaltic wave (uncommonly)

TABLE 6.2: Potentially helpful laboratory test

BMP	Hypochloremia
	Metabolic alkalosis

Bedside and Abdominal Ultrasound

Bedside ultrasound by emergency physicians increasingly utilized but insufficient experience to recommend its use as definitive study

- Imaging modality of choice
  - Sensitivity 97–100%
  - Specificity 99–100%
- Measurements:
  - Pyloric channel length: >15–19 mm
  - Muscle thickness: >3.5–4 mm (more sensitive and specific)
  - Younger infants: pyloric length 17 mm ± 1.7, muscle thickness 3.6 mm ± 0.42
- Stable patients with inconclusive studies may be followed clinically and ultrasound repeated
- All patients with negative ultrasounds do not require upper gastrointestinal (GI) series

Classic Images

TABLE 6.3: Abdominal ultrasound technique: pyloric stenosis

High-frequency linear probe
Scan supine or in right lateral decubitus position
Transverse or oblique plane with the probe marker toward right shoulder
Small sips of liquid may help to visualize the stomach
Locate pyloric channel and then align probe with its long axis
Muscle: hypoechoic compared to parallel hyperechoic mucosal lines
Cervix sign: hypertrophied muscle mass indents duodenal bulb and bulges into antrum
Measure muscle: outer edge muscle to outer edge mucosa
Nipple sign: pseudomass of redundant mucosa prolapsing into antrum

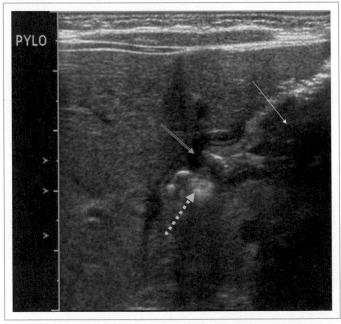

FIGURE 6.1: Normal pylorus on ultrasound. The double-lined arrow points to the normal pylorus, the thin white arrow corresponds to milk within the lumen of the stomach, and the dotted arrow points to air entering the first part of the duodenum from the stomach during normal peristalsis. (*Courtesy of Rajesh Krishnamurthy, Radiologist, Texas Children's Hospital, Houston, TX.*)

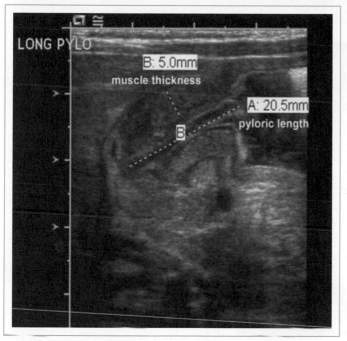

FIGURE 6.2: Hypertrophied pylorus on ultrasound. The pyloric channel as measured is >20 mm in length and the muscle thickness of the channel diameter >4 mm (*Courtesy of Rajesh Krishnamurthy, Radiologist, Texas Children's Hospital, Houston, TX.*)

Upper GI Series
- Previously the standard imaging procedure for PS
  - Sensitivity 90–100%
  - Specificity 99–100%
- Scout film
  - Nonspecific findings
  - Distended stomach bubble, little bowel gas, increased peristalsis
- Contrast material is instilled into the stomach through an orogastric tube
- Contrast is observed passing through the pylorus using fluoroscopy
- Diagnoses other causes of vomiting, such as gastroesophageal reflux or small bowel obstruction more readily

TABLE 6.4: Classic signs: upper gastrointestinal series for pyloric stenosis

Caterpillar	Wave of gastric peristalsis on scout film
Shoulder	Antrum filling defect created by prolapse of the hypertrophied muscle
Mushroom	Thickened muscle indents the duodenal bulb
Double track	Elongated and narrowed channel appears as a double track of contrast squeezed into separate compartments due to mucosal redundancy
String	Elongated and narrowed channel

 TABLE 6.5: Upper gastrointestinal series: pyloric stenosis

IV contrast	No
PO contrast	Yes
Amount of radiation	6.0 (includes fluroscopy)*

*Approximate dose.

Classic Images

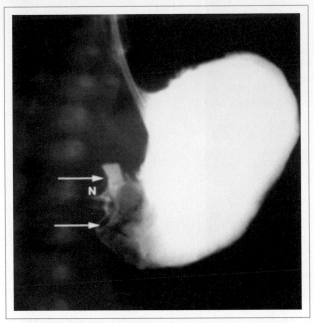

FIGURE 6.3: Infantile hypertrophic pyloric stenosis demonstrated by barium upper gastrointestinal series showing pyloric channel narrowing (N) and elongation with shoulder sign (*arrows*). (From Mulholland MW, Maier RV, et al. Greenfield's Surgery: Scientific Principles and Practice, 4th ed. Philadelphia: Lippincott Williams & Wilkins, 2006.)

Basic Management
- NPO
- Volume resuscitation for infants with severe dehydration
  - 20 mL per kilogram bolus of normal saline solution
  - Repeat as needed based on improvement in peripheral perfusion (quality of pulses, capillary refill), mental status, and heart rate
- Correction of electrolyte abnormalities with intravenous fluid replacement
  - D5 0.45% saline at 1.5 times maintenance
  - Add 10–20 mEq/L of KCl once urine output is noted
- General surgery consultation
- Definitive management: pyloromyotomy—open or laparoscopic

Summary

TABLE 6.6: Advantages and disadvantages of imaging modalities in pyloric stenosis

Imaging modalities	Advantages	Disadvantages
Ultrasound	Readily available Noninvasive No radiation	Operator-dependent
Upper gastrointestinal series	Readily available Less operator-dependent Able to make other diagnoses	Orogastric tube for contrast Radiation exposure

7

Intussusception

Sarah Nowygrod and Richard Bachur

Background

Intussusception is the most common cause of intestinal obstruction in infants and young children. It occurs when one segment of the intestine telescopes into an adjacent segment, most commonly at the ileocolic junction. Approximately 75% of cases are idiopathic, and the remaining cases are caused by an underlying condition which creates a pathologic lead point for the intussusception (e.g., Meckel's diverticulum, polyp). Eighty percent of cases occur under the age of 2 and it rarely occurs over the age of 6 without a pathologic lead point. The diagnosis can be difficult to make because of the nonspecific presentation and young children's inability to describe their symptoms. Delayed diagnosis may lead to bowel necrosis and perforation.

TABLE 7.1: Classic history and physical

Classic triad: (i) abdominal pain, (ii) currant-jelly (red) stool, (iii) palpable abdominal mass	Present less than 50% of the time
Sudden onset of intermittent severe pain drawing of legs to chest and/or inconsolable crying	
Abdominal pain alternating with lethargy	Rarely lethargy alone
Vomiting	⊥ Bilious
Abdominal tenderness, distention, or mass	variably present
Heme positive or bloody stools	Present 50% of the time

TABLE 7.2: Potentially helpful laboratory tests

None are diagnostic	
Chemistry panel	Assess for dehydration
Complete blood count	Assess degree of gastrointestinal blood loss or if considering other diagnoses

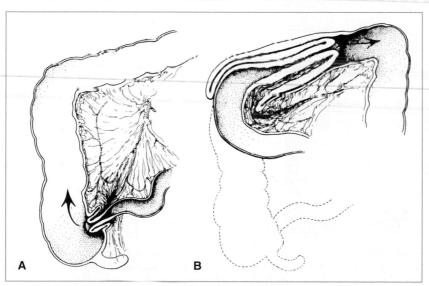

FIGURE 7.1: Ileocolic intussusception. **A:** Beginning of an intussusception in which terminal ileum prolapses through ileocecal valve. **B:** Ileocolic intussusception continuing through the colon. This can often be palpated as a mass in the right upper quadrant. (From Fleisher GR, Ludwig S, and Henretig FM. Textbook of Pediatric Emergency Medicine, 5th ed. Philadelphia: Lippincott Williams & Wilkins, 2005.)

KUB X-ray

- High false negative rate
- Normal (early presentation)
- Small bowel obstruction (advanced presentation)
- Left lateral decubitus view helps bring air from the transverse colon into the ascending colon and cecum
- Prone views may allow air to fill cecum to rule out ileocolic intussusception
- Positive signs:
  - Absence of air in the right upper and lower quadrants
  - Soft tissue density in the right upper quadrant
  - Crescent sign (semilunar lucency) represents intestinal gas trapped between the two intestinal walls
- Negative signs:
  - Air or stool in the *ascending* colon and cecum
- Distal colonic air is not useful to rule out intussusception

 TABLE 7.3: KUB x-ray: intussusception

IV contrast	No
PO contrast	No
Amount of radiation	0.7 mSv per view*

*Approximate dose.

Classic Images

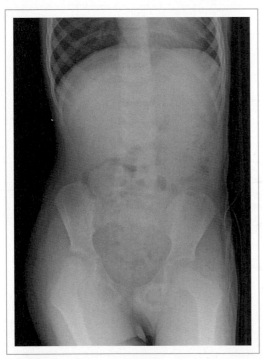

FIGURE 7.2: Lateral decubitus view: A soft tissue mass is evident in the right lower quadrant. Crescent sign demonstrated with air trapped between the bowel walls of the intussusception. (*Courtesy of Children's Hospital Boston, Boston, MA.*)

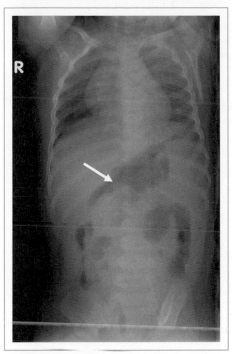

FIGURE 7.3: Lateral decubitus view: There is an intraluminal soft tissue mass (*arrow*) in the region of the transverse colon which represents an intussusception. (*Courtesy of Children's Hospital Boston, Boston, MA.*)

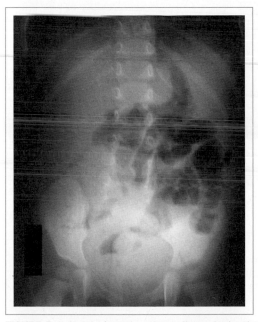

FIGURE 7.4: A plain frontal supine radiograph showing no obstruction but a soft-tissue density in the right lower abdomen. (From Fleisher GR, Ludwig S, and Baskin MN. Atlas of Pediatric Emergency Medicine. Philadelphia: Lippincott Williams & Wilkins, 2004.)

Abdominal Ultrasound
- Using a high-frequency linear transducer, apply slow and steady downward pressure to displace bowel gas from the right upper quadrant down to the right lower quadrant
- Move the probe caudad from the right upper to the right lower quadrant
- Psoas muscle must be visualized to exclude intussusception
- "Target" sign: ("Donut" sign): several hypoechoic rings surrounding a hyperechoic center on transverse view
- "Pseudokidney" sign: reniform appearance of bowel wall with central hyperechoic region surrounded by a hypoechoic region on longitudinal view

Classic Images

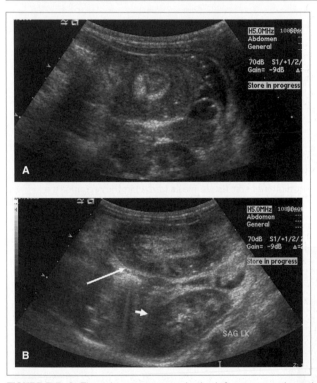

FIGURE 7.5: A: There is a mass seen in the left upper quadrant that contains alternating concentric hypoechoic and hyperechoic rings. **B:** The "pseudokidney" sign: a mass representing the intussusception (*long arrow*) displaces the left kidney inferiorly (*short arrow*). (*Courtesy of Children's Hospital Boston, Boston, MA.*)

Barium or Air Enema
- Gold standard for diagnosis of ileocolic intussusception
- Sensitivity 100%, specificity 100%
- Fluoroscopy confirms the intussusception and monitors for reduction
- Reduction can also be performed under sonographic guidance
- Contraindications: unstable patient, shock, or free air
- Risk of perforation with reduction: ~1%
- Successful reduction rate: 80–90%

TABLE 7.4: Fluoroscopy for barium or air enema: intussusception

IV contrast	No
PO contrast	No
PR contrast	Yes
Amount of radiation	2–8 mSv*

*Approximate dose.

Classic Images

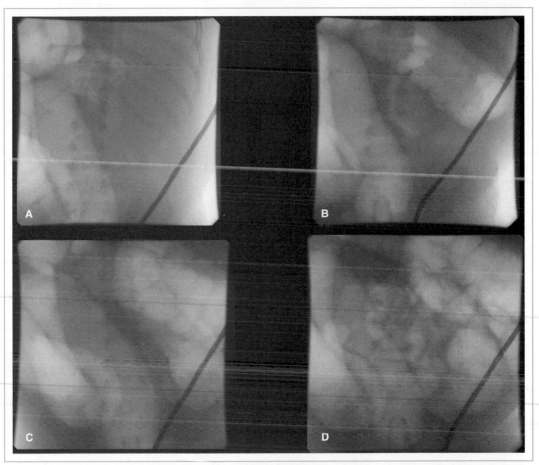

FIGURE 7.6: Four images of an ileocolic intussusception reduction by air enema. Viewed clockwise: (**A**) Air reduction shows an ileocolic intussusception extending to the transverse colon. (**B**) Air seen flowing across the transverse colon after successful reduction. (**C**) Air seen going through the ascending colon. (**D**) Air passing into the ileum. (*Courtesy of Children's Hospital Boston, Boston, MA.*)

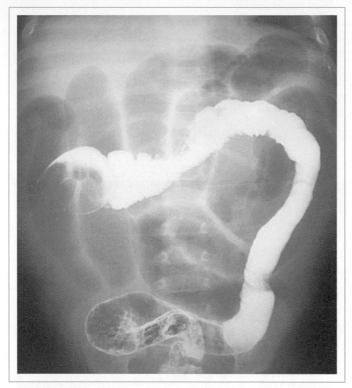

FIGURE 7.7: Ileocolic intussusception. Barium enema shows the intussusception as the filing defect within the hepatic flexure surrounded by spiral mucosal folds. Significant distended small bowel represents distal small bowel obstruction. (From Fleisher GR, Ludwig S, and Baskin MN. Atlas of Pediatric Emergency Medicine. Philadelphia: Lippincott Williams & Wilkins, 2004.)

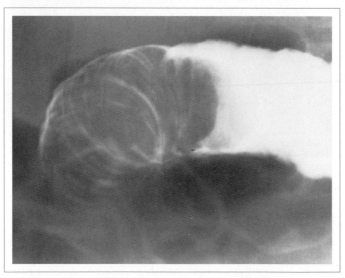

FIGURE 7.8: Barium enema demonstrating intussusception. Obstruction of the colon at the hepatic flexure. Note the characteristic coiled-spring appearance. (From Eisenberg RL. An Atlas of Differential Diagnosis, 4th ed. Philadelphia: Lippincott Williams & Wilkins, 2003.)

Abdominal CT Scan

- Not a first-line imaging modality
- May be used to characterize a pathologic lead point previously detected by ultrasound
- May be identified incidentally when CT is obtained for other reasons (e.g., appendicitis evaluation)
- Sensitivity and specificity for diagnosis have not been well studied
- Look for a round soft tissue mass with concentric rings, "target sign" representing loops of small bowel most likely in the area of the ileum

 TABLE 7.5: Abdominal/pelvic CT: intussusception

IV contrast	Yes
PO contrast	Yes
Amount of radiation	10–14 mSv*

*Approximate dose.

Classic Images

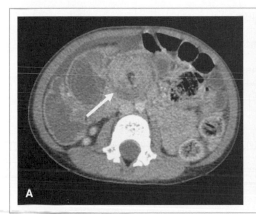
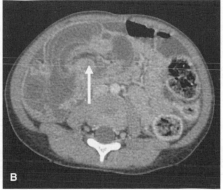

FIGURE 7.9: Two images of intussusception seen on contrast CT scan: **A:** There is a mass within the mid abdomen demonstrating an internal swirled appearance with central low attenuation likely representing mesenteric fat within an ileocolic intussusception (*arrow*). **B:** The intussusception is also captured on longitudinal view (*arrow*). The surrounding loops of small bowel are dilated and filled with gas and stool likely secondary to obstruction and reactive ileus. (*Courtesy of Children's Hospital Boston, Boston, MA.*)

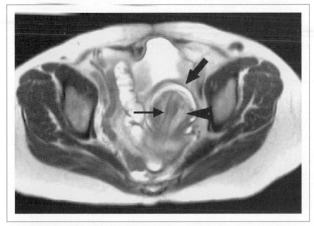

FIGURE 7.10: Colonic intussusception. Axial T2-weighted image demonstrating layers of sigmoid colonic intussusception with outer colon wall (*arrow*), pericolonic fat (*arrowhead*), and inner colon wall (*thin arrow*). (From Leyendecker JR and Brown JJ. Practical Guide to Abdominal and Pelvic MRI. Philadelphia: Lippincott Williams & Wilkins, 2004.)

Basic Management

- NPO
- Intravenous hydration
- Pain control
- General surgery consultation
  - Surgeon present during air enema reduction in case of perforation or massive pneumoperitoneum
- Reduction via enema
  - Barium was previously used, but now air is used more commonly
  - Safer, cheaper, and more effective
  - In the prone position, an uninflated balloon catheter is placed into the rectum; buttocks are taped together
  - Air is introduced into the rectum with monitored pressure
  - Reflux of air from cecum into ileum confirms complete reduction
  - Patients should not be sedated for pressure reduction enemas
- Antibiotics
  - With peritoneal signs
  - Prophylactically for potential perforation during pressure reduction procedure
- Admission Post-reduction
  - There is a 10% recurrence usually within 24–48 hours
- Surgical treatment
  - Suspected intussusception in those who are acutely ill
  - Evidence of perforation
  - Patients in whom nonoperative reduction is unsuccessful
  - Resection of a pathologic lead point

Summary

TABLE 7.6: Advantages and disadvantages of imaging modalities in intussusception

Imaging modalities	Advantages	Disadvantages
KUB	Quick Universally available Low radiation	Low sensitivity (~45%) Low specificity High false negative rate
Ultrasound	Low cost High sensitivity (98–100%) High specificity (88–100%) Minimal patient discomfort No radiation	Availability Operator-dependent Body habitus limitations
Contrast enema	Gold standard Diagnostic and therapeutic	Limited availability Requires skilled personnel Radiation exposure Requires on-site surgeon for reduction
CT scan	Used more for adult diagnosis Identification of lead points	Radiation exposure Not well studied in children

8

Necrotizing Enterocolitis

Catherine E. Perron

Background

Necrotizing enterocolitis (NEC) is a disorder characterized by mucosal or transmucosal ischemic necrosis of a part of the intestine, and is associated with inflammation, invasion of enteric gas forming organisms, and dissection of gas into the muscularis and portal venous system. With severe NEC, bowel perforation may occur. NEC occurs in 1–3 per 1,000 births and is one of the most common abdominal emergencies in the neonate. The incidence decreases with increasing gestational age and birth weight. Although the majority of NEC cases are found in premature infants, with rates as high as 7% in neonatal intensive care unit admissions, approximately 10% of identified cases are found in term infants, typically in those with predisposing illnesses such as congenital heart disease, respiratory distress, birth anoxia, seizures, sepsis, history of umbilical catheter, hypercoagulable states, or abdominal wall defects such as gastroschisis. Males and females are affected equally. NEC usually develops in the first 3–10 days of life, but can occur in preterm infants in the first several months of life. Mortality rates, which are also related inversely to gestational age and weight, range from 5% in term infants to 50% in very premature infants (less than 1,000 g). The estimated yearly infant death rate in the United States from NEC is approximately 12 per 100,000 live births. Long-term morbidity from NEC is substantial in neonatal intensive care survivors.

TABLE 8.1: Classic history and physical

Premature infant or infant with predisposing illness
Feeding intolerance, vomiting
Apnea, lethargy, temperature instability
Abdominal distension
Gross blood or occult blood in stool

TABLE 8.2: Potentially helpful laboratory tests

CBC	Leukopenia (absolute neutrophil count <1,500 carries poor prognosis)
	Leukocytosis
	Thrombocytopenia (correlates with necrotic bowel)
BMP	Acidosis
	Hyponatremia
Coagulation panel	Prolonged PT/PTT (with disseminated intravascular coagulopathy)
Blood and CSF cultures	20–30% of cases have bacteremia
	Sepsis evaluation should be performed
Nonspecific labs (C-reactive protein)	Elevated

BMP, Basic Metabolic Panel; CBC, Complete Blood Count; CSF, Cerebrospinal Fluid; PT, Prothrombin Time; PTT, Partial Thromboplastin Time.

Multiview Abdominal X-rays

- Test of choice: Anteroposterior (AP) supine view, and either supine cross table (x-table) lateral or lateral decubitus with left side down
- Confirms the diagnosis and are used to follow the course of the disease
- Less useful, although still indicated, in very premature infants where classic radiographic signs may be absent

TABLE 8.3: X-ray findings: necrotizing enterocolitis

Ileus (dilated bowel)	Most common finding Nonspecific Present in early necrotizing enterocolitis (NEC) Diffuse or focal Edematous thickened bowel wall Visible also in low birth weight infants with intestinal inertia, prolonged crying, or breathing with CPAP (Continous Positive Airway Pressure).
Abnormal distribution of bowel gas	Paucity of gas in one area and dilatation of bowel in another Shift from generalized distension to unevenly distributed dilatation is a more useful sign
Fixed loops of bowel	Indicates lack of peristalsis, necrosis, or even perforation A fixed dilated loop present and unchanged for 24–36 hr indicates advanced disease
Pneumatosis intestinalis	Pathognomonic Small gas bubbles (submucosal) or linear streaks of air (subserosal) in bowel wall Focal or diffuse usually distal small intestine or colon Can be confused with stool in colon; premature infants <2 weeks old do not show this air in stool pattern, so must be considered pneumatosis Prone films or serial films with movement of stool may help differentiate pneumatosis from air in stool Present in 75% of infants with NEC Commonly seen in infants >37 weeks gestation and less common in infants <26 weeks gestation
Portal venous gas	Severe disease finding Radiolucent linear streaks over the liver—better seen on x-table lateral than anteroposterior film 10–30% of infants with NEC Commonly seen in infants >37 weeks gestation (40%) and less common when <26 weeks (10%)
Free intraperitoneal air	Small and localized or large and diffuse Over liver on lateral decubitus film In Morrison's pouch (posterior hepatorenal space) appears as triangular lucency projecting over liver in supine film Rigler sign: air on either side of bowel wall Football sign: large amounts of air create a hypolucent area in the central portion of a supine film with the falciform ligament creating markings or "laces" Tell-tale triangle: triangular lucencies between bowel loops below the anterior abdomen wall on supine film
Ascites or focal fluid collections	Indicates perforation or impending perforation May precede free air

 TABLE 8.4: Abdominal x-rays: necrotizing enterocolitis

IV contrast	No
PO contrast	No
Amount of radiation	0.7 mSv per view*

*Approximate dose.

Classic Images

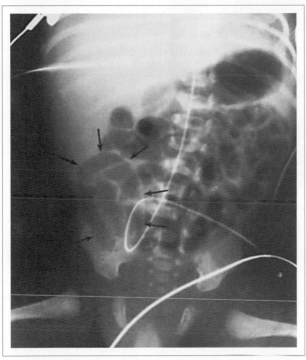

FIGURE 8.1: Distended focal bowel loops in necrotizing enterocolitis. (From Kirks DR. Practical Pediatric Imaging: Diagnostic Radiology of Infants and Children, 3rd ed. Philadelphia: Lippincott Williams & Wilkins, 1998.)

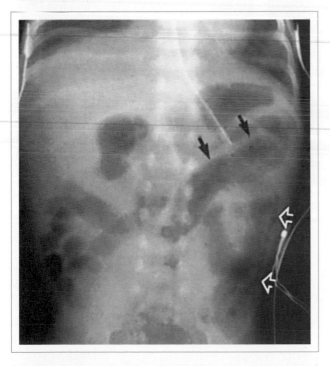

FIGURE 8.2: Pneumatosis intestinalis. (From Kirks DR. Practical Pediatric Imaging: Diagnostic Radiology of Infants and Children, 3rd ed. Philadelphia: Lippincott Williams & Wilkins, 1998.)

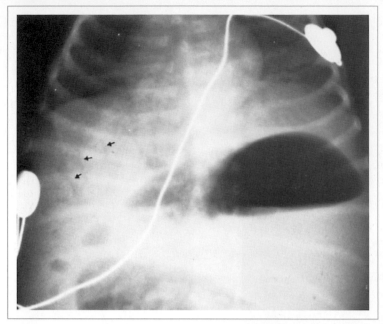

FIGURE 8.3: Portal vein gas (*arrows*) in an infant with necrotizing enterocolitis. (From Eisenberg RL. An Atlas of Differential Diagnosis, 4th ed. Philadelphia: Lippincott Williams & Wilkins, 2003.)

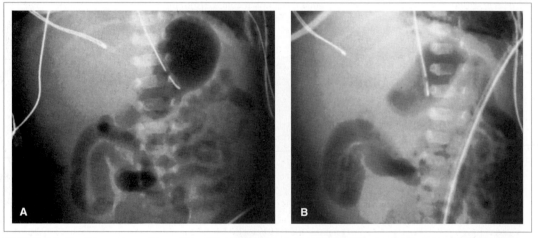

FIGURE 8.4: Fixed bowel loop. (From Kirks DR. Practical Pediatric Imaging: Diagnostic Radiology of Infants and Children, 3rd ed. Philadelphia: Lippincott Williams & Wilkins, 1998.)

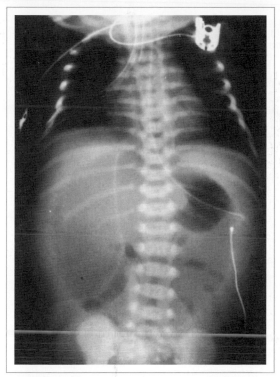

FIGURE 8.5: Supine abdominal x-ray film demonstrating a massive intraperitoneal air collection. The air is seen as a large central bubble on which is superimposed a dense linear opacity produced by the falciform ligament. The falciform ligament forms the lace for the football sign. (From MacDonald MG, Mullett M, Seshia MMK, et al. Avery's Neonatology: Pathophysiology and Management of the Newborn, 6th ed. Philadelphia: Lippincott Williams & Wilkins, 2005.)

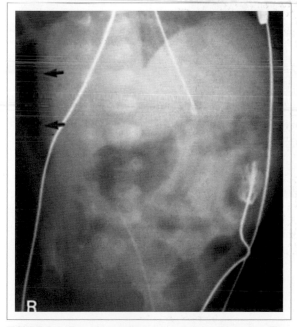

FIGURE 8.6: Free air over liver on lateral decubitus film. Fixed bowel loop. (From Kirks DR. Practical Pediatric Imaging: Diagnostic Radiology of Infants and Children, 3rd ed. Philadelphia: Lippincott Williams & Wilkins, 1998.)

Abdominal Ultrasound

- More recent modality to diagnose and serially examine cases of suspected NEC; color Doppler ultrasonography may be more sensitive for bowel wall necrosis or subtle changes

TABLE 8.5: Abdominal ultrasound: necrotizing enterocolitis

Pseudokidney sign	Kidney-like appearance of bowel wall with central hyperechoic region surrounded by a hypoechoic region on longitudinal view Indicates bowel necrosis and perhaps evolving perforation Not pathognomonic
Focal fluid collections or ascites	Dependent portion of peritoneal cavity, likely indicates perforated bowel.
Portal venous gas	Bubbles or moving foci in the liver and venous system
Free air	Either side of bowel wall Morrison's pouch

 TABLE 8.6: Abdominal ultrasound: necrotizing enterocolitis

IV contrast	No
PO contrast	No
Amount of radiation	None

Classic Images

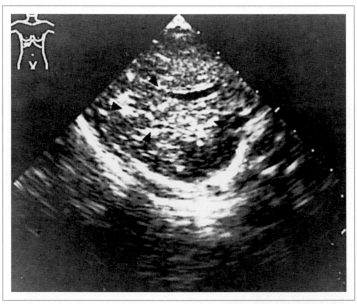

FIGURE 8.7: Portal venous gas on ultrasound. (From Kirks DR. Practical Pediatric Imaging: Diagnostic Radiology of Infants and Children, 3rd ed. Philadelphia: Lippincott Williams & Wilkins, 1998.)

Other Imaging Studies

Abdominal CT scan and contrast enema are not routinely performed because of radiation exposure, risk of perforation, and extravasation of contrast into abdominal cavity.

Basic Management

- Surgical intervention is reserved for infants with intestinal perforation
- Medical management
  - Orogastric tube
  - Bowel rest
  - Fluid resuscitation
  - Broad-spectrum antibiotics
  - Correction of metabolic and hematologic abnormalities
- Serial abdominal radiographs, physical examination, and laboratory studies are used to follow the clinical course

Summary

TABLE 8.7: Advantages and disadvantages of imaging modalities in necrotizing enterocolitis

Imaging modalities	Advantages	Disadvantages
Abdominal x-rays	Easily obtained	Premature infants may not have classic signs
	Diagnostic if classic signs are present	Radiation exposure
Ultrasound	May be more sensitive	Less well studied
	Bedside	Operator experience
	Noninvasive	Air obscures anatomy

9 Salter-Harris Fractures/Triplane Fracture

Lois K. Lee

Background

Physeal (growth plate) injuries are common in children and account for about 20–30% of all childhood fractures. These injuries occur secondary to the vulnerability of the pediatric musculoskeletal system since the physes are biomechanically weaker than the ligaments and their insertion sites. The physis is cartilaginous; and therefore, it remains radiolucent until skeletal maturation when the physis closes. The Salter-Harris classification is the most commonly used system to describe physeal fractures.

A type I fracture is a complete fracture through the physis, which separates the epiphysis (bulbous end of the long bone and includes the physis) from the metaphysis. These fractures may be difficult to identify radiographically except for some soft tissue swelling due to the radiolucency of the physis. A type II fracture extends from the physis into the metaphysis. In a type III fracture, the fracture extends from the physis into the epiphysis and often into the articular surface. In a type IV fracture, the fracture proceeds from the articular surface into the epiphysis, through the physis, and then into the metaphysis. A type V fracture is considered to be a crush injury to the physis, which may initially appear to have a normal radiograph. The diagnosis may be made retrospectively when a growth disturbance is recognized.

A triplane fracture is a complex fracture pattern of the distal tibia epiphysis. It was given this name because there are fractures in the sagittal, transverse, and frontal planes, classically described as a three-pointed star configuration. This fracture pattern occurs most commonly between the ages of 12 and 15 years when adolescents are transitioning to skeletal maturity. The fibula is also fractured in about 50% of cases.

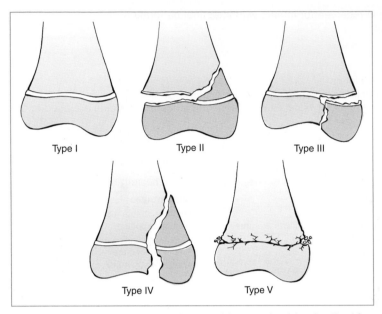

Type I   Type II   Type III

Type IV   Type V

FIGURE 9.1: The Salter-Harris classification of fractures involving the distal femoral physis. (From Bucholz RW, Heckman JD, Court-Brown C, et al., eds. Rockwood and Green's Fractures in Adults, 6th ed. Philadelphia: Lippincott Williams & Wilkins, 2006.)

TABLE 9.1: Classic history and physical

History of direct trauma to the area of fracture
History of twisting injury to foot/ankle (triplane)
Soft tissue swelling over physeal area
Focal tenderness over physeal area
Decreased range of motion of the joint

Extremity X-ray
- Obtain anterior-posterior and lateral views
- Image the joints above and below the fracture
- Oblique views may also be used to evaluate nondisplaced and minimally displaced fractures
- Contralateral extremity view may be helpful for comparison if there is an unusual finding in the injured extremity
- Triplane fractures may have the appearance of a Salter-Harris type III fracture on the anterior-posterior view and a Salter-Harris type II fracture on the lateral view

TABLE 9.2: Extremity x-ray: Salter-Harris or triplane fracture

IV contrast	No
PO contrast	No
Amount of radiation	0.001 mSv per view*

*Approximate dose.

Classic Images

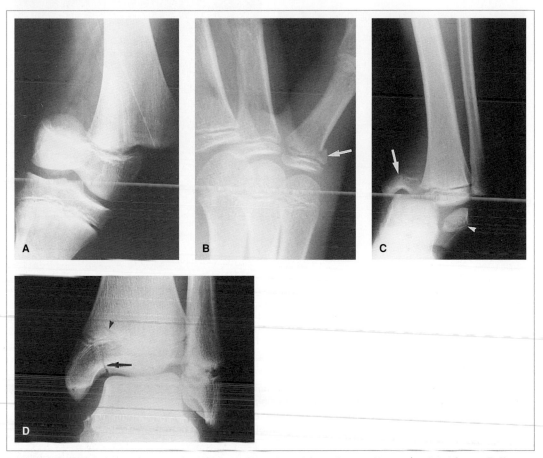

FIGURE 9.2: A: Type I, anterior-posterior (AP) knee. Note the epiphyseal separation at the distal femur. **B:** Type II, fifth digit of the hand. Observe the epiphyseal separation with an additional metaphyseal fragment (Thurston-Holland fragment) (*arrow*). **C:** Type III, AP ankle. Note the separation of the medial distal epiphysis (*arrow*) of the distal tibia, with an associated type I separation of the lateral malleolus (*arrowhead*). **D:** Type IV, AP ankle. Note the fracture lines extending through the medial aspect of the tibial epiphysis (*arrow*), with extension into the adjacent metaphysis (*arrowhead*). A type I epiphyseal separation is present, affecting the distal fibula. (From Yochum TR and Rowe LJ. Yochum and Rowe's Essentials of Skeletal Radiology, 3rd ed. Philadelphia: Lippincott Williams & Wilkins, 2004.)

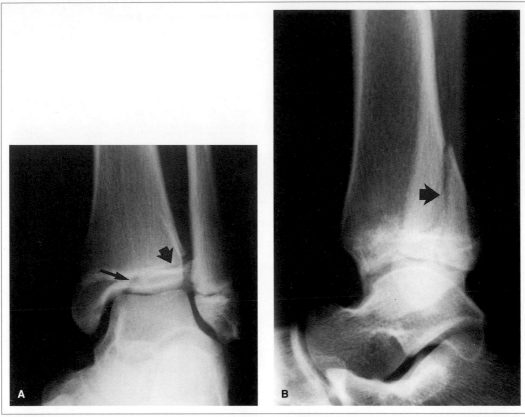

FIGURE 9.3: Triplane fracture of the distal tibia. **A:** Frontal radiograph shows fractures through the epiphysis (*thin arrow*) and the lateral physis (*fat arrow*). **B:** Lateral radiograph shows a coronal fracture of the posterior tibia (*arrow*). (From Daffner RH. Clinical Radiology: The Essentials, 3rd ed. Philadelphia: Lippincott Williams & Wilkins, 2007.)

CT Scan

- CT scans using reconstructed images can be helpful in the assessment of complex injuries, e.g., triplane fractures or highly comminuted fractures.
- For triplane fractures, a CT scan must be obtained to fully evaluate the number and configuration of fracture fragments and the amount of displacement as well as for preoperative planning.

 TABLE 9.3: CT scan: Salter-Harris fractures

IV contrast	No
PO contrast	No
Amount of radiation	3.5 mSv*

*Approximate dose.

Classic Images

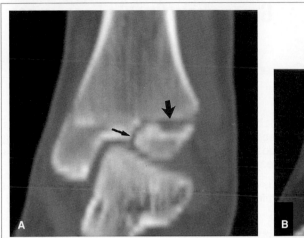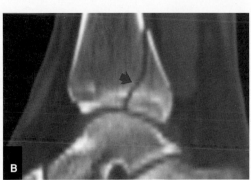

FIGURE 9.4: Triplane fracture of the distal tibia. **A:** Coronal tomographic reconstructed CT image shows the epiphyseal (*thin arrow*) and the physeal (*fat arrow*) fractures. **B:** Sagittal tomographic reconstructed CT image shows the coronal fracture (*arrow*) actually extends to the joint surface. (From Daffner RH. Clinical Radiology: The Essentials, 3rd ed. Philadelphia: Lippincott Williams & Wilkins, 2007.)

Basic Management

- For nondisplaced Salter-Harris type I or II fractures, the patient may be splinted and sent for urgent orthopedic referral.
- For any displaced Salter-Harris type fractures or nondisplaced Salter-Harris type III or IV fractures, the patient should have an emergent orthopedic referral for reduction and immobilization.
- Any open physeal injuries, those with neurovascular compromise or any concern for impending compartment syndrome should be managed emergently.
- Nondisplaced (<2-mm displacement) triplane fractures may be managed with closed reduction under general anesthesia and a long leg cast for immobilization.
- Displaced triplane fractures will require either open or closed reduction.

Summary

TABLE 9.4: Advantages and disadvantages of imaging modalities in Salter-Harris fractures

Imaging modality	Advantages	Disadvantages
X-ray	Low cost Availability Limited radiation exposure	Patient discomfort during manipulation May not show all triplane fracture fragments
CT scan	Multiplanar reconstruction (for triplane) Minimal patient discomfort	Availability Radiation exposure

10 Greenstick/Buckle Fractures

Lois K. Lee

Background

Forearm fractures account for about 45% of all childhood fractures. Of these, the most common are greenstick and buckle (or torus) fractures. Greenstick fractures are incomplete fractures occurring through only one side of the bone with the opposite cortex and periosteum intact. Buckle fractures occur when the bone is compressed and appears as a buckling of the bone at the metaphysis.

The forearm comprises two bones, the radius and the ulna. Often both bones are injured. If a fracture is apparent in only one bone, a possible additional injury should be suspected and evaluated for in the proximal or distal joint.

TABLE 10.1: Classic history and physical

Mechanisms of injury
Fall onto outstretched hand
Direct blow to the extremity (e.g., forearm or femur)
Extremity trapped between two objects (e.g., crib rails)
Mechanism may not always be apparent in young children
Pain of distal aspect of extremity
If injury is to arm, the child may not be using it
If injury is to leg, child may refuse to bear weight
Focal tenderness at site of fracture
Swelling and/or deformity at site of injury

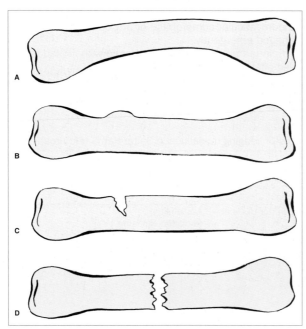

FIGURE 10.1: Common fractures in children. (**A**) Plastic deformation (bend). (**B**) Buckle (torus). (**C**) Greenstick. (**D**) Complete. From Nettina SM. The Lippincott Manual of Nursing Practice, 7th ed. Lippincott, Williams & Wilkins, 2001.

Extremity X-ray

- Obtain anteroposterior and lateral views of extremity
- Image the joints proximal and distal to the fracture with concern for dislocation or other injury
- Look for a buckle fracture as an incomplete linear fracture appearing as an outward bulge or buckling of the cortical margin on the concave side of the bone metaphysis
- Look for a greenstick fracture as an incomplete linear fracture appearing as an angulated break on the convex compression side of the bending bone cortex
- Look for a plastic bowing deformity of the metaphyseal cortex and observe for fracture in a companion bone

TABLE 10.2: Forearm x-ray

IV contrast	No
PO contrast	No
Amount of radiation	0.001 mSv per view*

*Approximate dose

Classic Images

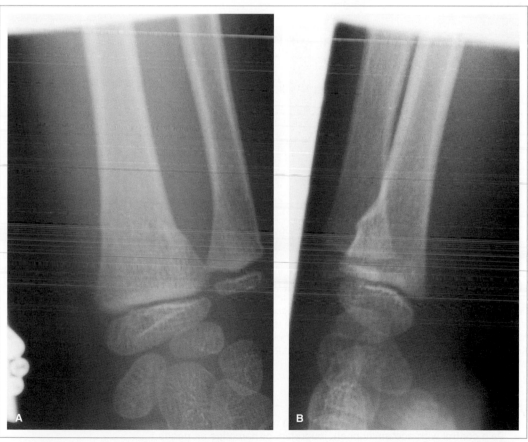

FIGURE 10.2: This buckle fracture of the distal radius is subtle on the anteroposterior view (**A**) but seen more clearly on the lateral view (**B**). (From Fleisher GR, Ludwig S, and Baskin MN. The Atlas of Pediatric Emergency Medicine. Philadelphia: Lippincott Williams & Wilkins, 2004.)

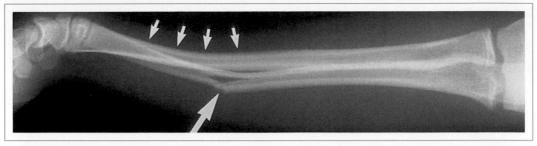

FIGURE 10.3: Greenstick fracture of the ulna (*large arrow*) and a bowing fracture (*small arrows*) of the radius. The extent of bowing can often be fully appreciated only with comparison views of the opposite extremity. (From Fleisher GR, Ludwig S, and Henretig FM. Textbook of Pediatric Emergency Medicine, 5th ed. Philadelphia: Lippincott Williams & Wilkins, 2005.)

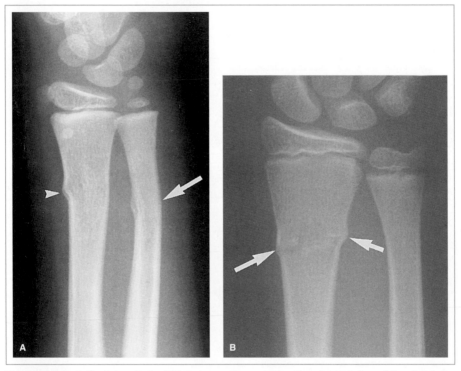

FIGURE 10.4: A: Posteroanterior (PA) forearm. Observe the altered angulation of the distal ulna, representing a greenstick fracture (*arrow*). A torus fracture of the radius is also seen (*arrowhead*). **B:** PA wrist. Note the bulging of the cortex of the distal radius consistent with a torus fracture (*arrows*). (From Yochum TR and Rowe LJ. Yochum and Rowe's Essentials of Skeletal Radiology, 3rd ed. Philadelphia: Lippincott Williams & Wilkins, 2004.)

Basic Management
- Splint extremity for comfort and protection of the injury
- Pain control with acetaminophen, ibuprofen, or narcotics as needed
- Buckle (or torus) fracture
  - Immobilize in either a splint or a short cast for 2–4 weeks
  - In cases of bicortical disruption, there is an increased risk of displacement; orthopedic referral for a long arm cast for 3–6 weeks is recommended
- Greenstick fracture
  - Immobilize in a splint
  - Refer to an orthopedic surgeon for closed reduction and casting

Summary

TABLE 10.3: Advantages and disadvantages of x-ray in greenstick fractures

Advantages	Disadvantages
Low cost	Need multiple views
Availability	Patient discomfort during manipulation for adequate x-ray
Minimal radiation exposure	views

11

Transient Synovitis

Rebecca L. Vieira

Background

Transient synovitis (TS), previously known as toxic synovitis, is a self-limited inflammatory process of the synovial lining of the hip that typically affects school-aged children. It is the most common cause of nontraumatic hip pain in children. The average annual incidence is approximately 0.2% with a cumulated lifetime risk of 3%. The etiology is not fully understood, although a postinfectious inflammatory response has been suggested. The diagnosis of TS is one of exclusion. The possibility of more serious hip pathology, such as septic arthritis, must be excluded through careful history, physical examination, and when indicated, laboratory and/or radiology studies. Patients with TS will often have an effusion of the affected hip with bilateral effusions present in up to 25% of cases of symptomatically unilateral transient synovitis. Prognosis is excellent, with most children making a full recovery with supportive treatment.

TABLE 11.1: Classic history and physical

Children 3–8 years old
Male > female (approximately 2:1)
Preceding viral illness common
Fever uncommon at presentation
Nontoxic appearing
Hip flexed, abducted, externally rotated; pain with internal rotation
Gait with limp, but usually able to bear weight

TABLE 11.2: Potentially helpful laboratory test

CBC	WBC usually <12,000 cells/mm^3
ESR	Usually <40 mm/hr
CRP	Usually <2 mg/dL
Elevated WBC, ESR, and/or CRP	Suspicious for septic arthritis, but not specific or sensitive
Lyme titers	Indicated in endemic areas if a hip effusion is present
Synovial fluid analysis	Indicated if effusion is present and concern for septic arthritis exists Gram stain: no organisms Cultures: no growth WBC: usually <50,000 per hpf

CBC, complete blood count; CRP, C-reactive protein; ESR, erythrocyte sedimentation rate; WBC, white blood cell.

Hip and Pelvis X-ray

- Perform AP and frog-leg views of the hip
- Consider imaging the contralateral hip for comparison
- Often no abnormal findings; an increase in the joint space suggests effusion
- Not sensitive for identifying effusions

TABLE 11.3: Hip x-ray: transient synovitis

IV contrast	No
PO contrast	No
Amount of radiation	0.6 mSv per view*

*Approximate dose.

Classic Images

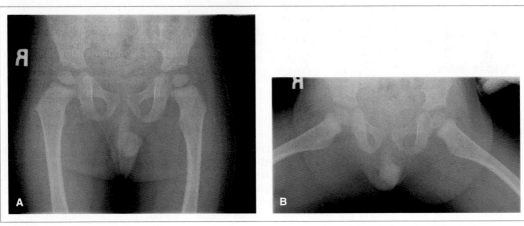

FIGURE 11.1: Normal AP (**A**) and frog-leg (**B**) views of the hips. (*Courtesy of The Children's Hospital, Boston, MA.*)

Hip Ultrasound
- Bedside ultrasound to identify hip effusions in children is poorly studied
- Use a 5–10 MHz high-frequency linear probe
- Image the child in a position of comfort (often with hip flexed, abducted, and externally rotated)
- Place the linear probe parallel to the femoral neck in the sagittal plane with the marker pointed toward the umbilicus
- Identify the joint capsule, including the femoral head and neck, acetabulum, and iliopsoas muscles
- Normal hips will have a negligible amount of anechoic fluid between the femoral neck and iliopsoas muscle
- Measure the distance between the anterior surface of the femoral neck and the posterior surface of the iliopsoas muscle for each hip (a measurement of ≥5 mm or a measurement of >2 mm difference from the contralateral hip is considered positive for an effusion)
- If anechoic fluid is present in the joint capsule, measure the largest distance between the femoral neck and iliopsoas muscle, positioning the calipers perpendicular to the femoral neck

TABLE 11.4: Helpful associated structures

Femoral head	Curvilinear hyperechoic (white) structure
Physis	Notch in anterior surface of femoral head (in growing child)
Iliopsoas muscle	Homogeneously striated echotexture anterior and parallel to femoral neck

Classic Images

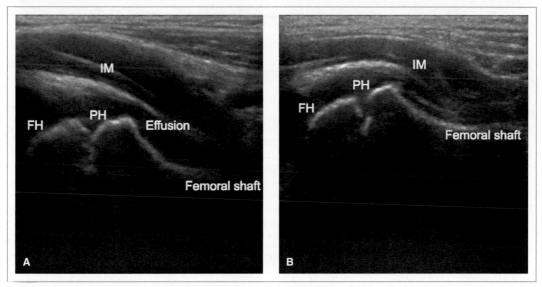

FIGURE 11.2. Bedside ultrasound showing right hip with effusion (**A**) and normal left hip (**B**). The femoral head (FH) is noted on the left side of the screen with the physis (PH) appearing as a notch. In image "A," anechoic fluid is noted between the femoral neck (FN) and iliopsoas muscle (IM). (*Courtesy of The Children's Hospital, Boston, MA.*)

Basic Management

- TS is a self-limited process
- Treatment is symptomatic with rest and nonsteroidal anti-inflammatory drugs (NSAIDs) to reduce synovial inflammation
- Activity can be gradually resumed as symptoms resolve, with full return to physical activity when the child is pain-free

Summary

TABLE 11.5: Advantages and disadvantages of imaging modalities in transient synovitis

Imaging modality	Advantages	Disadvantages
X-rays	■ Useful for identifying other diagnoses (e.g., fracture)	■ Not sensitive for effusion ■ Radiation exposure
Ultrasound	■ Gold standard for identifying hip effusion ■ Minimal patient discomfort ■ No radiation	■ Variable availability of official ultrasound ■ Operator dependent ■ Patient cooperation necessary ■ Presence of effusion not sensitive or specific for diagnosis

12 Slipped Capital Femoral Epiphysis

Theresa Becker

Background

Slipped capital femoral epiphysis (SCFE) is a hip disorder typically of adolescents in which the femoral epiphysis slips posteriorly, resulting in limp and impaired internal rotation. The etiology of SCFE is unknown but biomechanical and biochemical factors play a role. The mean age of presentation is 12 years in girls and 13.5 years in boys, near the time of peak linear growth, and the male-to-female ratio is approximately 1.5:1. Obesity is a significant risk factor, and the prevalence of SCFE is increased among Pacific Islanders and African Americans. SCFE is bilateral in 20–40% of cases at presentation. Associated risk factors are renal failure, history of radiation therapy, endocrine abnormalities, and various genetic disorders.

Early recognition is important, since delayed or missed diagnosis may result in progression of the slip, increasing the potential for complications including avascular necrosis of the femoral head and chondrolysis.

TABLE 12.1: Classic history and physical

Obese adolescent
Nonradiating, dull, aching pain in the hip, groin, thigh, or knee
May be acute (<3 weeks), chronic (>3 weeks) or acute on chronic with or without h/o trauma
Pain of hip, groin, or thigh which is increased by physical activity
Isolated knee pain (15% cases)
Altered gait
Guarding and decreased range of motion of the hip, especially internal rotation

TABLE 12.2: Potentially helpful laboratory tests (none needed routinely—only if atypical presentation*)

BUN/creatinine	Evaluate for renal failure
Endocrine studies (e.g., thyroid)	

*Age <10 or >16 years, weight <50th percentile, height <10th percentile for age and gender.

Pelvis and Hip X-rays

- Order an anterior-posterior view (AP) of the pelvis and "frog leg" lateral (hips flexed and externally rotated) views of both hips
- Consider a true cross-table lateral with acute onset of symptoms, as the frog-leg position may displace the physis in these unstable slips
- Radiographic changes are minimal before the slip occurs and are best seen with lateral (frog-leg) views; two radiographic views are 80% sensitive for SCFE
- Look for widening and irregularity of the physis, with thinning of the proximal epiphysis
- Earlier slip: blurring of the junction between the metaphysis and growth plate
- Later slip: posterior displacement of the femoral epiphysis (classic "ice cream slipping off a cone" appearance)
- The height of the epiphysis may be diminished because the femoral head rotates posteriorly
- Metaphyseal blanch sign of Steel: semicircular area of increased density on the proximal part of the femoral neck, created by the posteriorly displaced epiphysis overlapping the medial metaphysis (seen on AP pelvis view)
- Klein's line, drawn along the superior lateral cortex of the femoral neck on the AP pelvis radiograph, should intersect with the epiphysis; in the patient with SCFE, the epiphysis is flush or below this line (see Figure 12.2)
- If plain radiographs are normal but suspicion for SCFE is high, consider MRI.

TABLE 12.3: Pelvic and hip x-rays: slipped capital femoral epiphysis

IV contrast	No
PO contrast	No
Amount of radiation	0.6 mSv per view*

*Approximate dose.

Classic Images

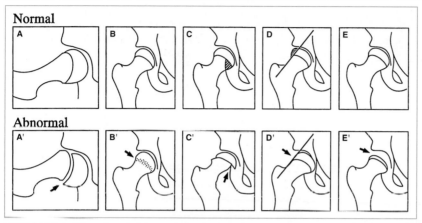

FIGURE 12.1: Slipped capital femoral epiphysis: radiographic signs. **A:** The femoral epiphysis normally sits upon the metaphysis like a scoop of ice cream on a cone. **A′:** The scoop (the femoral head) has slipped part way off the cone (the femoral neck). **B:** The normal femoral physis is sharply marginated. **B′:** There is blurring of the proximal femoral physis. **C:** The medial femoral neck normally overlaps the posterior part of the acetabulum forming a dense triangle (Capener triangle). **C′:** This triangular density is lost by the lateral displacement of the femoral neck. **D:** A line drawn along the femoral neck normally intersects at least the lateral sixth of the femoral epiphysis. **D′:** With displacement, no part of the epiphysis lies lateral to the line. **E:** The femoral epiphysis is of normal height. **E′:** With posterior slippage, there is apparent decrease in the height of the epiphysis. Modified from Bloomberg (496). (From Kirks DR. Practical Pediatric Imaging: Diagnostic Radiology of Infants and Children, 3rd ed. Philadelphia: Lippincott Williams & Wilkins, 1998.)

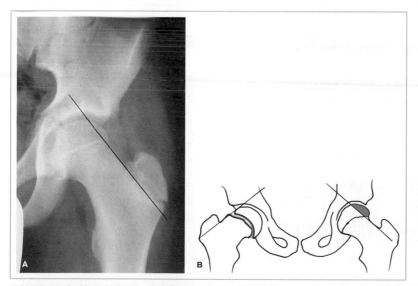

FIGURE 12.2: Slipped femoral capital epiphysis (SCFE): Klein's line. **A:** Normal Klein's line, anteroposterior hip. **B:** Note the abnormal Klein's line associated with SCFE, showing no intersection with the femoral epiphysis on left of diagram. (From Yochum TR and Rowe LJ. Yochum and Rowe's Essentials of Skeletal Radiology, 3rd ed. Philadelphia: Lippincott Williams & Wilkins, 2004.)

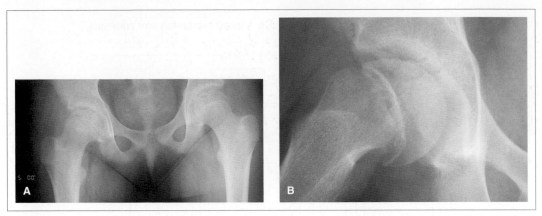

FIGURE 12.3: This 12-year-old boy had knee and thigh pain for 2 weeks; however, on examination, he had pain with internal hip rotation. **A:** His anteroposterior films show subtle signs of slipped capital femoral epiphysis on the right. **B:** The frog-leg views show the slip clearly. (From Fleisher GR, Ludwig S, and Baskin MN. Atlas of Pediatric Emergency Medicine. Philadelphia: Lippincott Williams & Wilkins, 2004.)

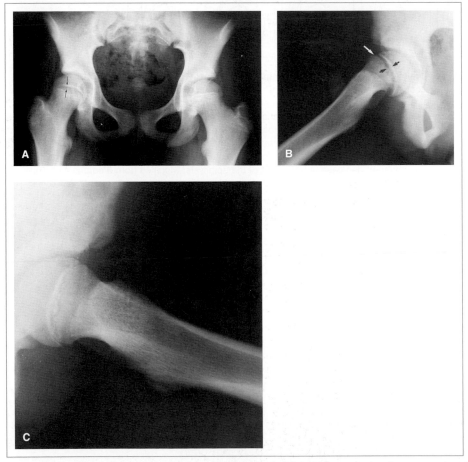

FIGURE 12.4: Slipped femoral capital epiphysis (SCFE). **A:** Pelvic radiograph showing asymmetry of the physis with widening on the right (*arrows*). **B:** Frog-leg lateral view of the right hip showing widening of the physis (*short arrows*) and malalignment of the epiphysis with the metaphysis laterally (*long arrow*). **C:** Frog-leg view of the left is normal. (From Daffner RH. Clinical Radiology: The Essentials, 3rd ed. Philadelphia: Lippincott Williams & Wilkins, 2007.)

Basic Management
- Non-weight bearing
- Urgent pediatric orthopedic consultation
- Surgical correction

Summary

TABLE 12.4: Advantages and disadvantages of x-ray in SCFE

Advantages	Disadvantages
Low cost	May miss diagnosis in early stages of disease
Readily available	

13

Legg-Calvé-Perthes Disease

Theresa Becker

Background

Legg-Calvé-Perthes disease (LCPD) is a childhood syndrome of avascular necrosis of the femoral head. It occurs between the ages of 3 and 12 years, with a peak onset at 5–7 years of age. The male-to-female ratio is 4:1. LCPD is bilateral in 10–15% of patients and if bilateral, it occurs sequentially. The etiology of LCPD remains unknown. LCPD has been associated with prenatal or secondhand smoke exposure, clotting abnormalities, low birth weight, maternal deprivation, and HIV infection. Avascular necrosis secondary to steroid use or an underlying disease may present similarly.

TABLE 13.1: Classic history and physical

Male 3–10 years old with insidious onset of hip or groin pain and/or limp
Pain is often present only during physical activity
Short-statured and/or overweight patient
History of delayed skeletal maturation
Decreased hip abduction and internal rotation
Limping gait
Leg length discrepancy and thigh muscle atrophy (severe cases)

TABLE 13.2: Potentially helpful laboratory tests (none needed routinely—only if other diagnoses considered)

CBC, ESR, CRP	Results expected to be normal

CBC, complete blood count; ESR, erythrocyte sedimentation rate; CRP, C-reactive protein.

Pelvis and Hip X-rays
- Order an anterior-posterior (AP) view of the pelvis and frog-leg lateral (hips flexed and externally rotated) views of both hips
- Often normal early in the disease process
- On the lateral view, look for widening of the articular cartilage with a small dense proximal femoral epiphysis
- On the lateral view, look for a subchondral fissure-fracture lucency along the anterolateral aspect of the epiphysis (crescent sign)

- Irregularity and flattening of the epiphysis develop over time
- Look for fragmentation and then healing of the femoral head, often with residual deformity on images later in the disease process
- Reduce radiation exposure by coning or by using a gonadal shield

 TABLE 13.3: Pelvic and hip x-rays: Legg-Calvé-Perthes disease

IV contrast	No
PO contrast	No
Amount of radiation	0.6 mSv per view*

*Approximate dose.

Classic Images

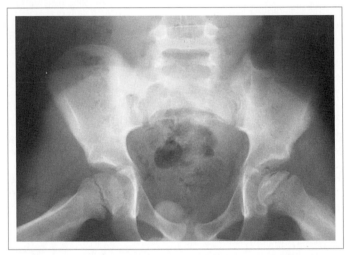

FIGURE 13.1: Legg-Calvé-Perthes disease of the left hip. Epiphysis is narrowed and radiodense. A subchondral fracture is also visible. (From Fleisher GR, Ludwig S, and Baskin MN. Atlas of Pediatric Emergency Medicine. Philadelphia: Lippincott Williams & Wilkins, 2004.)

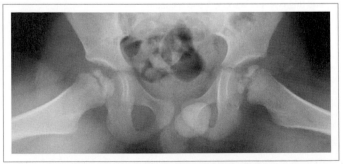

FIGURE 13.2: A 3-year-old with abnormal gait for 1 month. Both femoral heads are irregular and sclerotic. (From Fleisher GR, Ludwig S, and Baskin MN. Atlas of Pediatric Emergency Medicine. Philadelphia: Lippincott Williams & Wilkins, 2004.)

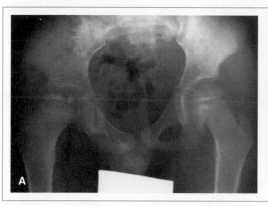
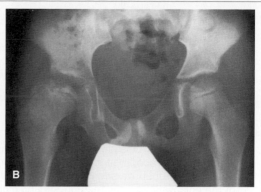

FIGURE 13.3: Progression of Legg-Calvé-Perthes disease. A 5-year-old boy with right hip pain. **A:** One year after presentation. The right proximal femoral epiphysis is fragmented and irregularly ossified. There is widening of the femoral neck and the metaphysis is lucent. **B:** Two years after presentation. The right proximal femur shows extensive deformity. A coxa magna deformity of the femoral head, a widened femoral neck, incomplete coverage (containment of the head), and evidence of physeal growth arrest are seen. (From Kirks DR. Practical Pediatric Imaging: Diagnostic Radiology of Infants and Children, 3rd ed. Philadelphia: Lippincott Williams & Wilkins, 1998.)

Hip MRI
- Sensitive for early detection of ischemia
- Useful when there is high suspicion for LCPD but x-rays are normal

 TABLE 13.4: Hip MRI: Legg-Calvé-Perthes disease

IV contrast	No
PO contrast	No
Amount of radiation	None

Basic Management
- Goal: Maintenance or restoration of the femoral head central position
- Pediatric orthopedic surgeon referral
- Non-weight bearing until outpatient follow-up
- Early treatment: nonsteroidal anti-inflammatory drugs (NSAIDs), physical therapy, and mechanical stress reduction

Summary

TABLE 13.5: Advantages and disadvantages of imaging modalities in Legg-Calvé-Perthes disease

Imaging modalities	Advantages	Disadvantages
X-ray	Low cost Readily available	May miss diagnosis in early stages of disease
MRI	May establish the diagnosis early in the course of the disease	Not readily available Expensive

14

Osgood-Schlatter Disease

Bridget J. Quinn and William P. Meehan III

Background

Osgood-Schlatter disease (OSD) is a common cause of anterior knee pain among adolescents. It is a traction apophysitis of the tibial tubercle where the patellar tendon inserts. Movements that place a repetitive stress on the developing tubercle's ossification center lead to separation of the epiphysis from the metaphysis and callous formation of the physis. In severe cases, it can lead to frank avulsion.

OSD occurs most commonly during periods of rapid growth in children aged 8–15 years old. Boys are affected at a later age (12–15 years) than girls (8–12 years) due to the different timing of the pubertal growth spurt. About 20–30% of cases are bilateral. There is no longer a gender discrepancy, as the number of girls participating in athletics has increased. It is estimated to occur in 20% of active adolescents versus 5% of nonathletes.

TABLE 14.1: Classic history and physical

Provoked by running, jumping, deep knee bends, stairs, kneeling with the knee fully flexed
Inability to participate in activities/sport without pain
Localized knee pain over the tibial tubercle that increases over time
Swelling over the tibial tubercle
Pain with resisted knee extension and/or squatting
Poor flexibility of the hamstrings and quadriceps

Knee X-rays: OSD

- AP and lateral knee radiographs may demonstrate
  - Soft tissue swelling anterior to the tubercle
  - Irregularity and/or fragmentation of the tibial tubercle
  - Ossicle within the patellar tendon
  - Calcification of the patellar tendon
  - Thickening of the patellar tendon
- Look for lesion on lateral image with the knee internally rotated at 10°–20°
  - Helps exclude, e.g., avulsion fracture of the tibial tubercle, tumor, or infection, particularly in unilateral presentations

 TABLE 14.2: Knee x-ray: Osgood-Schlatter disease

IV contrast	No
PO contrast	No
Amount of radiation	0.005 mSv per view*

*Approximate dose.

Classic Images

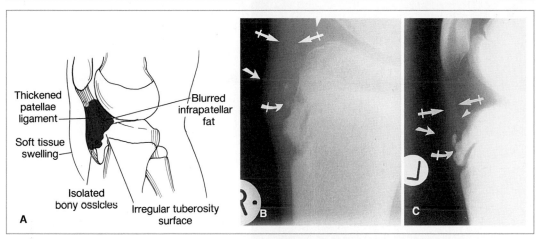

FIGURE 14.1: Osgood-Schlatter disease characteristic features. **A:** Diagram. **B** and **C:** Lateral knee. Observe the edema over the tibial tuberosity (*arrows*), blurred infrapatellar fat (*arrowhead*), thickened patellar ligament (*crossed arrows*), and fragmentation of the tuberosity (*curved crossed arrows*). (From Yochum TR and Rowe LJ. Yochum and Rowe's Essentials of Skeletal Radiology, 3rd ed. Philadelphia: Lippincott Williams & Wilkins, 2004.)

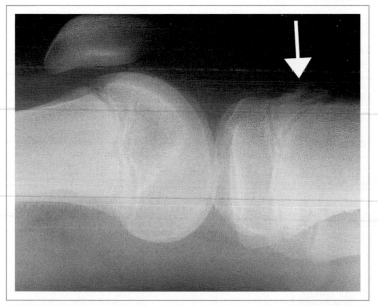

FIGURE 14.2: Radiographs are usually normal, but mild irregularities of the tibial tubercle (*arrow*) are often present. (From Fleisher GR, Ludwig S, and Baskin MN. Atlas of Pediatric Emergency Medicine. Philadelphia: Lippincott Williams & Wilkins, 2004.)

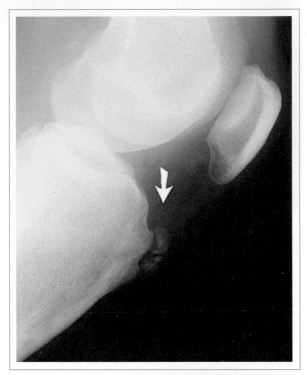

FIGURE 14.3: A protuberance on the tibia is visible, and the blurry area indicated by the arrow shows where inflammatory edema has accumulated. (From Yochum TR and Rowe LJ. Yochum and Rowe's Essentials of Skeletal Radiology, 3rd ed. Philadelphia: Lippincott Williams & Wilkins, 2004.)

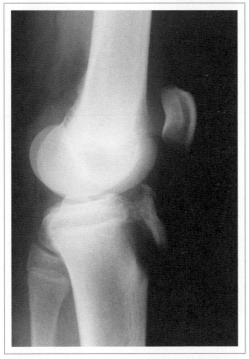

FIGURE 14.4: Acute tibial tubercle avulsion fracture in a child with history of Osgood-Schlatter disease. (From Fleisher GR, Ludwig S, and Henretig FM. Textbook of Pediatric Emergency Medicine, 5th ed. Philadelphia: Lippincott Williams & Wilkins, 2005.)

Knee MRI

In rare instances, MRI may be requested by the consultative service and used to define fracture patterns and aid in preoperative planning.

 TABLE 14.3: MRI: Osgood-Schlatter disease

IV contrast	No
PO contrast	No
Amount of radiation	None

Basic Management

- 90% of patients improve with conservative treatment
- Apply ice for 20 minutes several times/day to alleviate pain and inflammation
- Administer an analgesic (e.g., acetaminophen) and/or nonsteroidal anti-inflammatory (e.g., ibuprofen)
- Participation in activity as limited by pain
- Physical therapy focusing on flexibility of the quadriceps and hamstring in addition to quadriceps strengthening
- Protective pad or brace with a donut hole to protect the tubercle
- Infrapatellar strap to apply a counterforce to the epiphysis
- Outpatient follow-up with primary care physician, sports medicine physician, or orthopedic surgeon
- Surgical options reserved for recalcitrant pain in the mature skeleton.

Summary

TABLE 14.4: Advantages and disadvantages of imaging modalities in Osgood-Schlatter disease

Imaging modality	Advantage	Disadvantage
X-ray	Fast Low cost Minimal radiation Evaluates other etiologies (e.g., fracture)	May not delineate etiology
MRI	Delineates extent of injury Preoperative planning	Expensive Time Availability

15 Radiation Considerations in Children

Sara Schutzman and Keith Strauss

Introduction

Computerized tomography (CT) is an extremely valuable diagnostic tool for a variety of disorders in children evaluated in the emergency department (ED), including trauma, abdominal pain, headache, inflammatory processes, and renal calculi. Its use has been increasing dramatically, likely due to increased availability and refinements in CT technology. Currently, ~7 million studies are done annually on children, with the rate increasing ~10% per year. Only relatively recently has attention been focused on the risks of the associated radiation and its potential to cause a small but significant increased risk of cancer and death.

Unique Considerations in Children

There are several unique considerations in children that make them more susceptible to the deleterious effects of radiation:

1. Growing children have more rapidly dividing cells, which are more sensitive to radiation.

2. Children have a longer lifetime to develop cancers resulting from radiation exposure. The latent period for the majority of radiation-induced cancers exceeds 25 years, resulting in a higher risk for children compared to older patients.

3. Children receive a greater radiation dose than adults from the same CT scan parameters (settings).

4. Facilities too often fail to adjust CT scan parameters for size that needlessly increases radiation doses for children.

It is therefore imperative that clinicians take into account radiation risks when assessing the benefit of an imaging study to their patients.

Radiation Dose

CT radiation doses can be estimated in several ways. Absorbed dose measures the energy transferred from the x-ray to the patient's body per unit mass and is expressed in units of grays (Gy). Effective dose, which is expressed in units of sieverts (Sv), estimates the whole-body dose based on individual organ doses and sensitivities of those organs. Effective dose, therefore, estimates the risk of harm to a patient from a diagnostic examination involving ionizing radiation. Table 15.1 lists the effective radiation doses for common diagnostic studies as well as their comparison to the annual background radiation exposure of 3 mSv.

TABLE 15.1: Effective radiation doses and comparison to background radiation

Examination	Effective radiation dose*	Comparable to natural background radiation
Chest PA	0.01 mSv	2 d
Head CT	2 mSv	8 mo
Chest CT	6 mSv	2 yr
Abdomen CT	6 mSv	2 yr
Pelvic CT	6 mSv	2 yr

PA, posteroanterior.
*Approximate dose.

The effective dose estimate for a PA chest examination is included to illustrate that CT examinations with reduced radiation doses still deliver 200–700 times more radiation dose to the patient than the single chest examination. These doses assume that all reasonable steps are taken to reduce the radiation dose delivered to the patient. If the scan parameters are not adjusted for patient size, the dose for the youngest, most sensitive pediatric patients can exceed three times the radiation dose delivered to the adult patients for the same study.

Radiation Effects and Risks

Since radiation-induced cancers can take decades to present much of our carcinogenic risk data comes from follow-up studies of the atomic bomb survivors, who were exposed more than 65 years ago. While high radiation doses are well known to be associated with the development of malignancy, even lower doses of radiation, in the ranges of 10–50 mSv, incur a small increased lifetime risk for fatal cancer. Although estimated effective doses of 5–10 mSv have not definitively been shown to increase the risk of lethal cancer, major national and international organizations responsible for evaluating radiation risks have agreed to assume no threshold below which radiation doses do not have the potential to induce cancers.

Table 15.2 estimates the probability of radiation-induced fatal cancers by age group, assuming the estimated effective doses from a single CT examination listed in Table 15.1. The increased risk in childhood is clearly reflected. While estimates vary, for a child undergoing a single CT of the abdomen/pelvis, the risk of cancer mortality is ~1:1,000. Since the overall risk of death from cancer is ~1:4–1:5, one CT causes only a modest increase in risk (from ~24% to 24.05%). However, the overall lifetime exposures are believed to be cumulative. Since each subsequent CT scan increases the risk, all reasonable efforts should be made to limit the number of CT scans the same patient receives. In addition, the risks listed in Table 15.2 do not include nonfatal cancers.

TABLE 15.2: Risk of death from a single CT scan

Examination	First decade 0–9 yr	Second decade 10–20 yr	Adults
Head CT	1:2,000	1:6,000	1:10,000
Chest CT	1:1,300	1:2,100	1:3,300
Abdominal CT	1:1,100	1:1,800	1:2,900
Pelvic CT	1:1,100	1:1,800	1:2,900

For comparison, the annual risk of death from an auto accident is 1:7,000 and the risk of death from all accidents is 1:1,600.

What Can the ED Physician Do?

CT provides valuable and even life saving medical information, which should provide more benefit than harm. Given the potential risks of radiation, however, physicians should minimize the amount of radiation a child is exposed to while maintaining efficacy and reliability of the diagnostic test. The concept of ALARA (radiation "as low as reasonably achievable") should be advocated by all physicians. There are a variety of ways the exposure to radiation can be limited:

1. *Make sure the study is necessary.* It is estimated that 10–30% of CTs may be unnecessary. For example, not all children with head injury require CT, and evaluation of the multiple trauma patient does not require head/neck/chest/abdomen/pelvis CT.

2. *Explore alternative modalities that do not use ionizing radiation (e.g., ultrasound, MRI).* Although not ideal in all cases, ultrasound may be used in many cases to evaluate children for appendicitis. Likewise, nonemergent head imaging may be done using MRI through outpatient follow-up (e.g., first time afebrile seizure with nonfocal examination).

3. *Scan the least possible to obtain clinically important information.*

   a. Perform focused/limited studies (e.g., for appendicitis evaluations, do not perform full abdominal/pelvic CT).

   b. Scan the area once. Discourage "repeat CTs," e.g., with and without contrast as they are often unnecessary and dramatically increase the radiation dose.

4. *Verify with questions whether steps to reduce the radiation dose for each pediatric study have been set up by the imaging department.*

   a. Is appropriate shielding used (e.g., breast, thyroid)?

   b. Are the CT scanners and imaging department accredited to perform pediatric CT?

   c. Does the imaging department employ size-based scan parameters for children?

   d. Is a qualified medical physicist available and used to reduce radiation dose while maintaining image quality?

Section Editor: Jonathan A. Edlow

16

Acute Cerebral Ischemia and Infarction

Jonathan A. Edlow and Magdy Selim

Background

More so now than in the past, transient ischemic attack (TIA) and infarction (stroke) are important neurological emergencies. Firstly, they are becoming more common as the population ages. Secondly, newer data on TIA shows that many of these patients have actually had small strokes (even though the symptoms have passed) and also that the risk of a second event, which is often a large stroke, is approximately 5% in the first 2 days after the initial event. Finally, evaluation of TIA patients and treatment of the underlying vascular mechanism reduces the high acute stroke risk by about 80%. For stroke patients, various interventions (intravenous and intra-arterial tissue plasminogen activator [tPA], mechanical clot retrieval devices, and antithrombotics based on stroke/TIA etiology) can improve outcomes.

The two cardinal parts of the history are the abrupt onset of localizing (focal) neurological symptoms. TIA and stroke begin suddenly; when multiple body parts are involved (such as face and arm), they often become involved simultaneously, not sequentially. The findings are focal, that is, attributable to a cerebrovascular territory. A third concept, which is often quite helpful, is that these symptoms are usually "negative" (absence of strength, vision, sensation, speech) rather than "positive" (abnormal movements, hallucinations, paresthesias, etc), which are more typical of seizure or migraine.

Standard practice is to obtain a noncontrast head CT; however, at stroke centers, patients are increasingly getting acute perfusion CT and angiography and/or MRI/magnetic resonance angiography (MRA) sequences to define three variables:

1 How much brain is already irreversibly infracted (the infarcted core)?

2. How much brain tissue is ischemic, not yet infracted but at risk for infarction (the ischemic penumbra)?

3. Is the relevant cerebral artery occluded or patent?

The priorities in the emergency department are to (a) stabilize the ABCs, (b) exclude a hemorrhage or other cause of the symptoms, (c) evaluate for potential time-critical treatments like tPA, and (d) identify TIA patients and find and treat any underlying vascular mechanism quickly to prevent a future acute stroke.

TABLE 16.1: Classic history and physical

Acute onset of new focal neurologic symptoms
Headache (usually mild, if present) may point to a large vessel occlusion, posterior circulation infarct, arterial dissection, venous infarction, or hemorrhage
Rarely a stroke will present with seizure at onset
Note that for TIA, the symptoms and signs are by definition transient and will often have resolved by the time the patient arrives in the ED
Determining the NIH Stroke Scale value is a good way to quantify the examination

ED, emergency department; NIH, National Institute of Health; TIA, transient ischemic attack.

TABLE 16.2: Potentially helpful laboratory tests

CBC, Chem7: can evaluate for anemia, platelet disorders, hypo- or hyperglycemia, sodium abnormalities, or renal dysfunction
Coagulation panel: useful baseline information with regard to antithrombotic therapy
CK-MB, troponin: screen for potential causes of thrombus in cardioembolic stroke
Lipid profile and hemoglobin A1C: screen for undiagnosed hyperglycemia or hyperlipidemia (need not be performed in the ED)
Blood cultures: screen if endocarditis is of concern given history/physical examination

ED, emergency department.

Noncontrast Head CT Scan

- Widely and rapidly available, but its purpose in patients with acute ischemic stroke is not to make the diagnosis of stroke but to exclude other causes for the symptoms, especially hemorrhage, which is an exclusion for tPA and might invoke other therapies (see Chapter 20, "Intracerebral Hemorrhage")
- Relatively low radiation exposure
- It is important to recognize that the sensitivity of noncontrast CT in acute ischemic stroke evolves over time from symptom onset and is often normal in the hyperacute patient (see below)
- **Within the first 6 hours, the scan is frequently normal**
- The sensitivity of CT scan for detecting posterior fossa strokes (cerebellum and brainstem) is poor, especially during the hyperacute phase
- CT is almost always normal in patients with TIA and therefore do not accept a negative CT as evidence that a patient does not have an acute ischemic stroke, especially in the posterior fossa, or a TIA
- By extension, if a patient whose reported time of onset is 2 hours ago has a large hypodensity that the early suspect that the history of the onset time may be inaccurate or that the hypodensity is due to another (nonstroke) process such as a tumor
- A large stroke on noncontrast CT is associated with higher bleeding risk after IV tPA; there is controversy as to whether or not tPA should be considered in these cases

TABLE 16.3: Key findings

Look for findings of ischemic stroke mimics:
Intracranial hemorrhage (any location)
Tumor, subdural hematoma, and abscess (and others)
Look for early, subtle signs of infarction:
Clot in a vessel (hyperdense artery sign)
Loss of grey white differentiation
Loss of insular ribbon
Focal hypoattenuation

 TABLE 16.4: Noncontrast CT scan: ischemic stroke

IV contrast	No
PO contrast	No
Amount of radiation	2 mSV

CT Angiography and Perfusion CT

- CT angiography (CTA) can rapidly and noninvasively assess the patency of major cerebral blood vessels. Look for abrupt cut-off of a vessel or signs of a dissection (caution: these studies are complex and often involve looking at reconstructions that may be processed after the source images have been acquired).
- With improving CT hardware and software, its accuracy is close to that of the gold standard (digital subtraction angiography, or DSA).

- Using software, the use of IV contrast can lead to CT "perfusion" imaging. This perfusion study helps to define the ischemic penumbra. Postprocessing can create maps of cerebral blood flow, mean transit time, and cerebral blood volume.
- In some stroke centers, CTA has become a standard study in order to help make decisions about acute treatments (e.g., no tPA if all vessels open, IV tPA for distal occlusions, and IV ± intra-arterial tPA or mechanical clot retrieval for major proximal occlusions). Note that this is not standard of care at this point in time, which only requires a noncontrast CT.

 TABLE 16.5: CTA scan: ischemic stroke

IV contrast	Yes
PO contrast	No
Amount of radiation	3–4 mSV

MRI

- MRI is much more sensitive than CT to show an acute infarction and is positive much earlier (see images/figures below)
- Not all sequences will show the infarction; diffusion-weighted imaging is particularly sensitive
- In patients with TIA, about 40–50% will show diffusion-weighted imaging lesions that account for the patient's symptoms
- There are also more sophisticated sequences including ADC (apparent diffusion coefficient) mapping that can be performed to distinguish acute from old infarction

 TABLE 16.6: MRI: ischemic stroke

IV contrast	No
PO contrast	No
Amount of radiation	None

MRA

- MRA is used similarly to CTA (see above)
- It has the advantage of not requiring IV contrast, although gadolinium administration enhances the resolution of MRA
- MRI with diffusion and perfusion images plus MRA can supply similar information as perfusion CT and CTA in defining the ischemic penumbra

TABLE 16.7: Magnetic resonance angiography: ischemic stroke

IV contrast	No*
PO contrast	No
Amount of radiation	None

*Gadolinium needed for the perfusion study.

Classic Images

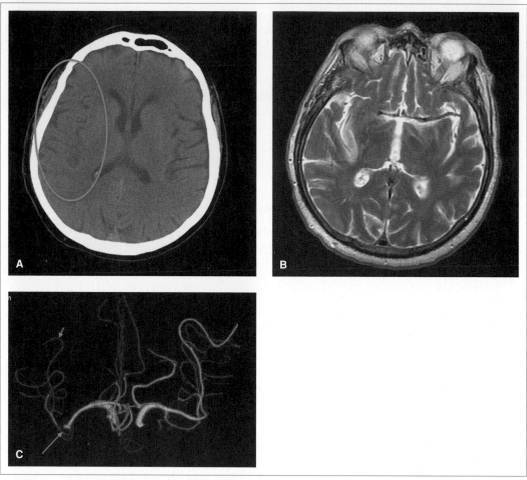

FIGURE 16.1: Right middle cerebral artery stroke. An 80-year-old man presented with hypertension and untreated atrial fibrillation presenting with the sudden onset (45 min before) of left-sided neglect, mild left-sided weakness, and dysarthria. Because of mild confusion, the time of onset was unclear. **A:** A noncontrast CT scan shows very minimal loss of sulcal markings (*green arrow*). **B:** A diffusion-weighted MRI image done within hours of the CT more easily illustrates the area of infarction. **C:** The CT angiogram shows markedly decreased flow in the right MCA (*small white arrows*).

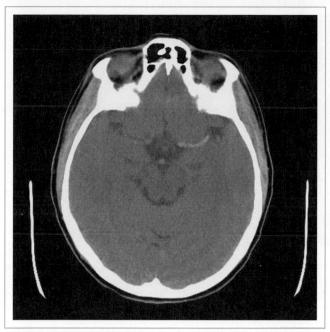

FIGURE 16.2: Left middle cerebral artery stroke. This noncontrast CT scan was taken from a 55-year-old man with the abrupt onset of severe right facial droop, right arm weakness, and inability to speak. It shows the "hyperdense MCA sign," which is a clot in the middle cerebral artery. His CT angiogram (not shown) showed a clot that was in the exact same area. At a community hospital, he was not treated with tissue plasminogen activator and when he arrived at the referral hospital (now at hour 5 after symptom onset), he underwent an endovascular clot removal.

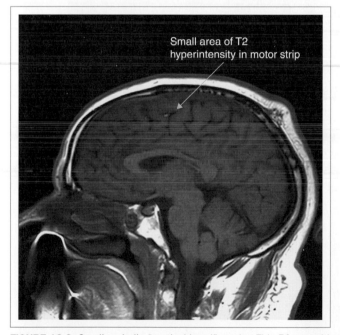

FIGURE 16.3: Small embolic "cortical hand" stroke. This 50-year-old woman presented to the emergency department with 1 day of weakness of several fingers on the left hand. She was thought to have a peripheral nerve or cervical nerve root injury and was referred to a neurologist 2 days later. The MRI was done then and shows a tiny area of T2 hyperintensity in the motor strip corresponding to the hand (on the homunculus). The concept of a "cortical hand" is important for emergency clinicians to know; such strokes are generally embolic to a very small branch of the MCA and an evaluation to identify and treat the embolic source must be undertaken.

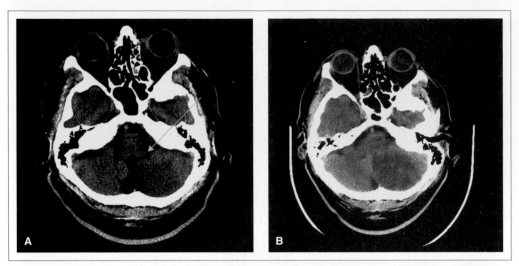

FIGURE 16.4: Cerebellar stroke. A 74-year-old man presented to the ED with 8 hours of sudden onset of vomiting and no other symptoms. On examination, he was unable to walk due to severe gait instability (but did not have nystagmus nor dysmetria). Hypodensity in his left cerebellar hemisphere (**A**). Note the wide open CSF filled space (*arrow*) around the brainstem. Two days later, the patient became drowsy and a repeat CT scan (**B**) shows edema in the area of infarction with obliteration of the previously patent space and brainstem compression.

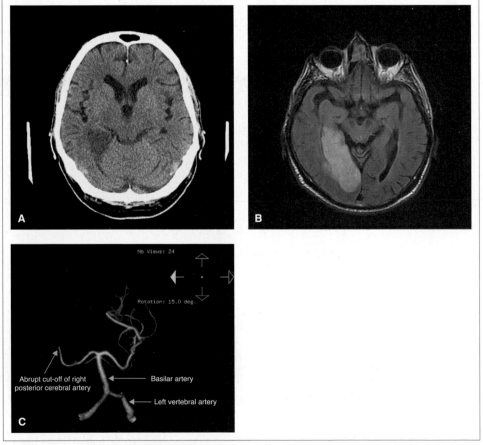

FIGURE 16.5: Right posterior cerebral artery stroke. This 70-year-old man presented with 1 day of left-sided visual field loss. His CT (**A**) shows hypodensity in the territory of the right posterior cerebral artery (PCA). An axial FLAIR MRI (**B**) done shortly afterward shows the stroke (at a lower cut of the brain) much more intensely than does the CT. The accompanying CT angiograph (**C**) shows an abrupt cut-off of the PCA.

Basic Management

- Airway management usually not necessary for anterior circulation strokes
- STAT blood glucose to exclude hypoglycemia
- Quick neurological examination to document the deficit, ideally using the National Institute of Health stroke scale
- Blood pressure control usually not indicated; allow the brain to "autoregulate" to maintain adequate cerebral perfusion pressure; if reducing the pressure pharmacologically, do so modestly
- Neurology consultation
- Neurointerventional consultation if an intra-arterial treatment is a possibility
- Admission to a stroke care unit—patients admitted to stroke units have better outcomes than those admitted to general medical units
- Hyperglycemia management
- Fever treatment
- A 12-lead EKG and cardiac monitoring
- Serial neurologic examinations to evaluate for neurologic deterioration

Summary

TABLE 16.8: Advantages and disadvantages of imaging modalities in ischemic stroke

Imaging modality	Advantages	Disadvantages
CT scan	Widespread availability Rapid Relatively low cost	Radiation Does not diagnose small strokes or stroke in the first 6–8 hr Subtle changes (of an early, large stroke or of a small bleed could be missed)
CT angiography (CT perfusion)	Rapid Highly accurate in evaluating an acute cut-off in a major cranial vessel Can be done with the CT scan	IV contrast Radiation
MRI	Can detect the actual stroke No radiation exposure	Cost, availability, time to perform Many patients have contraindications or claustrophobia
MR angiography	Can detect underlying vascular lesion Can be done with the MRI scan	Cost, availability, time to perform Many patients have contraindications or claustrophobia

17 Brain Mass Lesions

Jonathan A. Edlow

Background

This chapter discusses brain abscess and tumor mass lesions (intracranial hemorrhage and extra-axial hematomas are discussed in another chapter). Masses can present in various ways, the symptoms being a function of location, size, rapidity of growth and secondary changes from elevated intracranial pressure (ICP), vasogenic edema as well as ischemia from impingement on adjacent vascular structures or acutely bleeding into the mass. For example, a frontal lobe tumor can grow to an extremely large size before causing symptoms, whereas a very small mass in the brainstem may cause symptoms. All things being equal, a slow growing mass will cause fewer symptoms than a rapidly growing one. However, a slow growing mass may still cause abrupt symptoms from a bleed within it or from acute elevation in ICP once compensatory mechanisms are overwhelmed. Any mass can cause a seizure. Finally, pituitary adenomas can present with symptoms relating to hormone production (e.g., Cushing's syndrome or acromegaly).

Brain abscess is an uncommon cause of a mass lesion. These lesions may relate to trauma (surgical or accidental), spread from contiguous head/eyes/ears/nose/throat (HEENT) infections or hematogenous spread from bacteremia. Tumors can be benign or malignant and primary or metastatic. Primary malignancies include various grades of glioblastoma, oligodendroglioma, lymphoma, and meningioma. An example of a benign primary tumor would be an acoustic schwannoma.

TABLE 17.1: Classic history and physical

Wide range of presentations
"Classic" presentation of headache worse upon awakening is uncommon

Symptoms related to:
    Location of the mass
    Size of the mass
    Rapidity of growth of the mass

Secondary findings from hydrocephalus, edema, impingement on adjacent vascular   structures, or bleeding into the mass
Symptoms from a seizure or postictal phenomenon
Symptoms from a hormone dysregulation

Specific (common) presenting symptoms include:
    Headache
    Seizure
    Confusion

Any focal neurological finding
Fever (though often absent) with brain abscess

Note: The pace at which these symptoms develop varies by pathophysiology, e.g., headache may be gradual from a slowly growing mass but could be abrupt if there is bleeding into the tumor.

TABLE 17.2: Potentially helpful laboratory tests

WBC: not particularly sensitive in cases of brain abscess
Blood cultures: should be drawn in cases of suspected brain abscess
LP and CSF analysis: potentially *harmful* in patients with brain abscess and often   does not yield the organism so the risk-benefit ratio usually does not favor an LP

LP, lumbar puncture; CSF, cerebrospinal fluid.

CT Scan

- ■ CT is not as sensitive as MRI for both tumor and abscess
- ■ The CT scan may be completely normal
- ■ Mass lesions large enough to cause symptoms typically demonstrate finding(s):
  - ● hydrocephalus
  - ● shift of normal position of intracranial structures
  - ● vasogenic edema
- ■ Abscess may show only edema; infusion of IV contrast often shows the capsule and will define the abscess with greater clarity

 TABLE 17.3: CT scan: brain abscess or tumor

IV contrast	Yes, helpful for deciphering type of mass
PO contrast	No
Amount of radiation	2 mSV

MRI Scan

- MRI has revolutionized the diagnosis of mass lesions because one can now better see the mass, as well as any associated edema or hydrocephalus, the effects of adjacent structures including vascular structures and in the case of metastatic tumor, see small, secondary lesions that are still asymptomatic
- A completely normal MRI with and without gadolinium enhancement essentially rules out tumor as a cause of a patient's symptoms
- Although not a mass per se, herpes encephalitis usually presents with temporal lobe lesions, sometimes bilaterally

 TABLE 17.4: MRI: brain abscess or tumor

IV contrast	Yes
PO contrast	No
Amount of radiation	None

Classic Images

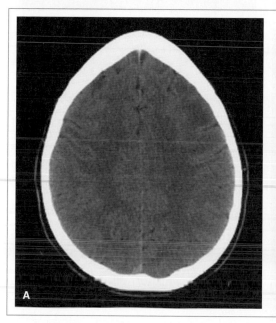 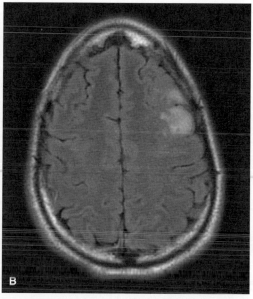

FIGURE 17.1: A and **B:** The same cut from a CT and an MRI of the same patient on the same day. The patient presented with a new seizure. The CT shows very mild edema that is easily seen on the T2-Flair MRI. The lesion is a low-grade glioma. These images illustrate how some tumors will be barely visible by CT but show up far better on MR sequences.

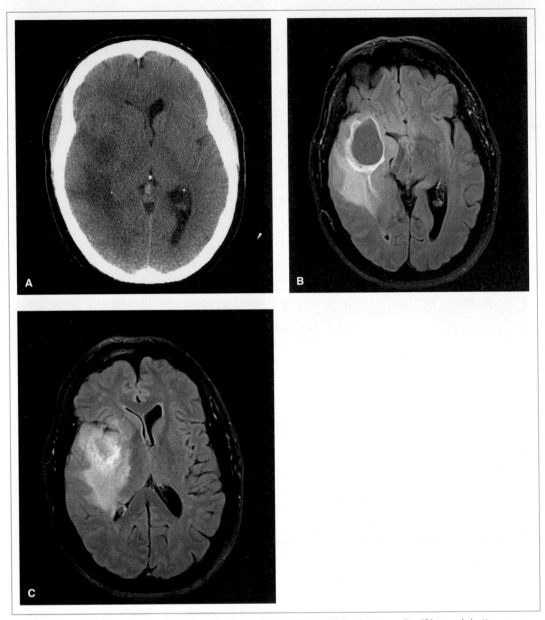

FIGURE 17.2: A and **B:** The same cut from a CT and MRI (T2-Flair). While the tumor itself is much better seen on MRI, the vasogenic edema (dark area on the CT, white area on MRI) is apparent on both. **C:** A cut from lower in the brain shows the tumor itself (dark area) in the temporal area. This patient presented with 1 month of temporal lobe seizures (episodic odd smells) and 3 days of increasingly severe headache. Decadron reduced the swelling; at surgery, a glioblastoma was found.

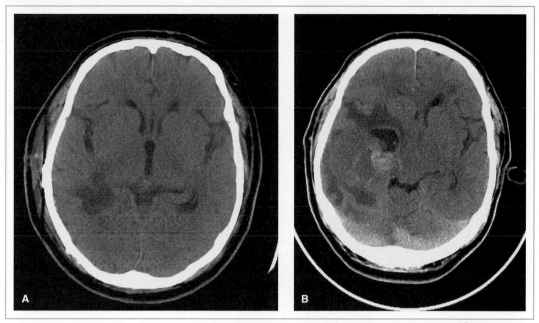

FIGURE 17.3: **A** and **B:** This patient with a history of renal cell carcinoma presented with 10 days of headache that got abruptly worse the day of the first CT scan, which shows hemorrhage into a complex tumor. Physical examination revealed a left homonomous hemianopsia of which the patient had been unaware. The second CT scan was done 5 weeks after surgical resection. The lesion was a metastatic lesion (the original renal cell carcinoma presented 7 years before the brain metastasis).

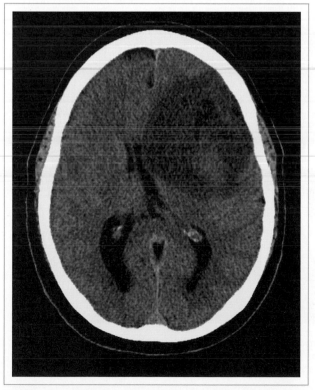

FIGURE 17.4: This patient presented with very mild aphasia and no headache. The tumor proved to be an oligoastrocytoma. Large tumors will sometimes present with remarkably minimal symptoms because they are so slow growing. The mild aphasia resolved postoperatively.

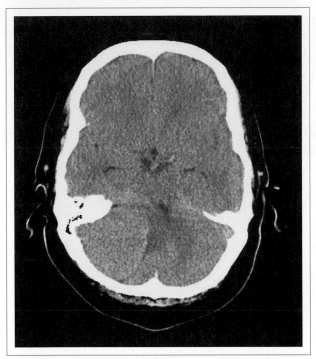

FIGURE 17.5: This patient presented with gradual onset of vertigo, nausea, and vomiting. The CT shows a right-sided cerebellar lesion, but it is subtle; IV contrast injection showed enhancement. A benign meningioma was found at surgery. IV contrast is a useful tool in patients who cannot tolerate MRI or if MRI is not available.

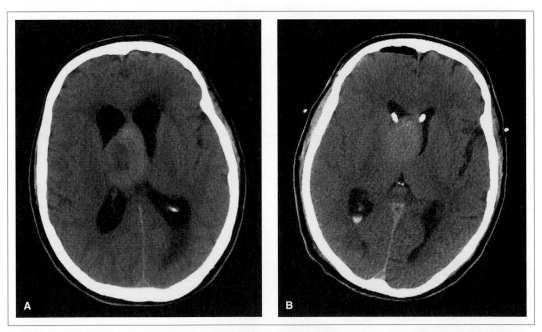

FIGURE 17.6: A and **B:** This patient with thalamic tumor presented with confusion and mild headache due to hydrocephalus from outflow obstruction from the lateral ventricles. Initial treatment was with external ventricular drains to treat the hydrocephalus and shows decreased hydrocephalus (B). The tumor was later shown to be a glioblastoma multiforme.

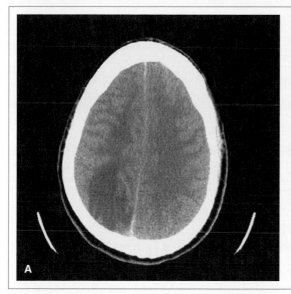 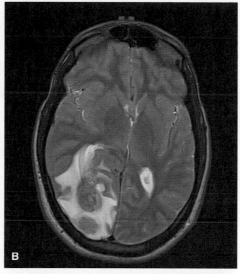

FIGURE 17.7: These images are of a 23-year-old non-immunosuppressed patient with several days of gradually increasing confusion and headache. Three weeks prior, he had a upper respiratory infection. **A:** CT scan shows some central hemorrhage in a lesion in the right parieto-occipital lobe that is mostly notable for the vasogenic edema that surrounds it. The CT was interpreted as consistent with mass, ruptured arterio-venous malformation (AVM) or venous thrombosis. **B:** MRI from the same days shows an enhancing mass with abundant vasogenic edema, thought to most likely represent tumor. At operation, this was a bacterial brain abscess.

Basic Management

- Assess ABCs
- Endotracheal intubation: consider if ICP is elevated and the patient is obtunded
- Early consultation with a neurologist and/or neurosurgeon
- Lumbar puncture: Caution in performing in cases of possible brain abscess; often does not yield the organism and may be harmful
- Steroid administration:
  - Reduces vasogenic edema (usually seen with tumor or abscess)
  - Give IV Decadron if patient is showing acute signs of herniation
  - Avoid in neurologically stable patients, in whom a new neoplasm Is a possibility as this may affect the results of a biopsy that will result in important information that guides treatment
- Antibiotic administration: in well-appearing clinically stable patients with possible brain abscess, discuss with consultant especially if early surgery or stereotactic drainage is planned as they may wish to wait to first obtain a tissue sample
- Patients presenting with obstructive hydrocephalus may benefit from early external ventricular drain placement
- Seizure treatment and prophylaxis: patients who have had a seizure should be treated with an anticonvulsant; prophylactic treatment is controversial

Summary

TABLE 17.5: Advantages and disadvantages of imaging modalities in brain mass

Imaging modality	Advantages	Disadvantages
CT scan	Low cost Minimal patient discomfort Availability Very sensitive for lesions large enough to cause compressive symptoms or headache	Lower sensitivity than MRI Radiation IV contrast dye reactions and side effects (if used)
MRI	Excellent sensitivity No radiation exposure Often helps with surgical planning	Cost, availability, time to perform Many patients have contraindications or claustrophobia Gadolinium reactions (if used)

18 Head Injury

Samuel Gross, Leah Honigman, and Carlo L. Rosen

Background

Head injury is responsible for approximately 5 million visits in the emergency department each year and is an important cause of morbidity and mortality. A large proportion of patients are males aged 15–40 years; however, the distribution of head injuries actually has peaks in the very young and the very old. The most common causes of traumatic head injuries include motor vehicle collisions and falls.

Common patterns of traumatic head injuries include:

- *Skull fracture:* Substantial blunt force causing one of three types of fractures—linear, depressed, basilar; this can also occur with penetrating injury
- *Epidural hematoma:* Damage to a vessel, usually an artery and often associated with skull fracture; classic presentation is head trauma and loss of consciousness followed by a lucid interval and then progressive decline
- *Subdural hematoma (SDH):* Often results from tearing of bridging veins, and patients with cerebral atrophy are at higher risk (e.g., elderly, alcoholics); it can be classified as acute (days), subacute, or chronic (>2 wk)
- *Subarachnoid hemorrhage (SAH):* Can be traumatic or spontaneous in origin
- *Diffuse axonal injury (DAI):* Results from high-speed injury with deceleration and rotational movement of the head; accounts for approximately half of parenchymal injuries
- *Cerebral/cortical contusion:* Common parenchymal injury in minor head trauma
- *Penetrating injury:* Gunshot wounds, stab wounds, and blast injuries

TABLE 18.1: Classic history and physical

History of direct head trauma (e.g., fall, automobile accident with or without loss of consciousness)
Altered mental status
Scalp hematomas, abrasions, lacerations, or step offs
Signs of basilar skull fracture: battle sign (postauricular hematoma), raccoon's eyes, hemotympanum, and clear rhinorrhea (evidence of CSF leak)

CSF, cerebrospinal fluid.

TABLE 18.2: Potentially helpful laboratory tests

Platelets, coagulation panel—assess increased bleeding risk
Toxicology screen, Chem7—medical etiology for altered mental status
Serum levels of any known antiepileptic medications

Head CT Scan

- Noncontrast head CT is first-line imaging for assessment of traumatic intracranial injury
- Most sensitive study for fractures, acute epidural or subdural hematoma
- Readily available and fast
- Can also evaluate for progression of hematoma over time
- Limitations: Basilar skull fractures may not be readily visible on head CT and instead rely on careful examination
- IV contrast is only useful if looking for underlying vascular abnormality or aneurysm as primary cause leading to trauma

TABLE 18.3: Key findings

Epidural hematoma

Typically hyperdense lens-shaped lesions as bleeding is restricted by dural attachments to skull at sutures

May cause shift, ventricular compression, and subfalcine or uncal herniation

Subdural hematoma (SDH)

Typically crescent-shaped lesions with sharp margins most often located at cerebral convexities, falx cerebri, or tentorium cerebelli

Acute SDH is hyperdense; subacute SDH is isodense; chronic SDH is hypodense relative to brain parenchyma

Subarachnoid hemorrhage (SAH)

Typically appears as clot or hemorrhage in the subarachnoid space, often with intercerebral extension; the location is typically higher on the convexities or at the anterior frontal or temporal fossae (not in the basilar cisterns where aneurysmal subarachnoid blood is found)

Also evaluate for intraventricular or subdural bleeding

Cerebral/cortical contusion

Half of lesions are hemorrhagic, which are typically round or oval hyperdensities at gyral surfaces with surrounding hypodense edema

May have mass effect or delayed hemorrhage

Commonly seen on inferior surface of frontal lobes and inferior/anterior temporal lobes from movement of brain over skull base

 TABLE 18.4: CT scan: head injury

IV contrast	No
PO contrast	No
Amount of radiation	2 mSv

Classic Images

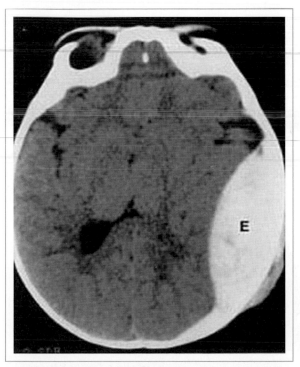

FIGURE 18.1: Axial noncontrast CT scan of the head showing a left parietal epidural hematoma. Note the high attenuation of blood as well as lenticular shape and compression of the brain parenchyma and ventricles. (*Courtesy of Beth Israel Deaconess Medical Center, Boston, MA.*)

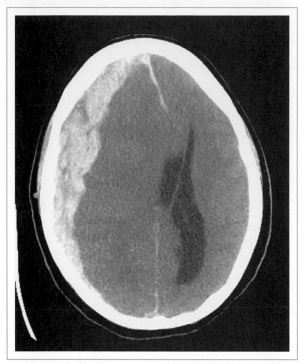

FIGURE 18.2: Axial noncontrast CT scan of the head with a large acute subdural hematoma with midline shift, compression of the ventricles, and herniation. (*Courtesy of Beth Israel Deaconess Medical Center, Boston, MA.*)

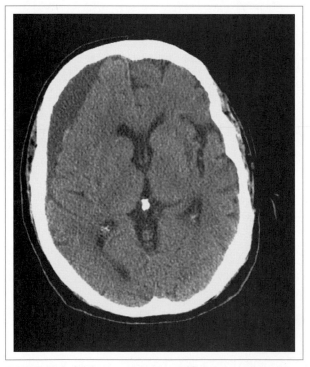

FIGURE 18.3: Axial non-contrast head CT demonstrating a chronic subdural hemorrhage. Note that the crescentic area of hemorrhage is hypodense relative to brain tissue. (From Harwood-Nuss A, Wolfson AB, Hendey GW, et al. The Clinical Practice of Emergency Medicine, 3rd ed. Philadelphia: Lippincott Williams & Wilkins, 2001.)

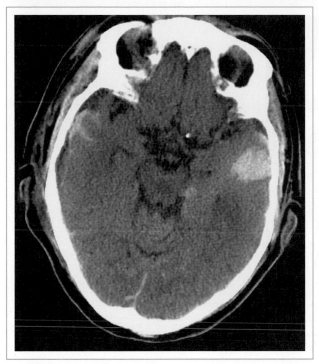

FIGURE 18.4: Axial noncontrast head CT scan. Patient has a small amount of subarachnoid blood on the right and a left-sided intraparenchymal bleed. *(Courtesy of Beth Israel Deaconess Medical Center, Boston, MA.)*

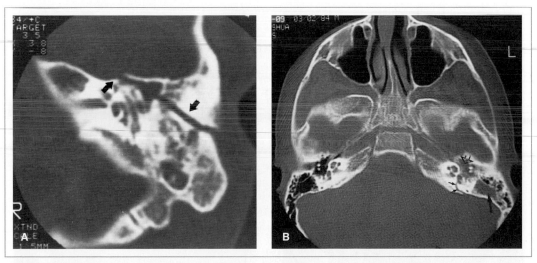

FIGURE 18.5: Basilar skull fracture. Patient was noted to have right hemotypanum on exam. CT reveals a fracture through the mastoid air cells. (From Harris J and Harris W. The Radiology of Emergency Medicine, 4th ed. Philadelphia: Lippincott Williams & Wilkins, 2000.)

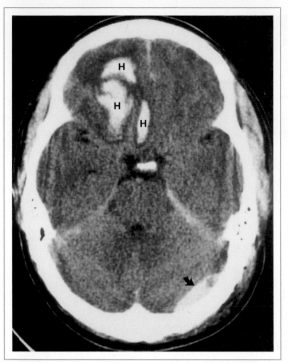

FIGURE 18.6: Cerebral contusions. The patient has hemorrhagic contusions on the base of the right frontal region with surrounding edema as well as a small left occipital epidural hematoma (*black arrow*). (From Harris J and Harris W. The Radiology of Emergency Medicine, 4th ed. Philadelphia: Lippincott Williams & Wilkins, 2000.)

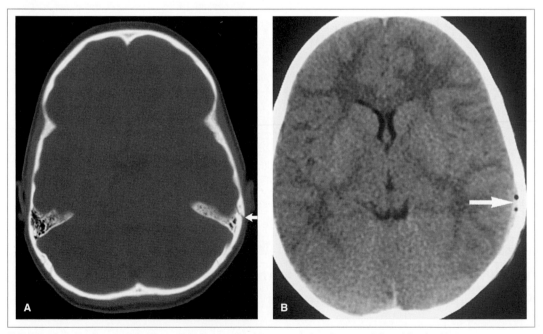

FIGURE 18.7: Basilar skull fracture. This 5-year-old girl was a pedestrian struck by a bicycle. Hemotympanum was noted on examination. **A:** The arrow indicates a fracture of the left temporal bone. The adjacent mastoid air cells are somewhat opacified. **B:** A small extra-axial hematoma with associated pneumocephaly is seen (*arrow*). (From Fleisher GR, Ludwig S, and Henretig FM. Textbook of Pediatric Emergency Medicine, 5th ed. Philadelphia: Lippincott Williams & Wilkins, 2005.)

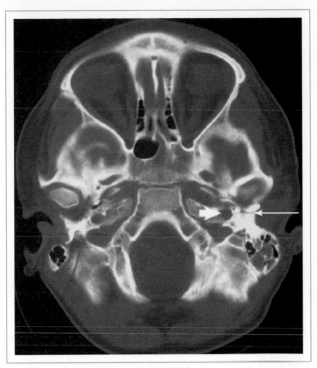

FIGURE 18.8: Basilar skull fracture. This 10-year-old male fell 10 feet to the ground. He had left hemotympanum. A head CT scan shows a fracture through the petrous portion of the temporal bone (*thin arrow*), extending toward the internal carotid canal (*thick arrow*). The left mastoid air cells are somewhat opacified. Other "cuts" of the CT confirm that the fracture involves the wall of the carotid canal. A cerebral angiogram was performed, which showed normal vascular integrity. (From Fleisher GR, Ludwig S, and Henretig FM. Textbook of Pediatric Emergency Medicine, 5th ed. Philadelphia: Lippincott Williams & Wilkins, 2005.)

Brain MRI
- Often difficult to obtain from the emergency department
- Limitations: long duration of study
- Helpful in assessment of DAI, tentorial or intrahemispheric SDH, SAH; also more sensitive for cerebral contusion

TABLE 18.5: Key findings

Cerebral/cortical contusion
Similar to appearance on CT, but more sensitive

Diffuse axonal injury
Typically located in parasagittal white matter, gray/white junction, corpus callosum, or brainstem
Lesions are hypointense on T1 and hyperintense on T2

 TABLE 18.6: MRI: head injury

IV contrast	No
PO contrast	No
Amount of radiation	None

Classic Images

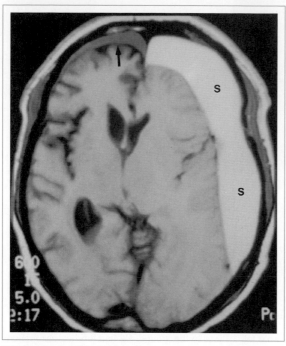

FIGURE 18.9: MRI with T1-weighted image showing a large acute left frontotemporal subdural hematoma with midline shift and subfalcine herniation. There is also a smaller subacute right frontal hematoma which is less intense (*arrow*). (From Harris J and Harris W. The Radiology of Emergency Medicine, 4th ed. Philadelphia: Lippincott Williams & Wilkins, 2000.)

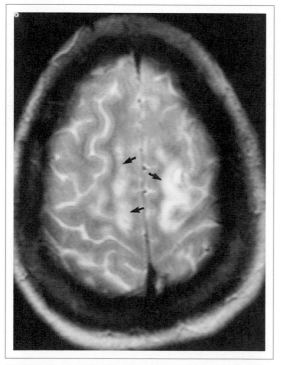

FIGURE 18.10: MRI with T2-weighted image demonstrating diffuse axonal injury in the frontal lobes. (From Harris J and Harris W. The Radiology of Emergency Medicine, 4th ed. Philadelphia: Lippincott Williams & Wilkins, 2000.)

Basic Management
- Assess and secure airway
  - Intubation required for the following: GCS <8, decreasing level of consciousness, patient is unable to protect the airway
- Immobilize cervical spine as there is often an associated injury
- Maintain SBP >90 with normal saline
- Consider neurosurgery consult for significant injuries, for example, epidural hematomas often require immediate evacuation and other lesions often require intervention
- Seizure prophylaxis: IV load with phenytoin for epidural hematoma, subdural hematoma, GCS <10, depressed skull fracture, penetrating injury, cerebral contusion, intracerebral hematoma, and seizures <24 hours from injury
- If the injured patient is anticoagulated:
  - Warfarin—give vitamin K and fresh frozen plasma; also consider specific clotting factors such as factor VII for IX
  - Aspirin or clopidogrel—platelet transfusion is an option, though it is still debated
- Consider osmotic diuresis (mannitol 0.25–1 g/kg) if there is evidence of elevated intracranial pressure

Available Imaging Decision Rules
Canadian Head CT Rule: This rule can be followed for patients with minor head injuries to determine risk for injuries requiring neurosurgical intervention. The rule suggests that patients with one high risk factor should get a head CT done, while patients with two medium risk factors should be considered for a CT scan or a period of clinical observation.

TABLE 18.7: Canadian Head CT Rule

High risk	GCS <15 2 hr after injury
	Suspected open or depressed skull fracture
	Evidence of basilar skull fracture
	More than two episodes of vomiting
	Age >65 years
Medium risk	Amnesia before impact >30 min
	Dangerous mechanism of injury:
	Pedestrian struck
	Ejection from MVC
	Fall >3 ft or down five stairs

GCS, Glasgow coma scale; MVC, motor vehicle collision.

New Orleans Criteria for CT: In patients with minor head injury and GCS of 15, no injury was found in patients who had none of the following characteristics (sensitivity 100%, 95% CI 95–100%):

- Headache
- Vomiting
- Age >60 years
- Intoxication
- Persistent anterograde amnesia
- Trauma above clavicles
- Seizure

On the basis of this observation, the New Orleans Criteria for CT suggest that patients without any of the above characteristics do not need a head CT.

Summary

TABLE 18.8: Advantages and disadvantages of imaging modalities in head trauma

Imaging modalities	Advantages	Disadvantages
CT scan	Rapid	Radiation
	Widespread	Difficult to see small hemorrhage
	First-line imaging	
MRI	Can detect underlying causes including tumor, stroke	Cost, availability, time to perform
	No radiation exposure	Many patients have contraindications or claustrophobia

Intracranial Pressure and Hydrocephalus

Scott G. Weiner

Background

Cerebrospinal fluid (CSF) is produced by the choroid plexus in the brain, circulates through the ventricular system, and is then absorbed back into the systemic circulation across the arachnoid villi and into the sagittal sinus. Approximately 150 mL is present and approximately 500 mL/day of CSF is produced, which results in complete turnover three to four times per day. There is a fixed volume of CSF in a finite volume of space and the normal intracranial pressure (ICP) is 5–15 mm Hg. Any blockage of normal CSF flow can cause hydrocephalus (literally "water on the brain").

The two main types of hydrocephalus are obstructive and nonobstructive. Obstructive hydrocephalus happens when the blockage occurs at the ventricular system by a tumor, colloid cyst, or primary stenosis. This blockage can also occur secondary to a congenital abnormality. Nonobstructive (communicating) hydrocephalus, often due to infection or subarachnoid hemorrhage, is caused by blockage outside of the ventricular system by either decreased flow through the basal cisterns or lack of absorption by the arachnoid villi. Additionally, it is possible to have hydrocephalus in the setting of normal ICP (normal pressure hydrocephalus) and elevated ICP without hydrocephalus (idiopathic intracranial hypertension, also known as pseudotumor cerebri).

TABLE 19.1: Classic history and physical of obstructive hydrocephalus

Headache
Nausea/vomiting
Decreased level of consciousness
Urinary incontinence
Ocular palsies, papilledema, decreased vision
Cushing response (raised systolic blood pressure and bradycardia)

TABLE 19.2: Classic history and physical of communicating hydrocephalus

Progressive (insidious) dementia, somnolence
Gait disturbance
Urinary incontinence
Impaired upward gaze
Notable absence of headache or papilledema

TABLE 19.3: Potentially helpful laboratory tests

CSF: Lumbar puncture is usually performed if a head CT does not elucidate the cause of symptoms, looking for elevated opening pressure. The CSF is then analyzed for infection or subarachnoid hemorrhage.

CSF, cerebrospinal fluid.

Noncontrast Head CT Scan

- Widely and rapidly available
- Relatively low radiation exposure
- Patients with brain atrophy can appear to have hydrocephalus; distinguish hydrocephalus from brain atrophy by noting that in atrophy the entire brain has become smaller, and the brain will be separated from the skull with enlarged ventricles and prominent sulci because of the decreased total size of the gyri
- The CT scan can also be used as part of a "shunt series" to ensure correct functioning of a ventriculoperitoneal (VP) shunt in patients with a history of hydrocephalus treated surgically

(note that plain films to follow the shunt may show a break in its continuity but do not play a role in the evaluation of the hydrocephalus itself)

TABLE 19.4: CT findings to evaluate for obstructive hydrocephalus and communicating hydrocephalus

Obstructive hydrocephalus	Communicating hydrocephalus
Caused by obstruction of CSF flow at the cerebral aqueduct. Therefore, look for: – enlarged lateral and third ventricles – small fourth ventricle and subarachnoid space In severe hydrocephalus, the brain tissue is compressed causing effacement of the gyri and sulci.	CSF is not reabsorbed from the subarachnoid space. Therefore, look for: – lateral and third ventricles not dilated out of proportion to the fourth ventricle and subarachnoid space

CSF, cerebrospinal fluid.

 TABLE 19.5: CT scan: hydrocephalus

IV contrast	No
PO contrast	No
Amount of radiation	2 mSV

Classic Images

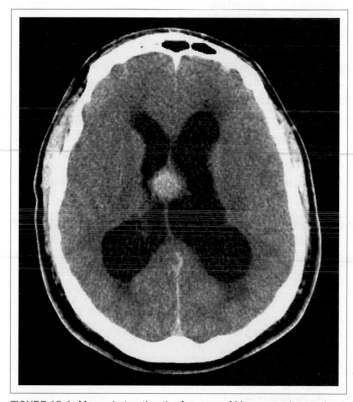

FIGURE 19.1: Mass obstructing the foramen of Monro causing moderate hydrocephalus.

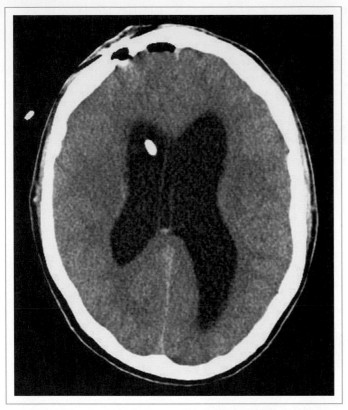

FIGURE 19.2: Marked hydrocephalus with a ventriculoperitoneal shunt visualized in the right lateral ventricle.

CT Angiography (CTA)

Can rapidly assess for underlying cause of hydrocephalus including brain tumor leading to obstructive hydrocephalus or aneurysmal bleeding causing nonobstructive hydrocephalus.

 TABLE 19.6: CTA scan: hydrocephalus

IV contrast	Yes
PO contrast	No
Amount of radiation	2 mSV

Classic Image

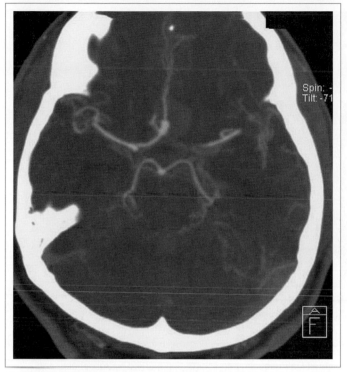

FIGURE 19.3: Reformatted CT angiogram demonstrating an aneurysm in the region of the anterior cerebral artery with surrounding subarachnoid blood.

MRI

- Used as an adjunct to CT and CTA in order to search for the underlying cause of hydrocephalus, such as tumor or hemorrhage
- With increased ICP, CSF is forced through gaps in the ependymal lining of the ventricles to be resorbed in the periventricular tissues
- Interstitial edema is seen on T2-weighted images as a smooth border of increased intensity along the edge of the ventricles; this may be seen on CT as well, but MRI is much more sensitive
- In obstructive hydrocephalus, the ventricles can be obstructed anywhere from the foramen of Monro to the outlet foramina of the fourth ventricle, and MRI can help determine the cause (e.g., gliomas, meningiomas, colloid, and cysticercus cysts).

 TABLE 19.7: MRI: hydrocephalus

IV contrast	Depends*
PO contrast	No
Amount of radiation	None

*Some MRI sequences require IV gadolinium contrast. Because there are so many different protocols for MRI, ideally, the clinician should speak to the radiologist to discuss the differential diagnosis and select the most useful sequences.

Classic Image

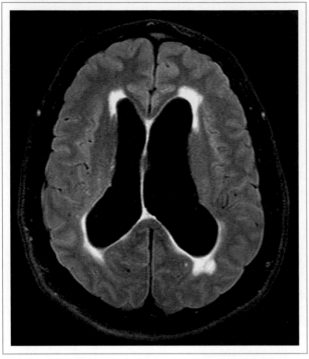

FIGURE 19.4: MRI using a modified T2-weighted Flair sequence demonstrating marked hydrocephalus and periventricular interstitial edema.

Basic Management

Intracranial pathology such as hemorrhage or mass can lead to brainstem herniation. In such cases, emergent airway management is indicated.

- *Obstructive hydrocephalus*: Search for and treat the underlying cause, which is usually a pathology causing a mass effect in the brain (e.g., tumor or cystic process)
- *Communicating hydrocephalus*: Search for and treat the underlying cause (e.g., meningitis or subarachnoid hemorrhage)
- *Normal pressure hydrocephalus*: There is no evidence that NPH can be treated with medications; response to VP shunting is variable
- *Idiopathic intracranial hypertension*: Usually treated by repeat lumbar punctures or the carbonic anhydrase-inhibiting diuretic acetazolamide

Summary

TABLE 19.8: Advantages and disadvantages of imaging modalities in hydrocephalus

Imaging modality	Advantages	Disadvantages
CT scan	Widespread availability Rapid Relatively low cost	Radiation Difficult to evaluate for underlying secondary cause
CTA	Widespread availability Rapid Can detect underlying causes of hydrocephalus much more readily than noncontrast CT	Administration of IV contrast can lead to allergic reaction or nephrotoxicity
MRI	Can detect underlying causes including tumor and stroke No radiation exposure	Cost, availability, time to perform Many patients have contraindications or claustrophobia

20 Intracerebral Hemorrhage

Joshua N. Goldstein

Background

Intracerebral hemorrhage (ICH) is the most devastating form of acute stroke, affecting approximately 65,000 people in the United States annually with an associated mortality of 30–50%. Even among survivors, morbidity remains high with many patients suffering permanent disability. No specific medical or surgical intervention has been shown to improve outcome. However, the repeated finding of lower morbidity and mortality after admission to a stroke or neuroscience intensive care unit suggests that a multifactorial approach by a multidisciplinary team likely offers the best hope of maximizing outcomes.

TABLE 20.1: Classic history and physical

Acute onset of focal or generalized neurologic symptoms
Headache and/or vomiting
Occasionally presents with seizure
New focal or generalized neurologic deficit

TABLE 20.2: Potentially helpful laboratory tests

CBC, Chem7: Can evaluate for anemia, thrombocytopenia, hyperglycemia, or renal dysfunction
Coagulation panel: Helpful in evaluation of metabolic or drug-related coagulopathy
Liver function tests: Can evaluate for a source of coagulopathy
CK-MB, troponin: Can screen for cardiogenic injury, which is relatively common after ICH

CBC, complete blood count; ICH, intracerebral hemorrhage.

Noncontrast Head CT Scan

- Widely and rapidly available; extremely sensitive for ICH
- Acute ICH typically appears as a bright white, high-density lesion
- Relatively low radiation exposure
- Can evaluate for mass effect or transtentorial herniation

TABLE 20.3: Key findings

Location
– Lobar: more likely to be due to cerebral amyloid angiopathy or secondary to a vascular abnormality
– Deep: thalamus, putamen (more likely to be due to longstanding hypertension)
– Cerebellar, brainstem: more likely to require neurosurgical intervention
Intraventricular extension (IVH) or hydrocephalus: IVH is associated with obstructive hydrocephalus and worse outcome; patients at risk for hydrocephalus may require external ventricular drain placement
Edema or heterogeneous appearance: large amounts of associated edema raise the concern for underlying tumor
Transtentorial herniation or mass effect: such patients may require emergency ICP management and neurosurgical consultation

- While most patients have primary intracranial pressure (ICH), many have underlying causes
- Secondary causes of ICH include aneurysm, arteriovenous malformation, Moyamoya disease, tumor, cerebral venous sinus thrombosis (CVST), or hemorrhagic transformation of ischemic stroke
- Maintain a high level of suspicion for these underlying causes—further imaging is often necessary to exclude an underlying (treatable) source

Classic Images

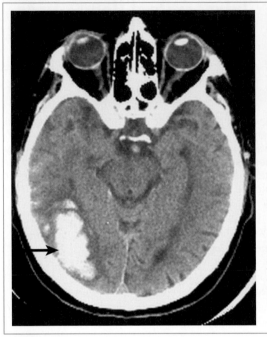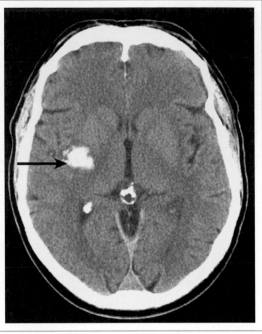

FIGURE 20.1: Lobar intracerebral hemorrhage (ICH) (**A**) and deep ICH (**B**).

☢ **TABLE 20.4:** CT scan: intracerebral hemorrhage

IV contrast	No
PO contrast	No
Amount of radiation	2 mSV

CT Angiography (CTA)

- Can rapidly and noninvasively assess for aneurysms, arteriovenous malformations, and other underlying causes of ICH
- Accuracy is close to that of the gold standard, digital subtraction angiography (DSA)
- Imaging with a venous phase (CTV) can evaluate for CVST
- Many patients will show "spots" of contrast within the hematoma after CTA, often termed the "spot sign"; this finding is a powerful predictor of ongoing bleeding and future hematoma expansion
- Reformatting images from the original source images takes some time to accomplish

☢ **TABLE 20.5:** CTA scan: intracerebral hemorrhage

IV contrast	Yes
PO contrast	No
Amount of radiation	2 mSV

Classic Images

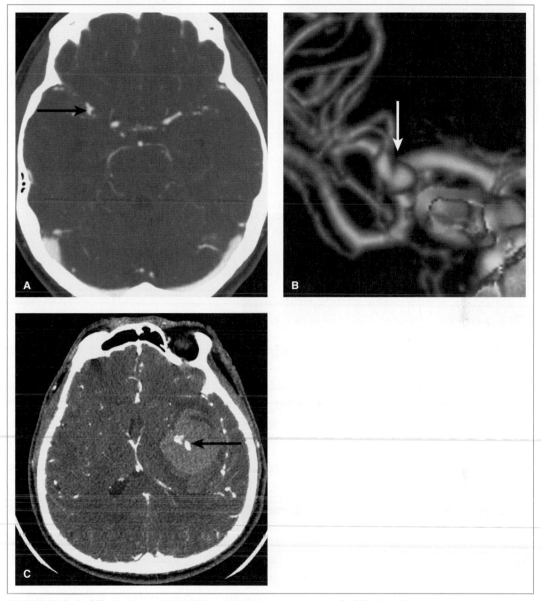

FIGURE 20.2: A: CTA showing a right middle cerebral artery aneurysm. **B:** CTA three-dimensional reconstruction showing the same aneurysm. **C:** Primary intracerebral hemorrhage with no underlying vascular malformation, but two large spots of contrast ("spot sign") are visible within the hematoma. (Parts A and B reprinted from Jagoda A, ed. *Emerg. Med. Pract.* 11(7): 2009.)

MRI

- When GRE (gradient recalled echo) sequences are used, this technique has been shown to be at least as sensitive, if not more sensitive, than CT for ICH
- Can detect "microbleeds"—evidence of subclinical ICHs in the past, considered a sign of underlying vasculopathy and possibly a risk factor for ICH
- Can be more sensitive and specific for diagnosis of underlying ischemic stroke, tumor, and other pathologies

- MR angiography is a noninvasive technique to evaluate the vasculature; time-of-flight sequences (TOF) can be performed without contrast, offering an option for those patients with renal disease or other contraindication to IV contrast
- MR venography can evaluate for CVST

 TABLE 20.6: MRI: intracerebral hemorrhage

IV contrast	Depends*
PO contrast	No
Amount of radiation	None

*Some MRI sequences require IV gadolinium contrast. Because there are so many different protocols for MRI, ideally, the clinician should speak to the radiologist to discuss the differential diagnosis and select the most useful sequences.

Classic Image

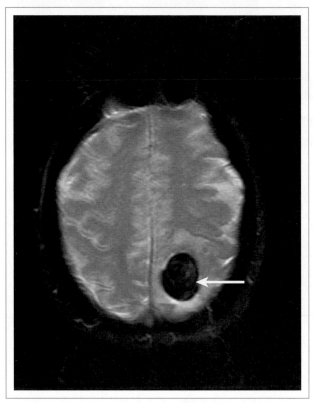

FIGURE 20.3: MRI using a susceptibility-weighted image (a modified T2-weighted GRE sequence) showing an intracerebral hemorrhage.

DSA (Digital Subtraction Angiography)
- Gold standard for evaluating vasculature for aneurysm, AV malformation
- If abnormalities are found, they can potentially be intervened upon with endovascular therapies (such as coils)
- Invasive: requires dedicated neurointerventional personnel and equipment

 TABLE 20.7: Digital subtraction angiography: intracerebral hemorrhage

IV contrast	Yes
PO contrast	No
Amount of radiation	0.8 mSV

Classic Image

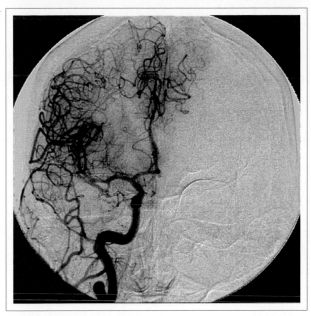

FIGURE 20.4: Normal digital subtraction angiogram of a patient with intracerebral hemorrhage.

Basic Management

- Airway management often necessary using standard indications
- Blood pressure control (though specific targets are controversial)
- Neurosurgical consultation for cerebellar or brainstem ICH
- Neurosurgical consultation for hydrocephalus and/or intraventricular hemorrhage
- Admission to a stroke or neurocritical care unit—patients are typically managed by neurologists, neurosurgeons, or neurointensivists depending upon the hospital
- Antiepileptic therapy for those who present with seizure
- Anticoagulation reversal for those on oral anticoagulants
- Platelet transfusion can be considered for those on oral antiplatelet agents
- Hyperglycemia management
- Fever management
- Cardiac monitoring
- Serial neurologic exams to evaluate for neurologic deterioration

Summary

TABLE 20.8 Advantages and disadvantages of imaging modalities in intracerebral hemorrhage

Imaging modality	Advantages	Disadvantages
CT scan	Widespread availability Rapid Relatively low cost	Radiation Difficult to evaluate for underlying secondary cause
CT angiography	Rapid Highly accurate in evaluating vascular abnormalities	IV contrast Radiation
MRI	Can detect underlying causes including tumor and stroke No radiation exposure	Cost, availability, time to perform Many patients have contraindications or claustrophobia
MR angiography	Can detect underlying vascular abnormalities	Cost, availability, time to perform Many patients have contraindications or claustrophobia
DSA	Gold standard for detecting vascular abnormalities	Invasive procedure, availability IV contrast

DSA, digital subtraction angiography.

21 Subarachnoid Hemorrhage

Lisa E. Thomas and Joshua N. Goldstein

Background

Trauma is the most common cause of subarachnoid hemorrhage (SAH). This chapter discusses nontraumatic SAH, which is seen in about 9 out of 100,000 people worldwide each year. Of all patients who present with spontaneous SAH, rupture of an intracranial aneurysm is the cause in 85%. Other causes include arteriovenous malformations, bleeding diathesis, hemorrhagic tumor, and perimesencephalic hemorrhage. It is estimated that 2% of the population harbor cerebral aneurysms. The risk of rupture leading to SAH is increased with factors such as autosomal dominant polycystic kidney disease, familial predisposition, hypertension, atherosclerosis, smoking, excessive alcohol intake, and advanced age. Many aneurysms do not rupture, but aneurysms >1 cm in size are more likely to rupture than smaller ones. Prognosis after SAH is poor with a 40% mortality rate and severe neurologic disability in more than 30% of survivors.

TABLE 21.1: Classic history and physical

Sudden-onset, severe, worst-of-life headache
Focal neurologic deficit, meningismus, or altered level of consciousness may be present
Physical examination may also be normal
Oculomotor nerve palsy (classically due to compression by posterior communicating artery aneurysm)

TABLE 21.2: Potentially helpful laboratory tests

Coagulation panel, platelet count: to screen for any coagulopathic state
Hemoglobin/hematocrit: if hematocrit less than 27–30%, blood may appear isodense on noncontrast head CT, thus decreasing imaging sensitivity for SAH
BUN/creatinine: To evaluate kidney function as patients may need contrast for vascular imaging
Troponin: To evaluate for cardiac involvement that can occur with SAH

BUN, blood urea nitrogen; SAH, subarachnoid hemorrhage.

Noncontrast Head CT

- CT scan without contrast is the first diagnostic study recommended in the evaluation of patients with suspected SAH
- Classic appearance on CT may be useful in distinguishing etiology of SAH
  - Aneurysmal: diffuse hyperdense blood surrounding basal cisterns
  - Traumatic: higher in cerebral convexities and coup/contrecoup lesions
  - Perimesencephalic (rarer, nonaneurysmal type): focal hyperdense blood anterior to midbrain, associated with excellent prognosis
- Higher sensitivity is seen in CT done earlier and in larger bleeds (spectrum bias)
- Sensitivity ranges from 93% to 100% when CT is obtained promptly within 24 hours of symptom onset
- By 1 week after symptom onset, CT is only 50% sensitive

TABLE 21.3: Limitations to sensitivity of noncontrast head CT

1. Sensitivity decreases with time after symptom onset
– Initially it is hyperdense compared to brain
– As blood is further degraded by circulating cerebrospinal fluid, CT sensitivity decreases as blood becomes isodense
2. Small volume bleeds may not be detected
3. Anemia, hematocrit <27–30, may be associated with a false-negative scan due to isodense blood on CT
4. Older technology, thicker CT slices, or motion artifact may reduce sensitivity

- The Fisher classification system uses increasing quantity of blood on CT scan to predict risk of symptomatic cerebral vasospasm

TABLE 21.4: Fisher classification

1. No blood
2. Diffuse SAH, no clots, no blood layering >1 mm
3. Local clots or blood layers ≥1 mm
4. Diffuse or no SAH, but + intracerebral/intraventricular clot

SAH, subarachnoid hemorrhage.

- If noncontrast CT is negative, a lumbar puncture may reveal red blood cells or xanthochromia indicating presence of SAH

 TABLE 21.5: Noncontrast CT scan

IV contrast	No
PO contrast	No
Amount of radiation	2 mSV

Classic Images

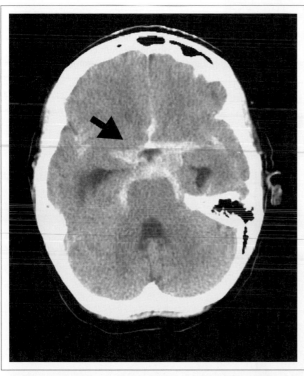

FIGURE 21.1: Aneurysmal subarachnoid hemorrhage (SAH). Noncontrast axial CT scan shows hyperdense blood near the base of the brain (*black arrow*) in the classic star-like pattern seen in aneurysmal SAH formed by blood radiating from the basilar cisterns into the sylvian fissures and the anterior interhemispheric fissure. This patient was found to have a ruptured anterior communicating artery aneurysm on angiography.

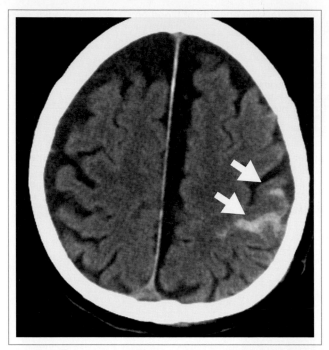

FIGURE 21.2: Traumatic subarachnoid hemorrhage (SAH). Noncontrast axial CT scan shows hyperdensities (*white arrows*) in the left frontotemporal sulci high in the cerebral convexities due to traumatic SAH in a patient who presented after a fall with head injury. Bilateral chronic frontal subdural hemorrhages/hygromas are also present.

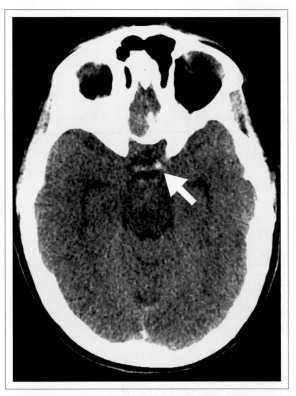

FIGURE 21.3: Perimesencephalic hemorrhage. Noncontrast axial CT scan shows hyperdense blood anterior to the midbrain (*white arrow*). This patient had a negative angiogram and excellent outcome.

Intra-Arterial Digital Subtraction Angiography (DSA)

- Once SAH has been found by noncontrast CT or lumbar puncture, conventional angiography is the gold standard for identifying the aneurysm, delineating its anatomical characteristics, and preoperative planning
- Invasive: 1% complication risk of permanent neurologic injury
- Angiography negative in 10–20% of cases due to:
  - perimesencephalic hemorrhage
  - vasospasm of the parent vessel (precluding aneurysm filling)
  - thrombosed aneurysm
  - rarer causes

 TABLE 21.6: Digital subtraction angiography: subarachnoid hemorrhage

IV contrast	Yes
PO contrast	No
Amount of radiation	0.8 mSV

Classic Image

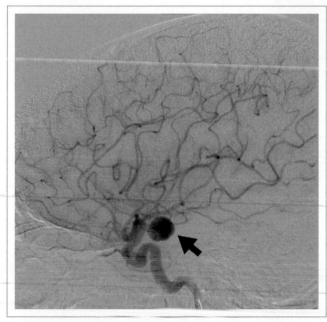

FIGURE 21.4: Lateral view from a digital subtraction angiogram of a patient with subarachnoid hemorrhage shows a large aneurysm (*black arrow*) in the posterior communicating artery.

CT Angiography

- CT angiography (CTA) is rapid, noninvasive, and in many centers the preferred alternative to traditional angiography for identification of an aneurysm
- IV contrast is injected through a vein
- Prospective studies show CTA may be used for preoperative planning
- Sensitivity is 95–100% and specificity is 87–100% compared to gold standard angiography
- Small aneurysms <3 mm may be missed by CTA
- Unruptured aneurysms may also be detected
- Reformats from source imaging require some time

 TABLE 21.7: CTA scan: subarachnoid hemorrhage

IV contrast	Yes
PO contrast	No
Amount of radiation	2 mSV

Classic Images

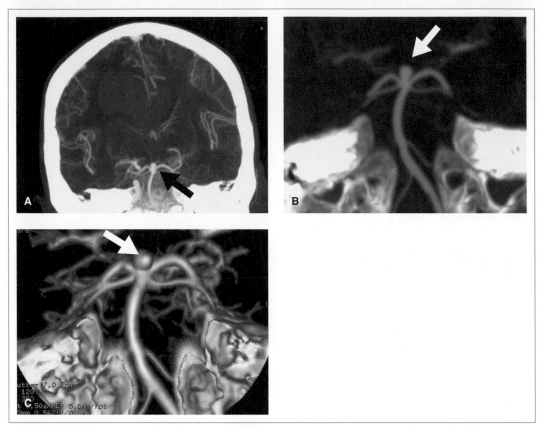

FIGURE 21.5: CTA shows a basilar tip aneurysm (*arrow*) in coronal two-dimensional reconstruction (**A**), maximum intensity projection (**B**), and three-dimensional reconstruction (**C**) images.

MRI

- MRI is often less readily available, more time consuming, and only a few limited studies have examined its use in diagnosing SAH
  - High oxygen levels in cerebrospinal fluid restrict the deoxygenation of hemoglobin and limit the sensitivity of conventional MRI sequences (T1- and T2-weighted imaging)
  - T2-fluid attenuated inversion recovery (FLAIR) is the most sensitive MR sequence for identifying SAH; hyperintense signal changes are seen in the sulci, but false positives may occur; false negatives may also occur from spectrum bias
- MRA may be used as an alternative to CTA or traditional intra-arterial angiography for identifying an aneurysm once SAH has been diagnosed; however, is it less studied and less sensitive than other modalities

 TABLE 21.8: MRI: subarachnoid hemorrhage

IV contrast	No
PO contrast	No
Amount of radiation	None

Classic Image

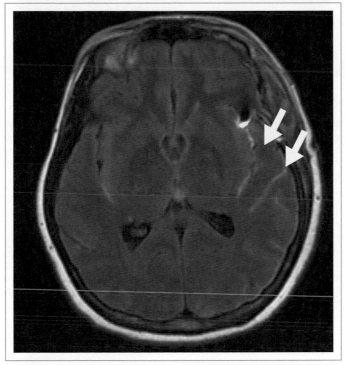

FIGURE 21.6: MRI T2-FLAIR shows hyperintense signal in the left temporal sulci indicating subarachnoid hemorrhage.

Basic Management

- NPO and bed rest
- Neurosurgical consultation
- Cerebrovascular imaging to assess for aneurysm (CTA, MRA, or conventional angiography)
- Avoid excessive hypertension to reduce risk of rebleeding
- Consider anticonvulsant
- Nimodipine (calcium channel blocker) for prevention of delayed vasospasm
- Admission, typically to an ICU, and ideally to an experienced neurovascular center where all the possible treatments and neurointensive care are available
- Definitive repair of aneurysm by surgical clipping or endovascular coiling

Summary

TABLE 21.9: Advantages and disadvantages of imaging modalities in subarachnoid hemorrhage

Imaging modality	Advantages	Disadvantages
Noncontrast CT	Rapid, widely available, inexpensive, sensitive, can reveal alternative diagnoses	Radiation exposure
CTA	Rapid, noninvasive Identifies the culprit vascular lesion	Radiation exposure, IV contrast
MRI MRA	Can reveal alternative diagnoses, avoids radiation	Time-consuming, less well studied, contraindications in many patients Spectrum bias still present
Digital subtraction angiography	Traditional gold standard, sensitive, and endovascular coiling can be performed	Invasive, IV contrast, some radiation exposure, restricted to centers with specialized teams

Multiple Sclerosis

Jonathan A. Edlow

Background

Multiple sclerosis (MS) is a disorder of inflammation and demyelinization of the central nervous system (CNS) predominantly affecting the white matter, but gray matter lesions are also found. Because it can affect any part of the brain or spinal cord, MS can present with a wide variety of symptoms, depending upon what part(s) of the CNS are involved. Furthermore, there are different temporal patterns such as relapsing remitting, progressive relapsing and primary progressive disease.

Some patients present with clinically isolated syndromes such as an internuclear ophthalmoplegia (INO) or optic neuritis, whereas others have widespread CNS lesions. Women are affected roughly twice as often as men and the disease usually begins in young adults. Individuals living in more northern latitudes are affected more than those in southern ones. Genetic factors also play a role. All that said, the cause of MS remains unknown. Despite all of the progress with MS, the diagnosis remains a clinical one and radiologic findings must be interpreted in the clinical context. *Dissemination of clinical events and lesions over space and time* is still a key principle of the classic diagnostic paradigm. MRI has become increasingly important because it can help establish the presence of this time and space dissemination.

TABLE 22.1: Classic history and physical

There is a wide range of presentations
Female patients aged 15–40 years are at highest risk
Rapidly diminished vision from optic neuritis
Diplopia from an INO
Lhermitte's phenomenon (electric shock in limbs with head or neck movement)
Episodic weakness, numbness, and incoordination that will vary based on what portion of the brain or spinal cord is involved
Almost any pattern of involvement can occur due to one or more (old and/or new) lesions

INO, internuclear ophthalmoplegia.

TABLE 22.2: Potentially helpful laboratory tests

Urinalysis: Spastic bladder of MS causes chronic infections often responsible for MS flares
CSF oligoclonal bands and IgG index: Useful but not required emergently

CSF, cerebrospinal fluid; IgG, immunoglobulin G.

CT Scan

CT is not a sensitive way to diagnose MS either in the brain or the cord and is not recommended if MS is the major reason for the imaging.

MRI Scan

- MRI has revolutionized the diagnosis of MS; in fact, diagnostic criteria increasingly use the functionality of MRI to find lesions that are new in time and space.
- An MRI for MS does not need to be ordered emergently; however, if ordering an MRI from the ED, it is important to inform the radiologist that MS is in the differential diagnosis so that the appropriate sequences can be obtained
  - A new T2-weighted lesion (not present on a scan >3 months prior) is adequate to diagnose a "new" lesion
  - Gadolinium enhancement also assists in distinguishing a new from an old lesion
  - The physical examination will guide what part of the CNS should be imaged

- Dawson's fingers are a finding that is fairly specific for MS; it consists of demyelinating plaques that radiate at right angles from the corpus callosum along the veins draining in this area
- Balo's concentric sclerosis is another finding seen in MS patients, sometimes thought to represent a clinical variant; concentric rings are seen on MRI and are thought to be due to layers of demyelinated tissue.
- MRI enhancement lasts approximately 1–2 months (but can be present for up to 5 months) and suggests active demyelination of the blood-brain barrier in those specific areas

TABLE 22.3: Common locations of MS lesions on MRI

Periventricular white matter (>80%)
Corpus callosum (50–85%)
Visual pathways (optic neuritis)
Posterior fossa (10%)
Brain stem (more common in younger patients)

 TABLE 22.4: MRI: multiple sclerosis

IV contrast	Yes, gadolinium is helpful
PO contrast	No
Amount of radiation	None

Classic Images

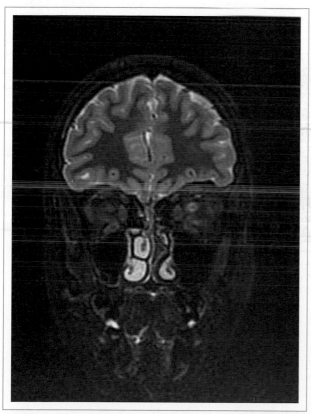

FIGURE 22.1: This is a coronal MRI image from a patient with retrobulbar optic neuritis. The image shows mild enhancement of the left optic nerve in a young patient with rapid onset of left eye blindness and a normal retinal exam.

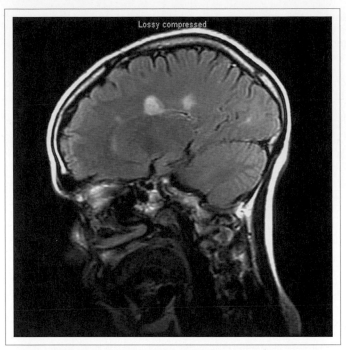

FIGURE 22.2: This MRI (of the same patient as in Figure 22.1) shows the classic finding known as "Dawson's fingers." These lesions are from the same patient as with the optic neuritis and were clinically silent.

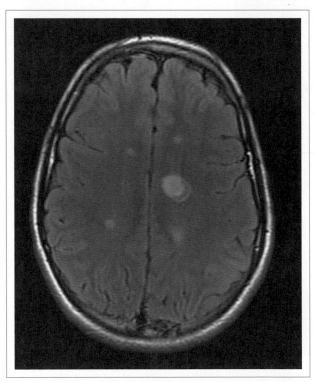

FIGURE 22.3: This finding of Balo's concentric sclerosis was also found on the initial MRI (of the same patient with retrobulbar neuritis). (Figures 22.1 to 22.3, which were obtained at the same time, show dissemination of lesions in space).

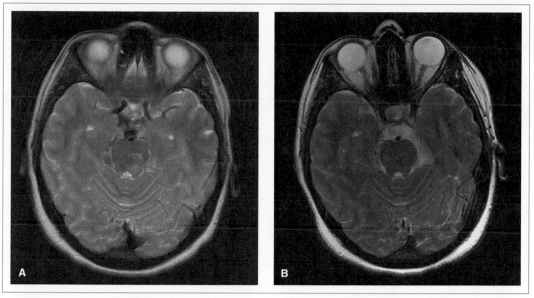

FIGURE 22.4: A: MRI scan shows two lesions in the left brainstem of a patient. **B:** Second MRI scan, taken 3 months later, of the same patient shows that the two lesions have largely resolved and there is a new one in the right brainstem. (Both episodes were symptomatic).

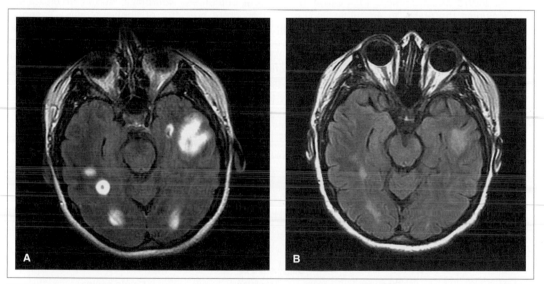

FIGURE 22.5: This is another example of MS plaques that are disseminated in time and space. Both of these axial flair images are at the same level, but (**A**) was obtained 6 months before (**B**).

Basic Management

- A neurologist who has experience in MS should manage these patients
- Since nerve conduction is slower with increasing temperature, fever should be managed aggressively, both with antipyretics as well as with antibiotics, to treat any underlying infection that is causing the fever
- Steroids:
  - Some patients are initially managed with large doses of "pulse" steroids
  - In patients with optic neuritis, steroids may improve the early regaining of sight, but this does not affect long-term outcomes

- Immune globulin and immune modulating agents such as interferons are beyond the scope of emergency medicine

Summary

TABLE 22.5: Advantages and disadvantages of MRI in MS

Advantages	Disadvantages
Shows old and new lesions	Cost, availability, time to perform
No radiation exposure	Many patients have contraindications or claustrophobia
Has prognostic value in patients with clinically isolated syndromes	

23 Spinal Cord and Cauda Equina Compression

Andrea Dugas

Background

Spinal cord and cauda equina compression are true neurologic emergencies requiring prompt diagnosis and treatment to improve neurological outcomes. Neurologic status at diagnosis, including the ability to ambulate, is the most accurate predictor of final outcome. Diagnosis of spinal cord compression can be difficult. Most adults have back pain during their lifetime but less than 5% of them have a serious underlying cause and even fewer have cord compression. Nontraumatic spinal cord and cauda equina compression can occur due to vertebral disk herniation, spinal or dural metastasis, infection (epidural abscess, osteomyelitis, or diskitis), or epidural hematoma. Older and osteopenic patients may have traumatic lesions with little or no overt trauma.

TABLE 23.1: Classic history and physical

Back pain
New neurologic deficits:
Impaired gait
Motor deficits
Sensory deficits
Urinary retention
Decreased rectal tone

TABLE 23.2: Back pain red flags

	Suggestive of		
Cancer	**Fracture**	**Infection**	**Cauda equina**
Age > 50 yr or < 17 yr	Age > 70 yr	Fever	Urinary retention
Duration > 1 mo	Trauma	IV drug use	Saddle anesthesia
Previous history of cancer	Midline tenderness	Recent bacterial infection	Decreased rectal tone
No relief with rest	Osteoporosis	Immunosuppression	Fecal incontinence
Unexplained weight loss	Prolonged use of corticosteroids	Recent spinal procedure	Bilateral LE weakness or numbness

TABLE 23.3: Potentially helpful laboratory tests

ESR, CRP: potential markers of inflammation
UA: to evaluate for pyelonephritis, hematuria, or other possible etiologies of back pain
Ca: if malignancy is suspected
PSA, SPEP, UPEP: to determine possible etiology if new malignancy is suspected
Coagulation panel: helpful if epidural hematoma is suspected
Blood cultures: if infection or epidural abscess is suspected

Ca, calcium; CRP, C-reactive protein; ESR, erythrocyte sedimentation rate; PSA, prostate-specific antigen; SPEP, serum protein electrophoresis; UA, urine analysis; UPEP, urine protein electrophoresis.

Spinal X-ray

- Plain films of the spine are economical, low in radiation, and rapidly available; however, they are neither sensitive nor specific for spinal cord compression
- They do not show soft tissue or spinal cord, but may show findings suspicious for bony changes from metastases, diskitis, or osteomyelitis
- Can show the bony anatomy: osteopenia, osteolytic masses, traumatic fractures, and vertebral alignment
  - CT of the spine is more sensitive for detection of fractures and other bony abnormalities
  - Shows abnormality only after 50–60% of the vertebral body has been destroyed
- In osteomyelitis, irregular vertebral end plates with decreased disk height and periosteal elevation may be seen
  - Lags behind clinical findings by 2–3 weeks
  - Not sensitive or specific
- False negative in 10–17% of patients with metastatic epidural spinal cord compression
- Not recommended to diagnose spinal cord compression

Classic Images

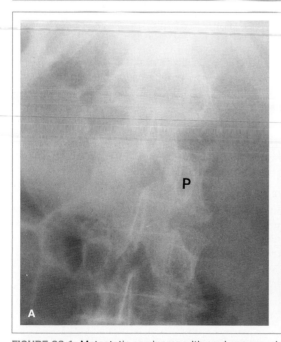
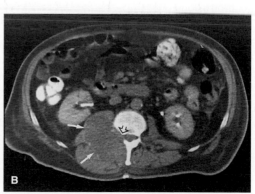

FIGURE 23.1: Metastatic carcinoma with cord compression. **A:** Frontal radiograph shows destruction of the pedicle and body of L2 on the right. Notice the normal pedicle (P) on the left. **B:** CT image through the same area shows a large paraspinal mass (*solid arrows*). Notice the destroyed pedicle on the right (*open arrow*). (From Daffner RH. Clinical Radiology: The Essentials, 3rd ed. Philadelphia: Lippincott Williams & Wilkins, 2007.)

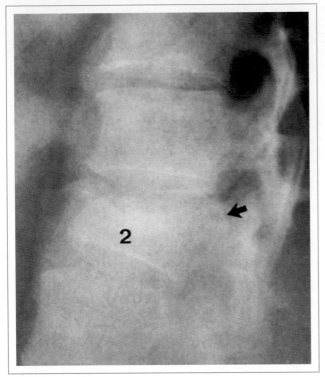

FIGURE 23.2: Lateral radiograph of a patient with a burst fracture of L2 shows compression of the body of L2 and posterior displacement of a large bone fragment (*arrow*) into the vertebral canal. (From Daffner RH. Clinical Radiology: The Essentials, 2nd ed. Philadelphia: Lippincott Williams & Wilkins, 1999.)

Spinal CT Scan

- Widely and rapidly available
- Shows bony anatomy far better than x-ray
- Shows cortical bone better than MRI, but MRI has improved evaluation of vertebral bone marrow, soft tissue, and the spinal cord
- Multiplanar reconstructions are essential to asses vertebral alignment and detect transverse fractures
- Test of choice in trauma cases; however, MRI can show if the fracture is compressing the cord as well as other nonbony traumatic injuries such as epidural hematomas and traumatic disc protrusions
- Less sensitive to patient movement than MRI

 TABLE 23.4: CT scan: spinal cord compression

IV contrast	Yes
PO contrast	No
Amount of radiation	6 mSv

Classic Image

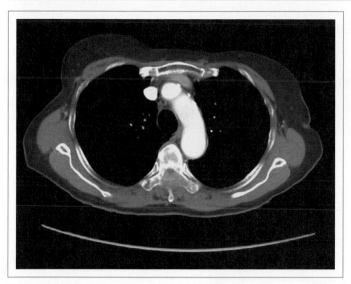

FIGURE 23.3: Expansile lytic metastasis in the spinous process and left lamina of T5 extending into the spinal canal and causing cord compression at this level.

Contrast Myelography

- Performed by lumbar puncture with infusion of contrast into the epidural space; the spinal canal is then imaged via x-ray or CT (most commonly CT)
- Cord compression is seen as indentations on the surface of the spinal cord; the sheaths of spinal nerve roots may be deviated, flattened, or obliterated
- Contrast shows outline of the spinal cord, but not soft tissue details of what is impinging on it
- Best test to evaluate for spine compression in patients who are unable to undergo MRI
- Cannot be done in patients with contraindications to lumbar puncture or those who are unable to tolerate the procedure

 TABLE 23.5: Myelography: spinal cord compression

IV contrast	Yes
Intrathecal contrast	Yes
PO contrast	No
Amount of radiation	6 mSv

Classic Image

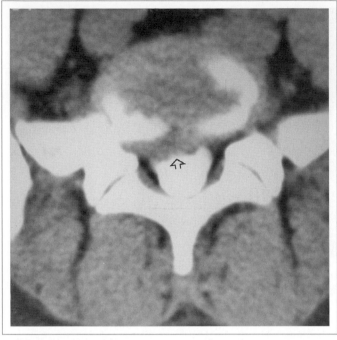

FIGURE 23.4: CT myelogram showing herniated disc compressing the contrast-filled thecal sac (*arrow*). (From Daffner RH. Clinical Radiology: The Essentials, 3rd ed. Philadelphia: Lippincott Williams & Wilkins, 2007.)

MRI
- Considered the gold standard for diagnosing cord compression
- The only imaging modality that shows the spinal cord parenchyma
  - Signal changes within the cord indicate edema, best seen on axial images
  - Excellent evaluation of the soft tissues
- Imaging modality of choice for spinal cord abscesses, tumors, vascular lesions, and epidural masses
- In spinal trauma, MRI not as accurate as CT in showing fractures, but can evaluate if fracture is compressing the spinal cord and show epidural hematomas, ligamentous injury, and traumatic disc protrusions
- Very sensitive (93%) and specific (97%) for metastatic cord compression
- Very sensitive (96%) and specific (94%) for osteomyelitis (which is seen as bright areas throughout vertebra on T2-weighted images)
- Noninvasive; no radiation
- Expensive and not available in all emergency departments
- Due to referred pain and incidence of multiple sites of tumor and abscess, it is recommended to image the entire spine, not just the location of the pain, in the absence of hard localizing neurological findings
- Discuss with the radiologist the clinical concerns, as gadolinium will likely be necessary

 TABLE 23.6: MRI: spinal cord compression

IV contrast	Yes, gadolinium is helpful
PO contrast	No
Amount of radiation	None

Classic Images

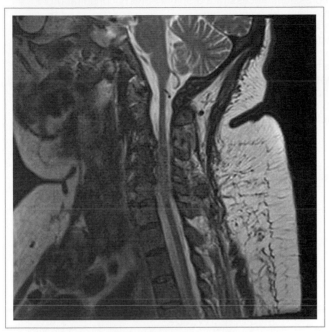

FIGURE 23.5: T2-weighted MRI showing epidural abscess extending from C3-C6. Hyperintensity of vertebral bodies C3 and C4 suggest osteomyelitis.

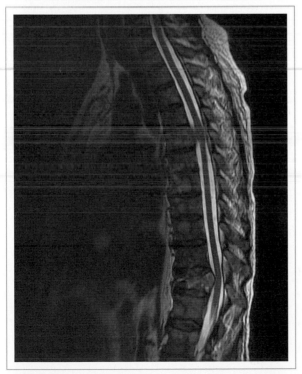

FIGURE 23.6: T2-weighted MRI showing complete marrow replacement of T5 with associated soft tissue component occupying much of spinal canal and causing cord compression. It also shows pathologic compression fracture of T11 with retropulsion of dorsal cortex that displace spinal cord.

Basic Management

- All spinal cord or cauda equina compressions necessitate a spinal surgery consultation to determine if the patient requires emergent decompression
- Metastatic cord compression
  - Often treated with steroids to reduce cord edema and alleviate pain
  - Radiation oncology consult to evaluate for possible radiation treatment
- Osteomyelitis and epidural abscess
  - Consider antibiotics based on patient's clinical situation and the knowledge that they will affect future culture data if the bone is biopsied or the abscess is drained (blood cultures will often demonstrate the organism)
- Epidural hematoma: consider reversing coagulopathy if one exists
- Pain management

Summary

TABLE 23.7: Advantages and disadvantages of imaging modalities in spinal cord compression

Imaging modality	Advantages	Disadvantages
X-ray	Low cost Low radiation Bedside availability	Not sensitive or specific for detecting spinal cord compression
CT scan	Availability Shows complex fractures	IV contrast Radiation exposure Poor soft tissue visibility
Myelography	Gold standard if unable to perform MRI Images obstruction of CSF	Time-consuming Invasive procedure IV contrast Radiation exposure No details of compressive mass
MRI	Gold standard Images spinal cord itself No radiation	Expensive Time consuming Availability IV contrast Does not show cortical bone Many contraindications

CSF, cerebrospinal fluid.

Section Editor: Ari Lipsky

24   Overview of Maxillofacial Trauma

Moses Graubard and Ravi Morchi

Background

There are more than 3 million facial injuries per year in the United States. Traumatic maxillofacial injuries are therefore frequently encountered in the emergency department (ED). The most commonly seen etiologies and fracture types tend to vary by practice location and type of hospital. Urban areas are more likely to see traumatic injuries from assaults, whereas rural areas will have more motor collisions and sports/recreational injuries.

TABLE 24.1: Most common maxillofacial fractures

Community EDs	Trauma center EDs
Nasal fractures	Zygomatic fractures
Mandibular fractures	Midface fractures

Falls are an especially common cause of facial injury in the very young and the elderly. **Syncope** should always be considered in cases of facial trauma resulting from a fall in an elderly patient. Syncope causing facial trauma—especially in an elderly patient—should raise a red flag because it often means the patient had no warning signs of his or her impending loss of consciousness. This increases the probability that the syncope was due to a life-threatening cause such as an unstable arrhythmia.

Domestic violence or **child abuse** should also be a consideration in the setting of facial trauma. The majority of domestic violence-related ED visits are for facial injury, and up to 25% of women who present with facial trauma are victims of domestic violence. *If a woman's injuries include an orbital fracture, the probability of sexual assault or domestic violence rises to more than 30%.*

Soft tissue structures in the face—especially nerves, salivary glands, and ducts—can be damaged by either penetrating or blunt injury. Penetrating injury may directly sever nerves and ducts, while blunt trauma may cause neuropraxia and fractures, which may lacerate nerves and ducts.

For specific signs and symptoms and their corresponding differential diagnoses and preferred imaging modalities, see Table 24.3.

Types of Imaging

Facial imaging techniques include plain x-ray, orthopantomogram ("panorex") films of the mandible, CT, ultrasound, and MRI.

Plain X-ray

- Because of its increased sensitivity and specificity, CT has largely supplanted plain x-ray in the assessment of bony injury of the face.
- Plain x-ray is still reasonable to use as the primary imaging test in patients in whom there is a low (but not negligible) suspicion of bony injury. Plain film series can be ordered for imaging the skull, face, zygoma, mandible, and sinuses.

113

Panorex

- A panorex uses a dedicated machine to take a 180° rotating plain film of the mouth and mandible.
- Panorex provides a full view of the upper and lower mandible, teeth, and temporomandibular joints.
- Panorex is an excellent test for suspected mandibular fracture.

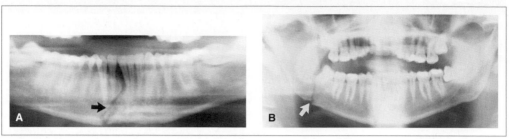

FIGURE 24.1: Multiple mandibular fractures demonstrated on panorex film. (From Harris J and Harris W. The Radiology of Emergency Medicine, 4th ed. Philadelphia: Lippincott Williams and Wilkins, 2000.)

Computed Tomography

- CT has many advantages over plain x-ray. It provides a good view of soft tissue, bone, acute hemorrhage, and foreign bodies. It is fast and readily available in most EDs and has become the preferred imaging modality. Its disadvantages are that it is much costlier than plain x-ray and that it delivers a higher dose of ionizing radiation to the patient.
- At most institutions, a facial CT scan will automatically be done with thin cuts since the objective of most of these scans is to finely image bony anatomy.
- It is important to be able to identify basic facial anatomy on CT images.

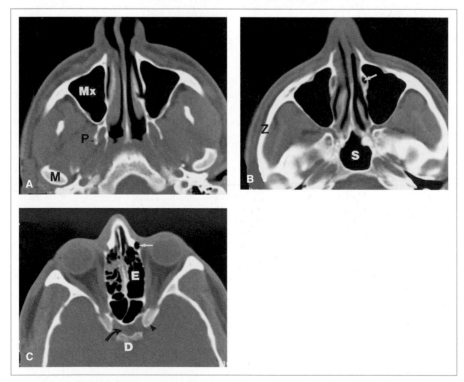

FIGURE 24.2: Normal facial anatomy by axial CT imaging. **A:** Image through the lower maxilla showing the maxillary sinus (Mx), pterygoid plates (P), and mandibular condyle (M). **B:** Image through the midmaxilla showing the zygomatic arch (Z), sphenoid sinus (S), and nasolacrimal duct (*arrow*). **C:** Image through the midorbits showing the nasolacrimal duct (*straight arrow*), ethmoid sinus (E), sella turcica (*curved arrow*), dorsum sellae (D), and anterior clinoid process (*arrowhead*). Also notice the excellent delineation of the extraocular muscles. (From Daffner RH. Clinical Radiology: The Essentials, 3rd ed. Philadelphia: Lippincott Williams & Wilkins, 2007.)

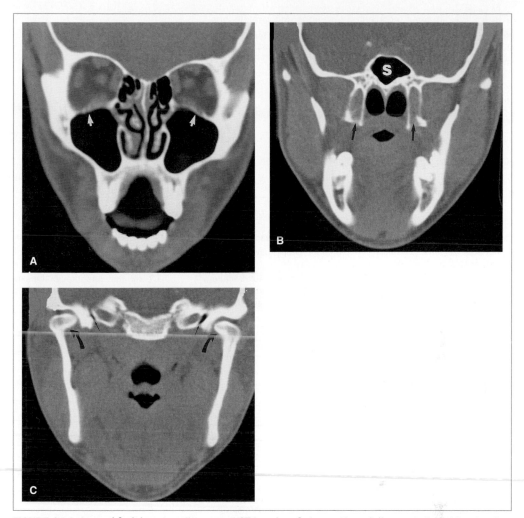

FIGURE 24.3: Normal facial anatomy by coronal CT imaging. **A:** Image through the posterior orbits showing the orbital floors (*arrows*). Also notice that the extraocular muscles are visible around the periphery of the orbits and the optic nerves can be seen centrally. **B:** Image through the posterior maxilla showing the pterygoid plates (*arrows*) and the sphenoid sinus (S). **C:** Image through the skull base showing the mandibular condyles (*curved arrows*) and Eustachian tubes (*small straight arrows*). (From Daffner RH. Clinical Radiology: The Essentials, 3rd ed. Philadelphia: Lippincott Williams & Wilkins, 2007.)

Magnetic Resonance Imaging

- MRI is generally superior to CT for imaging soft tissue. However, it is time-consuming and is often less readily available than CT.
- It is generally not useful in acute facial trauma, as it is inferior to CT for imaging bony anatomy.

TABLE 24.2: Imaging techniques: strengths and weaknesses

Imaging modality	Visualizes well	Visualizes poorly	Useful for fractures	Useful for foreign bodies	Contraindications
Plain x-ray	Bone, radio-opaque foreign bodies	Soft tissue	Yes	Yes	None
Panorex	Mandible, teeth	Soft tissue	Yes	Yes	None
CT	Soft tissue, blood, bone, air		Yes	Yes	None
Ultra-sound	Globe, fluid collec-tions	Bone, air	No	Yes	Open globe injury
MRI	Soft tissue, air	Bone	No	Yes for organic material and plastic, but con-traindicated with metal	Metallic foreign bodies, aneurysm clips, severe claustrophobia

TABLE 24.3: Choosing the best initial imaging technique based on physical findings

Physical exam finding	Suspected injury/condition	Preferred initial imaging modality
Orbital bony tenderness, diplopia, enophthal-mos, or subcutaneous emphysema	Orbital blowout fracture	CT with thin cuts through the orbits
Bilateral periorbital ecchymoses ("raccoon eyes")	Basilar skull fracture or ethmoid fracture	CT with thin cuts through the skull base
Proptosis	Retrobulbar hematoma	Ultrasound or CT
Limitation of extraocular movements	Entrapment of extraocular muscles	CT
Nasal bone tenderness, crepitus, or obvious deformity (isolated injury)	Nasal bone fracture	No imaging needed
Focal mandibular tenderness, malocclusion, sublingual hematoma, positive tongue blade test	Mandibular fracture	Panorex, plain x-ray (mandibular series), or CT
Missing tooth that is unaccounted for	Aspiration of tooth	Chest x-ray
Hemotympanum, ruptured tympanic membrane, blood in external canal, CSF otorrhea, posterior auricular hematoma (Battle's sign), facial nerve palsies (other than isolated V2), acute sensorineural hearing loss	Temporal bone fracture or basilar skull fracture	CT
Focal muscular weakness or focal numbness ▪ Facial nerve: inability to wrinkle forehead (temporal branch), shut eyes tightly (zygomatic branch), smile (buccal branch) or pucker or hold cheeks full of air (marginal mandibular branch) ▪ Trigeminal nerve: sensory deficit to unilateral face or upper neck ▪ Lingual nerve: sensory loss to anterior two-thirds of tongue	Acute nerve injury likely due to facial fracture	CT

Basic Management and Disposition
- Follow ATLS protocol
- Emergent versus urgent consultation, e.g., trauma surgery, oromaxillofacial surgery, etc.
- Administer analgesia, antibiotics, and/or tetanus prophylaxis as indicated
- Patients with open fractures and virtually any significant injury to the eye, ear, or salivary gland should be hospitalized and treated by the appropriate specialty
- Patients with uncomplicated fractures, simple lacerations, and contusions can be safely discharged with appropriate follow-up
- Social work, advocate services, police, or other designated consultants should be notified in cases of suspected or known abuse or violence

25

Mandibular and Maxillary Fractures

Samuel Clarke and Timothy Horeczko

Background

Injury to the midface and jaw is a common presenting complaint to the emergency department (ED) and constitutes approximately 2% of hospital admissions in the United States. Trauma to the midface resulting in fractures to the maxillary bone or mandible is more common among young male patients and is most frequently the result of motor vehicle accidents or interpersonal violence. It is essential to diagnose these fractures because of their potential for causing airway compromise, facial nerve palsies, and dural tears, as well as lasting facial deformity.

Fractures to the midface have traditionally been described using the **Le Fort classification**. Le Fort fractures more commonly occur in combination with other complex facial fractures (e.g., zygomatico-maxillary complex or ZMC, orbital blowout, or mandibular fracture) than in isolation.

TABLE 25.1: Classic history and physical

Physical assault to face

"LIPS-N" mnemonic—physical findings correlating with a positive facial CT
   Lip laceration
   Intraoral laceration
   Periorbital contusion
   Subconjunctival hemorrhage
   Nasal laceration

Numbness of the face—cheek or teeth (infraorbital nerve); lower jaw or chin (mandibular nerve)
Inability to open the mouth or tolerate secretions
Malocclusion—(mandibular fracture)
Tongue blade test—unable to break with twisting (mandibular fracture)

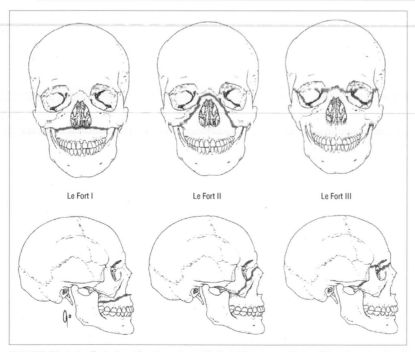

Le Fort I   Le Fort II   Le Fort III

FIGURE 25.1: Le Fort classification of maxillofacial fractures. The red line denotes the fracture line. (From Snell RS. Clinical Anatomy, 7th ed. Lippincott, Williams & Wilkins, 2003.)

117

TABLE 25.2: Le Fort fracture patterns

Le Fort I: fracture of pterygoid plates and all walls of the maxillary sinuses (well visualized in coronal CT)
Le Fort II: fracture of pterygoid plates, medial orbital, and lateral maxillary walls; the zygomatic arch and lateral orbital walls are left intact
Le Fort III: fracture of pterygoid plates, nasal septum, medial and lateral maxillary walls, and zygomatic arches (i.e., complete craniofacial disjunction)

Plain X-ray

- Largely replaced by CT
- The traditional plain films are the Waters (zygomatico-alveolar arch and orbits), panoramic (mandible), submentovertex or occlusal/axial (zygomatic arch fractures), and lateral (nasal bone, posterior displacement of midface) views
- Isolated fractures of the body of the mandible without high-risk features can be imaged with plain films (panoramic and PA views with maximal mouth opening)

 TABLE 25.3: Plain film: mandible/maxillary fractures

IV contrast	No
PO contrast	No
Amount of radiation	0.1 mSv per view

Classic Images

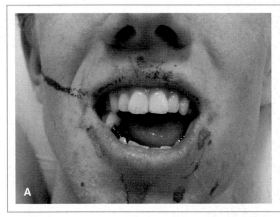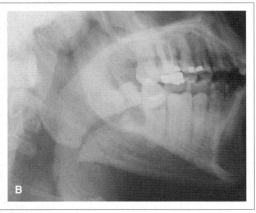

FIGURE 25.2: Open mandibular fracture as seen clinically (**A**) and radiographically (**B**). (*Part A courtesy of Madelyn Garcia, MD. Part B courtesy of Robert Hendrickson, MD.*) (From Greenberg M. Greenberg's Text-Atlas of Emergency Medicine. Philadelphia: Lippincott Williams & Wilkins, 2005.)

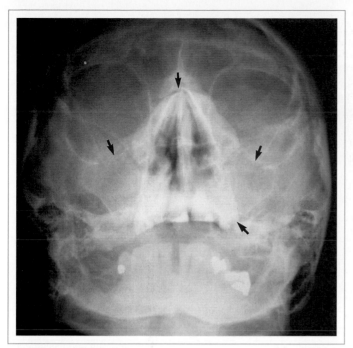

FIGURE 25.3: Waters view demonstrates extensive soft tissue swelling and distortion of the facial anatomy. Fractures are visible through the floors of both orbits, bridge of the nose, and lateral maxillary wall on the left (*arrows*). In addition, note the malocclusion between the maxilla and the mandible. (From Richard H. Daffner, Clinical Radiology: The Essentials, 3rd ed. Philadelphia: Lippincott Williams & Wilkins, 2007.)

CT Scan

- CT (ordered with "fine cuts" through the face) has been shown to have greater sensitivity than plain x-ray in identifying nondisplaced mental fractures (due to overlap with the spine on plain films) as well as mandibular ramus fractures (due to inadequate visualization of the condyle if the patient is unable to open his/her mouth completely)
- CT provides a rapid diagnosis, requires only one patient position as compared to plain films, and can guide surgical management
- If there is clinical suspicion for complicated injury to the midface or to the mandibular rami or condyles, CT is indicated
- CT coronal and sagittal reconstructions may elucidate fractures missed by plain films and conventional CT

TABLE 25.4: CT: mandibular/maxillary fractures

IV contrast	No
PO contrast	No
Amount of radiation	1–2 mSv

Classic Images

Le Fort I:

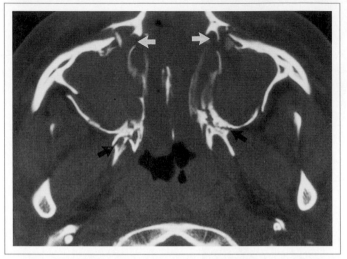

FIGURE 25.4: Le Fort I fracture. Axial CT scan demonstrates comminuted fractures involving all walls of both maxillary sinuses, with associated fractures through the pterygoid plates (*black arrows*). Both nasolacrimal ducts are also disrupted (*white arrows*). Both maxillary antra are completely opacified. (Reprinted with permission from Gean AD. Imaging of Head Trauma. Philadelphia: Lippincott Williams & Wilkins; 1994:456.)

Le Fort II:

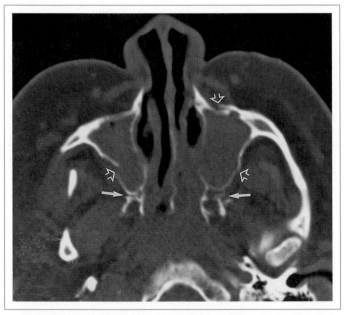

FIGURE 25.5: Axial CT image shows bilateral maxillary fractures (*open arrows*) as well as fractures through the pterygoid plates (*solid arrows*). Notice the opacification of the maxillary sinuses. (From Daffner RH. Clinical Radiology: The Essentials, 3rd ed. Philadelphia: Lippincott Williams & Wilkins, 2007.)

Le Fort III:

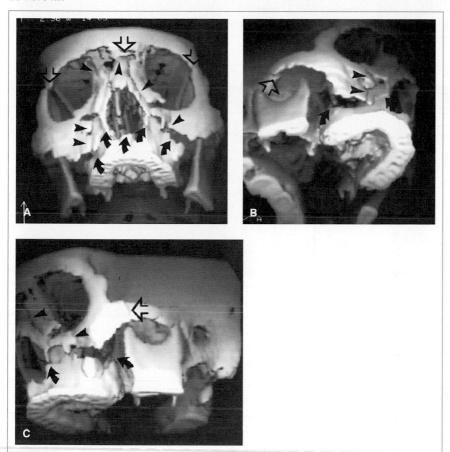

FIGURE 25.6: Le Fort III ("total facial smash") injury as portrayed on straight frontal (**A**) and each lateral oblique (**B** and **C**) 3D CT images. Le Fort I fracture distribution is indicated by *curved arrows*, Le Fort II by *arrowheads*, and Le Fort III by *open arrows*. (From Harris J and Harris W. The Radiology of Emergency Medicine, 4th ed. Philadelphia: Lippincott Williams and Wilkins, 2000.)

Magnetic Resonance Imaging

- Rarely used as a first-line diagnostic modality in maxillofacial fractures, but should be considered a useful adjunct in the context of concomitant soft-tissue pathology
- Patients presenting with cranial nerve deficits (e.g., traumatic Bell's palsy) not explained by fracture patterns seen with CT may benefit from MRI to identify potential causes of nerve pathology (e.g., compression by adjacent hematoma, nerve transaction, or axonal injury)
- MRI is also considered superior to CT for identifying damage to the articular surface of the condyles of the mandibular ramus

TABLE 25.5: Test characteristics of imaging modalities in midface and mandibular fractures

	Sensitivity	Specificity	Comments
Plain films			
Face series	87–91%	95–97%	For suspected midface fracture
Mandible series	77–89%	88–96%	For suspected isolated jaw fracture
Panoramic film (Panorex)	74–83%	92–100%	For suspected isolated jaw fracture
Computerized Tomography (CT)			
Head	90%	95%	Nondedicated study for facial fractures
Face	>90%	>90%	Dedicated study specifically for midface
Mandible	92%	87%	Dedicated mandible study

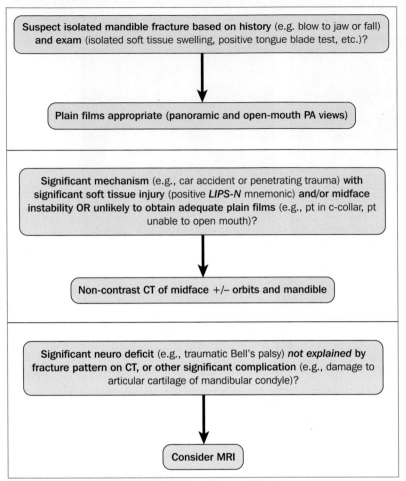

FIGURE 25.7: Clinical decision tree.

Basic Management
- ATLS guidelines
- Patients with injuries likely to require surgery should be kept NPO
- No established evidence to support the use of routine antibiotics for facial fractures
- Analgesia tailored to the individual patient should be titrated to comfort
- Frequent reevaluation of the patient with maxillofacial and mandibular trauma is important to monitor and potentially manage the airway
- Subspecialty consultation with oral and maxillofacial surgery or head and neck surgery is warranted in all Le Fort-type midface and mandibular fractures

Summary

TABLE 25.6: Advantages and disadvantages of imaging modalities in mandibular and maxillary fractures

Imaging modality	Advantages	Disadvantages
Plain x-ray	Inexpensive	Decreased sensitivity, need for exact patient positioning
CT scan	Fast, high degree of sensitivity and specificity, patient positioning less problematic	Greater cost and radiation exposure than plain films
MRI	Greater sensitivity for soft-tissue and nerve injuries	Time and cost intensive; inappropriate for unstable patients

26

Orbital and Zygomatic Fractures

Pranav Shetty and Timothy Horeczko

Background

Orbital and zygomatic fractures are increasingly common today; they present not only as isolated injuries as seen in assault, but also in the setting of multitrauma, such as in motor vehicle collisions. Careful attention to the mechanism of injury, the patient's airway and cervical spine, and neurologic examinations, as well as evaluation for concurrent injuries, will guide initial management, imaging, and definitive care.

The orbit is a bony cavity within the facial skeleton, which houses and protects the eyeball and associated structures. The frontal bone and the lesser wing of the sphenoid form the roof of the orbit, while the maxillary and zygomatic bones comprise its floor. The greater wing of the sphenoid and the zygomatic bone join to form the lateral wall, and the ethmoid and lacrimal bones form the medial wall. A unique feature of the medial wall is the *lamina papyracea* of the ethmoid—the thinnest portion of bone in the body. While the orbit provides reasonable protection to the eye and neurovascular structures, its relatively fixed volume can contribute to ischemia and mechanical damage, especially to the retina and extraocular muscles.

General inspection of the face for symmetry is best performed from the head of the bed (**bird's eye view**) or the foot of the bed (**worm's eye view**). Any concerning abnormalities in history or physical examination mandate further testing, primarily imaging studies and subspecialty consultation.

TABLE 26.1: Classic history and physical

Diplopia (binocular)—entrapment of extraocular muscle (usually inferior or medial orbital wall fracture)
Anesthesia/paresthesia—eyebrow/forehead (supraorbital nerve); maxilla/upper lip (infraorbital nerve)
Trismus—(zygomatic fracture)
Periorbital ecchymosis, exophthalmos, enophthalmos, hypoglobus, hyphema, telecanthus

Plain X-ray

- Used primarily when CT is not available
- Waters (occipitomental), Caldwell (posteroanterior), and "jug-hangle" (zygomatic arch) views may provide preliminary information such as the extent and type of fracture
- Sensitivity ranges from 64% to 78%

 TABLE 26.2: Plain film: orbital/zygomatic fractures (three views)

IV contrast	No
PO contrast	No
Amount of radiation	0.1 mSv per view

Classic Images

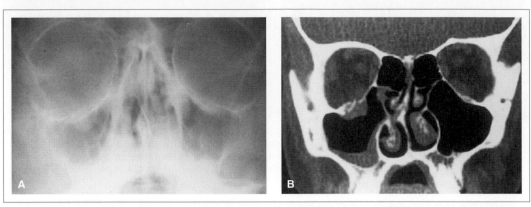

FIGURE 26.1: A: Blowout fracture. The plain film shows a teardrop configuration of the blowout fractures involving the right orbit. Note the associated fracture through the orbital floor and an air-fluid level in the maxillary sinus. **B:** CT section (of the same patient in part **A**) more clearly demonstrates the multiple fragment fracture through the orbital floor. Teardrop sign and an air-fluid level are evident in the right maxillary sinus. (From Fleisher GR, Ludwig S, and Henretig FM. Textbook of Pediatric Emergency Medicine, 5th ed. Philadelphia: Lippincott Williams & Wilkins, 2005.)

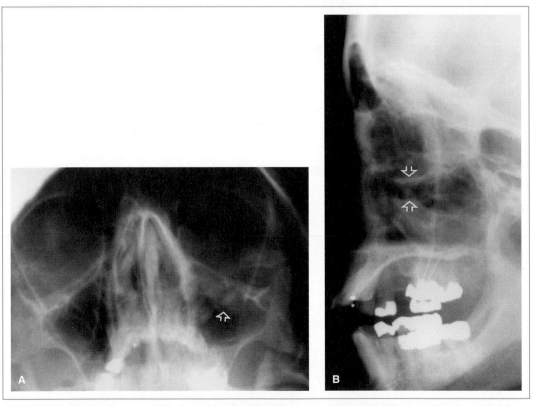

FIGURE 26.2: Blowout fracture of the left orbital floor. **A:** Waters view shows a double density at the roof of the left maxillary sinus (*arrow*) as well as an air-fluid level. **B:** Lateral facial radiograph shows a "double floor sign" (*arrows*). The lower arrow points to the depressed floor of the left orbit. (From Daffner RH. Clinical Radiology: The Essentials, 3rd ed. Philadelphia: Lippincott Williams & Wilkins, 2007.)

CT Scan

- Gold standard for imaging the facial skeleton.
- The sensitivity of CT scan for orbital fractures ranges from 79% to 96%.
- The order should request the thinnest cuts possible in order to optimize definition of the facial bones. This is generally requested as a facial CT *with thin cuts through the orbit* (the specific CT protocol and the "thinness" or resolution of the sections are institution- and scanner-dependent).
- No IV contrast is needed to evaluate the bony anatomy, and any fluid collection seen on CT in the setting of trauma should be assumed to be hemorrhage.
- A complete radiologic evaluation includes coronal and sagittal reconstructions, which can assist in fracture detection and surgical planning.
- An orbital CT scan exposes a patient to a radiation level of 0.6 mSv, or 2–4 months of background radiation, a relatively small dose when compared to CT scans of the chest, abdomen, or pelvis.
- Orbital wall (blowout) fractures are usually through the medial or inferior wall. Orbital contents may herniate into the ethmoid sinuses following a medial wall fracture, or into the maxillary sinus after an orbital floor fracture. Fractures involving the roof of the orbit more commonly occur in pediatric trauma due to the lack of pneumatization of the frontal sinus and are highly associated with intracranial injuries and skull fractures. Lateral orbital wall fractures do not often occur in isolation and are more commonly present as part of a zygomatico-maxillary complex "tripod" fracture.
- Zygomatic fractures rarely occur in isolation, commonly presenting as zygomatico-maxillary complex fractures. The most common fracture is the tripod fracture, which involves the three major attachments of the zygoma to the frontal, maxillary, and sphenoid bones.

☢ TABLE 26.3: CT: orbital/zygomatic fractures

IV contrast	No
PO contrast	No
Amount of radiation	1 mSv

Classic Images

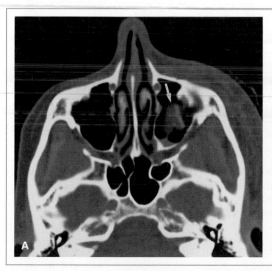 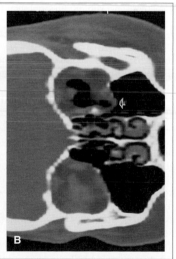

FIGURE 26.3: A: Axial CT image shows a soft-tissue density (*arrow*) projecting into the maxillary sinus on the left. This represents the orbital content herniated through the fracture. **B:** Coronal tomographic reconstruction shows the fractured orbital floor and the downward herniation of orbital contents (*arrow*). (From Daffner RH. Clinical Radiology: The Essentials, 3rd ed. Philadelphia: Lippincott Williams & Wilkins, 2007.)

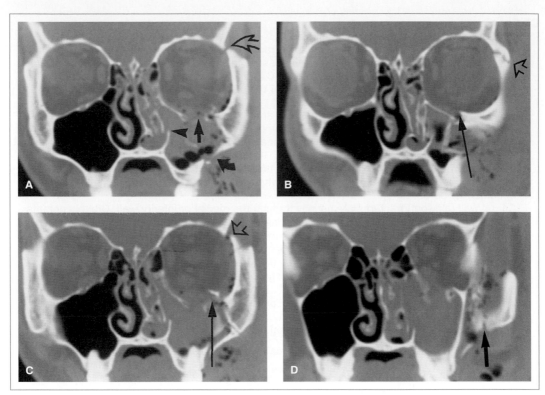

FIGURE 26.4: Comminuted, displaced left zygomatico-maxillary complex fracture as shown on coronal CT images from anterior (**A**) to posterior (**D**). **A:** Disruption of the "friendly line" (*curved arrow*); the medial wall (*arrowhead*) of the antrum; the inferior orbital rim (*arrow*); and separation of the left zygomaticofrontal suture (*curved open arrow*). **B** and **C:** The same findings and, in addition, fracture of the orbital floor (*long stemmed arrow*) and the lateral orbital wall (*open arrow*) posterior to the rim. **D:** The zygomatic arch fracture (*arrow*). In all images, the left antrum and the left ethmoidal air cells are almost completely opacified by blood and/or edema. (From Harris J and Harris W. The Radiology of Emergency Medicine, 4th ed. Philadelphia: Lippincott Williams and Wilkins, 2000.)

Magnetic Resonance Imaging
- Contraindicated if there is a possibility of a metallic foreign body
- Has improved evaluation of soft tissue structures: better at identifying entrapment of muscles/ nerves, but worse at identifying all fractures
- MRI may be better than CT at identifying subtle "trapdoor" orbital floor fractures in children due to soft tissue entrapment

Basic Management
- Follow ATLS guidelines to prioritize life-threatening conditions. Facial trauma is often associated with other high-risk complications, such as airway obstruction and spinal cord injury.
- Orbital fractures may result in a retro-orbital hematoma and exophthalmos, which can be vision-threatening due to ischemia of the retina and optic nerve; see Chapter 22.
- Although controversial, prophylactic antibiotics are indicated for open fractures and fractures that violate a sinus cavity.
- Other orbital fractures, even those causing entrapment and diplopia, are not considered ophthalmologic emergencies unless accompanied by globe injury or visual impairment. In general, these may be managed with patching for comfort, special precautions (no nose blowing, sneezing), and urgent (within 48 hours) subspecialty consultation.
- Zygomatic fractures are often displaced and may require delayed surgical intervention for pain, trismus, or for cosmetic purpose; patients should have urgent subspecialty follow-up.

Summary

TABLE 26.4: Advantages and disadvantages of imaging modalities in orbital fractures

Imaging modality	Advantages	Disadvantages
Plain x-ray	Inexpensive, universally available	Lower sensitivity (64–78%), difficult to interpret
CT scan (face)	Increased sensitivity (79–96%)	Costly, difficult in unstable patient, higher radiation exposure

27

Nasal Fractures

Nicholas Drakos and Ari M. Lipsky

Background

Nasal bone fractures are the most common site-specific bone injuries of the facial skeleton, accounting for approximately 40% of all facial fractures. The epidemiology of nasal fractures parallels the epidemiology of facial trauma. The highest incidence is seen between 15 and 30 years of age with a male-to-female ratio of greater than 2:1. There is also a small but significant increase in nasal fractures seen in the elderly population secondary to their higher rate of falls.

Nasal bone fractures should always be suspected in the setting of facial trauma. However, because isolated nasal bone fractures are rarely an emergent issue, the foremost goal of the emergency physician should be to recognize, manage, and appropriately disposition associated complications and injuries that place the patient at increased risk for morbidity and mortality.

TABLE 27.1: Nasal fractures: complications and associated injuries

Cosmetic deformity
Septal deviation with resultant breathing difficulty
Nasal septal hematoma with resultant abscess formation or necrosis of septal cartilage leading to a saddle nose deformity
Naso-orbital-ethmoid fractures ■ Lacrimal duct injury ■ Ocular compromise ■ Cribriform plate fracture with potential dural tears and cerebrospinal fluid (CSF) leak
Le Fort II and III fractures.

The diagnosis of isolated nasal bone fractures is primarily ascertained by a careful history and physical examination. Radiographic imaging should be used when there is a suspicion for associated injury requiring further delineation. Furthermore, imaging will rarely change management in the case of isolated nasal bone fracture.

TABLE 27.2: Classic history and physical

Blunt force trauma to nasal region
Difficulty breathing through nose
Deformity noted by patient
Epistaxis or nasal discharge
Crepitus

Plain X-ray

■ Bony facial structures may be evaluated using plain films, though additional facial fractures and soft-tissue injuries are much better visualized using CT.

- The sensitivity is 53–90%, depending upon the combination of plain films used. Old fractures, vascular markings, cartilage fractures, midline nasal sutures, nasomaxillary sutures, and thinning of the nasal wall all contribute to difficulty in interpreting plain film imaging of the nasal bones.
- Plain films of the face may be used to screen for fractures in cases where a low suspicion exists for periorbital, zygomatic, or mandibular fractures.

 TABLE 27.3: Plain film: nasal fracture (two views)

IV contrast	No
PO contrast	No
Amount of radiation	0.1 mSv per view

Classic Images

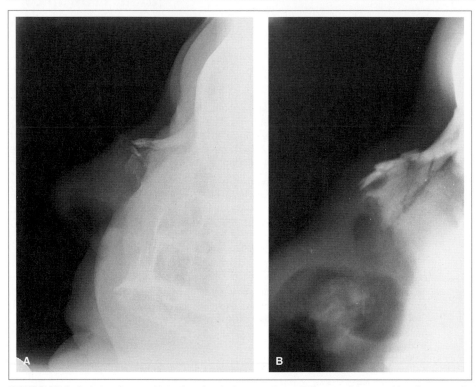

FIGURE 27.1: A: Lateral nose. Note the simple fracture through the nasal bone, with adjacent soft tissue swelling. **B:** Lateral nose. Observe the comminuted fracture of the nasal bone. (From Yochum TR and Rowe LJ. Yochum and Rowe's Essentials of Skeletal Radiology, 3rd ed. Philadelphia: Lippincott Williams & Wilkins, 2004.)

Orbital CT
- Noncontrast CT of the face with fine cuts of the area of concern, such as the orbits, is currently the most sensitive and widely available modality for evaluation of bony facial structures.
- CT also visualizes soft tissue structures, which can be helpful in evaluating associated injury such as extraocular muscle entrapment in the case of orbital fractures.
- Three-dimensional CT facial reconstructions may be considered in the evaluation and management of nasal fractures to better elucidate associated facial bone injuries.
- It is important to consider a noncontrast CT of the head in patients who have had a confirmed or suspected loss of consciousness associated with trauma.

 TABLE 27.4: CT scan: nasal fracture (orbital CT)

IV contrast	No
PO contrast	No
Amount of radiation	1 mSv

Classic Images

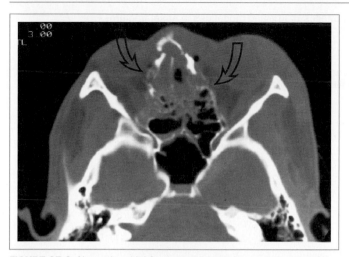

FIGURE 27.2: Nasoethmoidal fracture with massive comminution of the nasal skeleton (*curved arrows*) including the nasal bones anteriorly, nasal process of maxillae, septum, ethmoid cell walls, and the medial orbital walls. Massive edema and/or hemorrhage occupies the nasal cavity and the ethmoidal sinuses. (From Harris J and Harris W. The Radiology of Emergency Medicine, 4th ed. Philadelphia: Lippincott Williams and Wilkins, 2000.)

TABLE 27.5: Basic management of nasal fractures and associated complications

Injury/ complication	H&P findings*	Work-up/ imaging†	Treatment	Inpatient consultation	Disposition
Isolated nasal bone fracture	(−) Breathing difficulty (−) Deformity	None indicated	Ice and analgesia	None indicated	Discharge home
	(+) Breathing difficulty and/or (+) Deformity and/or (+) Open internal fracture	None indicated	Ice and analgesia ±Prophylactic antibiotics for open fracture	None indicated	Discharge home with outpatient follow-up. Open reduction typically performed within 5–7 d
Naso-orbito-ethmoid (NOE) fractures (associated with lacrimal duct injury, ocular compromise, and cribriform plate fractures with potential dural tears and CSF leak)	(+) Telecanthus (+) Enophthalmos (+) Epiphora (+) Nasal discharge	1. Test nasal discharge for presence of CSF (halo sign, glucose content) 2. Assess EOM and perform slit lamp examination 3. CT face with 2 mm cuts; consider 3D reconstructions if available	1. CSF leak: Emergent reduction 2. Open-globe injury: Eye shield and antibiotics	1. OMFS or ENT: all NOE fractures 2. Neurosurgery: suspected or confirmed CSF leak or findings of cribriform plate fracture on CT 3. Ophthalmology: open-globe injury, entrapment, lacrimal duct injury	Admit for appropriate surgical management
Le Fort II and III fractures	(+) Midface mobility	CT face with 2 mm cuts Consider 3D recons if available		OMFS or ENT	Admit for appropriate surgical management

*Findings listed in the table are in addition to the swelling, crepitus, and/or nasal bone mobility characteristic of nasal bone fractures.
†Plain films may be considered as a screening tool if there is low suspicion for associated injury.
CSF, cerebrospinal fluid; ENT, ear, nose & throat surgery; EOM, extraocular movements; OMFS, oral and maxillofacial surgery.

Summary

TABLE 27.6: Advantages and disadvantages of imaging modalities in nasal fractures

Imaging modality	Advantages	Disadvantages
Plain x-ray	Inexpensive Low radiation Can be performed at bedside Can be used as a screening modality for associated fractures	Fair sensitivity (53–90%) and specificity Difficult to identify associated soft tissue injuries or fractures Does not alter management in cases of isolated nasal fractures
CT scan	High sensitivity and specificity Ability to identify associated soft tissue injuries or fractures	Increased cost Increased radiation Does not alter management in cases of isolated nasal fractures

28

Overview of the Eye

Sarah Battistich and Ari M. Lipsky

Background

It is estimated that 1 in 50 patients presenting for evaluation in emergency departments (EDs) has an eye-related complaint. Approximately half of emergent eye complaints are related to trauma or foreign bodies.

The use of imaging techniques, primarily ultrasound and CT scan, can often be helpful in establishing a particular diagnosis or ruling out concerning conditions. Early recognition of a potentially sight-threatening disorder may maximize the potential for salvage of the patient's vision.

This chapter presents an overview of and offers general guidelines regarding emergent imaging of the eye. For more information on specific conditions, please see the subsequent chapters.

TABLE 28.1: Key historical elements

Past ophthalmic history (e.g., prior visual acuity, use of corrective lenses, medications, surgeries)
History of trauma, chemical exposure, risk for foreign body
Current visual acuity
Pain, itching
Redness
Drainage, discharge
Diplopia, visual field cuts
Tetanus status

TABLE 28.2: Key examination elements

Visual acuity (best corrected; use pinhole if needed)
Visual fields
Ocular motility
Pupils
External examination (lids, lashes, lacrimal apparatus, conjunctiva, sclera, cornea)
Slit lamp examination (as above; also consider fluorescein, anterior chamber, iris, lens)
Direct ophthalmoscopy (retina, including optic disc and fundus)
Ocular tonometry (contraindicated if globe rupture suspected)

Imaging of the Eye

Often, one of the more challenging elements of the eye examination is deciding whether the patient requires imaging. Presence or suspicion of any of the following is an absolute indication for radiographic imaging:

- Deep penetrating wound
  - Determine the extent of eye injury and assess adjacent involvement
- Intraocular foreign body
  - Localize the foreign body and assess injury extent
- Significant blunt trauma
  - Identify lens displacement, intraocular hemorrhage, vitreous and retinal detachment, optic nerve compromise, extraocular muscle injury, and orbital wall fractures

Below are guidelines for choice of initial imaging modality; additional modalities may be required. These guidelines are not exhaustive and should be considered within the context of the individual patient.

TABLE 28.3: Preferred initial modalities for suspected injuries

Physical examination finding	Suspected injuries/conditions	Preferred initial imaging modality
Periorbital emphysema	Orbital wall fracture (usually medial)	CT
Limitation of extraocular movements	Entrapment of extraocular muscles	CT
Edema, erythema, pain with eye movement	Orbital cellulitis	CT or MRI
Proptosis	Retrobulbar mass, bleeding, or infection	CT or US
Unilaterally fixed and dilated pupil after trauma	Traumatic mydriasis, optic nerve damage, retained foreign body, early tentorial herniation	CT
Sudden, atraumatic monocular visual loss with no external or anterior chamber abnormality	Vitreous hemorrhage, retinal detachment	US
Visual loss with no external or anterior chamber abnormality, +/− headache	Stroke, cavernous sinus thrombosis, intracranial process causing optic nerve compression	MRI or CT
Moderate to severe trauma	Fracture, globe rupture, hemorrhage	CT
Intraocular foreign body by history; scleral or corneal laceration on examination	Retained foreign body, injury to orbital contents	US or CT

Types of Imaging

Ultrasound

Over the past decade ophthalmic ultrasound has been increasingly used in the ED evaluation of suspected intraocular pathology. The eye is a fluid-filled structure and as such is an ideal acoustic window to obtain excellent images. Studies of ED physician's use of ultrasound have found excellent sensitivity and specificity after appropriate training. Ultrasound is useful for evaluating intraorbital structures, including the anterior and posterior chambers (e.g., for foreign bodies), lens, fundus, optic disc, as well as the retrobulbar space. Ultrasound can be a useful adjunct to the physical examination. However, it cannot evaluate the bony orbit. It is relatively contraindicated in suspected globe rupture, as it requires applying pressure to the eye with the ultrasound probe.

Your ophthalmologic consultant may use the terms "A-scan" (or "amplitude scan") and "B-scan" (or "brightness scan"), which, when combined, give the practitioner a two-dimensional picture of the eye. If your ED, like most, does not have a dedicated ophthalmologic ultrasound with a small cylindrical probe, any high frequency (usually 5–10 MHz) probe can be used.

The eye should be scanned in both the transverse and sagittal planes. Figure 28.1 demonstrates a typical acoustic window and visible orbital structures. The anterior chamber should be clear and full. You might appreciate flattening of the anterior chamber in the setting of globe rupture, and a hyphema may be visible as a bright spot within the anterior chamber. The lens is visible as a bright, or hyperechoic, structure. The vitreous should be clear and dark. Any heterogeneous, hyperechoic densities are abnormal and usually represent vitreous hemorrhage or foreign bodies. The fundus should be smooth and bright. The optic disc may be seen but should not protrude into the vitreous space (this out-pouching would be consistent with papilledema). Any flap or smooth "line" attached to the retina but within the vitreous should alert the physician to a possible retinal detachment. Hypoechoic densities posterior to the retina suggest a retrobulbar hemorrhage.

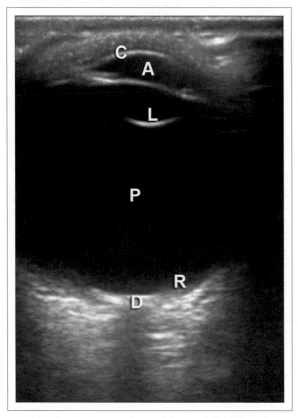

FIGURE 28.1: Normal ultrasound of the eye. A, anterior chamber; P, posterior chamber; D, optic disc; C, cornea; R, retina; L, lens. (*Courtesy of Bret Nelson, MD, Mt. Sinai Medical Center, New York, NY.*)

CT Scan

CT is readily available in most EDs and provides good imaging of soft tissue, bone, acute hemorrhage, and most foreign bodies. This is the preferred modality if you are also concerned about intracranial pathology, as it is relatively easy to obtain a CT scan of the orbits or face in conjunction with a CT scan of the brain. Consult with your radiologist about the best protocol to order; usually a CT scan with orbital fine cuts is preferred.

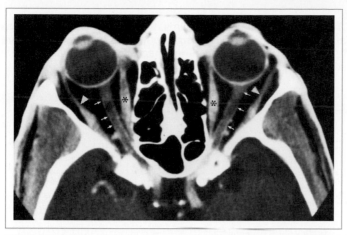

FIGURE 28.2: Axial CT section through the midportion of the orbits shows the aqueous and the vitreous chambers. Notice that the lens is biconvex and slightly flattened anteriorly. The lateral (*arrowhead*) and medial (*asterisks*) rectus muscles are also clearly seen. The midportion of the muscle is termed the belly. The optic nerves (*arrows*) are low density and are surrounded by the high-density meningeal sheath. (From Harris J and Harris W. The Radiology of Emergency Medicine, 4th ed. Philadelphia: Lippincott Williams and Wilkins, 2000.)

Magnetic Resonance Imaging

MRI is occasionally important for emergent ophthalmologic evaluation, such as when small masses or hemorrhage around the optic nerve is suspected. As compared to CT, MRI provides superior visualization of tissue and blood, but relatively poor imaging of bone. Importantly, if there is a concern for a metallic foreign body, MRI is contraindicated.

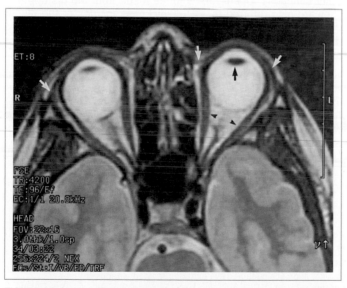

FIGURE 28.3: Axial T2-weighted MR image through midglobe shows linear low-signal orbital septum (*white arrows*) at its origin near the periosteum of the lateral and medial orbital walls between the higher signal preseptal and posterior orbital fat. The vitreous fluid is of high-signal intensity, and the lens (*arrow*) and extraocular muscles (*black arrowheads*) are of low-signal intensity. (From Harris J and Harris W. The Radiology of Emergency Medicine, 4th ed. Philadelphia: Lippincott Williams and Wilkins, 2000.)

Plain X-ray

Although ultrasound and CT have largely replaced plain films, they may be useful in the case of suspected displaced orbital wall fracture or metallic foreign body if the other modalities are not available. The superior sensitivity of CT and ultrasound has made the use of plain films rare in many departments in the setting of eye trauma.

TABLE 28.4: Appropriateness of imaging modalities for eye injuries by modality

Indication	Ultrasound	CT	MRI	Plain x-ray
Intraocular hemorrhage	+	+	+	−
Retrobulbar hemorrhage or mass	+	+	+	−
Foreign body	+	+	+ (organic/plastic) − (metallic)	+/−
Fracture	−	+	−	+/−
Contraindications (eye-specific)	Globe rupture	None	Metallic object	None

29

Open-Globe Injury

Jonie Hsiao and Cori Poffenberger

Background

Approximately 2.4 million eye injuries occur in the United States annually, making traumatic injury the leading cause of monocular blindness. Open-globe injuries result from the disruption of the outer integrity of the eye. They are also referred to as full-thickness injuries of the eye wall at the cornea and/or sclera. Open-globe injuries are often devastating and can lead to permanent vision loss; therefore, prompt diagnosis and emergent ophthalmology consultation are essential to optimizing patient outcomes.

Penetrating injuries result from sharp or high-speed projectile objects and may result in retained foreign body; the globe is lacerated at the site of the penetration. In contrast, injuries from blunt trauma result due to a dramatic initial increase in the intraocular pressure. As the internal fluid of the eye is incompressible, the globe will actually rupture at the weakest site, not at the site of direct impact. These weak sites occur at areas where the sclera is thinnest, such as the insertion sites of the extraocular muscles, at the limbus, around the optic nerve, and in areas of previous surgical incisions.

TABLE 29.1: Classic history and physical

Severely decreased vision and pain
Deflated appearance of globe
Extrusion of intraocular contents
Irregular-shaped pupil
Decreased intraocular pressure (DO NOT TEST)
Positive Seidel's sign: fluorescein-stained eye extrudes stained vitreous in "waterfall" pattern
Associated hyphema, vitreous hemorrhage, subconjunctival edema, chemosis, lens subluxation, and change in depth of anterior chamber
If occult, may present with only mild pain or mild change in acuity

Orbital CT

- The imaging modality of choice due to high accuracy and availability
- Axial and coronal images with thin cuts, typically 1.25–3 mm, without contrast

- In one study, orbital CT demonstrated a sensitivity of 75% and a specificity of 93% in the absence of clinical information
- For "occult" injuries, studies suggest a sensitivity ranging from 55–68% and specificity of 86–100%
- Allows for simultaneous assessment of damage to adjacent structures, especially associated fractures, and identification of foreign bodies

TABLE 29.2: Common CT findings

Intraocular foreign body
Intraocular emphysema
Irregular contour of sclera
Volume loss of globe
Possible associated findings: altered lens position, change in anterior chamber depth compared to unaffected eye

 TABLE 29.3: CT: Open-globe injury

IV contrast	None
PO contrast	None
Amount of radiation	1 mSv

Classic Images

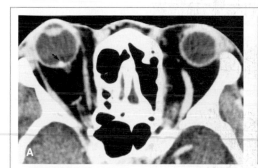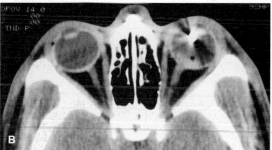

FIGURE 29.1: A: Axial CT with metallic foreign body in the right eye. **B:** Axial CT with opaque foreign body and gas within left globe. (From Harris J and Harris W, The Radiology of Emergency Medicine, 4th ed. Philadelphia: Lippincott Williams and Wilkins, 2000.)

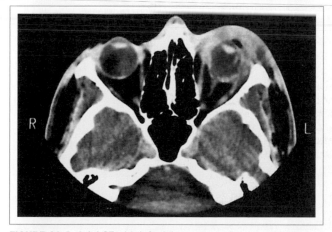

FIGURE 29.2: Axial CT with left globe rupture after blunt trauma not evident on clinical examination with disruption of corneoscleral contour. (From MacCumber MW and Bauer BA. Management of Ocular Injuries and Emergencies, 4th ed. Philadelphia: Lippincott Williams and Wilkins, 1998.)

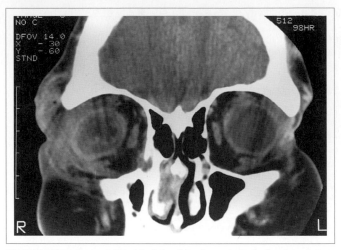

FIGURE 29.3: Coronal CT with right globe irregularity indicative of rupture and hyperdense areas indicative of intraocular hemorrhage. (From Harris J and Harris W. The Radiology of Emergency Medicine, 4th ed. Philadelphia: Lippincott Williams and Wilkins, 2000.)

MRI
- Contraindicated if metallic foreign body suspected
- Sensitivity and specificity not well studied, but likely highly sensitive in delineating soft-tissue structures
- Usually impractical and time-consuming in the acute setting with delay in definitive diagnosis; intraoperative examination is preferred to rule in the diagnosis

Ultrasound
- A high suspicion for an open-globe injury is at least a relative contraindication to ocular bedside ultrasound in the ED setting
- May be used by specialist to detect occult injuries
- Can visualize discontinuity of sclera

Classic Images

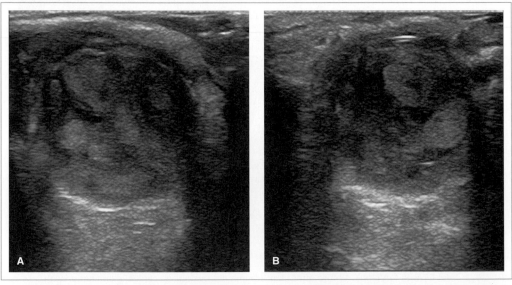

FIGURE 29.4: Ultrasound images (**A, B**) of a ruptured globe. Note that the normal eye contains hypoechoic fluid whereas the ruptured globe contains blood seen as hyperechoic material within the eye. (*Courtesy of Penelope Chun, New York Hospital Queens, Flushing, NY.*)

Basic Management

- Check visual acuity and perform slit lamp examination
- Shield the eye as soon as diagnosis of open-globe injury is made or suspected
- Emergent ophthalmology consultation
- IV antiemetics as necessary to prevent Valsalva and further extrusion of intraocular contents
- Prophylactic antibiotics to prevent endophthalmitis
- Update tetanus
- NPO for likely surgical intervention
- Pain management

Summary

TABLE 29.4: Advantages and disadvantages of imaging modalities in open-globe injuries

Imaging Modalities	Advantages	Disadvantages
CT scan	Availability Good sensitivity/specificity Concomitant identification of other injuries Identification of foreign bodies	May miss occult injuries
MRI	Likely high sensitivity	Time-consuming Limited ED availability Contraindicated with possible metallic foreign body
Ultrasound		May exacerbate injury by extruding intraocular contents and is thus essentially contraindicated

30 Retrobulbar Hemorrhage

Brecken Armstrong-Kelsey and Ravi Morchi

Background

Retrobulbar hemorrhage is an ophthalmologic emergency that can result in permanent visual loss unless it is diagnosed and treated promptly. Hemorrhage into the potential space that surrounds the globe causes damage to the orbital vessels. This condition most commonly occurs because of blunt facial trauma causing a nondisplaced orbital fracture, but can also occur after retrobulbar anesthesia or other orbital/ocular instrumentation.

Two separate mechanisms act together to cause ocular damage. First, hemorrhage behind the globe causes increased intra*orbital* pressure, compromise of the ophthalmic artery, and, subsequently, an orbital compartment syndrome. Secondly, hemorrhage also causes the globe to be forced against the eyelids, which are strongly attached to the orbital rim by the medial and lateral canthal ligaments. This causes an increase in the intra*ocular* pressure and a subsequent decrease in the perfusion pressure to the optic nerve and retina. Central retinal artery insufficiency and optic nerve ischemia result in visual loss if the pressure is not relieved within 90–100 minutes of the initial insult.

TABLE 30.1: Classic history and physical findings

History of blunt facial trauma or recent retrobulbar anesthesia
Decreased visual acuity in the affected eye
Proptosis of the affected eye
Limited extraocular movements
Afferent pupillary defect in the affected eye
Blanched ophthalmic artery on ophthalmoscopic examination
Increased intraocular pressure

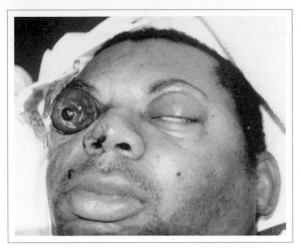

FIGURE 30.1: Retrobulbar hemorrhage demonstrating dramatic proptosis and subconjunctival hemorrhage after a fist strike in a patient on warfarin. (From Harwood-Nuss A, Wolfson AB, et al. The Clinical Practice of Emergency Medicine, 3rd ed. Philadelphia: Lippincott Williams & Wilkins, 2001.)

Orbital CT Scan
- Gold standard imaging modality for the diagnosis of retrobulbar hemorrhage
- Thin-slice helical CT with coronal reconstructions is the optimal study, producing the best image quality and reduced radiation to the lens over standard CT
- CT will demonstrate a fluid collection posterior to the globe on the affected side

 TABLE 30.2: CT scan: retrobulbar hemorrhage

IV contrast	No
PO contrast	No
Amount of radiation	1.0 mSv*

*In patients with trauma mechanism, head CT (in addition to orbital cuts) will likely be necessary increasing the radiation dosage to approximately 2–2.5 mSv.

Classic Images

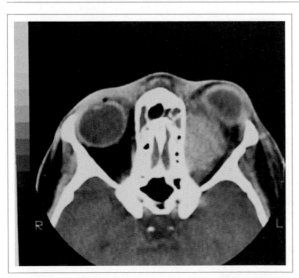

FIGURE 30.2: CT demonstrates a large subperiosteal hemorrhage along the medial orbital wall, compressing the optic nerve and distorting the globe. (From Tasman W and Jaeger E. The Wills Eye Hospital Atlas of Clinical Ophthalmology, 2nd ed. Lippincott Williams & Wilkins, 2001.)

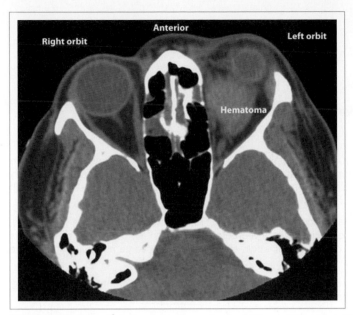

FIGURE 30.3: Left retrobulbar hematoma clearly visible on CT imaging. (*Courtesy of David Thompson MD, Denver Health Medical Center, Denver, CO.*)

Basic Management

- Emergent ophthalmology consult
- Administer pain medication
- Any compromise to the retinal circulation by retrobulbar hemorrhage requires immediate decompression by an ophthalmologist. Because of the rapid progression of this condition to permanent visual loss, temporizing measures, e.g., lateral canthotomy, may need to be taken by the emergency physician prior to both the radiologic diagnosis and the arrival of the ophthalmologist to the ED:
- Lateral canthotomy and cantholysis
  - Temporizing measure
  - Releases pressure on the globe, thereby decreasing intraocular pressure and restoring blood flow to the retinal artery
  - Indications: proptosis and a significant decrease in visual acuity with or without IOP >40 mm Hg and afferent pupillary defect
  - Contraindications: ruptured globe
- Medications to decrease intraocular pressure (temporizing measures to help improve perfusion pressure to the optic nerve until definitive treatment is available)
  - Carbonic anhydrase inhibitors
  - Topical beta-blockers
  - IV mannitol

Summary

TABLE 30.3: Advantages and disadvantages of CT in retrobulbar hemorrhage

Advantages	Disadvantages
Easily available	Time consuming
Not operator dependent	Radiation exposure
Diagnose concurrent disease	

31 Retinal Detachment

Elga Tinger and David Burbulys

Background

It is estimated that 1–2 in 10,000 people per year develop a retinal detachment. The lifetime risk is nearly 1 in 300 and higher in patients with risk factors, such as history of cataract surgery or high myopia. Without early diagnosis and treatment, the likelihood of vision loss is high with retinal detachment and may be irreversible and complete.

The diagnosis on funduscopic examination alone is challenging and often difficult even for an experienced ophthalmologist. This is especially true if the detachment is small, peripheral, or if there is facial or eye trauma preventing a careful examination. Ultrasound has become an integral tool in the diagnosis of retinal detachments.

Retinal detachment occurs when there is a separation of the sensory retina from the underlying pigment epithelium with accumulation of subretinal fluid.

TABLE 31.1: Classic history and physical

Painless unilateral decreased visual acuity
Increased age
History of cataract surgery, head trauma, myopia, diabetic retinopathy, or uveitis
Family history of retinal detachment
Near normal visual acuity if the macula is not involved
Visual field deficit
Sensation of floaters
Sensation of flashing lights or colors
Normal direct ophthalmoscopy is common
Billowing forward of the hazy gray membranous retina

Bedside Ultrasound

Technique

- A standard 10 MHz linear array transducer, or vascular probe, is commonly used.
- A sonolucent adhesive barrier, such as Tegaderm, may be used over the eyelid to increase patient comfort and decrease the risk of conjunctival irritation from ultrasound conducting gel. A liberal amount of water-soluble, warmed gel is applied to minimize pressure and improve image quality.
- The examiner's hand is stabilized on the forehead and bridge of the patient's nose to avoid excessive pressure to the eyes. Scanning is done in a slow cephalad to caudad motion followed by a lateral to medial motion. As an alternative, it may also be helpful to keep the probe stationary while the patient slowly moves his or her eyes under a closed lid from side to side and up and down. Both eyes should be examined for comparison.
  - Retinal detachments appear as bands of echogenic material within the vitreous body, in the posterior or lateral globe.
  - Small detachments appear as convex domes and larger detachments are cone shaped.
  - The detached retina may be attached anteriorly to the ora serrata and posteriorly to the optic disc giving the appearance of a funnel on axial imaging and a circular image on coronal sections.
  - With real-time evaluation, a recent detachment frequently has undulating motion, whereas a chronic, older, stiffer detachment has less motion due to the formation of adhesions and scar tissue.
- The duration of the examination should be limited as the eyes are theoretically ultrasound sensitive and there is a potential risk of high-energy exposure.

TABLE 31.2: Ultrasonographic appearance of possible diagnoses

Diagnosis	Ultrasonographic appearance
Retinal detachment	Band of echogenic material within the vitreous body
Vitreous detachment	Collection of echogenic material between the vitreous body and the retina
Vitreous hemorrhage	Echogenic material within the vitreous body
Retrobulbar hemorrhage	Hypoechoic lucency deep to the retina

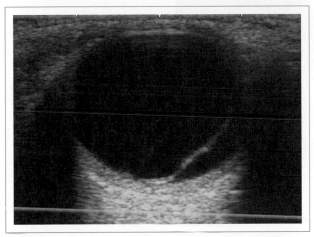

FIGURE 31.1: Retinal detachment seen by ultrasound. (*Courtesy of Timothy Jang, MD, Harbor-UCLA Medical Center Torrance, California.*)

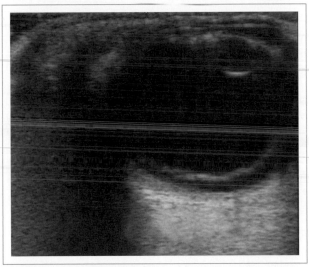

FIGURE 31.2: Convex-shaped smaller retinal detachment. (*Courtesy of Timothy Jang, MD, Harbor-UCLA Medical Center Torrance, California.*)

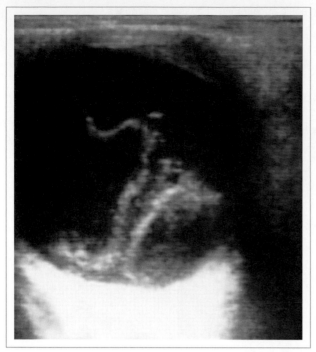

FIGURE 31.3: Funnel-shaped larger retinal detachment. (*Courtesy of Mike Peterson, MD, Harbor-UCLA Medical Center Torrance, California.*)

Computed Tomographic Scan

Currently, there are case reports in the literature demonstrating the utility of high-resolution CT to detect retinal detachments. These are largely incidental findings and no well-controlled studies to date demonstrate their sensitivity or specificity.

Basic Management

- Emergent ophthalmologic consultation
- Definitive therapy generally involves mechanically apposing the sensory retina and retinal pigment layer to close the break, followed by retinopexy to create an adhesion of the retina to the pigment epithelium and prevent the retinal break from reopening

Summary

TABLE 31.3: Advantages and disadvantages of ultrasound in retinal detachment

Advantages	Disadvantages
Low cost	Operator dependent
Minimal patient discomfort	Difficult to discern vitreous body from retinal detachment
No ionizing radiation	
Bedside availability	
Rapid	

32 Intraocular Foreign Bodies

Mark Deaver and Ari M. Lipsky

Background

Ophthalmologic emergencies represent 3% of all ED visits in the United States. Many of these injuries involve the presence of one or multiple intraocular foreign bodies (IOFB). IOFBs can penetrate anywhere within the globe, with most located posterior to the lens (64%). Other locations include anterior to the lens (32%) and intralenticular (4%). Although the presentation of an IOFB can be dramatic, physicians must maintain a high degree of suspicion in all patients with a concerning history. Approximately 20% of patients with penetrating foreign bodies of the globe report no pain or apparent visual changes. This represents a true diagnostic challenge, as retained IOFB can lead to complications including endophthalmitis, retinal damage, and partial or complete vision loss.

TABLE 32.1: Classic history and physical

Foreign body sensation
Recent exposure to high velocity projectiles (hammering, sawing, drilling, etc.)
No use of protective eyewear
Conjunctival edema and erythema
Altered or asymmetric pupil
Positive Seidel fluorescein test: indicates globe injury

Plain X-rays

- Plain films (usually Caldwell and Waters' views) are not the optimal studies, as nearly 60% of penetrating objects are missed and therefore cannot be effectively used to rule out the presence of IOFB.
- Normal structures such as the ophthalmomeningeal foramen can be mistaken for an IOFB and may lead to delays in final diagnosis and disposition.
- Although plain films can detect radiopaque materials, they cannot be used to determine whether these materials are metalic.
- Plain films have poor sensitivity for radiolucent materials such as graphite, plastic, and other organic materials (wood, plant matter, etc.).
- Even when plain films do identify an IOFB, they do not provide sufficient information about the foreign body's location with respect to the surrounding soft tissues to appropriately guide further management of the injury.

 TABLE 32.2: Plain film: intraocular foreign bodies (three views)

IV contrast	No
PO contrast	No
Amount of radiation	0.1 mSv per view

Orbital CT Scan

- CT is the imaging modality of choice for suspected penetrating injuries to the eye with a 98% sensitivity for both metallic and nonmetallic objects.
- CT can be completed quickly with minimum discomfort to the patient.
- The exact location of the object within the eye can be determined by obtaining coronal and sagittal reconstruction images. This information can then be communicated to the consultant for better preoperative assessment.
- The CT images can also be used to determine whether coexistent injuries are present, such as orbital fractures and lens disruption.
- The nature of the IOFB (glass, metal, stone, plant matter, wood, etc.) can be determined by the attenuation level of the object (i.e., number of Hounsfield units).

- CT scan can miss nonmetallic, very low density objects such as dry wood or other plant matter. If wood is the likely foreign body, view images using bone windows, which allows better identification because the inner structure of the wood is visualized (see image below).
- Additional concerning features on CT include blood-vitreous humor level, air within the globe, and flattening of the globe suggestive of globe rupture and leakage of aqueous or vitreous humor.

 TABLE 32.3: CT scan: intraocular foreign body

IV contrast	No
PO contrast	No
Amount of radiation	1 mSv

Classic CT Images

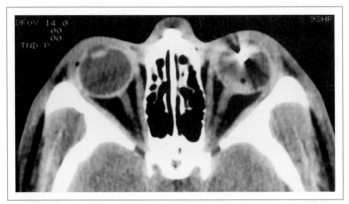

FIGURE 32.1: Axial CT scan through the midorbits demonstrates a small high-density foreign object located within the vitreous of the left globe. There is gas in the vitreous. Lower velocity objects tend to lodge anteriorly as this one did. Note streaking artifacts from metal. (From Harris J and Harris W. The Radiology of Emergency Medicine, 4th ed. Philadelphia: Lippincott Williams and Wilkins, 2000.)

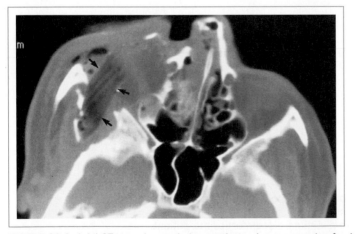

FIGURE 32.2: Axial CT scan, bone window settings, shows a wooden foreign body (*arrows*) containing typical striations. Bone windows are needed for identification of wood. There are multiple fractures involving the right side of the face. (From Harris J and Harris W. The Radiology of Emergency Medicine, 4th ed. Philadelphia: Lippincott Williams and Wilkins, 2000.)

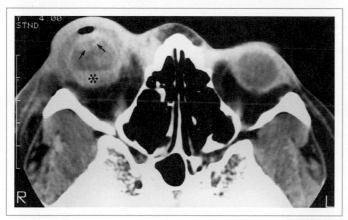

FIGURE 32.3: Axlal CT scan through the inferior aspect of the orbits shows extensive right preorbital soft tissue swelling and air beneath the inferior eyelid. The right globe has been lacerated and is slightly elongated, indicating loss of pressure. The lens (*small arrows*) is disrupted, and there is a high-density blood-vitreous level (*asterisk*) within the dependent portion of the eye. (From Harrls J and Harris W. The Radiology of Emergency Medicine, 4th ed. Philadelphia: Lippincott Williams and Wilkins, 2000.)

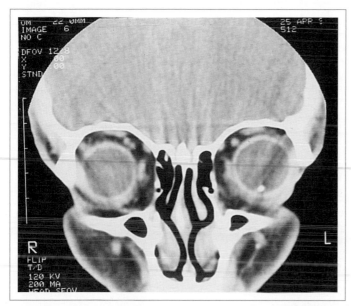

FIGURE 32.4: A small pellet in the inferior left eye. (From Tasman W and Jaeger E. The Wills Eye Hospital Atlas of Clinical Ophthalmology, 2nd ed. Philadelphia: Lippincott Williams & Wilkins, 2001.)

Bedside Ocular Ultrasound

- Bedside ultrasound can be used to diagnose both metallic and nonmetallic foreign bodies with a sensitivity of 93%; this modality is a useful adjunct if CT imaging is delayed or there is a particular concern about radiation exposure
- To obtain the best image quality, a linear 10-mHz transducer probe should be used with the operator applying gel to the patient's closed eye prior to use
- Related lesions such as vitreous hemorrhages and retinal detachments can be evaluated in real-time
- Ultrasound can be time-consuming as the patient must cooperate and be able to perform repeated ocular movements to allow the operator to better visualize the globe
- Ultrasound is contraindicated in patients with open ("ruptured") globes
- Ultrasound cannot determine the nature of the foreign body and small amounts of intraocular air can be mistaken for an IOFB

Classic Ultrasound Images

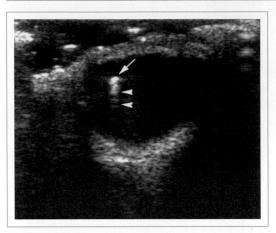

FIGURE 32.5: Ultrasound image of the eye demonstrating a foreign body. (*Courtesy of Michael Blaivas, MD, Northside Hospital, Georgia, Atlanta, GA.*)

Magnetic Resonance Imaging
- MRI has a lower detection rate for IOFB than either CT or ultrasound
- MRI is considered superior to CT for detecting porous, low-density objects such as dry wood
- If a metallic foreign body is suspected, then obtaining an MRI is contraindicated given several case reports of blindness in patients with metallic IOFB who underwent MRI
- MRI should be considered in patients where there is a high degree of suspicion for nonmetallic, low-density IOFB and prior imaging modalities have been negative (both ultrasound and CT scan)

 TABLE 32.4: MRI: intraocular foreign body

IV contrast	No
PO contrast	No
Amount of radiation	None

Basic Management
- NPO with IV maintenance hydration
- Avoid increases in intraocular pressure
  - Keep patient calm
  - Elevate head of bed to 30 degrees
  - Administer anti-emetics as needed
- IV antibiotics
- Ophthalmology consultation
- Admission for surgical removal of foreign body

Summary

TABLE 32.5: Advantages and disadvantages of imaging modalities in intraocular foreign bodies

Imaging modality	Advantages	Disadvantages
Plain film	Low cost Availability	Low sensitivity
CT scan	Gold standard Availability Other diagnoses also possible	Radiation exposure
Ultrasound	Low cost No radiation Bedside availability	Contraindicated in open globes Time-consuming Requires patient cooperation
MRI	Detection of low-density IOFB Other diagnoses also possible No radiation	Absolutely contraindicated with metallic IOFB Availability Time-consuming Cost

IOFB, intraocular foreign bodies.

33

Orbital Cellulitis

Stephanie Donald and Cori Poffenberger

Background

Orbital cellulitis, also known as postseptal cellulitis, refers to an infection of the orbital contents surrounding the globe, posterior to the orbital septum. The orbital septum is a thin membrane that serves as a barrier between anterior and posterior orbital structures.

Orbital cellulitis is a relatively rare entity that most commonly affects children. This is believed to be due to their higher incidence of upper respiratory infections in combination with decreased integrity of their orbital septa. The most frequent cause of orbital cellulitis is local spread of a sinusitis. With only the thin lamina papyracea separating the orbit from the ethmoid sinuses, the vast majority of these cases originate in the ethmoid sinuses. Consistent with this process of local spread, the bacterial pathogens most frequently isolated are *Staphylococcus aureus,* nontypeable *Haemophilus influenzae*, *Moraxella catarrhalis*, and *Streptococcus pneumoniae*. Other causes of orbital cellulitis include extension of other orbital infections (e.g., dacryoadenitis, dacryocystitis, or panophthalmitis), orbital fracture, dental infection, eye surgery, trauma, and bacteremia, resulting in seeding of the orbital contents.

Orbital cellulitis can usually be differentiated from periorbital (or preseptal) cellulitis based on history and physical examination; however, the emergency physician should be familiar with the imaging modalities that can be used to confirm or exclude the diagnosis.

TABLE 33.1: Classic history and physical

History of sinusitis and/or upper respiratory infection, trauma, or recent eye surgery
Unilateral eye involvement
Decreased vision
Chemosis
Proptosis
Pain with, and limited, extraocular muscle movement
Increased intraocular pressure
Fever: absent in about one-fourth of cases

TABLE 33.2: Potentially helpful laboratory tests

CBC: Usually requested, but not generally useful
Blood cultures: Obtained as part of the standard evaluation

CBC, complete blood count.

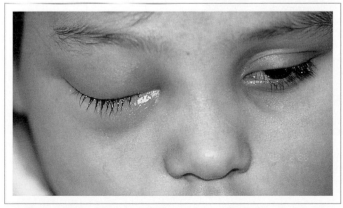

FIGURE 33.1: Photograph of a 9-year-old girl with orbital cellulitis. (From Fleisher GR, Ludwig S, and Baskin MN. Atlas of Pediatric Emergency Medicine, Philadelphia: Lippincott Williams & Wilkins, 2004.)

147

Computed Tomographic Scan

- CT is the imaging modality of choice to confirm the diagnosis of orbital cellulitis, with a sensitivity of 84–100%
- While IV contrast is not necessary to visualize most of the findings of orbital cellulitis, it does aid in identifying complications such as orbital abscesses and therefore is generally used
- Both axial and coronal views with thin cuts through the orbits should be obtained, as axial views alone may miss associated orbital or subperiosteal abscesses
- Proptosis or sinusitis with bony invasion or spread into the orbit may be seen on CT
- CT may also demonstrate displacement and destruction of the extraocular musculature

TABLE 33.3: Common CT findings

Proptosis of the affected globe compared to the unaffected side
Increased density of retro-orbital fat
Edema of extraocular muscles
Paranasal sinus infections
Erosion of sinus contents into affected orbit

 TABLE 33.4: CT: orbital cellulitis

IV contrast	Yes
PO contrast	No
Amount of radiation	1.0 mSv

Classic Images

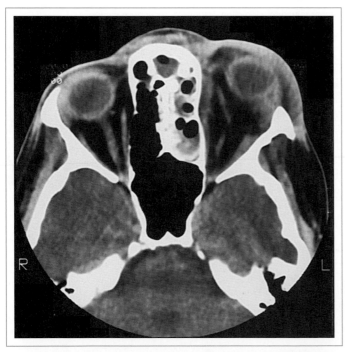

FIGURE 33.2: CT scan showing pansinusitis and diffuse orbital swelling involving the left eye consistent with orbital cellulitis. (From Tasman W and Jaeger E. The Wills Eye Hospital Atlas of Clinical Ophthalmology, 2nd ed. Philadelphia: Lippincott Williams & Wilkins, 2001.)

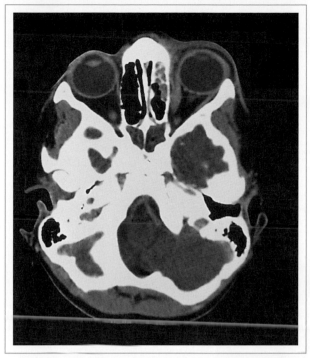

FIGURE 33.3: CT scan showing thickening of the left medial rectus muscle and a small subperiosteal fluid collection as well as adjacent sinus disease. (From Fleisher GR, Ludwig S, and Baskin MN. Atlas of Pediatric Emergency Medicine, Philadelphia: Lippincott Williams & Wilkins, 2004.)

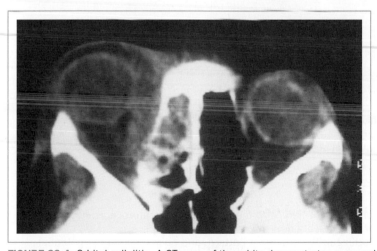

FIGURE 33.4: Orbital cellulitis. A CT scan of the orbits demonstrates a mass lesion along the medial wall of the orbit in a child with ethmoid sinusitis and orbital infection. No abscess cavity is seen, suggesting that the infection is at the stage of a cellulitis that will respond to IV antibiotic therapy without drainage. (From Fleisher GR, Ludwig S, and Baskin MN. Atlas of Pediatric Emergency Medicine, Philadelphia: Lippincott Williams & Wilkins, 2004.)

Magnetic Resonance Imaging

- MRI is a time-consuming and often not readily available modality in the ED setting
- Its utility lies primarily in its ability to detect complications such as optic nerve ischemia and/or infarction, and cavernous sinus thrombosis

 TABLE 33.5: MRI: orbital cellulitis

IV contrast	Yes, gadolinium is helpful
PO contrast	No
Amount of radiation	None

Classic Images: MRI

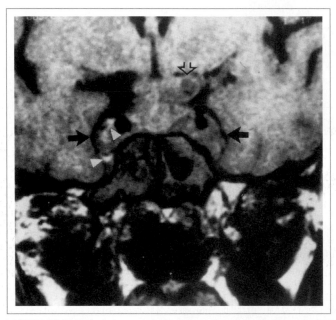

FIGURE 33.5: MRI of cavernous sinus thrombosis (complication of orbital cellulitis): MRI without gadolinium shows distention of the right cavernous sinus with high-density clot (*arrowhead*). (From Scheld WM, Whitley RJ, and Marra CM. Infections of the Central Nervous System, 3rd ed. Philadelphia: Lippincott Williams & Wilkins, 2004.)

Bedside Ultrasound

- Quick, portable study, but only useful when performed by skilled operators; currently rarely utilized in the ED setting for this indication
- Will demonstrate diffuse mottling of the orbital fat pattern, and edema within the potential space of Tenon, within the orbital fat
- Is limited by the fact that it cannot differentiate between causes of inflammation
- May show a discrete cavity of infection or abscess that can be acoustically outlined

Classic Images: Ultrasound

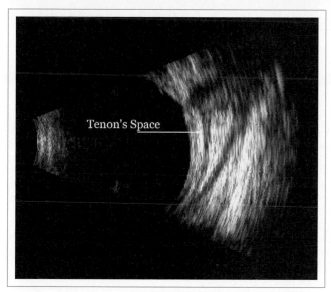

FIGURE 33.6: Ultrasound of the orbit demonstrating mottling of the orbital fat pattern and edema in the space of Tenon. (From Coleman DJ, Silverman RH, Lizzi FL, and Rorden MJ. Ultrasonography of the Eye and Orbit, 2nd ed. Philadelphia: Lippincott, Williams, and Wilkins. 2006.)

Basic Management

- Administration of IV antibiotics is the first management step, with broadened coverage for MRSA depending on patient population
  - First-line treatment is usually a penicillinase-resistant penicillin such as nafcillin or a second- or third-generation cephalosporin
  - In the penicillin-allergic patient, vancomycin or clindamycin is a useful alternative
- Blood cultures may be obtained if systemically ill, but are usually negative
- Admission to the hospital is recommended in all cases
- Ophthalmology consultation, with other subspecialty consultations (especially ENT if a contiguous sinusitis/abscess is present) as needed
- Anticoagulation is indicated if cavernous sinus thrombosis is present

Summary

TABLE 33.6: Advantages and disadvantages of imaging modalities in orbital cellulitis

Imaging modality	Advantages	Disadvantages
CT scan	Gold standard Rapidly available	Radiation exposure Repeated CT scans can damage lens
MRI	Excellent imaging of orbital structures Can visualize structures such as optic nerve and cavernous sinus	Time-consuming Limited availability in the emergency setting
Ultrasound	Low cost Portable	Requires high level of operator training and comfort May miss associated abscess

34

Acute Mastoiditis

Casey Buitenhuys

Background

Acute mastoiditis, an inflammatory process of the mastoid air cells, is a fairly uncommon pediatric clinical problem, though it is the most common intratemporal complication of acute otitis media (AOM). The mastoid air cells are contiguous with the middle ear cleft and may become inflamed from direct extension of AOM via the emissary veins. If not treated, mastoiditis can extend intratemporally, leading to tympanic membrane perforation, conductive hearing loss, and cranial nerve palsies, or extratemporally, leading to intracranial and extracranial abscess, meningitis, and cerebral venous sinus thrombosis. Adjunctive testing and imaging may be important in the emergency department to help identify acute mastoiditis, often in the setting of recent AOM. The imaging may further help to identify the specific complication(s), as they tend to require different degrees of invasive and noninvasive treatment.

TABLE 34.1: Classic history and physical

Greater incidence in age <12 yr (especially <2 yr)
Antecedent history of acute otitis media
High fever, otalgia, malaise, upper respiratory infection
Tympanic membrane erythema and middle ear effusion
Postauricular swelling, edema, erythema, and tenderness
Pinna may be displaced forward

TABLE 34.2: Potentially helpful laboratory tests

CBC: may demonstrate leukocytosis
Blood culture: to assist in identification of bacterial pathogen

CBC, complete blood count.

Computed Tomographic Scan

- Expert opinion currently recommends CT as the initial imaging study in suspected mastoiditis. The CT is a contrast study with fine cuts through the temporal bone.
- If altered mental status or focal neurologic findings are seen, then a noncontrast study of the brain should be performed first.
- The sensitivity of CT for the diagnosis of acute mastoiditis is 87–100%.
- CT is effective in differentiating between uncomplicated (incipient) and complicated (coalescent) mastoiditis.
- Incipient mastoiditis appears as fluid-filled mastoid air cells in the clinical picture of mastoiditis. This entity can be indistinguishable radiographically from AOM and must be distinguished on clinical criteria.
- Coalescent mastoiditis demonstrates bony erosion of the mastoid air cells so that all cells appear to coalesce into larger cells. Coalescent mastoiditis may lead to additional intratemporal and extratemporal complications of mastoiditis.
- Erosion into the apex of the petrous bone may cause Gradenigo's syndrome: otorrhea, headache, and abducens nerve palsy.
- The routine use of CT in the diagnosis of acute mastoiditis has come into question. For well-appearing children with a bulging tympanic membrane, postauricular edema, and erythema, conservative treatment with antibiotics and close follow-up could possibly be considered. Those that fail to defervesce should receive imaging for possible surgical treatment.

TABLE 34.3: CT scan: mastoiditis

IV contrast	Yes
PO contrast	No
Amount of radiation	2 mSv

Classic Images

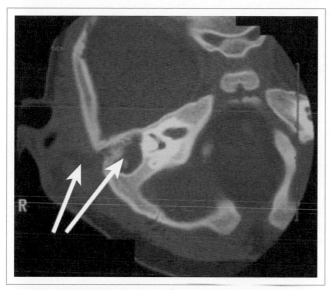

FIGURE 34.1: Acute coalescent mastoiditis with subperiosteal abscess (*arrows*). (*Courtesy of John S. Oghalai, MD, Baylor College of Medicine, Houston, TX.*)

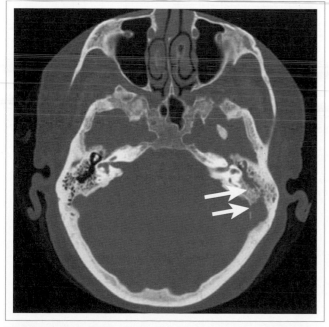

FIGURE 34.2: CT image of mastoiditis with sigmoid sinus thrombus (*arrows*). (*Courtesy of John S. Oghalai, MD, Baylor College of Medicine, Houston, TX.*)

Magnetic Resonance Imaging
- Magnetic resonance imaging is not the initial test of choice in acute mastoiditis.
- When the diagnosis of venous sinus thrombosis is considered (i.e., there are signs or symptoms of intracranial hypertension, toxemia, or hydrocephalus), magnetic resonance venogram is a more sensitive test than CT.
- Usually, venous sinus thrombosis results from direct extension of an extradural abscess.
- MRI will usually require sedation for pediatric patients.

 TABLE 34.4: MRI: mastoiditis

IV contrast	Yes, gadolinium is helpful
PO contrast	No
Amount of radiation	None

Plain X-ray
- Plain radiographs may demonstrate opacification of the mastoid region but are not reliable in making the diagnosis of mastoiditis.

Basic Management
- Incipient mastoiditis
  - May be managed with outpatient antibiotics for select cases (e.g., nontoxic appearing, no intracranial complications).
  - Otolaryngology follow-up: may need daily for intramuscular antibiotics.
- Coalescent mastoiditis (and admitted incipient mastoiditis)
  - NPO plus maintenance IV fluids.
  - IV antimicrobials: it is recommended to start a beta-lactam covering pneumococcus in addition to staphylococcal coverage (e.g., clindamycin and vancomycin).
  - ENT surgery consultation should be requested.
  - Myringotomy is usually performed for all types of mastoiditis, and additional surgical management depends on extent of disease.
  - Intracranial complications of mastoiditis should be managed with neurosurgical consultation.

Summary

TABLE 34.5: Advantages and disadvantages of imaging modalities in mastoiditis

Imaging modality	Advantages	Disadvantages
CT scan	Readily available No discomfort Usually does not require sedation Identifies complications requiring surgical management	May require sedation in very young patients Radiation exposure May require IV contrast
MRI	Identifies complications requiring surgical management Preferred for dural venous disease Identifies labyrinthitis	Usually requires sedation Time-consuming Not readily available

35

Sinusitis

Jason J. DeBonis and Amy H. Kaji

Background

The defining feature of rhinosinusitis is inflammation of the lining of the paranasal sinuses, generally thought to be due to obstruction of the draining pathways of the sinuses. Since rhinitis almost invariably accompanies sinusitis, the current preferred nomenclature for this condition is *rhinosinusitis* and not *sinusitis*. The duration of symptoms subdivides rhinosinusitis into acute (<4 weeks), subacute (4–12 weeks), and chronic (>12 weeks) conditions. Acute rhinosinusitis is further classified as acute viral rhinosinusitis (AVRS) or acute bacterial rhinosinusitis (ABRS), with the latter occurring in only 0.5–2.0% of cases.

If untreated, rhinosinusitis may lead to acute orbital complications (e.g., orbital cellulitis, orbital abscess, and subperiosteal abscess), intracranial complications (e.g., subdural abscess, meningitis, encephalitis, and cavernous and sagittal sinus thrombosis), as well as osteitis and osteomyelitis.

Rhinosinusitis affects approximately 30 million people per year in the United States and accounts for close to 16 million office visits per year. Direct costs, from emergency department and outpatient visits, diagnostics, medications, and procedures have been estimated at $3.5–5.8 billion per year. It is the fifth most common diagnosis for which antibiotics are prescribed. In half of the instances, the diagnosis—and hence the treatment—is incorrect.

TABLE 35.1: Classic history and physical*

Feature	Viral	Bacterial
Duration (symptoms)	1–10 d	Usually > 10 d or worsening symptoms within 10 d after initial improvement
Color change (nasal discharge)	+/−	+++, quality usually yellow-green and thick
Hyposmia/anosmia	+/−	More common
Postnasal drip	+/−	More common
Fever, cough, fatigue	+/−	More common
Maxillary dental pain / Facial pain/pressure / Ear pain/pressure	+/−	+++, often unilateral and associated with a particular sinus

*Purulent nasal/pharyngeal secretions, mucosal erythema, periorbital edema, facial erythema, sinus tenderness, and absence of maxillary sinus transillumination

TABLE 35.2: Potentially helpful laboratory tests

Generally: None
Specifically: CBC, ESR, CRP, and cultures of nasal secretions are of limited value and not generally indicated

CBC, complete blood count; ESR, erythrocyte sedimentation rate; CRP, C-reactive protein.

Imaging

Plain Films

- Plain radiographs are generally obsolete due to their relatively poor accuracy; however, they may be useful in some parts of the world where CT and MRI are not available
- Sinus plain film radiography includes a lateral, a Caldwell (P/A), and a Waters' (occipitomental) view with the patient sitting upright; adding a base (submentovertex) view enables visualization of the sphenoid sinus
- Sinus opacification, air-fluid level, or marked or severe mucosal thickening is consistent with rhinosinusitis

- While the reported specificity is fair (up to 80%), the sensitivity is low except for imaging of the maxillary sinus (sensitivity 80%)
- The high false-negative rate is attributable to poor visualization of the ethmoid sinuses
- False positives result from artifact and the inability to distinguish polyps and nasal masses from fluid or mucosal edema

 TABLE 35.3: Plain film: rhinosinusitis (three views)

IV contrast	No
PO contrast	No
Amount of radiation	0.1 mSv per view

Classic Images

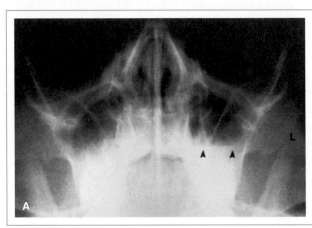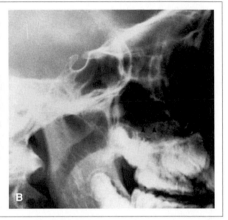

FIGURE 35.1: Anteroposterior (**A**) and lateral (**B**) radiographs show an air-fluid level in the left maxillary sinus (*arrowheads*) and mucoperiosteal thickening on the right side. (From Fleisher GR, Ludwig S and Henretig FM. Textbook of Pediatric Emergency Medicine, 5th ed. Philadelphia: Lippincott Williams & Wilkins, 2005.)

Computed Tomographic Scan
- CT noncontrast scan of the sinuses is the imaging procedure of choice for imaging all of the sinuses (especially the sphenoid and ethmoid sinuses)
- Coronal views are particularly helpful as these display the anatomy in a plane identical to that seen during endoscopy
- Signs of rhinosinusitis include air-fluid levels, total sinus opacification, and mucosal thickening >5 mm
- CT *with* contrast should only be used when there is concern for sinusitis with complications
- CT provides more information about the surrounding anatomy, especially the frontal recess, orbital contents, and the brain
- The sensitivity and specificity of CT scan for diagnosis of rhinosinusitis varies considerably in the literature; in general, CT is sensitive but not specific for sinusitis
- In one study, 42% of healthy, asymptomatic individuals were found to have some form of mucosal abnormality and 87% of patients with a URI were found to have abnormalities of a maxillary sinus
- CT is not useful for distinguishing between viral, bacterial, fungal, and allergic rhinosinusitis
- It may also be difficult to distinguish advanced malignancy from rhinosinusitis, and in immunocompromised patients with early invasive rhinosinusitis, CT may be negative
- The radiation exposure of CT is obviously higher than that of plain films; however, the degree of radiation varies with the imaging protocol ordered (i.e., CT sinuses vs CT face)

TABLE 35.4: CT scan: rhinosinusitis

IV contrast	No, except if assessing potential complications
PO contrast	No
Amount of radiation	1–2 mSv

Classic Images

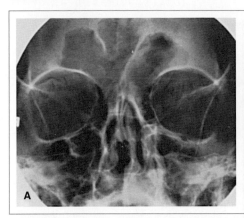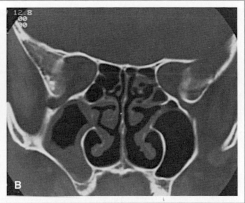

FIGURE 35.2: Imaging studies of sinusitis. **A:** Caldwell view of the frontal and ethmoidal sinuses. Note partial opacification of both frontal sinuses with mucosal thickening in the left frontal sinus and associated sclerosis in the left frontal bone. **B:** Coronal CT view of the ethmoidal and maxillary sinuses. Note mucosal thickening in the right maxillary sinus. (*Parts A and B courtesy of Dr. W. D. Robertson.*) (From Gorbach SL, Bartlett JG, and Blacklow NR. Infectious Diseases, 3rd ed. Philadelphia: Lippincott Williams & Wilkins, 2003.)

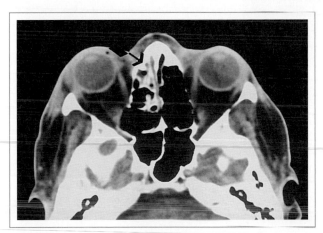

FIGURE 35.3: The axial CT scan of a patient with mucormycosis shows clouding and mucosal thickening in the right ethmoid sinus (*arrow*). (From Tasman W and Jaeger E. The Wills Eye Hospital Atlas of Clinical Ophthalmology, 2nd ed. Philadelphia: Lippincott Williams & Wilkins, 2001.)

Magnetic Resonance Imaging
- MRI with gadolinium can provide soft tissue detail superior to other imaging modalities
- MRI is used in conjunction with CT for the evaluation of complications of acute rhinosinusitis when extrasinus involvement is suspected (e.g., superior sagittal venous thrombosis or cavernous sinus thrombosis)
- Signal intensity from the high-fat content of bone marrow can be confused with fluid retained in the sinuses
- MRI is not indicated for the routine evaluation of rhinosinusitis

 TABLE 35.5: MRI: rhinosinusitis

IV contrast	Yes, gadolinium is helpful
PO contrast	No
Amount of radiation	None

Classic Images

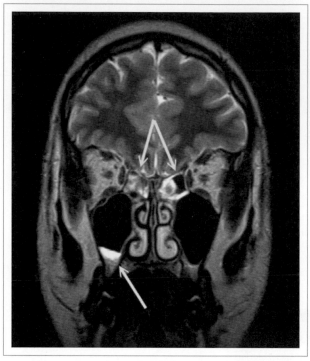

FIGURE 35.4: T2-weighted MRI of paranasal sinuses reveals fluid in the ethmoid air cells and the right maxillary sinus (*arrows*). (*Courtesy of Vivek David, MD, Progressive Radiology, Washington, DC.*)

Basic Management
- Symptomatic relief may include, but is not limited to:
  - analgesics
  - mechanical irrigation with buffered, hypertonic saline
  - topical glucocorticoids
  - topical decongestants (e.g., oxymetazoline for no more than 3 days)
  - antihistamines
  - mucolytics
- After 10 days, or if the patient gets better and then worsens again ("double sickening"), either another 7 days of observation (in mild ABRS when pain is mild and temperature is <38.3°C) or antibiotics (in severe ABRS when pain is moderate-severe or temperature is ≥38.3°C) may be indicated
- If the patient is immunocompromised, has an underlying or complicating condition, or fails observation, antibiotics are indicated
- If initial antibiotic failure occurs, consider further workup (e.g., CT scan) and/or further treatment with either amoxicillin-clavulanate or a respiratory fluoroquinolone
- Nosocomial acute bacterial rhinosinusitis can occur (e.g., after prolonged nasotracheal intubation) and often is associated with gram-negative organisms; remove foreign bodies and use culture-directed antibiotic therapy
- Immunocompromised hosts are at risk for acute fulminant fungal rhinosinusitis—treat accordingly

Summary

TABLE 35.6: Advantages and disadvantages of imaging modalities in sinusitis

Imaging modality	Advantages	Disadvantages
Plain films	Low cost Less radiation Less time-consuming	Soft tissue limitations Ethmoid sinuses not well-visualized Poor sensitivity/specificity
CT scan	Best choice Availability Other diagnoses also possible	More radiation exposure False positives
MRI	Soft tissue accuracy	Time-consuming Expensive False positives
Ultrasound	Low cost No radiation Bedside availability	Cannot visualize all sinuses Operator dependent Interuser variability

36

Acute Myocardial Infarction

Jessica Klausmeier and Shamai A. Grossman

Background

Chest pain is one of the most common presenting complaints to the emergency department. The challenge for the emergency physician is to rapidly recognize when chest pain represents an acute myocardial infarction (AMI) in order to initiate interventions aimed at improving myocardial perfusion. Time correlates directly with myocardial survival. While history, physical examination, and electrocardiographic evaluation are essential to the diagnosis of an acute coronary event, these elements often are unable to discern the etiology of a patient's chest pain. In this circumstance, additional diagnostic methods including laboratory tests and imaging studies may be useful.

TABLE 36.1: Classic history and physical

Left-sided or substernal chest pain or pressure radiating to the left arm or neck
Radiating pain to left chest, right chest, shoulders, neck, jaw, arms, epigastrium, or upper back
Nausea
Diaphoresis
Shortness of breath
Deep, visceral, and intense discomfort often described as pressure or tightness
Pain lasting minutes, not seconds, precipitated by exertion or emotional stress and relieved by resting or by taking a sublingual nitroglycerin
Elderly or female patient with atypical symptoms, e.g., shortness of breath (most common), fatigue, or nausea
Pale, diaphoretic patient with left fist over precordium
Lungs clear
Diminished S1 and S2
Audible S3 (15–20%)
S4 gallop with jugular venous distension and rales (congestive heart failure)

TABLE 36.2: Potentially helpful laboratory tests

Chemistry panel
Cardiac enzymes
Complete blood count (CBC)
Coagulation panel

Chest X-ray

- Obtain posteroanteior and lateral views if possible
- Look for noncardiac chest pain etiologies, e.g., pneumonia or pneumothorax
- Look for a widened mediastinum if concern for aortic dissection
- Most commonly normal
- Look for evidence of underlying cardiac disease
  - Cardiomegaly
  - Pulmonary edema or cephalization of the vessels, pleural effusions
  - Enlarged left ventricle

TABLE 36.3: Chest x-ray (PA and Lateral): acute myocardial infarction

IV contrast	No
PO contrast	No
Amount of radiation	0.10 mSv

Classic Images

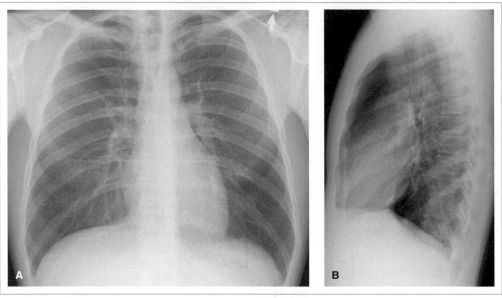

FIGURE 36.1: Normal posteroanterior **(A)** and lateral **(B)** chest radiographs. (From Collins J and Stern EJ. Chest Radiology: The Essentials, 2nd ed. Philadelphia: Lippincott Williams & Wilkins, 2008.)

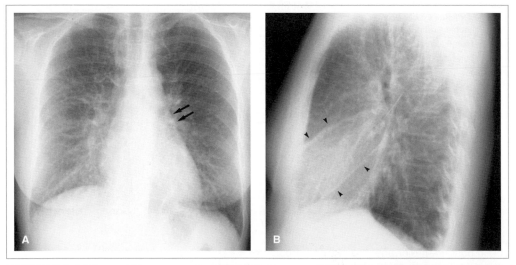

FIGURE 36.2: A 52-year-old woman experiencing an acute myocardial infarction. **A:** The heart is not enlarged. The left atrial appendage segment of the left heart contour (*arrows*) is straightened. Notice the moderate to severe bilateral interstitial edema obscuring the pulmonary vascular markings and the increase in caliber of upper lobe vessels. **B:** In lateral view, all vascular markings are indistinct and the interlobar fissures are thickened (*arrowheads*), containing edema fluid. The left ventricle is not dilated. Although the left atrial appendage segment is straightened on the posteroanterior view, the left bronchus is not posteriorly displaced in lateral, indicating the mildness of left atrial enlargement. (From Topol EJ, Califf RM, et al. Textbook of Cardiovascular Medicine, 3rd ed. Philadelphia: Lippincott Williams & Wilkins, 2006.)

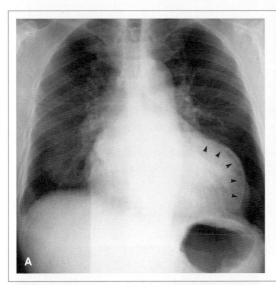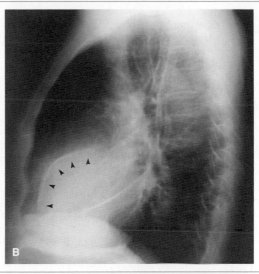

FIGURE 36.3: A 53-year-old man with chronic stable angina. **A:** Posteroanterior view of the chest shows mild pulmonary venous hypertension and enlargement of the left ventricular contour. Curvilinear calcification of the distal interventricular septum (*arrowheads*) defines the extent of a previous myocardial infarction. **B:** In lateral view, the calcification (*arrowheads*) is superimposed on the cardiac mass. (From Topol EJ, Califf RM, et al. Textbook of Cardiovascular Medicine, 3rd ed. Philadelphia: Lippincott Williams & Wilkins, 2006.)

Transthoracic Cardiac Ultrasound

- Technique
  - Four views: subxiphoid, parasternal long, parasternal short, apical four chamber (and apical two chamber)
  - Patient supine or in left lateral decubitus position
  - Small footprint transducer with frequency range of 2–5 MHz, allowing visualization between the ribs
  - Transesophageal imaging also frequently employed by consultants but invasive and time-consuming
  - Bedside cardiac ultrasound
    - ▶ Screening examination
    - ▶ Look for dilated ventricles or hypocontractility in any of the views
    - ▶ Look for pericardial effusions
- Information
  - Some measurements and calculations are obtained using machine-specific software
    - ▶ Presence of effusion and tamponade physiology
    - ▶ Cardiac output
    - ▶ Valve function
    - ▶ Ventricular and septal wall motion
    - ▶ Detection of papillary muscle disruption
    - ▶ Detection of ventricular dilation/aneurysm
    - ▶ Aortic root anatomy
    - ▶ Stress echocardiography gives additional information regarding dynamic changes related to increasing cardiac demand

- Limitations
  - Operator dependent
  - May be limited by patient's body habitus (transesophageal echocardiography helps to circumvent this problem but can be logistically difficult to obtain)
  - Availability of cardiologists or technicians to perform a complete study
  - Bedside focused echocardiography may not detect subtle wall motion abnormalities
- Pearls
  - Segmental wall motion abnormalities are highly suggestive of AMI
  - Useful in identifying acute injury in patients who have had prior MI, chronically elevated troponins, or an abnormal EKG at baseline
  - Not every patient will have adequate images in each window; placement of the ultrasound probe will vary between patients depending on anatomic differences such as the orientation of the heart in the chest

Classic Images

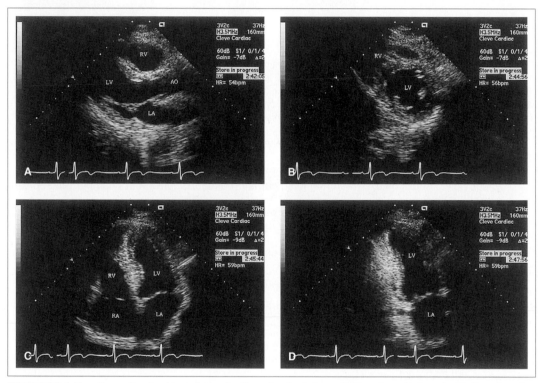

FIGURE 36.4: Two-dimensional echocardiography. Four standard views. **A:** Parasternal long axis. **B:** Parasternal short axis. **C:** Apical four chamber. **D:** Apical two chamber. AO, aorta; LA, left atrium; LV, left ventricle; RA, right atrium; RV, right ventricle. (From Topol EJ, Califf RM, et al. Textbook of Cardiovascular Medicine, 3rd ed. Philadelphia: Lippincott Williams & Wilkins, 2006.)

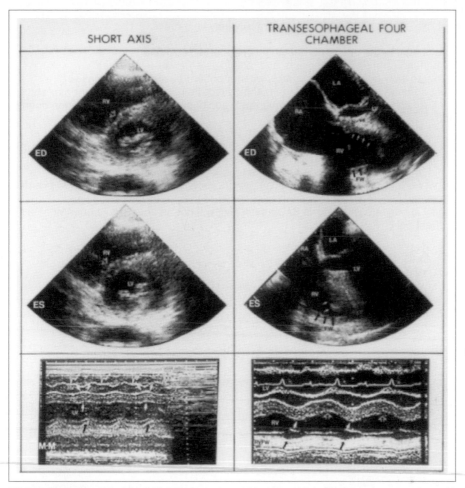

FIGURE 36.5: Transthoracic, transesophageal, and M-mode echocardiograms from a patient with right ventricle (RV) infarction, refractory shock, and right atrium (RA) infarction. In short axis at end diastole (ED), the RV is markedly dilated and the interventricular septal curvature is reversed (*open arrow*) with a shift into the left ventricle (LV). The four-chamber view demonstrates marked RA enlargement as well as severe RV dilation and bowing of the septum into the LV (*white arrows*). At end systole (ES), the septum bulges paradoxically into the RV in both short-axis (*open arrow*) and four-chamber views (*white arrows*). RV free wall (*FW, dark arrows*) was dyskinetic in four-chamber view. These findings are confirmed in the M-mode views from the transthoracic and transesophageal images. Excess volume administration can cause RV dilatation, septal shift into the LV with impairment of LV filling, and paradoxic decrease in cardiac output despite an increase of pulmonary capillary wedge pressure. (Reproduced with permission from Goldstein JA, Barzilai B, Rosamound TL, et al. Determinants of hemodynamic compromise with severe right ventricular infarction. *Circulation* 1990;82:359–368.)

Cardiac CT Angiography
- Technique
  - Heart rate is slowed via beta-blockade
  - CT angiography is performed
- Information
  - Evaluate for presence of significant calcification of coronary arteries
  - Evaluate patency of coronary arteries
  - Evaluate for dissection of coronary arteries
  - Evaluate patency of previously placed stents
  - Evaluate for aneurysm or anomalous anatomy
  - May provide incidental information about other intrathoracic processes that could lead to chest pain (pneumonia, pericardial effusion/pericarditis, pneumothorax, aortic dissection)

- Limitations
  - IV contrast dye—kidney dysfunction or contrast allergy limitations
  - Cost
  - Images are limited in the presence of ectopic beats or dysrhythmia
  - Limited experience among technologists and radiologists (newer technique)
  - Must be able to slow heart rate adequately without patient becoming hypotensive
  - If significant coronary artery disease found, AMI cannot be ruled out and patient may still need stress testing or cardiac catheterization with additional contrast administration during angiography
- Pearls
  - Computed tomography angiography (CTA) is a less invasive alternative to angiography in patients who have a low likelihood of needing a percutaneous intervention
  - Most helpful in ruling out coronary artery disease in low-risk patients
    - ▷ If coronary arteries are clear of significant calcification and are widely patent, myocardial ischemia can essentially be ruled out as a cause of the patient's chest pain
  - Limited utility in patients with known CAD as imaging will **not** be able to rule out AMI as a cause of chest pain

 TABLE 36.4: Coronary CTA: acute myocardial infarction

IV contrast	Yes—needed to delineate vasculature
PO contrast	No
Amount of radiation	16.00 mSv

Classic Images

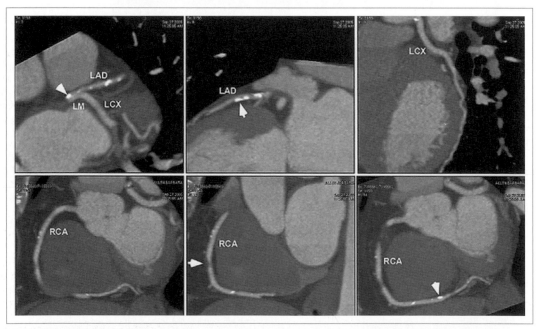

FIGURE 36.6: Curved multiplanar reconstructions and multiple-intensity projection CTA. The left main (LM) coronary artery shows a calcified plaque with ~50% stenosis. The left anterior descending artery (LAD) shows calcified plaque in its proximal and mid segments with apparent moderate to severe stenosis. The distal segment of the left circumflex artery (LCX) is free of disease. The dominant right coronary artery (RCA) shows a noncalcified plaque in its mid segment with moderate stenosis and a small calcified plaque in its distal segment with _50% stenosis. (From Di Carli MF and Hachamovitch R. New technology for noninvasive evaluation of coronary artery disease. *Circulation*. 2007;115;1464–1480.)

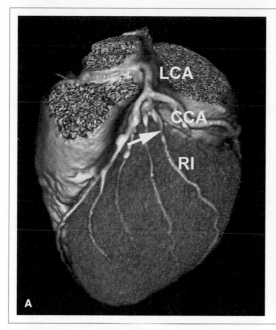
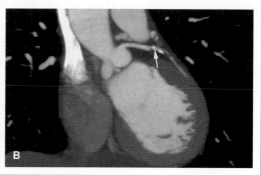

FIGURE 36.7: A 63-year-old woman with atypical chest pain and a negative nuclear stress test. **A:** Volume-rendered image from a 64-slice cardiac CT angiogram shows the left main coronary artery (LCA) arising from the aortic root (cut away). The circumflex coronary artery (CCA) in the atrioventricular groove and a large ramus intermedius (RI) branch have been outlined in gray in this image. A mixed calcified and soft plaque is present in the proximal portion of the ramus intermedius, causing significant stenosis (*arrow*). **B:** Coronal maximal intensity projection image of the left main coronary artery shows the lesion in the proximal segment of the ramus intermedius (*arrow*). (*Courtesy of H. Scott Beasley, MD, Department of Radiology, Western Pennsylvania Hospital, Pittsburgh, PA.*) From Daffner RH. Clinical Radiology: The Essentials, 3rd ed. Philadelphia: Lippincott Williams & Wilkins, 2007.

Basic Management

- Assess and stabilize airway, breathing, and circulation
- IV, oxygen, and cardiac monitor
- Institutional chest pain protocol and guidelines
- Prompt cardiac consultation

Summary

TABLE 36.5: Advantages and disadvantages of imaging modalities in acute myocardial infarction

Imaging modality	Advantages	Disadvantages
Chest x-ray	Minimal radiation Fast, noninvasive Inexpensive May find other important causes of non-AMI chest pain	Nonspecific findings Cannot diagnose AMI by CXR
Cardiac ultrasound	No radiation Fast, noninvasive, can be performed at bedside Gives information regarding cardiac function May be able to identify aortic dissection	Operator-dependent Not sensitive or specific Limited in patients with obesity Difficulty in detecting subtleties on bedside emergency echocardiogram
Coronary CTA	If normal, can essentially rule out coronary artery disease as a cause of chest pain (potentially eliminates need for admission for ROMI) Can detect other pathology that may be causing patient's chest pain	Time-consuming Requires additional training for radiologist and technician Requires contrast Significant radiation exposure Must be able to sufficiently slow heart rate without patient developing hypotension

AMI, acute myocardial infarction; CTA, computed tomography angiography; CXR, chest X-ray; ROMI, rule out myocardial infarction.

37

Congestive Heart Failure

Dana A. Stearns and Vicki E. Noble

Background

Congestive heart failure (CHF) is a cardiac syndrome in which the ventricles are either contracting/emptying poorly (systolic dysfunction) or inadequately filling (diastolic dysfunction). This leads to progressive vascular congestion and interstitial edema in the pulmonary as well as systemic circulation. The prevalence of CHF increases dramatically with age, from 1–2% in the 50–59 age group to more than 20% in persons aged 75 and older. It is the most common admitting diagnosis in individuals older than 65 years. Annual mortality ranges from 10% in stable patients with mild symptoms to 50% in patients with advanced symptoms.

TABLE 37.1: Classic history and physical

History	
Dyspnea on exertion (DOE), paroxysmal nocturnal dyspnea (PND), orthopnea, and nocturnal angina	
Signs (left-sided CHF)	**Signs (right-sided CHF)**
Tachycardia at rest	Jugular venous distention
Alveolar rales	Hepatojugular reflux
Paradoxical splitting S2	Hepatomegaly
S3 S4 gallop	Peripheral edema
Valvular murmur (Aortic/Mitral Stenosis/Insufficiency)	Ascites
Displaced apical lift	Peripheral cyanosis
Tachypnea	
Hypoperfusion	
CNS: somnolence, confusion	
Cardiac: angina, hypotension with exertion	
Renal: oliguria, elevated blood urea nitrogen (BUN), creatinine	
GI: anorexia	
Musculoskeletal: fatigue	
Skin: poor capillary refill, cool, clammy	

TABLE 37.2: Physical findings in cardiogenic versus noncardiogenic CHF

Cardiogenic	Noncardiogenic
Pulmonary edema/alveolar crackles	Clear lungs
S3 gallop	Absent gallop
Jugular venous distention	Normal jugular venous pressure
Cool, clammy extremities	Warm, perfused extremities

TABLE 37.3: Potentially helpful tests

CPK/troponin	Creatinine
Beta-natriuretic peptide (BNP)	Blood urea nitrogen (BUN)
Electrolytes	Liver function tests
ECG	TSH

Chest X-ray

Plain radiographs remain a first-line radiographic test.

- The modality may be obtained quickly at the bedside and with minimal disruption in patient management
- Elevated pulmonary vascular pressure in CHF commonly manifests as a diffuse and progressive series of densities and patterns that help to distinguish pulmonary edema from other conditions that cause radiographic infiltrates
- Enlargement of the cardiac silhouette may suggest cardiomegaly and assist with management decisions
- Pleural effusions can be easily detected and corroborate physical examination findings

TABLE 37.4: Chest x-ray findings in cardiogenic and noncardiogenic CHF

Cardiogenic CHF	Noncardiogenic CHF
CHF severity related to pulmonary venous hypertension (measured by pulmonary arterial wedge pressure [PAWP])	No cephalization
Grade I PVH (PAWP 15–20 mm Hg) vascular redistribution bases = apices (cephalization); vessels >3 mm diameter at first intercostal space	Edema does not spare periphery or upper fields
Grade II PVH (PAWP 20–25 mm Hg) Kerley B lines (peripheral interlobar septal fluid markings), peribronchial cuffing; hazing of hilar vascularity; costodiaphragmatic pleural effusions	Interstitial appears more consolidative
Grade III PVH (PAWP >25 mm Hg) alveolar fluid; basilar/perihilar infiltrates (butterfly/bat wing perihilar pattern)	

 TABLE 37.5: Chest x-ray (AP Portable): CHF

IV contrast	No
PO contrast	No
Amount of radiation	0.02 mSv

Classic Images

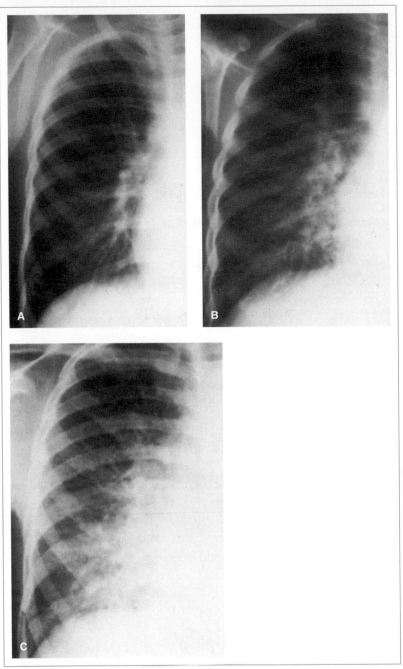

FIGURE 37.1: Pulmonary edema: interstitial stage. **A:** Note early development of streaky white lines (interstitial septal edema) radiating from the hilar region. In this case, the lines primarily are Kerley A lines. This patient had acute glomerulonephritis. **B:** More extensive reticular pattern of pulmonary interstitial edema in a patient with cardiac failure secondary to aortic stenosis. **C:** Very extensive interstitial edema producing pronounced reticulation through the lung and some underlying parenchymal haziness. Kerley A and B lines are present. This patient had acute glomerulonephritis. (From Swischuk LE. Emergency Radiology of the Acutely Ill or Injured Child, 2nd ed. Philadelphia: Lippincott Williams & Wilkins, 1986:85.)

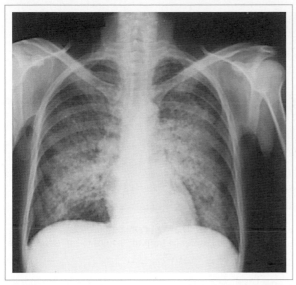

FIGURE 37.2: Typical bat wing (outer one third of lungs) or butterfly (inner two thirds of lungs) appearance in uremic pulmonary edema. Note sparing of both costophrenic angles. (From Crapo JD, Glassroth J, Karlinsky JB, et al. Baum's Textbook of Pulmonary Diseases, 7th ed. Philadelphia: Lippincott Williams & Wilkins, 2004.)

Chest Ultrasound

- With the patient sitting upright, a low-frequency (2–5 MHz) transducer is used to image the lungs in both the sagittal and transverse planes
- When the lung tissue is well aerated, sound only transmits as far as the pleura and a reverberation pattern ("A-line") of horizontal lines is created
- As lung tissue starts to fill with fluid, hyperechoic bright lines that originate at the pleura and extend to the edge ("B-lines") are visible
- Parenchymal fluid is directly proportional to the amount of transmission and thus the number of B-lines
- B-lines correlate with chest x-ray and computed tomographic findings of lung water as well as thermodilution assessments with Swan-Ganz catheters, natriuretic peptide levels, pulmonary artery wedge pressures, and other echocardiographic findings of heart failure
- Recent studies suggest that patients pre- and postdialysis resolve B-lines in real time with volume removal; this is an advantage over chest radiography

Classic Images

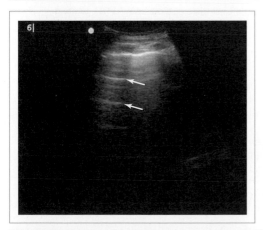

FIGURE 37.3: "A-lines" or horizontal reverberation artifacts; the bright white line at the top is the pleura. (*Courtesy of Vicki Noble, MD, Massachusetts General Hospital, Boston, MA.*)

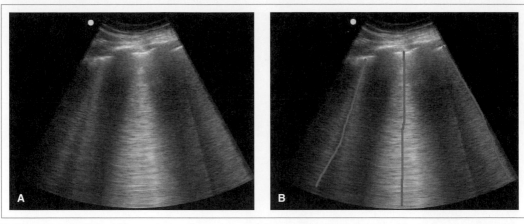

FIGURE 37.4: **A:** "B-lines" or vertical artifacts that mark interstitial fluid. The bright white horizontal line at the top is the pleura. **B:** "B-lines" are highlighted with vertical grey lines extending from the pleura to the edge of the image. (*Courtesy of Vicki Noble, MD, Massachusetts General Hospital, Boston MA.*)

Cardiac Ultrasound
- Doppler and 2-D cardiac ultrasonography can be used to assist in the evaluation of systolic and diastolic ventricular performance, valvular integrity, estimate ejection fraction, as well as evaluate global and regional left ventricular function

Classic Images

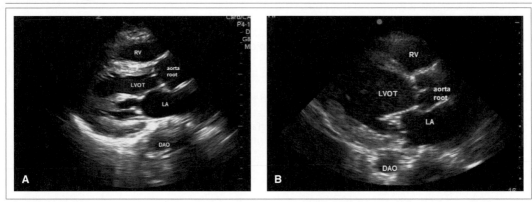

FIGURE 37.5: **A:** Parasternal long view with the RV, aorta root, left ventricle outflow tract (LVOT), LA, and descending thoracic aorta (DAO) marked. **B:** Parasternal long view with the same chambers marked but the left ventricle here looks enlarged.

Chest CT Scan
- May provide a rapid and accurate assessment of the heart, mediastinal contents, and the pulmonary vasculature
- Excellent visualization of the hemithoraces and reveals the nature and distribution of pulmonary edema
- Multichannel CT scanning is useful in the assessment of valvular abnormalities and may identify irregular hypertrophic ventricular wall segments and wall motion dynamics commonly associated with CHF

TABLE 37.6: Chest CT: CHF

IV contrast	Yes
PO contrast	No
Amount of radiation	7 mSv

Classic Images

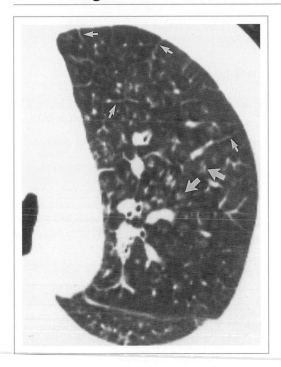

FIGURE 37.6: Pulmonary edema. Thickening of the interlobular septa (small arrows) and ill-defined centrilobular opacities (large arrows). Note also the thickening of the peribronchovascular interstitium, with peribronchial cuffing. (From Eisenberg RL, An Atlas of Differential Diagnosis 4th Ed. Philadelphia: Lippincott Williams & Wilkins, 2003.)

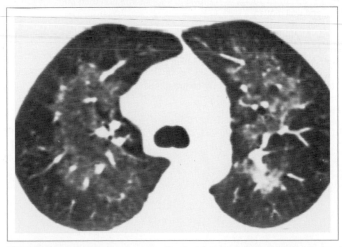

FIGURE 37.7: Pulmonary edema. Central "ground-glass," low-grade lung opacification persists 3 weeks after myocardial infarction. (From Eisenberg RL. An Atlas of Differential Diagnosis, 4th ed. Philadelphia: Lippincott Williams & Wilkins, 2003.)

Basic Treatment

- Obtain IV access, place on oxygen and cardiac monitoring.
- CHF caused by left ventricular systolic dysfunction: afterload and preload reducing agents followed by a loop diuretic; reserve digitalis glycosides or dobutamine for conditions of severe failure refractory to first-line agents
- CHF caused by diastolic dysfunction: rate controlling agents, judicious afterload reduction and diuretic use.
- Identify and treat precipitating factors (e.g., dietary salt indiscretion, medication noncompliance,anemia, infection, and obstructive sleep apnea)

Summary

TABLE 37.7: Advantages and disadvantages of imaging modalities in CHF

	Advantages	**Disadvantages**
Chest radiograph	Helps distinguish CHF from other causes of hypoxia	Inaccurately measures systolic function when radiographic findings of congestion and edema are absent
	Cardiac silhouette (specific but insensitive for cardiomyopathy)	Unable to differentiate type of LV dysfunction
	Identifies interstitial edema	Findings lag behind clinical improvement
		Frequent false negatives
		Radiation exposure
Chest ultrasonography	Repeatable	Requires equipment and training of clinicians
	No radiation exposure	False positives—other pathologic lung processes that thicken interstitium
	Identifies interstitial edema	
	Inexpensive	
	Steep learning curve	
	Resolution of findings in real time with diuresis	
Cardiac ultrasonography	Identifies global/regional ventricular function	Operator dependent
	Cardiac output/ejection fraction calculation	Inadequate results 10%
	Determines systolic/diastolic LV function abnormalities	Underlying lung disease makes interpretation difficult
	Assess pulmonary arterial and ventricular filling pressures	
	Assess valvular function	
	Assess pericardial space, pericardial effusion, and tamponade risk	
	Low false-positive and false-negative rates	
Chest computed tomography	Evaluation of ventricular wall hypertrophy, apical morphology, and wall motion dynamics (LV wall thickness >13 mm = hypertrophy is an RV wall thickness >6 mm = hypertrophy)	Provides less information than MRI
	Delineates valvular and congenital cardiac abnormalities	Radiation exposure
	Excellent views of heart, mediastinal, and pulmonary vasculature	IV contrast reaction
	Pulmonary interstitium is easily visualized	
	Low false-positive and false-negative rates	

38

Pericarditis/Pericardial Effusion

Zoe D. Howard and Emily L. Senecal

Background

Acute pericarditis is a relatively benign disease; however, it can be associated with the accumulation of nonphysiologic fluid in the pericardial space, which has the potential to cause tamponade. An effusion confirms the diagnosis of pericarditis; its absence does not exclude it. Cardiac tamponade occurs when the pericardial fluid accumulates faster than the pericardium can stretch, resulting in the compression of the cardiac chambers and hemodynamic instability. Prompt diagnosis of pericardial effusion or tamponade expedites early mobilization when life-saving interventions are indicated.

TABLE 38.1: Classic history and physical of pericarditis

Sharp, pleuritic, retrosternal chest pain
Radiation to trapezius
Relieved with sitting forward
Pericardial friction rub
Nonproductive cough
Dyspnea
Tachycardia
Possible fever

TABLE 38.2: Classic history & physical of tamponade

Hypotension
Tachycardia
Dyspnea
Elevated JVP
Distant heart sounds
Pulsus paradoxus
Shock

TABLE 38.3: Potentially helpful laboratory tests

CBC, ESR, CRP	Nonspecific marker of inflammation, limited diagnostic utility
Cardiac biomarkers	Elevation suggests possible myocarditis

CBC, complete blood count; CRP, C-reactive protein; ESR, erythrocyte sedimentation rate.

TABLE 38.4: EKG changes with of pericarditis and tamponade

Pericarditis
Stage 1: Diffuse ST segment elevation with concomitant PR segment depression
Stage 2: Normalization of ST segment elevation and PR segment depression
Stage 3: Diffuse T-wave inversion
Stage 4: EKG normalization

Tamponade
Tachycardia, low voltage, electrical alternans (classic)

Chest X-ray

- Posteroanterior chest shows a heart width > half the thoracic cage width
- New cardiomegaly with clear lung fields is suggestive of acute effusion
- To enlarge cardiac silhouette on radiograph, 200–250 mL fluid is required

 TABLE 38.5: Chest x-ray (PA and Lateral): pericarditis

IV contrast	No
PO contrast	No
Amount of radiation	0.1 mSv

Classic Images

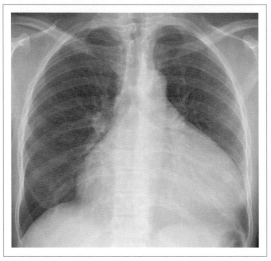

FIGURE 38.1: Chest radiograph demonstrating clear lung fields with cardiomegaly. (From Collins J and Stern EJ. Chest Radiology: The Essentials, 2nd ed. Philadelphia: Lippincott Williams & Wilkins, 2008.)

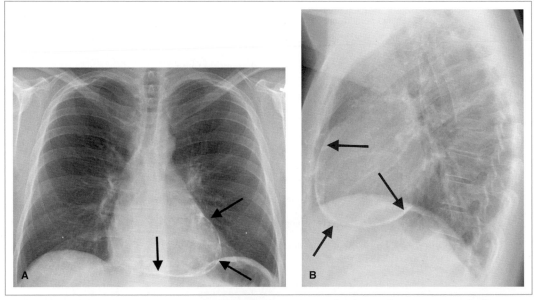

FIGURE 38.2: Constrictive pericarditis. Posteroanterior (**A**) and lateral (**B**) chest radiographs show curvilinear calcification conforming to the anatomy of the pericardial sac (*arrows*). (From Collins J and Stern EJ. Chest Radiology: The Essentials, 2nd ed. Philadelphia: Lippincott Williams & Wilkins, 2008.)

Bedside Cardiac Ultrasound/Echocardiography

- The pericardial cavity contains 15–50 mL of physiologic fluid
- On ultrasound, 25–50 mL of fluid can be seen
- Parietal pericardium is highly echogenic and appears bright white
- An effusion is an echo-free (anechoic or black) space between visceral and parietal pericardium
- Technique for bedside cardiac ultrasound:
  - use the curvilinear lower frequency (2–5 mHz) or phased-array probe
  - begin with the parasternal long axis, positioning the probe from atria to apex, or the subxiphoid view, placing the probe under the costal margin aiming toward the left shoulder
  - use the parasternal, subxiphoid, and apical views to visualize the heart in various planes
  - angle the probe obliquely to image through the intercostal space, decreasing rib shadows
  - adjust the depth on the screen to visualize the posterior pericardium as this is the most dependent area in a supine patient and is where fluid will accumulate first
  - anechoic area anterior to the right ventricle may not be an effusion, but an epicardial fat pad; perform more than one view to eliminate this misinterpretation
- Transesophageal echocardiography (TEE) is indicated:
  - when TTE is nondiagnostic
  - when TTE fails to achieve optimal images
  - in postoperative cardiac surgery patients
  - in patients concerning for localized effusions or valvular abnormalities
- Tamponade on ultrasound:
  - systolic collapse of the right atrium
  - diastolic collapse of the right ventricle
  - septal bowing toward the left ventricle during inspiration
  - mitral and tricuspid valve flow velocity paradoxus
  - inferior vena cava (IVC) and hepatic vein dilation with minimal respiratory variation
  - "swinging heart"

TABLE 38.6: Helpful associated structures

Liver	Acoustic window
	Landmark in subxiphoid view
Descending thoracic aorta	Differentiate pericardial (anterior) from pleural (posterior) effusion
	Landmark in parasternal long view

TABLE 38.7: Characterizing Pericardial Effusions

Pericardial effusion	Small	Moderate	Large
Size (width)	<5 mm	5–20 mm	>20 mm
Volume	<100 mL	100–500 mL	>500 mL
Location	Posterior/inferior to LV, loculated	Apex, circumferential	Circumferential, swinging heart

Classic Images

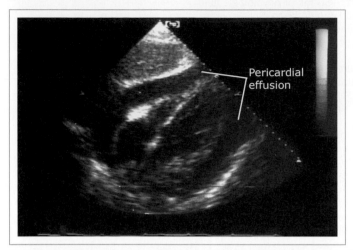

FIGURE 38.3: Subxiphoid view demonstrates pericardial effusion. (From Cosby KS and Kendall JL. Practical Guide to Emergency Ultrasound. Philadelphia: Lippincott Williams & Wilkins, 2006.)

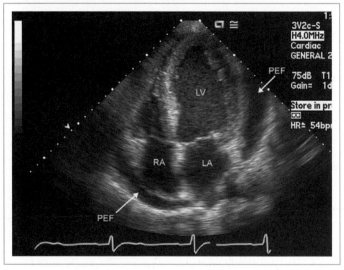

FIGURE 38.4: Apical four-chamber view recorded in a patient with a moderate, predominantly lateral pericardial effusion (*arrow*). Note also that a smaller fluid collection behind the right atrium (RA). LA, left atrium; LV, left ventricular. (From Feigenbaum H, Armstrong WF, and Ryan T. Feigenbaum's Echocardiography, 6th ed. Philadelphia: Lippincott Williams & Wilkins, 2005.)

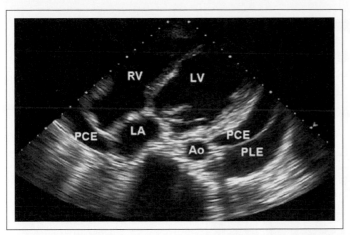

FIGURE 38.5: Pleural and pericardial effusion, low parasternal view. The circular structure is the descending aorta (Ao), sitting on the thoracic spine. The line on the right side of the screen is the pericardium, separating pericardial (PCE) from pleural fluid (PLE). Note how the pericardial fluid is beginning to interpose itself between the heart and descending aorta, while the pleural effusion is lateral to the aorta. (From Cosby KS and Kendall JL. Practical Guide to Emergency Ultrasound. Philadelphia: Lippincott Williams & Wilkins, 2006.)

Chest CT Scan

- Further characterizes pericardial disease, more specifically localizes pericardial fluid, and is useful when echocardiogram is equivocal
- Detects loculated effusions
- Tamponade findings:
  - bowing of intraventricular septum
  - superior vena cava/IVC distention
  - contrast reflux into IVC
  - compression of cardiac chambers
  - renal/hepatic congestion

 TABLE 38.8: Chest CT scan: pericardial effusion

IV contrast	Yes (characterization and identification of local tissue)
PO contrast	No
Amount of radiation	7 mSv

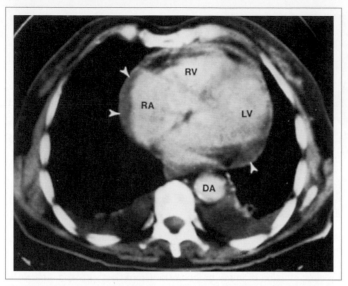

FIGURE 38.6: Pericardial effusion. CT scan made after the injection of intravenous contrast material shows the pericardial effusion as a low-density area (*arrowheads*) that is clearly demarcated from the contrast-enhanced blood in the intracardiac chambers and descending aorta. Note the bilateral pleural effusions posteriorly. (DA, descending aorta; LV, left ventricle; RA, right atrium; RV, right ventricle.) (From Eisenberg RL. An Atlas of Differential Diagnosis, 4th ed. Philadelphia: Lippincott Williams & Wilkins, 2003.)

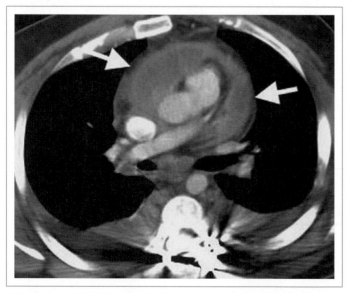

FIGURE 38.7: CT shows high-density pericardial fluid and thickening and enhancement of the pericardium (arrows). (From Collins J and Stern EJ. Chest Radiology: The Essentials, 2nd ed. Philadelphia: Lippincott Williams & Wilkins, 2008.)

Chest MRI

- Superior for determining composition of pericardial fluid
- Further characterizes pericardial disease, more specifically localizes pericardial fluid, and is useful when echocardiogram is equivocal

 TABLE 38.9: MRI: pericardial effusion

IV contrast	No
PO contrast	No
Amount of radiation	None

Classic Images

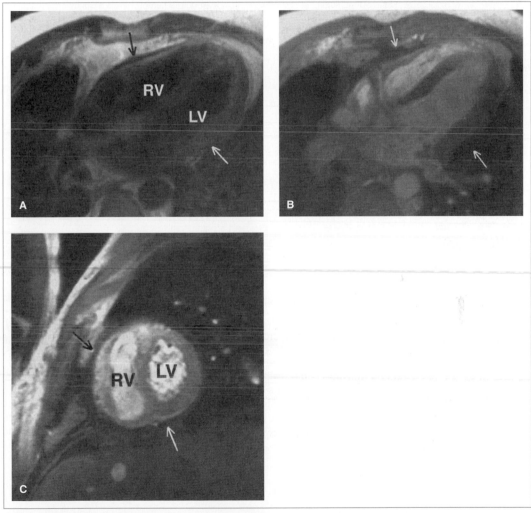

FIGURE 38.8: Constrictive pericarditis. Spin-echo and cine magnetic resonance imaging; horizontal long-axis and short-axis views. On the "dark blood" image (**A**), thickened pericardium is represented by a curvilinear signal void (*arrows*) separated by the bright signal of the epicardial and pericardial fat. There is an associated conical/tubular compression deformity of the basal and middle portions of the right ventricle (RV) and left ventricle (LV). On the "bright blood" images (**B** and **C**), the fibrous/calcified nature of the pericardium is confirmed by the dark appearance of the pericardium (*arrows*). The abnormal pericardium caused abrupt limitation of diastolic filling of the ventricles on the cine image loops. (*Courtesy of R. D. White, MD, Cleveland Clinic Foundation.*) (From Topol EJ, Califf RM, et al. Textbook of Cardiovascular Medicine, 3rd ed. Philadelphia: Lippincott Williams & Wilkins, 2006.)

Summary

TABLE 38.10: Advantages and disadvantages of imaging modalities in pericarditis

Imaging modality	Advantages	Disadvantages
Chest x-ray	Fast, noninvasive Inexpensive	Nonspecific findings
Echocardiography	Modality of choice Fast, noninvasive, at bedside Highly sensitive and specific Can see effusions with as little fluid as 25 mL	Operator dependent Limited in patients with obesity/obstructive lung disease Difficult to distinguish if loculation/hematoma present Limited window—cannot image entire pericardium
CT scan	Less false positives, less operator dependent Detects <50 mL fluid Detects loculated effusions Detects pericardial calcifications (essential to the diagnosis of constrictive pericarditis)	Requires contrast Radiation exposure Requires hemodynamic stability
MRI	Highly sensitive Can detect <30 mL of fluid Can characterize fluid/mass No contrast or radiation exposure	Less available Longer image acquisition time Requires hemodynamic stability Arrhythmias can significantly decrease image quality

39

Infective Endocarditis

Keith A. Marill

Background

Infective endocarditis (IE) is defined as an infection of the endocardial surface of the heart, which may include the heart valves, mural endocardium, or a septal defect. Endocarditis can cause a number of abnormalities potentially visible on cardiac imaging including valvular vegetations, regurgitation, or deformity, and perivalvular abscess or pseudoaneurysm. Embolic phenomenon from right heart infection may be visible on pulmonary imaging, and emboli from left-sided disease may be visualized in the central nervous system and throughout the body. Over the past two decades, the primary imaging modality used to diagnose and to assess IE has been transesophageal echocardiography (TEE). However, new techniques and technology have improved the performance of transthoracic echocardiography (TTE), multislice CT, and MRI (rarely used) for the diagnosis of IE and its complications.

TABLE 39.1: History and physical

Fever and chills	Most common: ~90% of patients develop fever
Constitutional complaints	Anorexia, weight loss, myalgias, night sweats, cough, and lower back and joint pains
Risk factors	Valvular disease, dental surgery, and injection drug use
Primary: cardiopulmonary	Heart murmur, new or changed (~85% of patients), shortness of breath, rales, jugular venous distention, and peripheral edema
Secondary: embolic phenomena Stroke syndromes	Cranial nerve deficits Focal weakness or numbness Roth spots
Secondary: embolic phenomena/autoimmune glomerulonephritis skin manifestations	Hematuria Fluid overload Splinter hemorrhages, petechiae, Janeway lesions, Osler nodes
Rapid or indolent pace	Infecting organism dependent

TABLE 39.2: Pathognomonic physical examination

Classic IE sign	Description	Test characteristics
Splinter hemorrhages	Dark linear red lesion in the nail beds	Nonspecific
Osler nodes	Tender subcutaneous nodules usually found on the distal pads of the digits	More common in chronic than acute cases 10–25% sensitivity
Janeway lesions	Nontender maculae on the palms and soles	~10% sensitivity
Roth spots	Retinal hemorrhages with small clear centers	~5% sensitivity
Petechiae	Small nonblanching red spots	20–40% sensitivity Nonspecific

IE, infective endocarditis.

TABLE 39.3: Potentially helpful laboratory tests

Blood cultures	Not helpful for initial evaluation Two sets: >90% sensitivity when bacteremia is present Three sets: improve sensitivity; potentially helpful with previous administration of antibiotics
Erythrocyte sedimentation rate	High sensitivity >90%, but not specific
Urinalysis	Proteinuria microscopic hematuria 50% of cases
Cell blood count	Anemia of chronic disease common in subacute endocarditis
Serology for fastidious organisms	*Chlamydia*, Q fever (*Coxiella*), *Legionella*, and *Bartonella* Culture-negative endocarditis

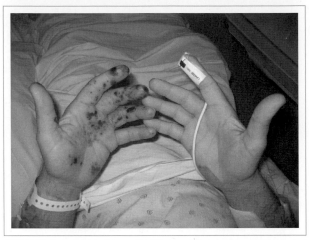

FIGURE 39.1: Adult with methicillin-sensitive native valve *Staphylococcus aureus* endocarditis, bacteremia, and multiple microabscesses. The reason for greater rash involvement of the left upper extremity as opposed to right was unknown. (*Courtesy of Massachusetts General Hospital, Boston, MA.*)

Chest X-ray

- Look for an enlarged heart or pulmonary congestion suggestive of congestive heart failure
- Pulmonary embolic phenomena strongly suggest tricuspid disease, which is most common in patients with a history of IV drug use

 TABLE 39.4: Chest x-ray (PA and Lateral): endocarditis

IV contrast	No
PO contrast	No
Amount of radiation	0.1 mSv

Classic Images

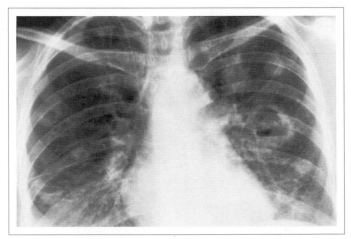

FIGURE 39.2: Septic pulmonary emboli. Several round lesions, many with cavitation, are seen throughout the lungs in this IV drug user with staphylococcal tricuspid endocarditis. (From Eisenberg RL. An Atlas of Differential Diagnosis, 4th ed. Philadelphia: Lippincott Williams & Wilkins, 2003.)

Bedside Cardiac Ultrasound and TTE

- Not as sensitive as TEE for valvular vegetations
- Sensitivity highest in right-sided disease because the pulmonic and tricuspid valves are closer to the chest wall
- Bedside ultrasound can be used by emergency physicians to assess for valvular abnormalities and vegetations but this is not yet standard of care
- Bedside technique:
  - Use the low-frequency curvilinear or a phase array probe and have a low threshold to move the patient into a left lateral decubitus position
  - Look for hyperechoic thickening or vegetations on the leaflets of the valves
  - Evaluate the aortic and mitral valves on long parasternal view
  - Evaluate the mitral valve and slide the probe cephalad in the same plane without rotating the probe on short parasternal view to evaluate the aortic valve
  - Perform the examinations in color Doppler mode to assess valvular flow.
  - Up to 20% of studies may be technically inadequate due to obesity, chronic obstructive pulmonary disease, or chest wall deformities
- Harmonic imaging (hTTE) has led to variably improved sensitivity (80–90% for vegetations >1cm), and this technique improves the signal-to-noise ratio by imaging the second harmonic frequency (twice the fundamental frequency)
- TTE may be limited in prosthetic valve endocarditis (especially mitral) due to shadowing from the prosthetic valve

Classic Images

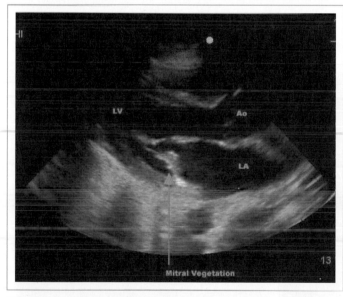

FIGURE 39.3: A 33-year-old male patient presented to the emergency department (ED) at the Juba Teaching Hospital in Juba, South Sudan, with 3 days of acute left-sided arm and leg weakness and inability to walk. In the ED, he was found to be febrile and tachycardic. Physical examination revealed complete left-sided hemiparesis. Bedside echocardiography revealed a hyperechoic vegetative lesion (*arrow*) on the mitral valve leaflet. The presentation was highly suggestive of IE with embolism. The resources for further diagnosis and therapy of such a patient are limited in Southern Sudan; cardiology and cardiothoracic surgery are not available, there are no neurologists, and diagnostic imaging is limited to x-ray or ultrasound. LA, left atrium; LV, left ventricle; Ao, aortic root. (*Courtesy of Dana Sajed, MD, Massachusetts General Hospital, Boston, MA.*)

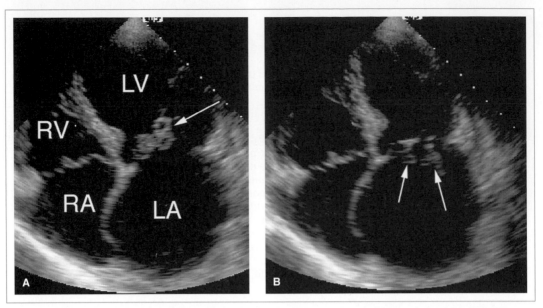

FIGURE 39.4: A large vegetation involving the anterior mitral leaflet is shown with four chamber view. **A:** The size and location of the mass is evident (*arrow*). **B:** During systole, the vegetation can be seen on the left atrial side of the mitral valve (*arrows*). LA, left atrium; LV, left ventricle; RA, right atrium; RV, right ventricle. (From Feigenbaum H, Armstrong WF, and Ryan T. Feigenbaum's Echocardiography, 6th ed. Philadelphia: Lippincott Williams & Wilkins, 2005.)

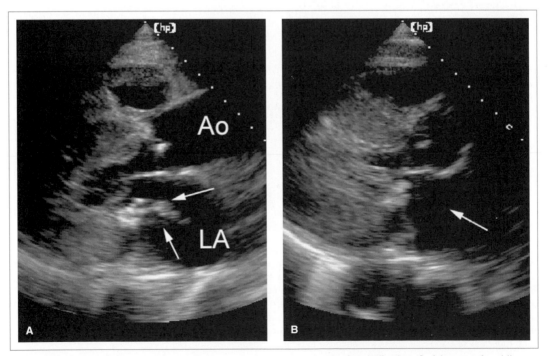

FIGURE 39.5: The appearance of a vegetation may change as a result of embolization. **A:** A large and mobile vegetation (*arrows*) can be seen attached to the left atrial (LA) side of the posterior mitral leaflet. **B:** An echocardiogram recorded 1 week later, after a stroke. Note that the vegetation (*arrow*) is much smaller, most likely the result of embolization. Ao, aorta. (From Feigenbaum H, Armstrong WF, and Ryan T. Feigenbaum's Echocardiography, 6th ed. Philadelphia: Lippincott Williams & Wilkins, 2005.)

Transesophageal Echocardiography

- Gold standard
  - Major Duke criteria for the diagnosis:
    - Oscillating intracardiac mass on valve or supporting structures or in the path of regurgitant jets, or on iatrogenic devices, in the absence of an alternative anatomic explanation
    - Abscess
    - New partial dehiscence of prosthetic valve
    - New valvular regurgitation
  - Requires clinical corroboration to diagnose IE
- Important for culture negative cases, e.g., fungal endocarditis, where large, friable vegetations are often observed.
- Visible vegetations suggest a worse prognosis with increased risk of embolic disease, chronic heart failure, and death.
- Larger left-side valvular vegetations (>1 cm) are associated with increased stroke risk; the degree of mobility of vegetations is associated with their size, but mobility is not independently associated with stroke risk.
- Highly sensitive for local complications such as valve ring abscess or fistula formation and for valvular perforation.

Classic Images

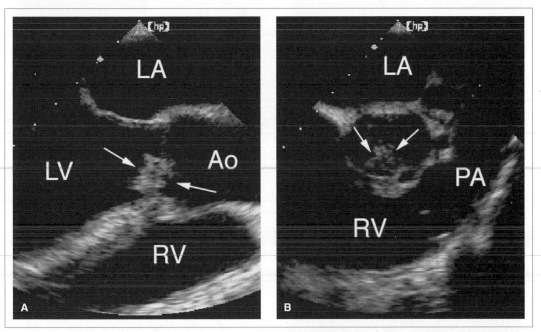

FIGURE 39.6: An aortic valve vegetation is demonstrated on this transesophageal echocardiogram (*arrows*). The mass was clearly seen from the long-axis (**A**) and short-axis (**B**) views. The mass was not detected on transthoracic imaging. Ao, aorta; LA, left atrium; LV, left ventricle; RV, right ventricle; PA, pulmonary artery. (From Feigenbaum H, Armstrong WF, and Ryan T. Feigenbaum's Echocardiography, 6th ed. Philadelphia: Lippincott Williams & Wilkins, 2005.)

Cardiac CT

- Advanced multislice and dual-source cardiac CT demonstrate excellent valvular vegetation, perivalvular abscess, and pseudoaneurysm detection
- Provides additional information useful for preoperative valvular surgery planning such as the extent of coronary artery disease
- Limitations: the contraindication of contrast injection in patients with renal insufficiency, the necessity of beta blocker pretreatment for a sufficiently slow heart rate, and the inability to examine patients with an irregular heart rhythm such as atrial fibrillation
- Detection of leaflet perforation is poor compared to TEE, which benefits from Doppler visualization of flow

 TABLE 39.5: Cardiac CT: endocarditis

IV contrast	No
PO contrast	No
Amount of radiation	5–20 mSv

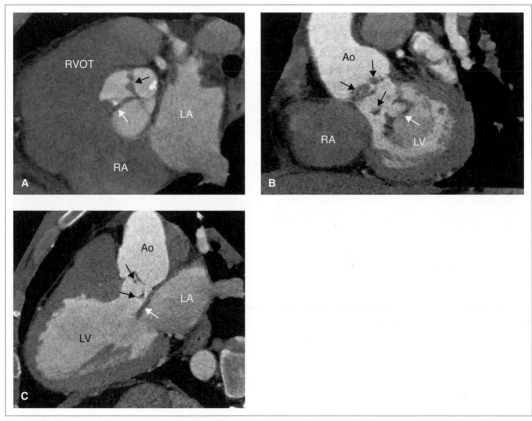

FIGURE 39.7: ECG-gated cardiac CT was performed in a 38-year-old male patient who was IV drug user and presented with fevers and bacteremia. **A:** Short-axis reconstruction of the aortic valve demonstrated a functionally bicuspid valve, with fusion of the right and left leafl ets. These fused commissures were thickened and contained a 6-mm vegetation (black arrow). A second vegetation is present on the commissure between the right and noncoronary leaflets (white arrow). Abnormal calcifications are present, which are consistent with valvulopathy. **B:** A MinIP slab reconstruction through the short axis of the mitral valve demonstrates irregularity and discontinuity of the anterior leaflet (white arrow), a 5 mm vegetation extending from the anterior leaflet into the left ventricular outflow tract (LVOT) (thick black arrow), and thickening of the aortic valve seen in profile (thin black arrows). **C:** Left-ventricular outflow tract (3-chamber) view MinIP slab reconstruction demonstrates abnormal thickening of the anterior leaflet of the mitral valve (thick white arrow), adjacent vegetation in the LVOT (thick black arrow), and a portion of an aortic valve vegetation (thin black arrow). Ao, aorta; LA, left atrium; LV, left ventricle; RVOT, right ventricle outflow tract. (*Courtesy of Dr. Brian B. Ghoshhajra, Department of Radiology, Massachusetts General Hospital, Boston, MA.*)

Basic Management

- Maintain a low threshold to consider IE as a diagnosis
- Obtain blood cultures prior to treatment
- Administer early empiric parenteral antibiotics directed at likely organisms
- Admit to hospital for continued treatment pending culture results
- Order appropriate imaging and consult cardiology

Summary

TABLE 39.6: Advantages and disadvantages of imaging modalities in endocarditis

Imaging modality	Advantage	Disadvantage
Chest x-ray	Identify secondary phenomena – Multiple pulmonary emboli suggest right heart disease with sensitivity >50% – Enlarged cardiac silhouette or pulmonary congestion suggest CHF	Neither sensitive nor specific
TTE	Availability Highly specific for valvular vegetations Positive test suggests IE	Sensitivity ~60% Negative test doesn't rule out IE
TEE	Gold standard Sensitivity >90% Highly specific for valvular vegetations	Sedation required Availability
Cardiac CT	High sensitivity and specificity Aids preoperative planning	Radiation Requires breath holding Requires IV contrast Requires a slow heart rate Requires a regular rhythm Availability of multislice CT scanner Availability of radiologic expertise

CHF, Chronic heart failure; IE, infective endocarditis.

40

Aortic Stenosis and Valvular Heart Disease

Pierre Borczuk

Background

Single valvular heart disease may be categorized as that caused by stenosis and or as disease caused by insufficiency. Stenosis causes a pressure overload and myocardial hypertrophy. Myocardial dilatation occurs only when heart failure has developed. In valvular insufficiency, both hypertrophy and dilatation occur due to volume overload. Most disease is chronic in nature, except for the rare acute valvular rupture, which presents more dramatically.

A careful history, physical examination, ECG, and radiographic imaging will help the emergency physician determine which valve(s) may be diseased as well as the potential etiology. The focus of this chapter will be aortic stenosis (AS) with brief description of aortic insufficiency (AI), mitral stenosis (MS), and mitral insufficiency (MI). Of particular note is mitral valve prolapse (MVP), the most common valvular disease in industrialized nations, which is associated with an increased incidence of exercise-related mitral regurgitation, sudden death, and dysrhythmias. A discussion of tricuspid and pulmonary valve disease, which are much less common, prosthetic heart valves, or multivalvular disease is beyond the scope of this imaging chapter.

Transthoracic ultrasonography is the noninvasive gold standard test to evaluate valvular heart disease. ED-based bedside ultrasonography curricula do not currently incorporate quantitative assessment of AS or other valvular disease pathologies. The average survival for the patient presenting with AS and angina is 5 years, with AS and syncope 3 years and with AS and congestive heart failure 2 years.

TABLE 40.1: Classic history and physical

AS	History of rheumatic heart disease or congenital bicuspid aortic valve; less commonly degenerative heart disease or calcified valve
	Chest pain, dyspnea, syncope
	Paroxysmal nocturnal dyspnea, exertional syncope, angina, myocardial infarction, atrial fibrillation (10%), and endocarditis (2%)
	Crackles at bases, peripheral edema, and/or jugular venous distention
	Pulse of small amplitude, normal or low blood pressure, and narrow pulse pressure
	Point of maximum impulse shifted to the left
	Harsh systolic ejection murmur best heard in the second right intercostal space and radiating to the right carotid
	Paradoxical splitting of S2
	Delayed carotid upstrokes (pulsus parvus et tardus)
	Delay between brachial and radial pulses (indicates severe AS)
	Dysrhythmia leading to sudden death
AI	*Acute*
	History of infective endocarditis or aortic dissection
	Dyspnea, pulmonary edema, and pink frothy sputum
	Fever and chills (endocarditis)
	Tearing chest pain, sweating, tachycardia, tachypnea, and rales (dissection)
	High-pitched blowing diastolic murmur heard after S2 at the right second or third intercostal parasternal space
	S3 with long diastolic murmur or systolic flow murmur possible
	Chronic
	History of congenital bicuspid valve, rheumatic heart disease, syphilis, Marfan syndrome, ankylosing spondylitis, relapsing polychondritis, or appetite-suppressing drugs, e.g., fenfluramine
	Gender: male
	Palpitations and premature ventricular contractions
	Stabbing chest pain, fatigue, or dyspnea
	Wide pulse pressure and prominent ventricular impulse (head bobbing)
	Peripheral pulse that has a quick rise in upstroke followed by a peripheral collapse (Water hammer pulse)
	Accentuated precordial apical thrust
	To and fro femoral murmur (Duroziez sign)
	Capillary pulsations visible at the proximal nail bed with pressure applied to the tip (Quincke's pulse)
	Peripheral vasodilation
MS	History of rheumatic heart disease, left atrial myxoma, thrombus, or tumor that prolapses through the orifice during diastole
	History of pulmonary hypertension or atrial fibrillation
	Exertional dyspnea
	Hemoptysis
	Paroxysmal nocturnal dyspnea
	Middiastolic rumbling murmur with crescendo toward the S2
	Loud S1 followed by a loud high-pitched opening "snap" heard at the apex
	Prominent a wave at the neck
	Normal or low blood pressure
	Rales
	Systemic emboli
MI	*Acute*
	History of inferior myocardial infarction, trauma, and infective endocarditis
	Shortness of breath, dyspnea, tachycardia, and pulmonary edema
	S3 and S4
	Harsh apical systolic murmur starting with S1, apical thrill, systolic thrust, and active apical impulse
	Cardiogenic shock or arrest
	Prominent a wave on jugular venous distension
	Chronic
	History of rheumatic heart disease, mitral valve prolapse, coronary artery disease or cardiomyopathy, and appetite-suppressing drugs, e.g., fenfluramine
	Exertional dyspnea
	Atrial fibrillation
	Late systolic left parasternal lift
	High-pitched holosystolic murmur at the fifth intercostal space
	Soft S1 and audible S3
	Systemic emboli
MVP	Gender: male; age >45 yr
	Short diastolic murmur
	Atypical chest pain, palpitations, fatigue, and dyspnea unrelated to exertion
	Pectus excavatum, scoliosis, or a straight thoracic spine
	Midsystolic click
	Late systolic murmur with crescendo into S2

AI, aortic insufficiency; AS, aortic stenosis; MI, mitral insufficiency; MS, mitral stenosis; MVP, mitral valve prolapse.

TABLE 40.2: Potentially helpful laboratory tests

Cardiac markers	Evaluate myocardial ischemia
Beta-natriuretic peptide	Evaluate pulmonary edema
CBC	Evaluate infection and anemia
TSH	Evaluate thyrotoxicosis
Blood cultures	Evaluate endocarditis

CBC, complete blood count; TSH, thyroid stimulating hormone.

Chest X-ray

- Obtain a posteroanterior (PA) and lateral view if possible
- Typically, the cardiac silhouette is normal; however, significant hypertrophy may manifest as an enlarged cardiac silhouette
- Lateral view: may demonstrate valve calcification
- Distinguish calcific mitral from aortic valve on lateral view by drawing a line from the inferior aspect of the right pulmonary artery along the right middle lobe branch to the tip of the xiphoid; the aortic valve is above this line and the mitral valve is below

 TABLE 40.3: Chest x-ray (PA and Lateral): valvular disease

IV contrast	No
PO contrast	No
Amount of radiation	0.1 mSv

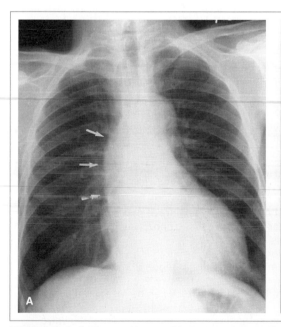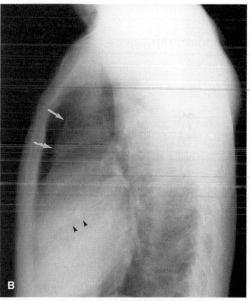

FIGURE 40.1: A 60-year-old man with degenerative calcific aortic stenosis. **A:** Posteroanterior examination shows increased rounding of the left ventricular portion of the left heart border and dilatation of the ascending aorta (*arrows*). **B:** Lateral examination shows aortic valvular calcification (*arrowheads*) in the center of the cardiac silhouette and filling of the retrosternal air space by the dilated, calcified (*arrows*) ascending aorta. The left ventricle is not dilated. (From Topol EJ, Califf RM, et al. Textbook of Cardiovascular Medicine, 3rd Edition. Philadelphia: Lippincott Williams & Wilkins, 2006.)

Classic Images

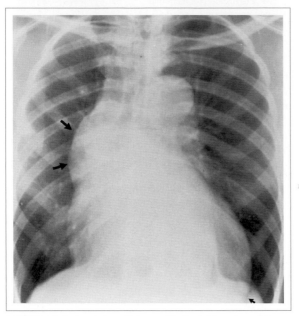

FIGURE 40.2: Aortic insufficiency. Marked dilatation of the ascending aorta (*arrows*), suggesting some underlying aortic stenosis. The left ventricle is enlarged with downward and lateral displacement of the cardiac apex. Note that the cardiac shadow extends below the dome of the left hemidiaphragm (*small arrow*). (From Eisenberg RL. An Atlas of Differential Diagnosis, 4th ed. Philadelphia: Lippincott Williams & Wilkins, 2003.)

Transthoracic Ultrasound

TABLE 40.4: Common transthoracic ultrasound views for specific anatomic evaluation

View	Best for visualizing
Parasternal long axis	Aortic valve, mitral valve, outflow tract, and LV contractility
Parasternal short axis	Measure mitral valve area, investigate aortic valve structure/vegetations
Apical four chamber	RV, LV function, and MR with Doppler
Subcostal	Part of FAST, pericardial effusion

FAST; LV, left ventricle; MR, mitral regurgitation; RV, right ventricle.

- Two-dimensional ultrasound can diagnose and estimate the severity of aortic stenosis, and can determine whether the patient has valvular pathology versus subvalvular (hypertrophic obstructive cardiomyopathy or HOCM) stenosis
- Aortic valve can be best seen in parasternal long axis view
- Look for calcifications of the valve, which will make them appear more prominent (whiter and thicker than the other valves)
- Using preset cardiac calculations, the left ventricular outflow track can be measured and valve area estimated
- Assess with color Doppler mode the severity of stenosis by measuring a mean aortic valve gradient
- If the aortic jet is not parallel to the Doppler beam or if the cardiac output is impaired, the mean gradient/severity will be underestimated
- Color Doppler image also identifies regurgitant flow

Classic Images

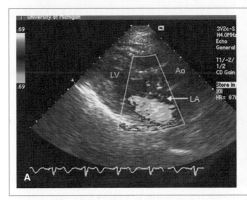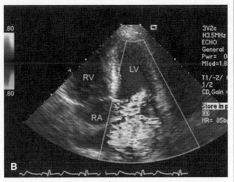

FIGURE 40.3: Parasternal long-axis view (**A**) and apical four-chamber view (**B**) recorded in a patient with mitral stenosis. **A:** Note the marked doming nature of the mitral valve opening in diastole with focal thickening at the tips of both the anterior and posterior leaflets. In the real-time image, note that pliability of the midportion of the mitral valve is preserved. **B:** Apical four-chamber view reveals a similar phenomenon with doming of the mitral valve in diastole toward the apex. Ao, aorta; LA, left atrium; LV, left ventricle; RA, right atrium; RV, right ventricle; RVOT, right ventricular outflow tract. (From Feigenbaum H, Armstrong WF, and Ryan T. Feigenbaum's Echocardiography, 6th ed. Philadelphia: Lippincott Williams & Wilkins, 2005.)

Basic Management
- Oxygen and continuous cardiac and hemodynamic monitoring
- ECG
- Be careful using certain classes of medications in patients with AS, e.g., nitrates and venodilators such as morphine, because of preload dependence
- Diagnosis-specific treatment for dissection, dysrhythmia, endocarditis, myocardial infarction, pulmonary edema, etc.
- Cardiology consultation
- Emergency cardiothoracic surgery consultation with acute valvular disease

Summary

TABLE 40.5: Advantages and disadvantages of imaging modalities in aortic stenosis

Imaging modality	Advantages	Disadvantages
X-ray	Portable, available	Nonspecific
Ultrasound	Gold standard, portable	Technical expertise needed

41

Hypertrophic Cardiomyopathy

William Binder

Background

Hypertrophic cardiomyopathy (HCM) is a relatively common form of genetic heart disease, with a prevalence estimated at 0.2% in the general population. HCM is defined clinically by the presence of left or right ventricular hypertrophy in the absence of other cardiac or systemic disease. It is often, but not always, asymmetric, and the hypertrophy can be segmental or diffuse.

In at least 25% of patients, asymmetrical septal hypertrophy, leads to a significant pressure gradient between the apical left ventricle and the left ventricular outflow tract, resulting in hypertrophic obstructive cardiomyopathy (HoCM). There are primarily two forms of obstructive cardiomyopathy: subaortic ventricle hypertrophy and midventricular obstruction. These two forms may coexist in one patient. A variant, apical hypertrophy, and other rarer forms of HoCM comprise the 25–30% of obstructive forms of HCM. The remainder of patients have the nonobstructive form of HCM. Currently, HCM is the term used in the medical literature that encompasses both the obstructive and nonobstructive forms of the disease.

TABLE 41.1: Classic history and physical

Family history of HCM
Dyspnea
Syncope or near syncope
Chest pain
Palpitations associated with lightheadedness and dizziness
Symptoms worsened by alcohol, heavy meal, or position changes
New murmur in adolescents
Provocable or resting harsh systolic murmur
LVH: Displaced PMI, fourth heart sound
RVH: prominent A wave in jugular venous pulse
ECG abnormalities

ECG, electrocardiogram; HCM, hypertrophic cardiomyopathy; LVH, left ventricular hypertrophy; PMI, point of maximum impulse; RVH, right ventricular hypertrophy.

TABLE 41.2: Risk stratification of sudden cardiac death in patients with HCM based on cardiac imaging findings

Echocardiography
  LV wall maximal thickness (≥30 mm)
  LV dilatation and decreased EF
  Reduced septal Ea in children
  LVOT gradient at rest ≥30 mm Hg (better predictor for overall mortality)

Nuclear imaging
  Perfusion defects
  Reduced coronary flow reserve
  Increased MIBG washout rate

Cardiac MRI
  LV wall maximal thickness (≥30 mm)
  LV dilatation and decreased EF
  Late enhancing areas with delayed gadolinium-enhanced images

LV, left ventricle; LVOT, left ventricle outflow tract; Ea, early diastolic velocity; MIBG, metaiodobenzylguanidine.
Adapted from Nagueh SF and Mahmarian JJ. Noninvasive cardiac imaging in patients with hypertrophic cardiomyopathy. *J Am Coll Cardiol* 48(12):2006;2410–2422.

TABLE 41.3: Potentially helpful laboratory tests

CPK-MB
Troponin
BNP

CPK-MB, creatine phosphokinase myocardial band; BNP, brain natriuretic peptide.

Chest X-ray

- Obtain both posteroanterior and lateral views when possible
- Often no abnormalities, but look for left ventricular, left atrial, or right atrial enlargement
- Bulge on the left heart border, between the left atrial appendage and left ventricular apex, may reflect anterolateral wall extension of anteroseptal hypertrophy
- Interstitial markings may be increased in the lung fields

 TABLE 41.4: Chest x-ray (PA and Lateral): hypertrophic cardiomyopathy

PO contrast	No
IV contrast	No
Amount of radiation	0.10 mSv

Classic Images

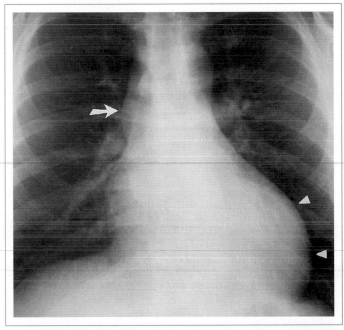

FIGURE 41.1: Left ventricular enlargement on posteroanterior chest radiograph. Prominence of the left ventricle with rounding along the inferior heart border and an apex that is pointing downward (*arrowheads*) are indicative of "left ventricular configuration." (From Brant WE and Helms CA. Fundamentals of Diagnostic Radiology, 3rd ed. Philadelphia: Lippincott Williams & Wilkins, 2007.)

Bedside Cardiac Ultrasound

- Bedside cardiac ultrasound may be performed by emergency physicians only for screening purposes, as this is not the standard for obtaining measurements
- Cardiac software packages on most ultrasound machines assist in making measurements
- Trans-thoracic echocardiogram
  - Most important diagnostic modality for identifying HCM
  - combination of M mode, Doppler, and two-dimensional delineates the nonobstructive and obstructive HM and can characterize the type, degree, and location of hypertrophy

- Use phased array sector probe (cardiac probe) or curved linear array probe with median frequency of 3.5 MHz (2.5–5 MHz); the smaller the footprint (area of contact) of the probe, the less likely rib shadows will hinder interpretation
- Some ultrasound machines, when in the "cardiac" setting or mode, may invert the image 180 degrees
  - This can be confusing when one is examining the heart during a FAST examination, when the machine will be in the abdominal or general mode, which does not flip invert the image
  - When examining the heart, the probe marker should be pointed to the patient's left.
- Consider placing the patient in the left lateral decubitus position to bring the mediastinal structures closer to the anterior chest wall
- Left ventricular (LV) wall thickness >13 mm suggestive of HoCM
- Left ventricle outflow tract gradient of >30 mm Hg is diagnostic of HoCM and is predictive of increased risk of death
- Doppler studies offer a more direct visualization of the presence, location, and degree of subaortic obstruction; parasternal and apical long axis views are best in this examination.
- Systolic anterior motion of the mitral valve occurs in 25% of patients with HCM and is seen well on the parasternal short axis view of the mitral valve
- M mode recordings may be helpful to visualize the difference between the rates of anterior leaflet motion compared to the anterior motion of the posterior wall in systole
- Parasternal long axis view offers the best view of the pattern of septal hypertrophy in relationship to the outflow tract
- Apical hypertrophy can be difficult to ascertain and additional imaging with cardiac MRI may be useful; color or pulsed Doppler examination may the best modality for demonstrating the absence of blood flow in the apical region
- Maneuvers that provoke outflow obstruction by changing preload and afterload can be used carefully

Classic Images

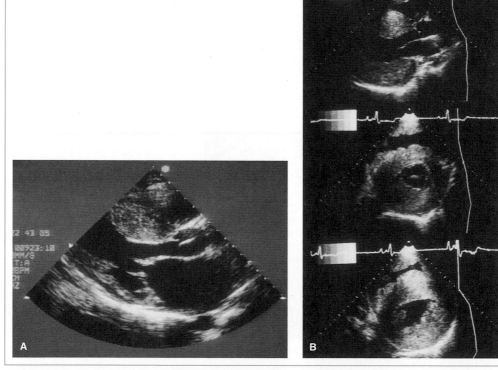

FIGURE 41.2: Two-dimensional echocardiogram in the parasternal (**A**) long-axis view demonstrating asymmetric septal hypertrophy and (**B**) long- and short-axis views demonstrating severe concentric hypertrophy. (From Topol EJ, Califf RM, et al. Textbook of Cardiovascular Medicine, 3rd ed. Philadelphia: Lippincott Williams & Wilkins, 2006.)

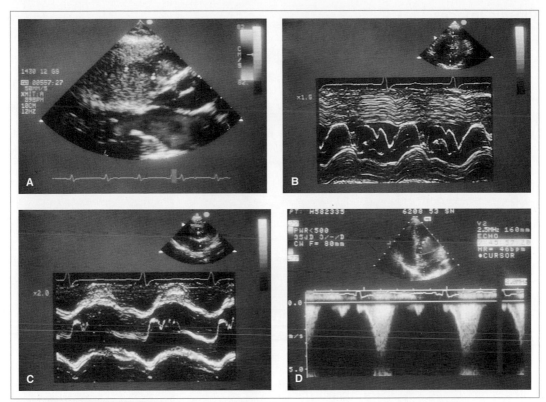

FIGURE 41.3: Parasternal long-axis view recorded in a patient with hypertrophic cardiomyopathy being considered for alcohol septal reduction therapy. Top: Image was recorded at baseline. Note the hypertrophy of the ventricular septum and the systolic anterior motion of the mitral valve. Bottom: Image was recorded after injection of a diluted perfluorocarbon-based contrast agent into a septal perforator artery. Note the absence of contrast effect in the ventricular septum but the appearance of contrast in the right and left ventricular cavity and the marked contrast effect in right ventricular muscle trabeculae (*arrow*). (Feigenbaum H, Armstrong WF, Ryan T. Feigenbaum's Echocardiography. 6th ed. Philadelphia: Lippincott Williams and Wilkins, 2005.)

Cardiac MRI

- Provides vivid images of both the pattern and degree of hypertrophy
- More accurate assessment of the LV wall and total cardiac mass than ultrasound
- Can diagnose HCM in patients with normal ultrasound (some studies have shown that echocardiography can underestimate LV wall thickness by 20% and in cases of extreme hypertrophy can underestimate by 10%)
    - Cine-CMR (Cardiac MRI) provides accurate quantification of the subaortic dynamic gradient
    - Late gadolinium enhancement allows deep tissue characterization of hypertrophied regions of the heart
    - Gadolinium injection in CMR can demonstrate patchy uptake consistent with focal areas of hypertrophy; it is a particularly useful modality in pre-HCM disease in mutation positive patients with relatively normal two-dimensional echocardiograms

 TABLE 41.5: Cardiac MRI: hypertrophic cardiomyopathy

PO contrast	No
IV contrast	Yes, gadolinium is helpful
Amount of radiation	None

Classic Images

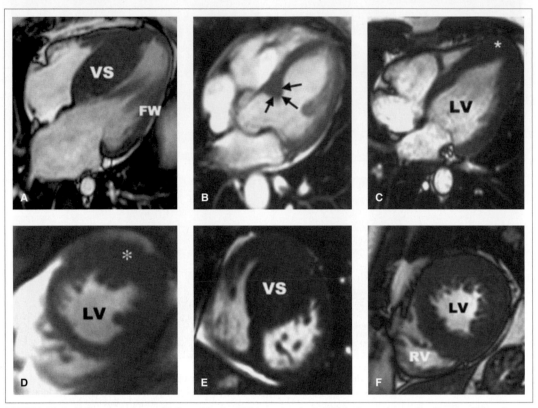

FIGURE 41.4: A diverse pattern of left ventricular (LV) hypertrophy in HCM. A spectrum of patterns of LV wall thickening constitutes the phenotypic expression of hypertrophic cardiomyopathy (HCM). Cardiovascular magnetic resonance end-diastolic short-axis and long-axis images demonstrate (**A**) hypertrophy involving the ventricular septum (VS), sparing the LV free wall (FW); (**B**) focal area of hypertrophy sharply confined to the basal anterior septum (*arrows*); (**C**) hypertrophy of the LV apex (*); (**D**) segmental hypertrophy predominantly of the anterolateral LV FW (*); contiguous anterior septum is normal thickness; (**E**) massive asymmetric hypertrophy of the anterior VS (wall thickness 48 mm) with sparing of hypertrophy in the posterior septum and LV FW; and (**F**) diffuse hypertrophy involving most of the septum and FW. RV, right ventricle. (From Maron MS, Maron BJ et al. Hypertrophic cardiomyopathy phenotype revisited after 50 years with cardiovascular magnetic resonance. *JACC* 54(3):2009;220–228.)

Cardiac CT

- Can complement invasive cardiac catheterization and can provide increasingly accurate information about forms of HCM that echocardiography can miss
- In comparison to MRI, which currently is the gold standard for imaging, patients who are claustrophobic, obese, or those with pacemakers and automatic implantable cardiac defibrillators can be imaged. Single photon emission computed tomography can also assess not just structural, but perfusion defects in patients with HCM

Basic Management

- Assess ABCs
- Hemodynamic and cardiac monitoring
- Admission is indicated for symptomatic presentation to the emergency department

Summary

TABLE 41.6: Advantages and disadvantages of imaging modalities in hypertrophic cardiomyopathy

Imaging modality	Advantages	Disadvantages
X-ray	Rapid Minimal radiation	Nonspecific
Echocardiography	Fast, noninvasive Defines disease No radiation	Misses some variants of HCM
MRI	Gold standard Very sensitive	Time consuming Unable to perform on all patients
CT	Can provide structural information and can be used in patients with pacemakers and AICDs Preoperation planning: increasingly useful in defining structural abnormalities	Radiation exposure Currently not as sensitive as MRI IV contrast

HCM, hypertrophic cardiomyopathy.

42 Pediatric Cardiomyopathy

J.E. Klig

Background

Pediatric cardiomyopathy can be primary (idiopathic) or secondary to a wide array of infectious, metabolic, nutritional, general systemic, heredo-familial, and toxicologic etiologies.

The primary pediatric cardiomyopathies are generally categorized as dilated, restrictive, hypertrophic (rare), and arrhythmogenic (very rare). The overall prevalence of cardiomyopathy increases from 10 to 36 per 100,000 live births from the newborn period to childhood and the teen years. Dilated cardiomyopathy is the most common form, and can present with marked cardiomegaly and dilatation of both ventricles along with impaired systolic function. Over 50% of pediatric patients with dilated cardiomyopathy present before 2 years of age.

The unexpected detection of an enlarged heart in an infant or child often occurs during radiographic evaluations for other noncardiac presentations or illnesses in the emergency department.

TABLE 42.1: Classic history and physical

Insidious onset of symptoms
Antecedent respiratory or gastrointestinal illness
Increasing dyspnea on exertion, exercise intolerance
Abdominal complaints, nausea, anorexia
Palpitations, syncope, or near-syncope
Fatigue or tachypnea during feedings, irritability (infants)
Wheezing (infants)
Failure to thrive (infants)
May be ill-appearing
Moderate-severe respiratory distress
Pallor
Weak pulses/pulsus alternans
Decreased air at lung bases (rales rare)
Muffled heart sounds, gallop, murmurs rare
Hepatomegaly
Older children: venous distension, peripheral edema

TABLE 42.2: Potentially helpful laboratory tests

CBC and differential
BMP
LFT
Cardiac enzymes
C-reactive protein, erythrocyte sedimentation rate
Urinalysis
Urine toxicology

BMP, basic metabolic panel; CBC, complete blood count; LFT, liver function tests.

Chest X-ray

- Deep inspiration needed to assess heart size accurately
  - Most children under 6 years of age often cannot/do not do this
  - Be aware of estimating falsely enlarged cardiac dimensions
- The cardiac silhouette is approximately 50% of chest width of infants and young children
- The cardiac silhouette is approximately 40% of chest width of older children
- Up to 6 years of age, the thymus, which joins as a silhouette with the upper margin of the heart (superior mediastinum) is prominent
- Cardiothymic silhouette in younger children can mistakenly lead to concern about an enlarged heart or mediastinal mass
- Ultrasound the thymus if in doubt
- Look for cardiomegaly, pulmonary venous congestion, and possibly pleural effusions and pulmonary edema
- Look for left lower lobe atelectasis due to compression of the left mainstem bronchus from left atrial enlargement

TABLE 42.3: Helpful associated structures

Chest wall/rib expansion	Assess heart size (no more than 50% of width)
Thymus	Until 5–6 yr of age
Diaphragm	Assess mid-phase (between inspiration-exhalation)

 TABLE 42.4: Chest x-ray (PA and Lateral): pediatric cardiomyopathy

IV contrast	No
PO contrast	No
Amount of radiation	0.10 mSv

Classic Images

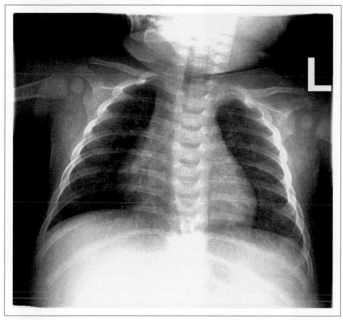

FIGURE 42.1: Normal chest radiograph of a 1 year old child. (*Courtesy of J.E. Klig, Massachusetts General Hospital, Boston, MA.*)

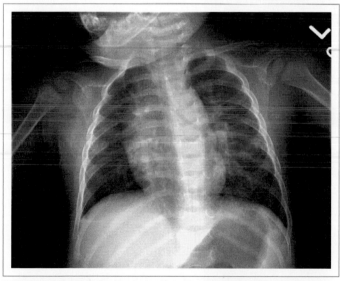

FIGURE 42.2: Chest radiograph of an 11-month-old child with a normal cardiothymic silhouette. (*Courtesy of J.E. Klig, Massachusetts General Hospital, Boston, MA.*)

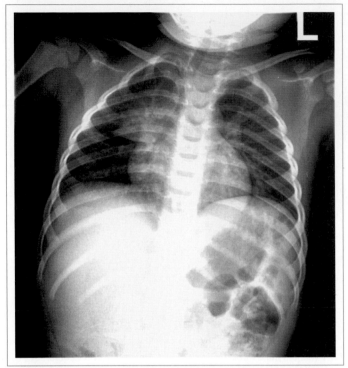

FIGURE 42.3: Chest radiograph of a normal thymus ("sail sign") in an 18-month-old child. (*Courtesy of J.E. Klig, Massachusetts General Hospital, Boston, MA.*)

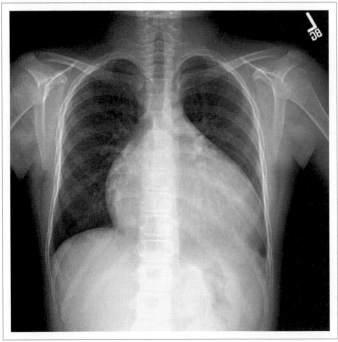

FIGURE 42.4: Chest radiograph of a 13-year-old boy with decreasing exercise intolerance and syncope. (*Courtesy of M.E. King, Massachusetts General Hospital, Boston, MA.*)

Transthoracic Cardiac Ultrasound

- Gold standard to establish the diagnosis
- Bedside ultrasound for screening purposes
  - 5–7.5 MHz curvilinear probe (3.5 MHz for adolescents)
  - Look for dilated ventricles and hypocontractility in any of the four views (subxiphoid, parasternal long, parasternal short, or apical four-chamber)
  - Look for pericardial effusion
  - Intracardiac thrombi may be seen
- Obtain formal transthoracic cardiac ultrasound

Classic Images

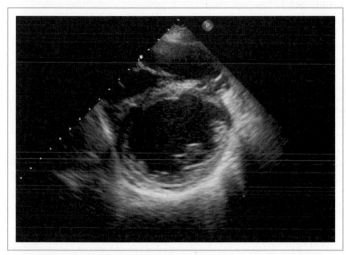

FIGURE 42.5: Two-dimensional echocardiogram (parasternal short-axis view) of a patient with idiopathic dilated cardiomyopathy showing a dilated left ventricle. (*Courtesy of M.E. King, Massachusetts General Hospital, Boston, MA.*)

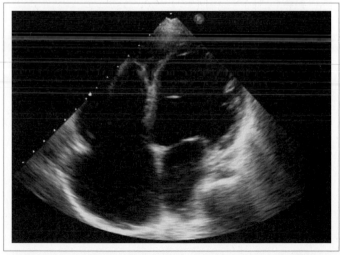

FIGURE 42.6: Two-dimensional echocardiogram (apical four-chamber view) of the same patient in Figure 42.5 with idiopathic dilated cardiomyopathy showing a dilated left ventricle, right atrium, and right ventricle. (*Courtesy of M.E. King, Massachusetts General Hospital, Boston, MA.*)

Basic Management

- Assess and stabilize airway, breathing, and circulation
- Oxygen and cardiac monitoring
- Hemodynamically unstable
  - Portable chest radiograph
  - Bedside ultrasound
- Hemodynamically stable
  - Routine chest radiographs
  - Bedside ultrasound and/or complete echocardiography
- Prompt pediatric cardiology consultation

Summary

TABLE 42.5: Advantages and disadvantages of imaging modalities in pediatric cardiomyopathy

Imaging modalities	Advantages	Disadvantages
Chest radiograph	Fast Inexpensive Low radiation exposure Diagnostic for cardiomegaly	Radiation exposure Subtle findings can be missed
Echocardiogram	Modality of choice Fully diagnostic No radiation exposure	Requires patient cooperation and/or sedation Operator-dependent

43

Asthma

Hector Rivera and Laura J. Bontempo

Background

Asthma is a chronic inflammatory disorder of the airways, which causes episodes of reversible airway obstruction. This obstruction is due to narrowing of the bronchi from a combination of inflamed tissue and bronchospasm. Patients experience symptoms that include dyspnea, wheezing, and coughing. It is estimated that 23.3 million Americans have asthma. Though a decrease in mortality since the 1980s has been promising, asthma was still responsible for 3,447 deaths in 2007. Females have a 44% higher mortality when compared to males, and blacks have two to three times higher mortality than whites. Low socioeconomic status, history of cocaine or heroin use, and comorbidities such as cardiovascular disease are risk factors for death from asthma.

TABLE 43.1: Classic history and physical

Cough, wheezing, and dyspnea
Mild: speaks in full sentences, patient may appear comfortable
Moderate: speaks in phrases, patient appears in moderate distress, signs of accessory muscle use are noted (retractions of intercostal and neck muscles), nasal flaring, tripod positioning
Severe: speaks words, patient is in severe distress, may show signs of altered mental status
Lung sounds may range from a prolonged expiratory phase in mild airway obstruction to decreased breath sounds indicating severe obstruction with or without wheezing

TABLE 43.2. Potentially helpful laboratory tests

None specific to asthma	
BMP	With frequent albuterol use, assess for hypokalemia
EKG, cardiac enzymes, BNP	Distinguish acute coronary syndrome from congestive heart failure in patients with cardiovascular comorbidities

BMP, basic metabolic panel; BNP, B-type natriuretic peptide; EKG, electrocardiogram.

Chest X-ray

- Often normal in asthma exacerbations
- Look for causes of the acute attack (e.g., pneumonia) or complications (pneumothorax, pneumomediastinum, atelectasis)

- Common features:
  - Pulmonary hyperinflation with increased lung lucency
  - Mild bronchial wall thickening
  - Note: Hyperinflated lungs from asthma maintain normal diaphragm contour; hyperinflation from chronic obstructive pulmonary disease classically is associated with flattened diaphragms

 TABLE 43.3: Chest x-ray (AP Portable): asthma

IV contrast	No
PO contrast	No
Amount of radiation	0.02 mSv

Classic Images

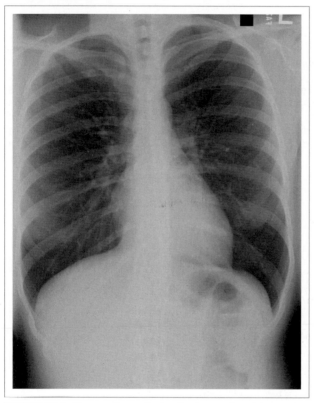

FIGURE 43.1: Chest radiograph showing hyperinflated lungs with normal diaphragm contour. (*Courtesy of Yale-New Haven Hospital, New Haven, CT.*)

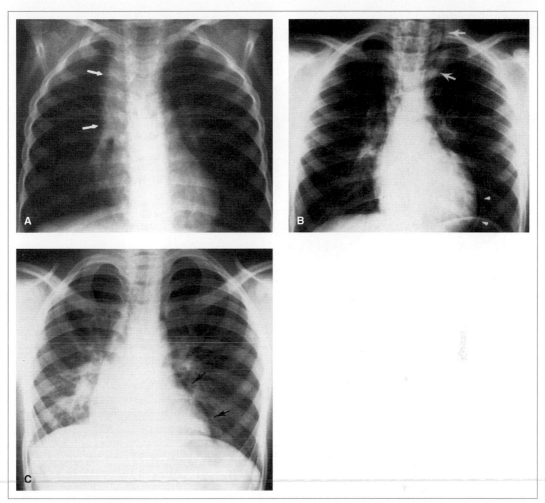

FIGURE 43.2: Pulmonary complications. **A:** Sublobar atelectasis. Asthmatic child with acute asthma attack. Note the area of apparent consolidation in the right paratracheal region (*arrows*). This represents collapse of one portion of the right upper lobe. A subtler finding assisting interpretation is that the minor fissure is slightly elevated. **B:** Pneumomediastinum. Asthmatic child with pneumomediastinum with air surrounding the small triangular thymus gland (T), extending as linear sheaths into the neck and superior mediastinum (*upper arrows*) and extending along the lower left cardiac edge (*lower arrows*). **C:** Medial pneumothorax. Note the thin strip of free air along the left cardiac border (*arrows*). The finding represents a medial pneumothorax and should not be confused with pneumomediastinum or pneumopericardium. (From Swischuk L. Emergency Radiology of the Acutely Ill or Injured Child, 2nd ed. Philadelphia: Lippincott Williams & Wilkins, 1986.)

Chest CT Scan

- Evaluates severity of disease as increased airway wall thickness has been associated with increased severity of illness
- Shows regional or diffuse air trapping
- May show abnormalities that chest x-ray does not (e.g., occult pneumothorax)
- Obtained if a change in medical management would be indicated (e.g., evaluating for aspergillosis or hypersensitivity pneumonitis)

 TABLE 43.4: Chest CT: asthma

IV contrast	No
PO contrast	No
Amount of radiation	7.0 mSv

Classic Images

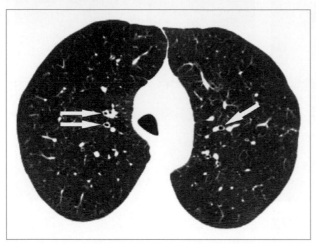

FIGURE 43.3: CT scan showing bronchial wall thickening (*white arrows*). (*Courtesy of Yale-New Haven Hospital, New Haven, CT.*)

Basic Management
- Oxygen supplementation to maintain saturation >90%
- Albuterol and ipratropium nebulized therapy are first-line for bronchodilation
- Corticosteroids reduce airway inflammation
- Magnesium sulfate IV is a smooth muscle relaxant and may be beneficial
- Adrenergic agents (e.g., epinephrine or terbutaline) may be helpful in severe asthma
- Heliox may be considered in severe asthma to decrease the work of breathing and increase the efficiency of gas exchange
- Noninvasive positive pressure ventilation may prevent intubation
- Patients with a severe asthma exacerbation with evidence of fatigue, severe distress, or mental status changes should immediately be intubated and mechanically ventilated
- Smoking cessation instructions if applicable

Summary

TABLE 43.5: Advantages and disadvantages of imaging modalities in asthma

Imaging modalities	Advantages	Disadvantages
Chest x-ray	Low radiation Portable Rapid acquisition	Nonspecific
CT scan	May identify associated pathology (e.g., small pneumothorax)	Radiation exposure Time-consuming Cost

44

Chronic Obstructive Pulmonary Disease

Mark F. Brady and Christopher Moore

Background

Chronic obstructive pulmonary disease (COPD) is characterized by progressive airflow limitation that is not fully reversible and encompasses the previously used subclassifications of emphysema, chronic bronchitis, and asthma. The prevalence increases with age, with more than 10% of the population over age 65 having COPD. Cigarette smoking is the most common risk factor: about 80% of those with COPD have a history of smoking and one fifth of smokers will be diagnosed with COPD in their lifetime. Approximately half of COPD exacerbations are due to respiratory infections, approximately 10% are secondary to environmental exposure to pollutants, and approximately one-third are idiopathic.

TABLE 44.1: Classic history and physical

Middle-aged smoker with chronic cough and insidious onset of dyspnea on exertion that may be masked by sedentary lifestyle
Dyspnea, productive cough, and wheezing
"Pink puffer" (emphysema)—thin, barrel chest, pursed lips, tripod sitting position
"Blue bloater" (chronic bronchitis)—obese, cyanosis, and lower extremity edema secondary to cor pulmonale
Use of accessory muscles to breathe and inward motion of lower rib cage with inspiration (Hoover's sign)
Prolonged expiratory phase, decreased breath sounds, hyperinflated lungs, rhonchi, crackles, and/or wheezing on lung auscultation
Low liver edge palpable secondary to hepatomegaly from right heart failure, or lung hyperinflation causing inferior displacement without true hepatomegaly

TABLE 44.2: Potentially helpful laboratory tests

ABG	Hypoxemia
	Hypercapnia
	pH near normal (renal compensation)
	pH <7.3: concern for an acute process
BNP	Combined with clinical picture
	Helps differentiate COPD from CHF
Cardiac markers	Helps differentiate COPD from acute coronary syndrome
Alpha-1 antitrypsin deficiency screening	Screening test

ABG, arterial blood gas; BNP, B-type natriuretic peptide; CHF, congestive heart failure; COPD, chronic obstructive pulmonary disease.

Chest X-ray

- Used to exclude other pulmonary processes
- Very low sensitivity (only about 50%) for moderate to severe COPD
- Classic findings related to emphysematous hyperinflation:
  - Flattened diaphragms
  - Hyperinflated lungs
  - Increased radiolucency
  - Increased anterior-posterior diameter
  - Increased retrosternal airspace on lateral view
  - Bullae
- Chronic bronchitis:
  - No typical image findings

- Pulmonary hypertension:
  - Prominent hilar vasculature
  - Exaggerated tapering of vessels toward the periphery
- Right-sided heart failure secondary to pulmonary hypertension:
  - Cardiomegaly
  - Vascular engorgement
  - Pleural effusions

 TABLE 44.3: Chest x-ray (PA and Lateral): COPD

IV contrast	No
PO contrast	No
Amount of radiation	0.10 mSv

Classic Images

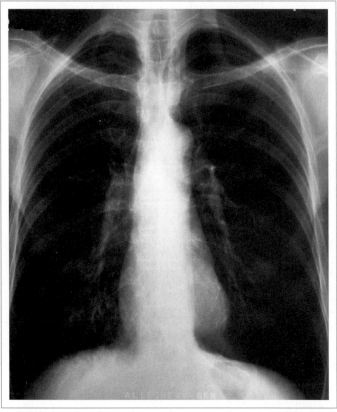

FIGURE 44.1: Posteroanterior chest x-ray of emphysema showing hyperinflated lungs, increased radiolucency, elongated heart shadow, flattened diaphragms, and a reduction in the prominence of peripheral pulmonary arteries. (From Daffner RH. Clinical Radiology: The Essentials, 3rd ed. Philadelphia: Lippincott Williams & Wilkins, 2007.)

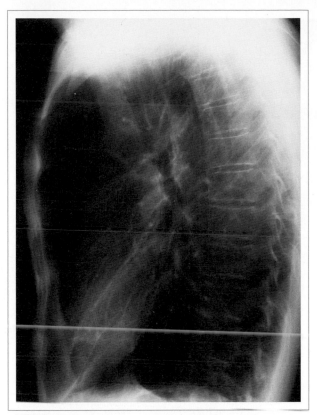

FIGURE 44.2: Lateral chest x-ray of emphysema showing increased anterior-posterior diameter and increased retrosternal airspace. (From Daffner RH. Clinical Radiology: The Essentials, 3rd ed. Philadelphia: Lippincott Williams & Wilkins, 2007.)

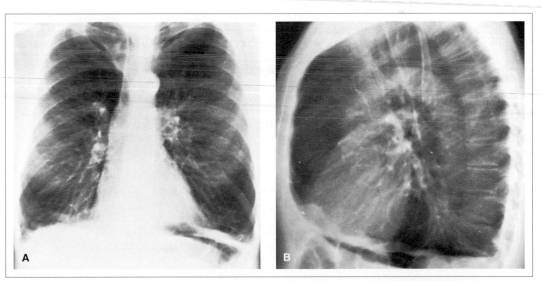

FIGURE 44.3: Pulmonary emphysema. (**A**) Frontal and (**B**) lateral views of the chest demonstrate severe overinflation of the lungs along with flattening and even a superiorly concave configuration of the hemidiaphragms. There is also increased size and lucency of the retrosternal airspace, an increase in the anteroposterior diameter of the chest, and a reduction in the number and caliber of peripheral pulmonary arteries. (From Eisenberg RL. An Atlas of Differential Diagnosis, 4th ed. Philadelphia: Lippincott Williams & Wilkins, 2003.)

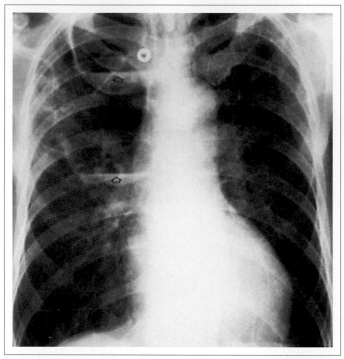

FIGURE 44.4: Pulmonary emphysema. Large bullae in the right upper lung. The presence of air-fluid levels (*arrows*) in the cystic spaces indicates superimposed infection. (From Eisenberg RL. An Atlas of Differential Diagnosis, 4th ed. Philadelphia: Lippincott Williams & Wilkins, 2003.)

Chest CT Scan

- More sensitive and specific for emphysema (especially with high-resolution CT)
- Not routinely recommended unless:
  - Diagnostic uncertainty
  - Suspicion of a secondary etiology
  - Evaluation for lung volume reduction surgery or bullectomy
- Provides descriptions of the extent and distribution (centriacinar or panacinar) of emphysema as well as airway diameters (high-resolution CT)
- Centriacinar: Look for round focal areas of low attenuation up to 1 cm in diameter amidst homogenous appearing lung parenchyma (Swiss cheese) in upper lung fields
- Panlobar: Look for lung simplification (large areas of uniformly low attenuation) predominantly with a lower lung distribution
- Note the presence of bullae (blebs): >1 cm thin-walled, air-filled structures located in the subpleural or intraparenchymal spaces
- Consider chest angiography with risk factors or concern for pulmonary embolus

 TABLE 44.4: Chest CT: COPD

IV contrast	No
PO contrast	No
Amount of radiation	7.0 mSv

Classic Images

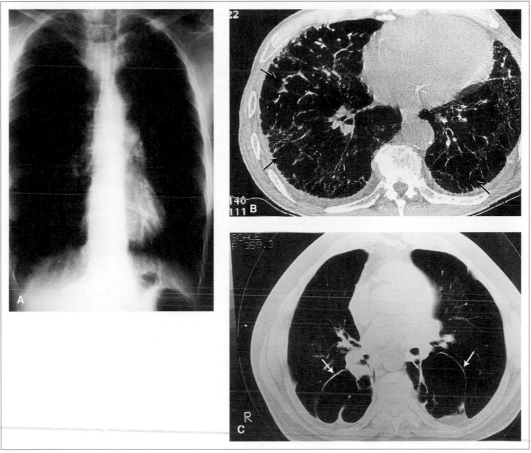

FIGURE 44.5: Pulmonary emphysema. **A:** Posteroanterior (PA) chest x-ray. Note that the hemidiaphragms are low in the chest, though not significantly flattened. The lung fields are overexposed relative to the mediastinum, and the heart is relatively small. **B:** High-resolution CT scan, axial chest. Multiple emphysematous bullae are readily identified (*arrows*). **C:** Bullous emphysema, CT scan, axial chest. Observe the large thin walled cystic air cavities in the superior segments of both lower lobes (*arrows*). (From Yochum TR and Rowe LJ. Yochum and Rowe's Essentials of Skeletal Radiology, 3rd ed. Philadelphia: Lippincott Williams & Wilkins, 2004.)

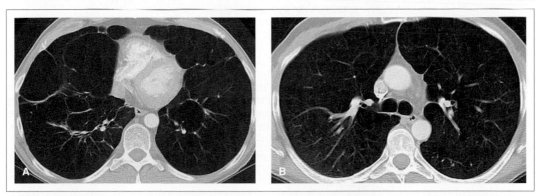

FIGURE 44.6: **A:** CT scan showing bullous emphysema in the lower lungs. **B:** CT scan at a more superior level shows less severe emphysema. (From Collins J and Stern EJ. Chest Radiology: The Essentials, 2nd ed. Philadelphia: Lippincott Williams & Wilkins, 2008.)

Basic Management

- Oxygen to maintain pulse oximetry >90% and PaO_2 >60 mm Hg
- Continuous pulse oximetry
- ECG—rule out cardiac involvement both as a cause of hypoxia and for ischemia secondary to hypoxia
- Avoid overoxygenation to prevent respiratory depression
- Continuous positive airway pressure (CPAP), biphasic positive airway pressure (BiPAP), mixed helium and oxygen (Heliox), or intubation may be considered
- Short-acting inhaled beta-agonists and short-acting anticholinergics
- Antibiotic use is controversial but may have benefit
- Magnesium may have a benefit in severe COPD exacerbations
- Hospital admission considerations:
  - Limitation of function at home
  - Significant dyspnea at home that puts the patient at risk for respiratory failure
  - Significant comorbid conditions
  - Failure to return to baseline pulmonary function tests (PFTs) and normal vital signs after treatment
- Smoking cessation counseling
- Pulmonary rehabilitation for select patients
- Home oxygen therapy for resting hypoxemia (PaO_2 ≤55 mm Hg)
- Outpatient pulmonary function tests

Summary

TABLE 44.5: Advantages and disadvantages of imaging modalities in COPD

Imaging modalities	Advantages	Disadvantages
Chest x-ray	Low cost Readily available Helps quickly assess for other processes, such as pneumonia and pneumothorax	Low sensitivity for COPD
CT scan	More sensitive and specific for emphysema Can identify many other non-COPD respiratory processes	No clear role if etiologies other than COPD are excluded Radiation exposure

COPD, chronic obstructive pulmonary disease.

45

Pneumonia

Khoshal Latifzai and Michael Osborne

Background

Pneumonia is an acute infection of the parenchyma of the lung that hinders appropriate gas exchange. In otherwise healthy individuals, it usually is overcome with proper antibiotic therapy. Comorbid conditions, however, complicate its clinical course, making pneumonia the sixth leading cause of death in the United States. The etiology of pneumonia (atypical bacterial organisms vs. typical; bacterial vs. viral) cannot be reliably determined from the imaging pattern of the infiltrate.

TABLE 45.1: Classic history and physical

Coughing, sputum production, pleuritic chest pain, rigors
Fever, tachypnea, hypoxemia
Diffuse fine crackles/rales or localized signs of consolidation (e.g., dullness to percussion, egophony)

TABLE 45.2: Potentially helpful laboratory tests

Sputum smear	Inflammation if ≥10 white blood cells per field. Gram stain may identify organism
Sputum culture	Tracheal or bronchial sample more accurate
Blood culture	In patients with infiltrates, it correlates well with the organism causing pneumonia, but is rarely useful
Pleural fluid analysis	(Smear and culture) Useful in pneumonia with empyema

Chest X-ray

- Findings range from patchy to dense and focal to diffuse infiltrates
- Lateral view to visualize retrocardiac infiltrates
- Cavitary infiltrates appear as a lucency (darkened area) within the lung parenchyma. It may have irregular margins that may be surrounded by consolidation, nodular or fibrotic (reticular) densities, or both. The wall surrounding the cavity may be thick or thin and calcification can exist around the cavity.
- For aspiration which occurs while sitting, look for involvement of the basal segments of the lower lobe
- For aspiration which occurs when recumbent, look for involvement of the posterior segments of the upper lobes and the apical segments of the lower lobes
- An abscess will appear as a solitary cavitary with an air-fluid level and is typically located in the dependent portions of the lung
- When empyema is present, there may be extension of the air-fluid level to the chest wall, extension of the air-fluid level across fissure lines, or a tapering border of the air-fluid collection
- Evaluate the costophrenic angle for fluid which suggests effusion or empyema
- Blunting of the costophrenic angle occurs with approximately 200 cc of fluid
- Obtain a lateral chest decubitus radiograph to assess pleural fluid; layering fluid is mobile, non-layering is loculated

TABLE 45.3: Helpful associated structures

Heart	
Right middle lobe: blurring of right heart border	
Left lingula: blurring of left heart border	
Diaphragm	
Lower lobe: blurring of hemidiaphragm	

 TABLE 45.4: Chest X-ray (PA and Lateral): pneumonia

IV contrast	No
PO contrast	No
Amount of radiation	0.10 mSv

Classic Images

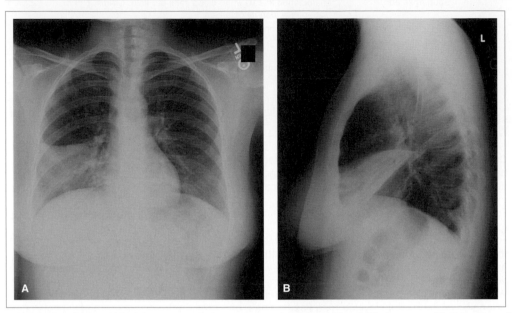

FIGURE 45.1: Right middle lobe pneumonia in posteroanterior (**A**) and lateral (**B**) chest x-ray. Right heart border is obscured by infiltrate as this lobe abuts pericardium. This demonstrates why auscultation posteriorly may not detect the consolidation, but listening in the right midlateral chest can. (*Courtesy of Yale-New Haven Hospital, New Haven, CT.*)

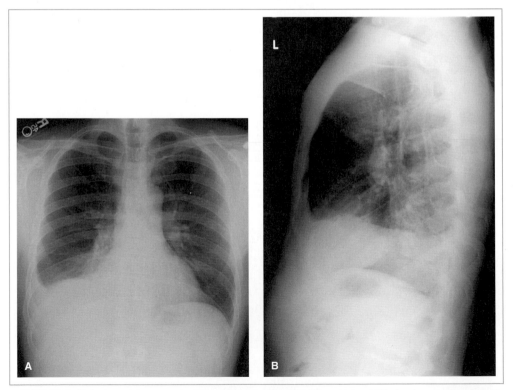

FIGURE 45.2: Right lower lobe pneumonia in posteroanterior (PA) (**A**) and lateral (**B**) chest x-ray. Right heart border is maintained since the infiltrate extends posterior to the heart border. Note the effusion blunting the right costophrenic angle in PA image (**A**) and posteriorly blunting in lateral (**B**). (*Courtesy of Yale-New Haven Hospital, New Haven, CT.*)

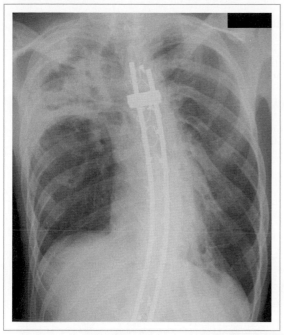

FIGURE 45.3: Right upper lobe cavitary pneumonia in anteroposterior chest x-ray. (*Courtesy of Yale-New Haven Hospltal, New Haven, CT.*)

Bedside Lung Ultrasound

- Low-frequency (3–5 MIlz) curvilinear or phased array probe placed in the coronal plane in the right or left upper quadrant
  - Right pleural spacc: place the probe in the right anterior to midaxillary line with indicator position toward the axilla; use the hyperechoic white diaphragm as a landmark and slide the probe cephalad to image the pleural space
  - Left pleural space: place the probe similarly but in the posterior axillary line
  - Useful for needle-guided aspiration and drainage of a potential pleural effusion or empyema
  - An anechoic (black) area may be seen above the diaphragm if pleural fluid is present
  - Tissue-like lung consolidation may be seen floating in the pleural fluid

Classic Images

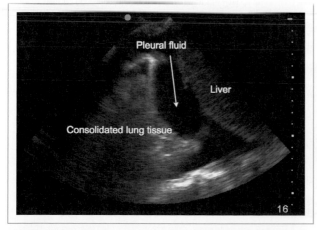

FIGURE 45.4: Coronal plane, low-frequency probe placed in the right upper quadrant demonstrates pleural fluid and lung tissue consolidation consistent with pneumonia. (*Courtesy of SLR Emergency ultrasound division, New York, NY.*)

CT Scan

- Can assess for pneumonia, lung abscess, tumor, pleural effusions and septations, pleural thickening, tumors, clots, aortic dissection or aneurysm, pneumothorax, pericardial effusion, small pleural effusions, and fractures
- Found more often than pulmonary embolus (PE) on CT for PE, in one study
- 5–10% of pneumocystis jiroveci (formerly known as pneumocystis carinii) pneumonia will only be evident on a CT scan
- Infiltrates appear as streaks in the lung field affected

 TABLE 45.5: CT scan: pneumonia

IV contrast	No
PO contrast	No
Amount of radiation	7.0 mSv

Classic Images

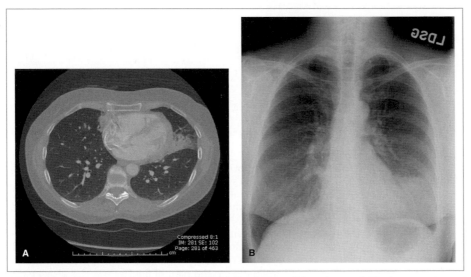

FIGURE 45.5: CT scan of chest with a lingular infiltrate seen (**A**), and same infiltrate on posteroanterior chest x-ray (CXR) (**B**). Note how on CXR the heart border is obscured. (*Image courtesy of Yale-New Haven Hospital, New Haven, CT.*)

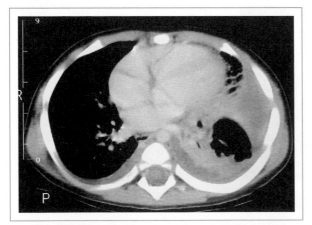

FIGURE 45.6: CT image demonstrates complicated pneumonia with loculated empyema. (From Mulholland MW, Maier RV, eds. Greenfield's Surgery: Scientific Principles and Practice, 4th ed. Philadelphia: Lippincott Williams & Wilkins, 2006.)

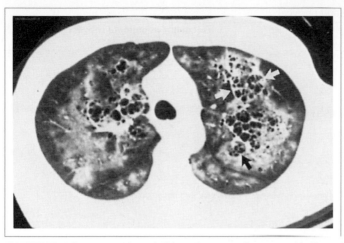

FIGURE 45.7: Pneumocystis carinii (now known as Pneumocystis jiroveci) pneumonia. Discrete thin- and thick-walled cysts occurring in association with consolidated lung. Coalescence of cysts results in the formation of a few bizarre-shaped cysts (*arrows*). Note that the intervening parenchyma appears grossly normal. (From Eisenberg RL. An Atlas of Differential Diagnosis, 4th ed. Philadelphia: Lippincott Williams & Wilkins, 2003.)

Summary

TABLE 45.6: Advantages and disadvantages of imaging modalities in pneumonia

Imaging modalities	Advantages	Disadvantages
Chest radiograph	Low cost Low radiation Fairly sensitive	May miss early pneumonia
Ultrasound	Low cost Rapid No radiation Assists thoracentesis	Difficult to differentiate location Difficult to differentiate type
CT scan	More sensitive than CXR May pick up alternate diagnoses	Cost Radiation exposure

CXR, chest x-ray.

46

Pulmonary Embolism

Nathan Teismann, Joshua Penn, and Christopher Kabrhel

Background

Acute pulmonary embolism (PE) is estimated to account for at least 1.5% of all deaths in the United States. Estimates of the overall incidence vary widely, and given the elusive nature of its diagnosis, most authorities believe that at least half of cases are clinically unrecognized. Adding to the complexity is the tremendous variability in severity, which ranges from asymptomatic and relatively benign to rapidly fatal. Given these factors, PE ranks among the most perplexing entities facing the practicing clinician.

No test for PE is perfectly sensitive or specific, so all results must be considered within the context of pretest probability assessment.

TABLE 46.1: Classic history and physical

	Frequency in patients with PE
Dyspnea	73%
Tachypnea	70%
Abrupt onset pleuritic chest pain	66%
Tachycardia	30%
Unilateral leg pain/swelling	26%
Hypotension, JVD and a right-sided S3 with right ventricular dysfunction	
Active malignancy, recent surgery or immobilization, history of VTE, and/or hypercoagulable state	
Additional risk factors for women include cigarette smoking, oral contraceptive use, and/or obesity	

PE, pulmonary embolism; JVD, jugular venous distension; VTE, venous thromboembolism.

TABLE 46.2: Potentially helpful laboratory tests

D-dimer: Test characteristics depend on the assay used
   Most have high sensitivity (90–95%), but low specificity (45–60%)
   Often elevated in patients at high risk for PE (pregnant/postpartum, postoperative, elderly, cancer)
   Extremely useful if negative in low-risk patients.

Creatinine: Impaired renal function can be a contraindication to imaging with IV contrast; calculating GFR is required for patients who need CT

ABG: To assess A-a gradient but now considered to be of limited diagnostic value

Troponin I: Elevated in 30–40% of patients with moderate to large PE; a risk factor for poor outcome

BNP and NT-proBNP: Limited sensitivity and specificity for PE but, as with troponin, may offer prognostic information as degree of elevation correlates with clinical severity

ABG, arterial blood gas; GFR, glomerular filtration rate; PE, pulmonary embolism.

Chest X-ray

- Initial chest x-ray findings may be normal
- Over a period of time, the lung fields may show atelectasis, infiltrate, pleural effusion, or elevated hemidiaphragm
- Can be useful by demonstrating alternative diagnoses (e.g., pneumothorax and pneumonia
- Westermark sign: is a dilatation of the pulmonary vessels proximal to the embolism with often a sharp cut off from collapsed distal vessels
- Hampton hump: a wedge-shaped infiltrate with the apex pointed toward the hilum (late finding)

 TABLE 46.3: Chest X-ray (Portable AP): pulmonary embolism

IV contrast	No
PO contrast	No
Amount of radiation	0.02 mSv

Classic Images

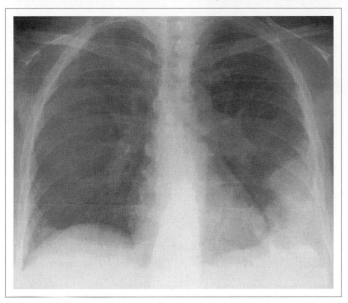

FIGURE 46.1: Parenchymal opacity in the left lower lung zone and prominent left pulmonary artery. (From Kahn GP and Lynch JP. Pulmonary Disease Diagnosis and Therapy: A Practical Approach. Philadelphia: Lippincott Williams & Wilkins, 1997.)

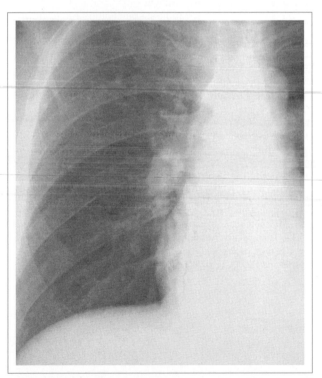

FIGURE 46.2: Enlargement of the right hilum from distention of the descending right pulmonary artery from a massive pulmonary embolus. The distention is not the result of raised pulmonary artery pressure proximal to the clot but of distention by the thrombus. Note the abrupt change of caliber in the descending pulmonary artery, which is accompanied by diminished vascularity in the lower lobe. (From Kahn GP and Lynch JP. Pulmonary Disease Diagnosis and Therapy: A Practical Approach. Philadelphia: Lippincott Williams & Wilkins, 1997.)

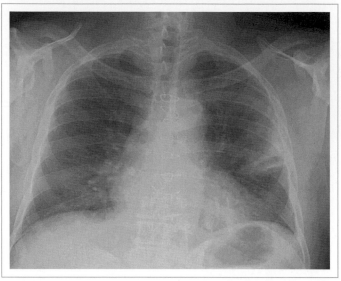

FIGURE 46.3: Hampton's hump. (*Image courtesy of James G. Smirniotopoulos, MD. Center for Neuroscience and Regenerative Medicine, Uniformed Services University, Bethesda, MD.*)

Chest CT Angiography

- CT angiography (CTA) has supplanted catheter-based pulmonary angiography as the standard imaging test of choice to diagnose PE
- One or more low-attenuation filling defects suggest the presence of PE
- The sensitivity of CTA has been shown to be 83–98% in most studies; specificities range from 90% to 96%
  - The sensitivity increases with concurrent use of CT venography (see below), and may increase further as CT scanner technology improves
- The largest study of CTA to date, PIOPED II, has demonstrated that diagnostic accuracy is improved when clinical risk assessment is combined with the results of CTA
  - The likelihood of PE in patients with a positive CTA and a high, intermediate, or low pretest risk was 96%, 92%, and 58%, respectively
  - The likelihood that PE was absent in patients with a negative CTA and a low, intermediate, or high pretest risk was 96%, 89%, and 60%, respectively
- Identifies or rules out other items in the differential diagnosis including pneumonia, aortic dissection, or malignancy
- The use of CTA is relatively contraindicated in pregnant women and in patients with renal failure or IV contrast allergies; in these patient populations, D-dimer may be useful in conjunction with another imaging modality such as lower extremity ultrasound
- Lower extremity CT venogram is almost always done in conjunction with the chest CTA; image acquisition is timed with venous run-off of IV contrast into the pelvis and legs (see chapter 65)

 TABLE 46.4: CTA: pulmonary embolism

IV contrast	Yes, to evaluate vasculature
PO contrast	No
Amount of radiation	15 mSv

Classic Images

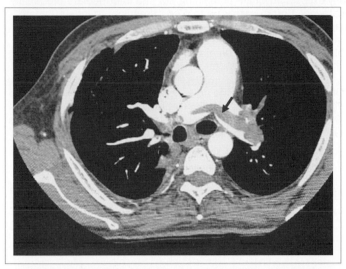

FIGURE 46.4: Massive pulmonary embolism shown by spiral CT. The low-density embolus is easily visualized "saddling" the left and right main pulmonary arteries (*arrow*) surrounded by the dense white contrast. The left pulmonary artery is the one most involved. (From Topol EJ, Califf RM, et al. Textbook of Cardiovascular Medicine, 3rd ed. Philadelphia: Lippincott Williams & Wilkins, 2006.)

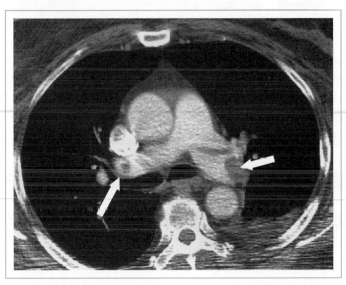

FIGURE 46.5: Bilateral pulmonary embolism (*arrows*) demonstrated by contrast-enhanced spiral computed tomography scan. (From Crapo JD, Glassroth J, Karlinsky JB, et al. Baum's Textbook of Pulmonary Diseases, 7th ed. Philadelphia: Lippincott Williams & Wilkins, 2004.)

Ventilation-Perfusion Scanning
- Ventilation perfusion (V/Q) scintigraphy has been replaced by CTA at most institutions; however
- Indicated when CTA is unavailable or contraindicated due to renal failure or contrast allergy
- To obtain the ventilation portion of the study, the patient inhales an aerosolized radiotracer (typically Technetium 99 or a xenon isotope) and is imaged with a high-resolution gamma camera. Either before or after the ventilation scan, an IV radiotracer is administered and the patient's lungs are imaged in multiple projections to create the perfusion scan. The images are compared, looking for an area that is ventilated but not perfused, suggesting the presence of a PE.

- Results are reported as normal, low probability, indeterminate, or high probability of PE. Because of poor sensitivity/specificity, many experts advocate combining low and intermediate probability results into an "indeterminate" category. Unfortunately, up to 67% of results are indeterminate.
- Although a normal V/Q scan reliably rules out the presence of PE, only a small percentage of patients (14% in PIOPED I) will have a normal study. Similarly, only a small number (13% in PIOPED I) will have a high-probability scan. Because the majority of patients will have a low probability or indeterminate result, this modality allows for a definitive diagnosis in a relatively small percentage of patients.
- While somewhat difficult to quantify, data support that the amount of radiation received by a fetus is greater with a V/Q scan than with a CT angiogram, regardless of trimester. The average fetal radiation of a CT angiogram is 0.01 mSV while the fetal exposure of a V/Q scan is 0.12 mSV. The actual amount of radiation varies by protocol, fetal size/gestational age, and shielding technique.

 TABLE 46.5: V/Q scan: pulmonary embolism

IV contrast	No, IV radiotracer for perfusion portion of study
PO contrast	No
Amount of radiation	2.2 mSv

Classic Images

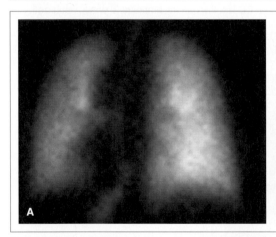 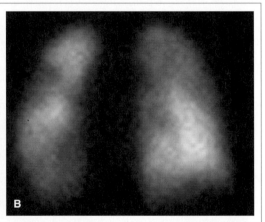

FIGURE 46.6: Ventilation-perfusion imaging in diagnosis of pulmonary embolism. **A:** Ventilation image, obtained with 99mTc pentetate aerosol, shows homogenous ventilation on posterior view. **B:** Matched perfusion image shows large (segmental) perfusion defects in the left midlung, and in the lateral segment of the left lower lobe. There is also decreased perfusion in the right upper lobe. The presence of unmatched segmental abnormalities indicates a high probability for pulmonary embolism. (From Crapo JD, Glassroth J, Karlinsky JB, et al. Baum's Textbook of Pulmonary Diseases, 7th ed. Philadelphia: Lippincott Williams & Wilkins, 2004.)

Pulmonary Angiography

- Considered the gold standard imaging test for PE, but because of its labor-intensive and invasive nature, it is rarely performed at most institutions.
- Contrast boluses are injected via a balloon-tipped catheter (typically placed percutaneously through the femoral vein) into the pulmonary artery. A filling defect obstructing a vessel or the outline of an embolus within a vessel indicates the presence of PE.
- Large, proximal PE are easily seen with this modality; however, considerable interobserver disagreement exists when evaluating subsegmental PEs isolated to the distal pulmonary arterial tree. Nonetheless, a normal pulmonary angiogram is felt to rule out clinically significant PE.

 TABLE 46.6: Pulmonary angiogram: pulmonary embolism

IV contrast	Yes, to evaluate vasculature
PO contrast	No
Amount of radiation	5 mSv

Classic Images

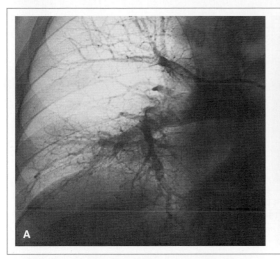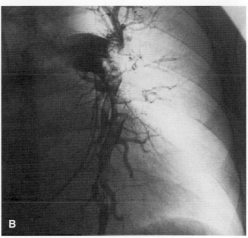

FIGURE 46.7: Angiograms demonstrate extensive intraluminal filling defects in both right (**A**) and left (**B**) pulmonary arteries. (From Baim DS. Grossman's Cardiac Catheterization, Angiography, and Intervention, 7th ed. Philadelphia: Lippincott Williams & Wilkins, 2005.)

Bedside Echocardiography

- Large PE can cause acute right-heart pressure overload. Resulting in right atrial (RA) and right ventricular (RV) enlargement, inferior vena cava (IVC) dilatation, increased tricuspid jet velocity, abnormal motion of the interventricular septum, and right ventricular free wall hypokinesis with preserved apical contractility ("McConnell's sign").
- Certain echocardiography findings may be easily apparent on bedside sonography, such as increased RV to LV ratio and abnormal appearance of the interventricular septum.
- Normally the RV diameter just below the tricuspid valve is less than 60% of the LV diameter just below the mitral valve. RV size greater than LV size is almost certainly abnormal and suggests markedly elevated right-heart pressures and possibly PE. This relationship is best visualized using the apical four-chamber view.
- In cases of PE with RV pressure overload, the septum, which normally assumes a convex shape arching away from the LV chamber, may bow inward toward the LV in the apical four-chamber view. From the parasternal short axis window, septal flattening may create a D-shaped (rather than O-shaped) appearance of the LV.
- No sonographic finding has adequate sensitivity or specificity to definitively rule in or rule out the diagnosis of PE.
- Occasionally, a clot may be visualized directly within the proximal pulmonary artery, RA, RV, or IVC (a so-called "thrombus-in-transit").

TABLE 46.7: Signs of right ventricular pressure overload on echo

RA and RV enlargement
IVC dilatation
Interventricular septum bowing inward toward LV
Increased tricuspid jet velocity
RV free wall hypokinesis with preserved apical contractility

IVC, inferior vena cava; LV, left ventricle; RA, right auricle; RV, right ventricle.

Classic Images

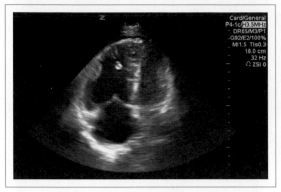

FIGURE 46.8: Apical four-chamber view of the heart in a patient with large pulmonary embolism. The right ventricle is dilated as a result of elevated pulmonary artery pressures. (*Courtesy of Justin Davis, MD, Kaiser Permanente: Oakland Medical Center, Oakland, CA.*)

Basic Management

- Assess airway, breathing, and circulation and provide initial stabilization
- Prompt anticoagulation with heparin or low-molecular-weight heparin is the mainstay of therapy
- If PE has been definitively diagnosed and the patient is unstable, treatment with thrombolytics is indicated
- The use of thrombolytics in patients with laboratory or echocardiographic evidence of RV dysfunction but with normal blood pressure remains controversial
- Alternative therapies include surgical or catheter-based embolectomy and IVC filter placement
- The clinical significance of small, subsegmental PE is unclear and in certain cases the risks of treatment with anticoagulation may outweigh the benefits

Summary

TABLE 46.8: Advantages and disadvantages of imaging modalities in pulmonary embolism

Imaging modality	Advantages	Disadvantages
Chest x-ray	Rapid Low radiation Sensitive and specific Widely available	Initial examination usually normal Most findings not specific Radiation exposure, especially in young women
CT angiogram (CTA)	Rapid Noninvasive Can detect alternative diagnosis	IV contrast Radiation exposure Contrast bolus must be timed accurately
CT venogram	Increases sensitivity of CTA Identifies blood clots in the pelvis that may not be detected by ultrasound	IV contrast Radiation exposure
V/Q scan	Can be used when IV contrast is contraindicated	Frequently does not provide definitive results May be difficult to obtain More radiation to fetus than CTA (pregnancy issue)
Lower extremity ultrasound	Limited examination can be done by emergency physicians Inexpensive	Diagnosis of PE is presumptive based on associated symptoms
Pulmonary angiography	Gold standard	Invasive Labor intensive Limited availability
Bedside sonography	Rapid Can be performed at bedside even in unstable patients No radiation	Cannot confirm or rule out PE Operator dependent Body habitus limitations

PE, pulmonary embolism; V/Q, ventilation-perfusion.

47 Acute Respiratory Distress Syndrome

Faizan H. Arshad and Christopher H. Lee

Background

Acute respiratory distress syndrome (ARDS) is recognized as the most severe manifestation of lung pathology on the spectrum of acute lung injury (ALI).

It is the result of increased pulmonary vascular permeability and develops in response to lung injury. ARDS is characterized by

- The rapid onset of diffuse, bilateral pulmonary infiltrates on chest x-ray (CXR)
- Noncardiogenic pulmonary edema
- Refractory hypoxia
- Decreased lung compliance ("stiff lungs")

In the United States, the incidence and mortality rates of both ALI and ARDS are similar. The age-adjusted incidence of ALI has been described as 86 per 100,000 person-years with an associated in-hospital mortality of 39%. Similarly, ARDS has an age-adjusted incidence of 64 per 100,000 person-years with an in-hospital morality of 41%. Additionally, 10–15% of patients admitted to an intensive care unit and 20% of mechanically ventilated patients meet the clinical criteria for ARDS.

TABLE 47.1: Classic history and physical

Pulmonary history
  Pneumonia
  Gastric aspiration
  Pulmonary contusion
  Fat emboli
  Near-drowning
  Inhalation injury
  Reperfusion pulmonary edema

Extra-pulmonary history
  Sepsis
  Severe trauma
  Multiple transfusions
  Cardiopulmonary bypass
  Drug overdose
  Acute pancreatitis
  Burns
  Trauma
  Respiratory distress
  Hypoxia

TABLE 47.2: Potentially helpful laboratory tests

ABG	Assess the PaO_2 and the alveolar-arterial O_2 gradient (elevated)
BNP	<100 pg/mL suggests noncardiac pulmonary edema Sensitivity 27%, specificity 95% Positive predictive value 90% Negative predictive value 44%

ABG, arterial blood gas; BNP, B-type natriuretic peptide.

Chest Radiograph

- Clinical symptoms often precede radiologic diagnosis
- Bilateral widespread patchy ill-defined opacities without cardiomegaly, vascular redistribution, or pleural effusions

- Diffuse ground glass opacification develops because of increased inflammatory fluid exudates into the interstitium and airspace and may lead to frank consolidation
- With disease progression, pulmonary vessels lose their margins, hazy opacities become more homogenous, and the hemidiaphragms and cardiac margins become blurred
- Findings plateau over a variable amount of time
- Any new consolidation may indicate a hospital-acquired infection
- As abnormalities on chest film begin to resolve, there may be residual coarse reticular opacities and cysts as a result of lung repair and barotrauma

 TABLE 47.3: Chest x-ray (Portable AP): ARDS

IV contrast	No
PO contrast	No
Amount of radiation	0.02 mSv

Classic Images

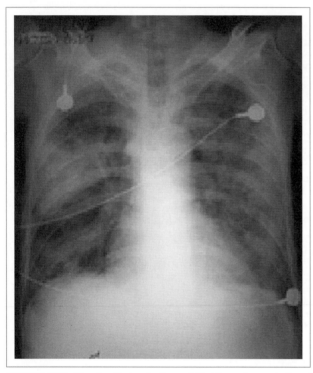

FIGURE 47.1: Chest radiograph of an adult with acute respiratory distress syndrome. (From American Association of Critical Care Nurses. Clinical Simulations: Shock Management. Philadelphia: Lippincott Williams & Wilkins, 2000.)

Chest CT Scan
- Heterogenous patchy distribution with regions of normal lung
- A single scan may demonstrate a near-normal area in nondependent lung zones (parasternal regions), ground glass opacification in the middle lung zones, and consolidated parenchyma in the most dependent zones (paravertebral regions)
- Ground glass opacification, though nonspecific, is the most common pattern
- Parenchymal opacification in a dependent lung represents compression atelectasis and rapidly resolves with repositioning of the patient
- Parenchymal opacification in a nondependent lung field may represent blossoming pneumonia or any other abnormality
  - Consolidation seems to be more prevalent in pulmonary ARDS whereas ground glass opacities are seen more commonly in extra-pulmonary ARDS, though both can be seen in either condition

- Bronchial dilation, thought to be secondary to the effects of inflammatory exudate on the airways, is also commonly seen

 TABLE 47.4: Chest CT ARDS

IV contrast	No
PO contrast	No
Amount of radiation	7.0 mSv

Classic Images

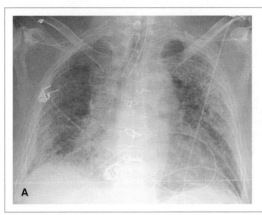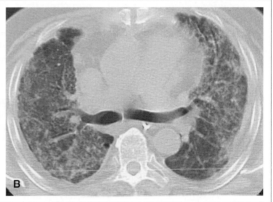

FIGURE 47.2: Acute respiratory distress syndrome (ARDS). This 69-year-old man had undergone a liver transplant several years earlier and developed ARDS as a result of herpes simplex virus pneumonia. **A:** Anteroposterior recumbent chest radiograph shows an endotracheal tube and bilateral interstitial and alveolar lung disease. **B:** Computed tomographic scan shows bilateral diffuse ground glass and reticular opacities. (From Collins J and Stern EJ. Chest Radiology: The Essentials, 2nd ed. Philadelphia: Lippincott Williams & Wilkins, 2008.)

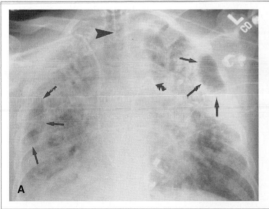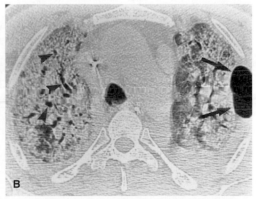

FIGURE 47.3: A: Anteroposterior recumbent chest radiograph shows bilateral alveolar lung disease (ALD). An endotracheal tube is in place (*arrowhead*). Oval collections of air are present in the periphery of the lungs, representing pneumatoceles from barotrauma (*arrows*). A right subclavian pulmonary artery catheter was placed to measure pulmonary capillary wedge pressure. The pressure was low, consistent with noncardiogenic pulmonary edema of acute respiratory distress syndrome. The tip of the catheter is projected over the left lower lobe pulmonary artery (*curved arrow*). **B:** Computed tomographic scan shows bilateral ALD, multiple abnormal rounded and tubular air collections within the lung representing dilated airways (*arrowheads*), and a peripheral pneumatocele on the left (*arrows*). (From Collins J and Stern EJ. Chest Radiology: The Essentials, 2nd ed. Philadelphia: Lippincott Williams & Wilkins, 2008.)

Bedside Lung Ultrasound

- Some studies have validated the ability to diagnose acute interstitial syndrome due to ARDS, cardiogenic pulmonary edema, pneumonia, and other interstitial syndromes with ultrasound
- Sensitivity and specificity are reportedly >90% for alveolar interstitial syndrome
- Utilize a 5–7 MHz microconvex phased-array probe in a longitudinal plane perpendicular to the ribs, with the probe indicator pointing cephalad
  - Linear and curvilinear probes may also be used
- Locate the pleural line: hyperechoic horizontal line approximately 0.5 cm below the chest wall tissues. Lung sliding in B-mode is visualized as the visceral pleura moves across the parietal pleura.
- Look for comet-tail artifacts that arise from the pleural line as sound waves reverberate between the pleural layers
- Look for A-lines: horizontal hyperechoic lines appearing parallel to and at regularly spaced intervals below the pleural line
- Look for B-lines: type of comet-tail artifact appearing as vertical hyperechoic lines arising from the pleural line, which erase A-lines and extend to the edge of the screen without fading
- Lung rockets: several B-lines visible between two ribs in one longitudinal view evoking the pattern of a rocket at liftoff
  - The number of B-lines may correspond to the degree of lung aeration loss
  - B-lines 7 mm apart represent interstitial edema caused by thickened interlobular septa
  - B-lines 3 mm apart or less represent alveolar edema caused by areas of ground glass
- A positive study is one in which there are at least two rib-spaces on each side of the thorax demonstrating at least three B-lines per field, excluding the last intercostal space (where B-lines may occur physiologically)

 TABLE 47.5: Lung ultrasound: ARDS

IV contrast	No
PO contrast	No
Amount of radiation	None

Classic Images

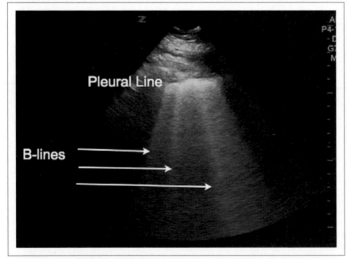

FIGURE 47.4: Classic portrayal of B-lines in a patient with acute respiratory distress syndrome. (*Courtesy of Yale New Haven Hospital, New Haven, CT.*)

Basic Management

- Oxygen
- Consider noninvasive versus mechanical ventilation
- Identification and treatment of the underlying condition
- Admission to an intensive care unit
- Mechanical ventilation with tidal volumes of 6 mL/kg of ideal body weight
- Increased use of positive-end expiratory pressure (PEEP) to increase alveolar recruitment

Summary

TABLE 47.6: Advantages and disadvantages of imaging modalities in acute respiratory distress syndrome

Imaging modalities	Advantages	Disadvantages
Plain film	Low radiation Portable Rapid acquisition	Variable quality Findings may lag behind clinical condition Findings may be nonspecific
CT scan	Gold standard Provides information regarding extent of ARDS Can modify management (e.g., ↑ PEEP to improve alveolar recruitment)	Radiation exposure Time-consuming
Ultrasound	Low cost Minimal patient discomfort No radiation exposure Bedside availability Rapid acquisition	Wide differential diagnosis Operator-dependent Technical and interpretive expertise

ARDS, acute respiratory distress syndrome; CT, computed tomographic; PEEP, positive-end expiratory pressure.

48

Pneumothorax

Glen D. Blomstrom and Michael J. Rest

Background

A pneumothorax occurs when gas replaces liquid in the pleural space, between the parietal and visceral pleura. This pathologic condition arises from one of the following mechanisms: (1) direct communication with the atmosphere (most common), (2) communication with the atmosphere via the alveoli (second most common), or (3) presence of gas producing organisms in the pleural space. Pneumothoraces are either spontaneous or traumatic. Spontaneous pneumothoraces can be further divided into primary, secondary, and catamenial. Traumatic pneumothoraces can be divided into iatrogenic and noniatrogenic. Tension pneumothorax describes a one-way valve in the pleural space with air entering from the atmosphere, either directly through the chest wall or via the airways/alveoli. Because air enters but cannot exit the pleural space, pressure increases. The tension pneumothorax compresses the lungs, the vasculature, and the mediastinum, causing hemodynamic compromise.

TABLE 48.1: Classic history and physical

Primary spontaneous
   Tall thin male
   Smoker or history of atmospheric pressure changes

Secondary spontaneous
   COPD, lung cancer, pulmonary metastases or HIV lung disease
   Barrel-chested, emphysematous body habitus
   Ill- or frail-appearing patient

Catamenial spontaneous
   Menstruating female
   Endometriosis

Iatrogenic traumatic
   History of lung biopsy, subclavian or internal jugular vein catheterization, or
     thoracentesis

Noniatrogenic traumatic   Chest trauma

Tension pneumothorax
   Tachypnea, hypotension, tachycardia, hypoxemia
   Cyanosis, a deviated trachea, and/or jugular venous distention

All pneumothoraces
   Sudden pleuritic chest pain
   Dyspnea
   Shortness of breath

COPD, chronic obstructive pulmonary disease; HIV, human immunodeficiency virus.

Chest X-ray
- Sensitivity 76% and specificity 100%
- Upright film
  - Look for a white margin of visceral pleura separated from parietal pleura, and absence of vascular markings beyond the visceral pleural margin; frequently seen at the apex
  - Size can be estimated by measuring the maximum apical interpleural distance; each centimeter approximates 10% collapse of the lung; that is, interpleural space of 3 cm indicates roughly 30% collapse of the lung
- Supine view
  - Relative lucency of the entire lung or an abnormally deep lateral costophrenic angle (deep sulcus sign)
  - A small contralateral or ipsilateral shift of the trachea and mediastinum can be a normal phenomenon not suggestive of tension pneumothorax
- Expiratory view
  - Questionable utility

TABLE 48.2: Helpful associated structures

Pleura	Thin white visceral pleural line shows the outline of the retracted lung
Diaphragm	Abnormally deep lateral costophrenic angle ipsilateral to the pneumothorax

 TABLE 48.3: Chest x-ray (Portable AP): pneumothorax

IV contrast	No
PO contrast	No
Amount of radiation	0.02 mSv

Classic Images

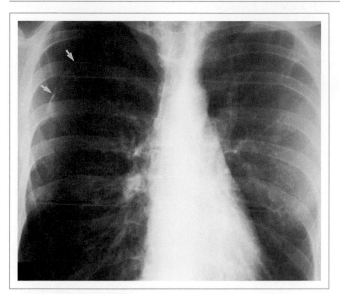

FIGURE 48.1: A subtle pneumothorax on right without mediastinal shift. (From Daffner RH. Clinical Radiology: The Essentials, 3rd ed. Philadelphia: Lippincott Williams & Wilkins, 2007.)

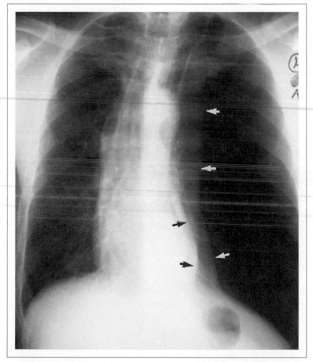

FIGURE 48.2: Tension pneumothorax in a 30-year-old man. The left ventricular contour is medial (*black arrows*) to the line of the pleura (*white arrows*) against the air-filled left chest. The heart and mediastinal structures are shifted toward the right. Notice the flattened left diaphragm. (From Topol EJ, Prystowsky EN, et al. Textbook of Cardiovascular Medicine, 3rd ed. Philadelphia: Lippincott Williams & Wilkins, 2006.)

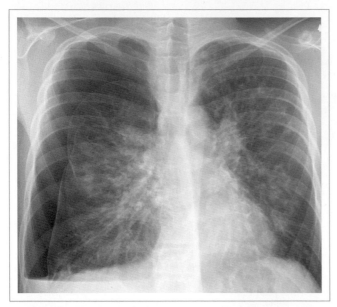

FIGURE 48.3: Posteroanterior chest radiograph of an 18-year-old man with cystic fibrosis shows a large right hydropneumothorax and severe bilateral cystic bronchiectasis. (From Collins J and Stern EJ. Chest Radiology: The Essentials, 2nd ed. Philadelphia: Lippincott Williams & Wilkins, 2008.)

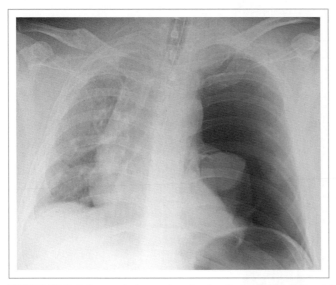

FIGURE 48.4: Anteroposterior supine chest radiograph of a 35-year-old man involved in a motor vehicle crash shows a large left pneumothorax, collapse of the left lung, and shift of the mediastinum to the right. The findings suggest a tension pneumothorax, which requires immediate decompression. (From Collins J and Stern EJ. Chest Radiology: The Essentials, 2nd ed. Philadelphia: Lippincott Williams & Wilkins, 2008.)

Chest CT Scan
- Gold standard for detecting and evaluating the size of a pneumothorax
- Sensitivity and specificity approaches 100%
- Differentiates pneumothorax from emphysematous-like changes or bullae
- In traumatic pneumothoraces, allows for evaluation of other traumatic injuries
- Can guide chest tube placement if there are pleural adhesions
- Can evaluate a chest tube, especially one that is not performing as anticipated

TABLE 48.4: Chest CT: pneumothorax

IV contrast	No
PO contrast	No
Amount of radiation	7.0 mSv

Classic Images

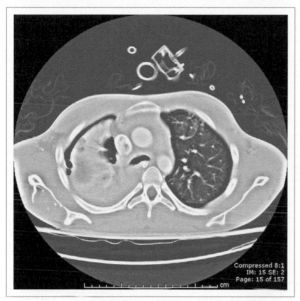

FIGURE 48.5: A small right pneumothorax with a chest tube in place. (*Courtesy of Yale-New Haven Hospital, New Haven, CT.*)

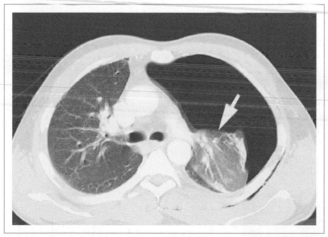

FIGURE 48.6: Large left pneumothorax with complete collapse of the left lung. (From Daffner RH. Clinical Radiology: The Essentials, 3rd ed. Philadelphia: Lippincott Williams & Wilkins, 2007.)

Bedside Lung Ultrasound
- In traumatic pneumothorax, sensitivity 68–98%, specificity 79–99%
- Highly sensitive in spontaneous pneumothorax
- Difficult to distinguish diseased lung versus bleb versus pneumothorax
- With the indicator pointed cephalad, place the probe in the second/third intercostal space in the midclavicular line and slide the probe caudally
- The upper rib-pleural line-lower rib profile is referred to as the bat sign

TABLE 48.5: Ultrasound findings

Normal lung findings	Visible sliding at the level of the pleura in B-mode
	Comet tail: vertical reverberation artifacts arising from the pleural line
	Seashore sign in M-mode
Lung findings suggestive of a pneumothorax	Loss of pleural sliding
	Absence of comet tails
	Stratosphere sign or bar code sign in M-mode
Other absent lung sliding etiologies	Patients who are not spontaneously breathing
	Complete atelectasis
	Apnea
	Pleural scarring
	Mainstem intubation on the contralateral side
Lung point	Transition between collapsed and normally expanded lung
	Difficult to locate, 100% specific for pneumothorax when identified

Classic Images

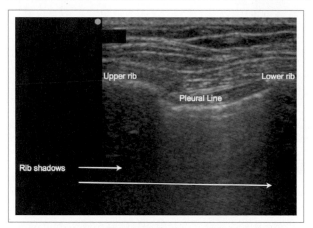

FIGURE 48.7: Normal lung. The bat sign (rib shadow, pleura, rib shadow). (*Courtesy of St. Luke's/Roosevelt emergency ultrasound division, New York, NY.*)

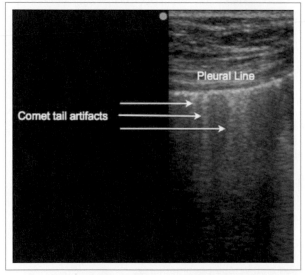

FIGURE 48.8: Normal lung. Bright white pleural line with comet-tail artifacts (*arrows*). (*Courtesy of St. Luke's/ Roosevelt emergency ultrasound division, New York, NY.*)

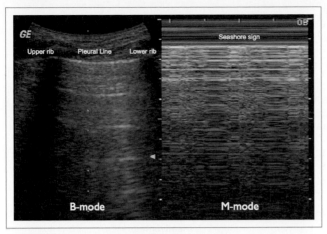

FIGURE 48.9: M-mode demonstrating the seashore sign seen in a normal lung; superficial parallel "waves" transitioning to diffuse scattered "sand." (*Courtesy of St. Luke's/Roosevelt emergency ultrasound division, New York, NY.*)

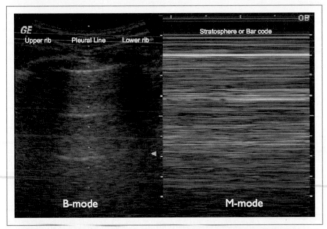

FIGURE 48.10: M-mode demonstrating the stratosphere sign/bar code sign consistent with pneumothorax. (*Courtesy of St. Luke's/Roosevelt emergency ultrasound division, New York, NY.*)

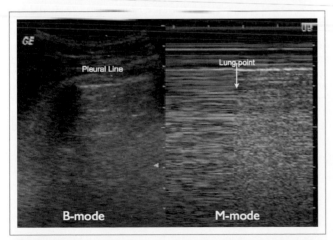

FIGURE 48.11: M-mode demonstrating the transition between seashore and bar code signs. The lung point is seen where normal lung meets collapsed lung. (*Courtesy of St. Luke's/Roosevelt emergency ultrasound division, New York, NY.*)

Basic Management
- Oxygen
- Pain control
- Tension pneumothorax
  - Emergent needle decompression over the second rib in the midclavicular line on the affected side
  - Once the tension has been released, insert a thoracostomy tube
- Nontension pneumothorax
  - Oxygen from a nonrebreather mask
- Optional treatments:
  - Conservative, aspiration, intercostal catheter, small bore/pigtail catheter, thoracostomy tube
- Consider follow-up radiograph to assess for size and stability

Summary

TABLE 48.6: Advantages and disadvantages of imaging modalities in pneumothorax

Imaging modalities	Advantages	Disadvantages
Chest x-ray	Portable possible Low radiation Low cost	Rapid Least sensitive
CT scan	Highly sensitive and specific (gold standard) May reveal other diagnoses	Time-consuming Expensive Radiation exposure
Ultrasound	Immediate Bedside Low cost No radiation Higher sensitivity than CXR	Operator-dependent Lower sensitivity and specificity than CT

49

Rib Fracture

Jonathan Fischer and Darrell Sutijono

Background

Rib fractures are the most common injury resulting from blunt chest trauma. Additional mechanisms of rib fractures include penetrating trauma and, on rare occasions, coughing spells, golfing, or rowing. The most commonly injured ribs are the fourth through ninth ribs. While an isolated rib fracture in a healthy host rarely causes significant morbidity, multiple rib fractures, especially in the elderly, often lead to significant morbidity and even death. This is a result of respiratory splinting and impaired cough secondary to pain, followed by development of pneumonia. The importance in diagnosing rib fractures is to alert the physician to potentially life-threatening complications, such as pneumothorax, hemothorax, vascular injuries, pulmonary contusions, and intra-abdominal injuries.

TABLE 49.1: Classic history and physical

Localized pain following blunt chest trauma
Sharp pain with inspiration
Respiratory splinting
Point tenderness on chest wall
Referred pain on chest compression
Ecchymosis
Bony crepitus
Muscle spasm over rib
Paradoxical chest wall excursion in the presence of a flail chest wall segment

Chest X-ray

- Primary imaging modality for detection of rib fractures
- Look for radiolucent line or step off in an otherwise radio-opaque bony rib
- Poor sensitivity: up to 50% of rib fractures and cartilaginous rib injuries are not apparent
- Sensitivity increases over time as callus forms
- May demonstrate pneumothorax, hemothorax, and/or pulmonary contusions
- Overpenetrated anteroposterior (AP), oblique, cone-down, or inspiratory/expiratory views improve sensitivity
- Assess for multiple rib fractures or segmental fractures of one rib
- Especially with fractures of the first three ribs, look for subcutaneous emphysema, widened mediastinum, apical capping, pleural effusion, tracheal deviation, left mainstem bronchus deviation, or esophageal deviation as signs of associated injuries.

 TABLE 49.2: Chest x-ray: rib fracture

IV contrast	No
PO contrast	No
Amount of radiation	0.02 mSv per view

Classic Images

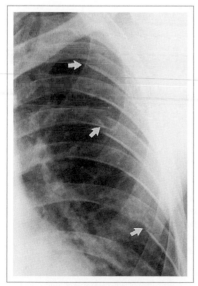

FIGURE 49.1: General features of rib fractures. Observe the multiple fracture sites (*arrows*). Rib fractures can be identified by searching for a fracture line, cortical offset, or altered rib angulation, and, when multiple, following along the line of injury, looking for additional lesions. (From Yochum TR and Rowe LJ. Yochum and Rowe's Essentials of Skeletal Radiology, 3rd ed. Philadelphia: Lippincott Williams & Wilkins, 2004.)

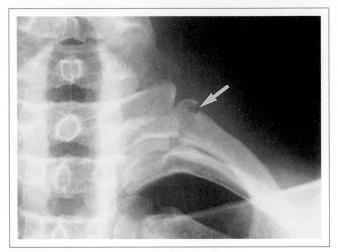

FIGURE 49.2: First rib fracture. Note the single fracture line traversing the first rib, just distal to the costotransverse joint (*arrow*). (From Yochum TR and Rowe LJ. Yochum and Rowe's Essentials of Skeletal Radiology, 3rd ed. Philadelphia: Lippincott Williams & Wilkins, 2004.)

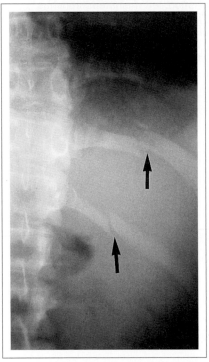

FIGURE 49.3: Lower rib fractures. Note the fracture lines through both the eleventh and twelfth ribs (*arrows*), with minimal displacement. *Comment:* The presence of fractures of the lower ribs warrants careful examination of the urinary system, especially renal function and structure. This may include an ultrasound or CT. (From Yochum TR and Rowe LJ. Yochum and Rowe's Essentials of Skeletal Radiology, 3rd ed. Philadelphia: Lippincott Williams & Wilkins, 2004.)

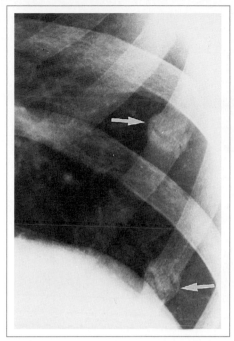

FIGURE 49.4: Healing rib fractures. Two sites of healing rib fractures are identified (*arrows*). Radiographic features consist of a localized region of increased density, bony expansion of the rib at the fracture site, and visualization of the fracture line. *Comment*: These rib fractures were not apparent on the initial radiographic examination after a chronic episode of coughing. Follow-up radiographs revealed callus formation, which now localizes the previously unrecognized fracture sites. (From Yochum TR and Rowe LJ. Yochum and Rowe's Essentials of Skeletal Radiology, 3rd ed. Philadelphia: Lippincott Williams & Wilkins, 2004.)

Bedside Soft-Tissue and Lung Ultrasound

- Sensitivity 80–87% and specificity 83–100%
- Place a high-frequency (i.e., 7–12 MHz) linear probe in the sagittal plane on the anterior chest
- Identify the anterior hyperechoic rib margin, its associated posterior acoustic shadowing, and adjacent pleural lines
- Rotate the transducer 90 degrees so that it is in-line with the longitudinal axis of the rib to visualize the bony cortex
- Sonography can also be used to diagnose fractures in the chondral rib segments; the anterior hyperechoic margin may not be as bright as in the ossified portion of the rib
- Rib segments shielded by the scapula and the clavicle are difficult to evaluate
- Fluid in the pleural space may be evaluated with a low frequency probe placed in the right or left upper quadrants of the abdomen in the mid or anterior axillary line with the indicator pointed toward the axilla
- A pneumothorax evaluation may also be performed

TABLE 49.3: Sonography: rib fracture

Discontinuity in hyperechoic (white) cortex
Hypoechoic (black) hematoma
Linear acoustic edge shadow
Reverberation artifact posterior to fracture
Localized pain with pressure applied by the probe
Indirect and associated finding: pleural effusion
Indirect and associated finding: pneumothorax

Classic Images

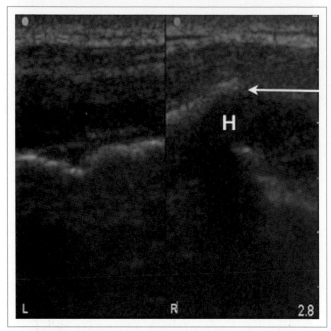

FIGURE 49.5: Normal left rib. Right rib with visible cortical discontinuity (*arrow*). (*Courtesy of SLR Emergency ultrasound division, New York, NY.*)

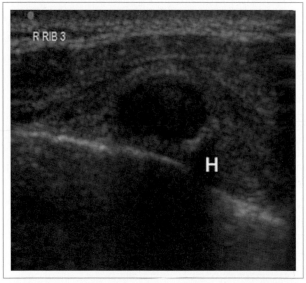

FIGURE 49.6: Right rib fracture transverse view with hematoma (H). (*Courtesy of SLR Emergency ultrasound division, New York, NY.*)

Chest CT Scan
- Diagnoses rib fractures and details intrathoracic contents (e.g., vascular, bony, and organ structures)
- Fractures of the cartilaginous rib segments more readily visualized
- Particularly indicated in the setting of fractures of the first three ribs.
  - Evaluates the trachea, major vascular structures, brachial plexus, and spine
- Indicated in the setting of lower rib fractures to evaluate for injury to the liver, spleen, kidneys, or diaphragm

 TABLE 49.4: Chest CT: rib fractures

IV contrast	Yes for vascular or solid organ injury evaluation
PO contrast	No
Amount of radiation	7.0 mSv

Classic Images

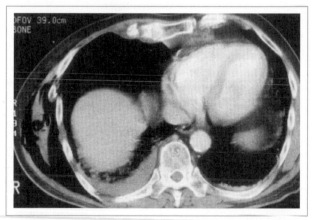

FIGURE 49.7: Rib fracture. Displaced fracture with extensive subcutaneous emphysema. There is also a sternal fracture with associated retrosternal hematoma. (From Eisenberg RL. An Atlas of Differential Diagnosis, 4th ed. Philadelphia: Lippincott Williams & Wilkins, 2003.)

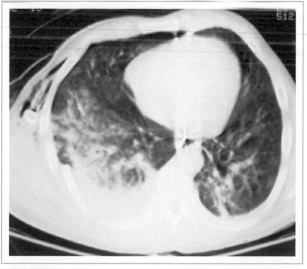

FIGURE 49.8: Pulmonary contusion. There are accompanying hemothorax, rib fractures, subcutaneous emphysema, and pleural drain. (From Eisenberg RL. An Atlas of Differential Diagnosis, 4th ed. Philadelphia: Lippincott Williams & Wilkins, 2003.)

Basic Management

- Oral anti-inflammatory analgesia for mild pain
- Oral or IV opioid analgesia for more severe pain
- Intercostal nerve block with a long active local anesthetic for severe pain or when opioid analgesia is not desired
- Epidural analgesia is highly effective and warranted in cases of severe pain
- Incentive spirometry
- Admission criteria:
  - More than three rib fractures
  - Flail chest
  - Severe pain associated with splinting or hypoxemia
  - Complications of rib fractures (i.e., pneumothorax)
  - Poor outpatient follow-up

Summary

TABLE 49.5: Advantages and disadvantages of imaging modalities in rib fractures

Imaging modalities	Advantages	Disadvantages
Radiography	Availability Familiarity Low cost Evaluation for associated pneumothorax and hemothorax	Poor sensitivity Poor visualization of chondral rib segments Radiation exposure
Ultrasound	Highly sensitive Low cost No radiation Bedside availability Visualization of chondral rib segments Evaluation for associated pneumothorax, hemothorax, and evidence of solid organ injury	Variable access to ultrasound machine and trained personnel Time-consuming
CT scan	Highly sensitive Detailed visualization of intrathoracic contents Visualization of chondral rib segments	Radiation exposure Costly

50

Tuberculosis

Caroline Pace and Reinier Van Tonder

Background

Tuberculosis (TB) is divided into primary and postprimary diseases. Primary pulmonary TB, forming soon after initial infection, is peripherally located and often accompanied by hilar and paratracheal lymphadenopathy. In the majority of cases, the lesions heal spontaneously and may be seen as small, calcified nodules (Ghon lesions). In an immunocompromised patient, primary pulmonary TB may progress to clinical illness. The primary lesion may enlarge rapidly and undergo central necrosis, thereby forming a cavitation. Postprimary disease is an endogenous reactivation of latent infection and is usually localized to the posteroapical segments of the lungs where higher oxygen tension favors mycobacterial growth. Although most patients who are infected with TB are asymptomatic, the likelihood of reactivation increases with HIV coinfection, immunosuppression, and advanced age.

TABLE 50.1: Classic history and physical

Fever and night sweats
Anorexia and weight loss
General malaise and weakness
Hemoptysis
Rales during inspiration, particularly notable after coughing
Amphoric breath sounds in areas of large cavitation

TABLE 50.2: Potentially helpful laboratory tests

CBC	Anemia (poor sensitivity and specificity)
	Leukocytosis (poor sensitivity and specificity)
BMP	Hyponatremia
	SIADH from pulmonary process
Induced sputum sample	Acid-fast bacilli staining and mycobacterial culture

BMP, basic metabolic panel; CBC, complete blood count; SIADH, syndrome of inappropriate antidiuretic hormone secretion.

Chest X-ray

- Normal in 90% of positive purified protein derivative skin tests
- Appearance of active TB is variable and can present in any lobe of either lung
- Primary TB
  - Look for a focal middle or lower lobe consolidation
  - Associated hilar lymphadenopathy (95% of cases)
  - Associated pleural effusion (10% of cases)
- Secondary reactivation TB
  - Look for upper lobe infiltrates described often as "fluffy," "soft," or "ill-defined"
  - Associated cavitation (40% of cases) appears as a central lucency because the cavity is filled with a caseous material
- Miliary TB
  - Look for small nodules scattered throughout both lung fields

 TABLE 50.3: Chest x-ray (PA and Lateral): pulmonary TB

IV contrast	No
PO contrast	No
Amount of radiation	0.10 mSv

Classic Images

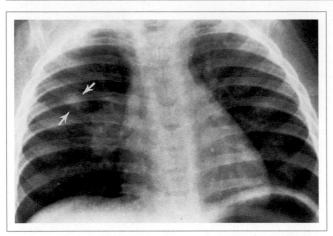

FIGURE 50.1: Primary tuberculosis. The combination of a focal parenchymal lesion (*arrows*) and enlarged right hilar lymph nodes produces the classic primary complex. (From Eisenberg RL. An Atlas of Differential Diagnosis, 4th ed. Philadelphia: Lippincott Williams & Wilkins, 2003.)

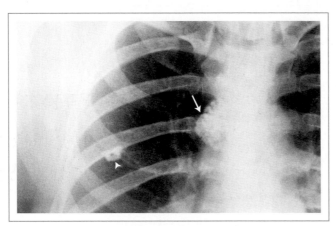

FIGURE 50.2: Ranke complex. Posteroanterior chest x-ray. Note the peripheral calcified granuloma (Ghon focus) (*arrowhead*) in combination with an ipsilateral calcified hilar lymph node (*arrow*). These tandem calcifications are signs of previous healed primary tuberculosis. (*Courtesy of James R. Brandt, DC, DABCO, Coon Rapids, MN.*) (From Yochum TR and Rowe LJ. Yochum and Rowe's Essentials of Skeletal Radiology, 3rd ed. Philadelphia: Lippincott Williams & Wilkins, 2004.)

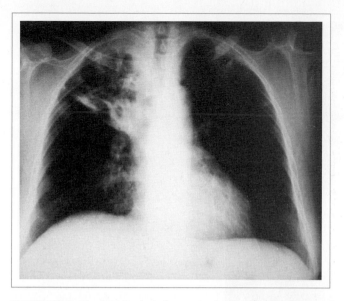

FIGURE 50.3: Chest radiograph demonstrating apical infiltrate with cavitation, typical of pulmonary tuberculosis. (From Harwood-Nuss A, Wolfson AB. The Clinical Practice of Emergency Medicine, 3rd ed. Philadelphia: Lippincott Williams & Wilkins, 2001.)

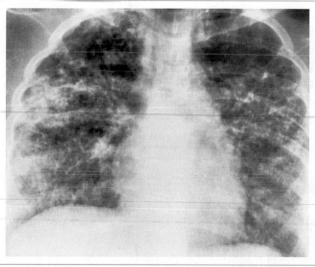

FIGURE 50.4: Secondary tuberculosis. Diffuse interstitial fibrosis pattern. (From Eisenberg RL. An Atlas of Differential Diagnosis, 4th ed. Philadelphia: Lippincott Williams & Wilkins, 2003.)

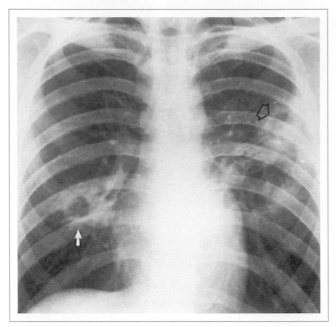

FIGURE 50.5: Secondary tuberculosis. Bilateral cavitary lesions (*arrows*) with relatively thick walls. (From Eisenberg RL. An Atlas of Differential Diagnosis, 4th ed. Philadelphia: Lippincott Williams & Wilkins, 2003.)

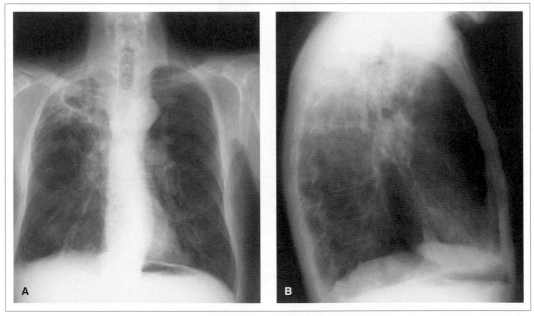

FIGURE 50.6: Chest radiographs (posteroanterior (**A**) and lateral (**B**) views) demonstrating cavitary reactivation of latent tuberculosis infection in the posterior apical segment of the right upper lobe. (From Crapo JD, Glassroth J, Karlinsky JB, et al. Baum's Textbook of Pulmonary Diseases, 7th ed. Philadelphia: Lippincott Williams & Wilkins, 2004.)

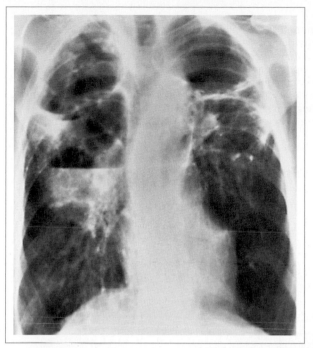

FIGURE 50.7: Tuberculosis. Multiple large cavities with air fluid levels in both upper lobes. Note the chronic fibrotic changes and upward retraction of the hila. (From Eisenberg RL. An Atlas of Differential Diagnosis, 4th ed. Philadelphia: Lippincott Williams & Wilkins, 2003.)

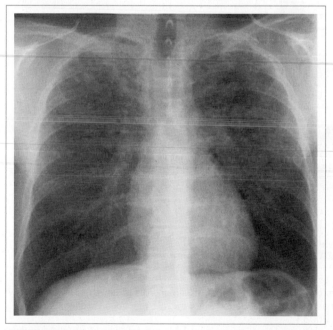

FIGURE 50.8: Chest radiograph (posteroanterior view only) demonstrating the radiographic presentation of miliary tuberculosis. (From Crapo JD, Glassroth J, Karlinsky JB, et al. Baum's Textbook of Pulmonary Diseases, 7th ed. Philadelphia: Lippincott Williams & Wilkins, 2004.)

Chest CT Scan

- In primary TB, look for hilar lymphadenopathy: the enlarged nodes have a low-density center with rim enhancement, are randomly distributed throughout the lungs and range in size
- Look for reactivation changes in the posterior segments of the upper lungs
- Cavitation is a distinguishing feature of postprimary TB and is evident in over 95% of cases: typically thick-walled and irregular, rarely containing air-fluid levels
- The associated complications of postprimary TB (erosion of vessels, rupture into the pleural space with hematogenous and bronchogenic spread) are better defined by a CT scan
- A tree-in-bud pattern of 5- to 10-mm nodules is associated with endobronchial spread on high-resolution CT

 TABLE 50.4: Chest CT: Tuberculosis

IV contrast	Yes
PO contrast	No
Amount of radiation	7.0 mSv

Classic Images

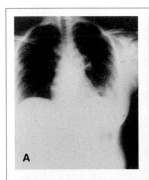
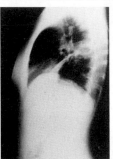
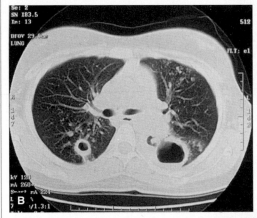
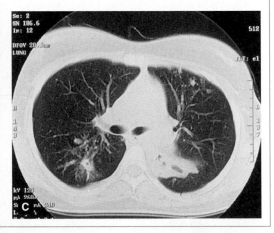

FIGURE 50.9: Chest radiograph (**A**) and CT scan (**B**), the latter of which more clearly demonstrates two cavitary lesions. A repeated CT scan (**C**) showed improvement after 1 month of treatment in a young woman with primary multidrug-resistant tuberculosis. (From Gorbach SL, Bartlett JG, and Blacklow NR. Infectious Diseases, 3rd ed. Philadelphia: Lippincott Williams & Wilkins, 2003.)

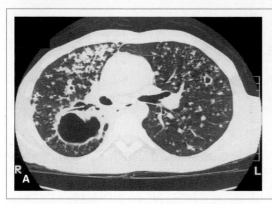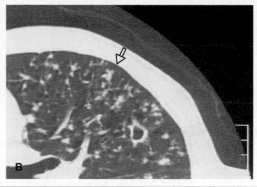

FIGURE 50.10: A: CT scan of a patient with extensive bilateral cavitary tuberculosis. **B:** Enhancement of the left anterior quadrant of the figure demonstrating the tree-in-bud pattern (*arrow*). (From Crapo JD, Glassroth J, Karlinsky JB, et al. Baum's Textbook of Pulmonary Diseases, 7th ed. Philadelphia: Lippincott Williams & Wilkins, 2004.)

Basic Management

- Place patients in negative pressure and adequate air exchange rooms
- The following are general guidelines (check the latest recommendations for updates on antimicrobial management)
  - Treat with four-drug regimen: isoniazid, rifampin, pyrazinamide, and either ethambutol or streptomycin
  - Pyridoxine should be coadministered with isoniazid
  - When sensitivity data is available, either ethambutol or streptomycin can be discontinued
- Consider infectious disease consultation
- Directly observed therapy is recommended
- HIV testing should be performed in patients with unknown status

Summary

TABLE 50.5: Advantages and disadvantages of imaging modalities in tuberculosis

Imaging modalities	Advantages	Disadvantages
Chest x-ray	Availability Low cost Portable if needed	Neither sensitive nor specific
CT scan	Availability Other diagnoses also possible	IV contrast Radiation exposure Costly

IV, intravenous.

51 Lung Cancer and Metastasis

Thomas E. Robey and Lara L. Bryan-Rest

Background

Lung cancer is the most common malignancy worldwide and is the most common cause of cancer-related death in the United States. It has a poor overall survival in both the United States (14% at 5 years) and globally (8% at 5 years). In 2009, deaths related to lung cancer were estimated at 157,910 and accounted for 28% of all cancer deaths. Smoking tobacco is the most common risk factor and is correlated to as many as 90% of all lung cancer cases. Toxin exposures, such as asbestos, second-hand smoke, and radon gas, as well as a history of radiation therapy to the chest, also confer increased risk.

Pulmonary metastases occur in 30% of all malignancies, primarily those spread hematogenously. Pulmonary nodules are the most common manifestation of metastatic disease to the lungs, owing to the lungs' large vascular bed. Patients may present to the emergency department with symptoms similar to those of a primary lung neoplasm. However, pulmonary symptoms may be absent in many patients with multiple lung metastases, so diagnosis may also be incidental.

TABLE 51.1: Classic history and physical

Chest pain
Cough
Dyspnea
Hemoptysis
Hypoxia
Pleural effusion
Postobstructive pneumonia
Wheezing
Superior vena cava syndrome (local spread)
Horner syndrome (local spread)
Cushing syndrome (paraneoplastic)
Bone pain (metastatic disease)
Intracranial hemorrhage (metastatic disease)

TABLE 51.2: Potentially helpful laboratory tests

BMP	Identify paraneoplastic syndromes (e.g., SIADH, Cushing syndrome)
CBC	Useful if hemoptysis is present
Sputum cytology	Quick and inexpensive; high specificity, but low sensitivity study
Pleural fluid	Laboratory analysis and cytology

BMP, basic metabolic panel; CBC, complete blood count; SIADH, syndrome of inappropriate antidiuretic hormone secretion.

TABLE 51.3: Primary tumors with high incidence of pulmonary metastasis

Source	Incidence of pulmonary metastasis
Choriocarcinoma	60%
Renal cell carcinoma	30%
Ewing sarcoma	18%
Osteosarcoma	15%
Testicular tumor	12%

Chest X-ray

- Universally accepted first-line imaging technique
- Identify either the original tumor or its sequela (e.g., pleural effusion)
- Look for a postobstructive pneumonia

TABLE 51.4: CXR findings in lung cancer and metastasis

Solitary nodule	May be seen in any region of the lung More common with a primary lung neoplasm
Multiple nodules	Common with lung metastases
Cavitary lesions	Common in rapidly growing tumors and those of squamous cell origin
Pleural effusion	Usually unilateral
Pneumothorax	Uncommon; may be seen as a consequence of pleural or chest wall invasion

 TABLE 51.5: Chest x-ray (PA and Lateral): lung cancer and metastasis

IV contrast	No
PO contrast	No
Amount of radiation	0.1 mSv

Classic Images

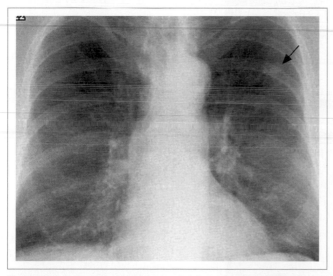

FIGURE 51.1: A solitary pulmonary nodule in the left upper lobe suggests the possibility of lung cancer. (From Crapo JD, Glassroth J, Karlinsky JB, et al. Baum's Textbook of Pulmonary Diseases, 7th ed. Philadelphia, PA: Lippincott Williams & Wilkins, 2004.)

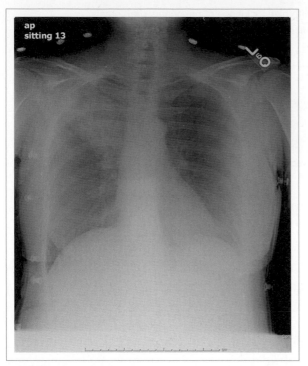

FIGURE 51.2: A large right upper lobe mass; later diagnosed as non-small cell carcinoma. (*Courtesy of Yale-New Haven Hospital, New Haven, CT.*)

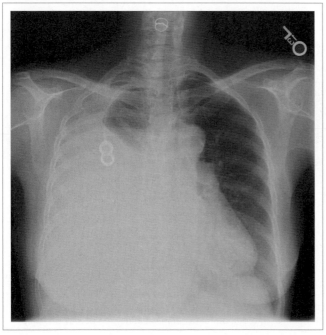

FIGURE 51.3: Large, malignant right-sided pleural effusion. Note that a double lumen porta-cath is already in place. (*Courtesy of Yale-New Haven Hospital, New Haven, CT.*)

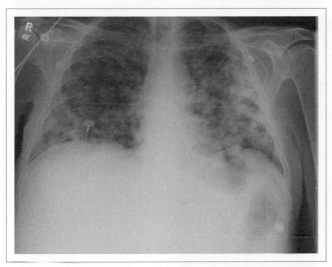

FIGURE 51.4: Multiple, variably sized lung nodules suggest hematogenous spread of an extrathoracic cancer, in this case colorectal cancer. (*Courtesy of Yale-New Haven Hospital, New Haven, CT.*)

Bedside Lung Ultrasound
- Bedside ultrasound is a quick way to identify associated findings of lung cancer (e.g., pleural effusion, pneumothorax, and metastasis to solid organs)
- Accessible, low cost, and no radiation exposure
- Diagnostic and therapeutic needle thoracentesis may be conducted under ultrasound (U/S) guidance
- Type and extent of tumor cannot be identified

Classic Images

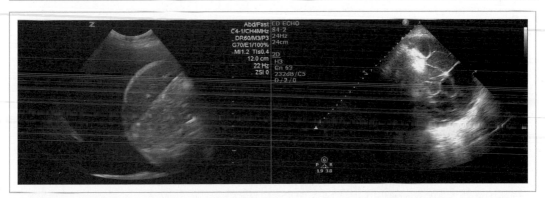

FIGURE 51.5: Pleural effusions are easily visualized by ultrasound. At left, the lung is shown floating in a large effusion using a sagittal midaxillary view. At right is a loculated pleural effusion visualized using a phased-array probe placed inferior to the costal margin in the midclavicular line. (*Courtesy of Yale-New Haven Hospital, New Haven, CT.*)

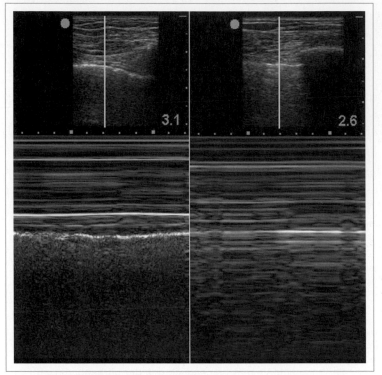

FIGURE 51.6: M-mode still images showing normal (left) and impaired (right) lung sliding visualized in a sagittal view of the intercostal space. M-mode at left shows classic seashore pattern seen in normal lungs with superficial parallel "waves" transitioning to diffuse scattered "sand." Only "waves" are seen at right suggesting pneumothorax. (*Courtesy of Yale-New Haven Hospital, New Haven, CT.*)

CT Scan

- A CT scan of the chest and upper abdomen is needed for staging lung cancer and is useful in correlating a patient's symptoms to local spread or mass effect
- Most common sites of lung cancer metastases include bone, adrenal glands, and brain (brain imaging should be done if there are any neurological signs or symptoms)
- Helical CT can acquire high-quality images in a single breath hold
- A CT scan cannot be relied upon to help differentiate between hyperplastic and malignant lymphadenopathy; false positives occur with inflammatory and infectious lymphadenopathy
- High radiation exposure: over 200 times that of a chest x-ray (CXR).

 TABLE 51.6: Chest CT: lung cancer and metastasis

IV contrast	No, unless mediastinal involvement is suspected
PO contrast	No
Amount of radiation	7 mSv

Classic Images

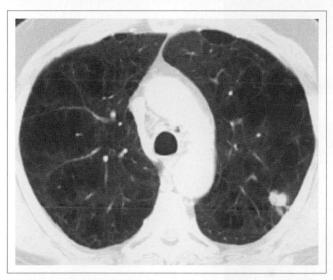

FIGURE 51.7: CT scan of a solitary lung nodule found on CXR demonstrating a noncalcified nodule in the posterior segment of the left upper lobe, with a tail extending to the pleura. The nodule is a non-small cell lung cancer. (From Crapo JD, Glassroth J, Karlinsky JB, et al. Baum's Textbook of Pulmonary Diseases, 7th ed. Philadelphia: Lippincott Williams & Wilkins, 2004.)

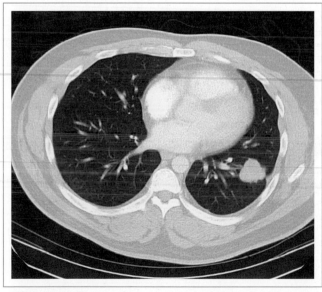

FIGURE 51.8: Left lower lung cancer that is tenting the adjacent pleura. (*Courtesy of Yale-New Haven Hospital, New Haven, CT.*)

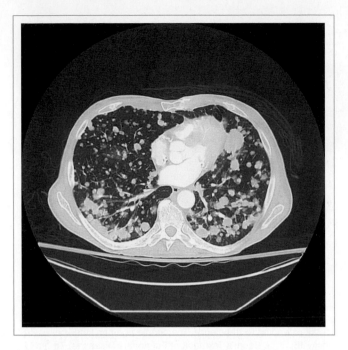

FIGURE 51.9: Innumerable pulmonary nodules of variable size. These nodules are metastatic colorectal cancer. (*Courtesy of Yale-New Haven Hospital, New Haven, CT.*)

Basic Management

- Symptomatic treatment and management, for example, oxygen, thoracentesis, chest tube placement (e.g., hypoxia, pleural effusion, pneumothorax)
- Consultation with a pulmonologist and oncologist for subsequent diagnostic evaluations (e.g., bronchoscopy and imaging modalities)
- Sputum cytology, bronchoscopy, or percutaneous biopsy is needed to diagnose primary pulmonary tumor or metastasis
- Admission is indicated if the patient's clinical condition warrants

Summary

TABLE 51.7: Advantages and disadvantages of imaging modalities in lung cancer and metastasis

Imaging modalities	Advantages	Disadvantages
CXR	Bedside availability Rapid Low radiation Low cost	Lower sensitivity Lower specificity
Bedside ultrasound	Bedside availability Low cost No radiation	Helpful for diagnosing associated findings, not the actual tumor
CT scan	Good availability Delineates other diagnoses	IV contrast Radiation exposure

Section Editor: Leon D. Sanchez

52

Appendicitis

Samantha F. Bordonaro and Robin B. Levenson

Background

Appendicitis is the most common surgical cause of right lower quadrant pain and necessitates prompt attention, diagnosis, and intervention. Each year, more than 250,000 cases of acute appendicitis require appendectomy in the United States. The lifetime risk of appendicitis for men and women is 8.6% and 6.7%, respectively. As imaging modalities have advanced and become more readily available, the ability to diagnose acute appendicitis, particularly in a patient who does not present with classic symptoms, has vastly improved. Appendicitis occurs when the appendix (a tubular structure that extends from the cecum) becomes obstructed, which typically results in bacterial colonization. The appendix becomes inflamed and dilated which can lead to ischemia. Ultimately, the appendix can rupture, resulting in peritonitis and possible abscess formation.

TABLE 52.1: Classic history and physical

Begins as periumbilical pain
Pain migrates to the right lower quadrant (RLQ)
Anorexia, nausea, vomiting
Low grade fever
Tenderness to palpation in the RLQ
May have rebound and guarding at McBurney's point (two-thirds distance from umbilicus to anterior superior iliac spine)
Rovsing's sign: remote palpation produces pain in the RLQ

TABLE 52.2: Potentially helpful laboratory tests

WBC: May be elevated with a left shift; specificity is ~76% for an elevated WBC and 62% for a left shift or neutrophils >75%
CRP: Has been studied as a potential marker, but similar to WBC is not particularly sensitive or specific

CRP, C-reactive protein; WBC, white blood cell count.

Ultrasound

- Ultrasound quality and usefulness is often operator-dependent.
- Bedside ultrasound in the emergency department may be performed but is not considered standard of care or sufficient to completely evaluate all abdominal and pelvic structures.
- Technique:
  - Keep the patient supine and use a linear-array, high-frequency transducer initially in a transverse orientation.
  - Identifying the point of maximal tenderness can often help locate the appendix.

- Appendix lies anterior to the psoas muscle and iliac vessels.
- Use graded compression to move bowel out of the field of view.
- Once the cecum and appendix are identified in the transverse orientation, it is important to obtain longitudinal images to differentiate the appendix (blind ending) from the terminal ileum as well as for assessment of the tip of the appendix.
- Ultrasound technique tips:
  - ▶ Use of the left hand behind the patient's back/flank to create pressure toward the probe may aid in appendix visualization.
  - ▶ If the appendix is deeper in the pelvis than is typical, it may be possible to apply upward pressure with the ultrasound probe in order to displace the cecum superiorly.
- Ultrasound appearance of the appendix:
  - Normally ≤6 mm in diameter when compressed (size can be controversial as a normal appendix can exceed 6 mm).
  - When inflamed, the appendix should be >6 mm, fixed and noncompressible.
  - Color Doppler may demonstrate hyperemia of the appendix wall.
  - Surrounding fat may be echogenic if inflamed, although this is a nonspecific finding.
  - An echogenic shadowing structure within the appendix suggests an appendicolith.
  - Fluid collection around/adjacent to the appendix or an irregular appendiceal border suggests perforation.
- Sensitivity is 91% in children and 86% in adults. Specificity is 97% (using graded compression) in children and 81% in adults.
- Ultrasound can be helpful in women of childbearing age who may have gynecologic emergencies that mimic appendicitis.
- Because ultrasound does not expose patients to radiation it can be useful in the pediatric or pregnant patient.
- Ultrasound evaluation can be useful for pregnant women, particularly in the first trimester. Ultrasound may be limited later in pregnancy because of displacement of the appendix by the growing fetus and enlarging uterus. MRI has now become the preferred modality later in pregnancy.

TABLE 52.3: Appendicitis findings on ultrasound

Target shape or bull's eye
Diameter >6 mm
Hyperechoic appendicolith (calcification within lumen) with associated posterior shadowing
Noncompressible
No peristaltic activity

TABLE 52.4: Helpful associated structures

Cecum
Surrounding periappendiceal fat
Psoas muscle
Iliac vessels

Classic Images

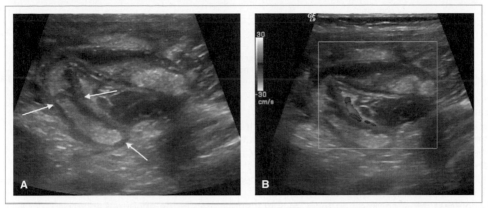

FIGURE 52.1: An 18-month-old male child with abdominal pain due to acute appendicitis. **A:** Ultrasound images of the right lower quadrant demonstrate a noncompressible, blind ending tubular structure representing the appendix, which is dilated at 7.7 mm. **B:** Ultrasound image of the right lower quadrant with color Doppler shows hyperemia of the wall of the appendix. Findings are consistent with acute appendicitis. (*Courtesy of Robin B. Levenson and Beth Israel Deaconess Medical Center, Department of Radiology, Boston, MA.*)

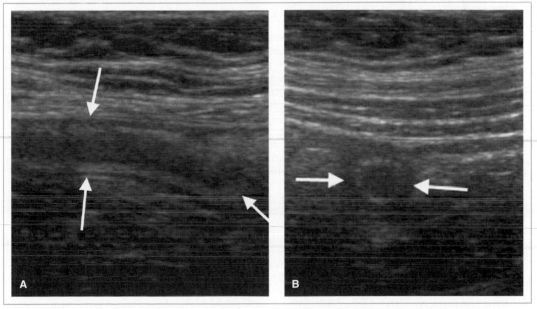

FIGURE 52.2: A 25-year-old woman, 22 weeks pregnant, presenting with right lower quadrant pain from acute appendicitis. Longitudinal (**A**) and transverse (**B**) ultrasound images of the right lower quadrant show a noncompressible dilated appendix, 8 mm in diameter, with a thickened wall. (*Courtesy of Robin B. Levenson and Beth Israel Deaconess Medical Center, Department of Radiology, Boston, MA.*)

TABLE 52.5: MRI: appendicitis

IV contrast	No*
PO contrast	Yes
Amount of radiation	None

*Gadolinium is contraindicated in pregnancy because it crosses the placenta and the true effect is unknown.

Computed Tomography (CT) Scan

- CT scan is the modality of choice in evaluation for acute appendicitis in the nonpediatric, nonpregnant patient. Its use has increased because of its high sensitivity and specificity as compared to ultrasound, its increased availability, and its strength in demonstrating alternative abdominopelvic pathology.
- Sensitivity is 95% in both children and adults. Specificity is 98% in children and 95% in adults.
- The CT protocol for acute appendicitis can vary:
  - IV contrast: Most common protocol. Aids in identification of the abnormal appendix, abscess, or in alternative diagnoses. Additionally, time to diagnosis is not delayed when using intravenous contrast without oral contrast.
  - Oral or rectal contrast: Administration of oral or rectal contrast varies by institution. With the latest generation of multislice scanners, intraluminal bowel contrast is usually not necessary, unless the patient is thin. Oral contrast allows for the visualization of the bowel which may be helpful in identifying the appendix, but often delays the time to diagnosis. Rectal contrast on the other hand is faster and may effectively opacify the cecum and appendix, but may be uncomfortable for the patient and can be technically cumbersome.
- Locating the appendix on CT scan:
  - Identify the ileocecal junction in the right lower abdomen.
  - Try to identify a blind-ending tubular structure that arises 1–4 cm caudad to the ileocecal valve, most often posteromedial, assuming standard cecal position.
  - The appendix usually arises from the same side of the cecum as the ileocecal valve which helps to identify it in cases of mobile cecum or atypical cecal orientation.
  - The course of the appendix varies in each patient; it can terminate as far superior as Morrison's pouch or the gallbladder fossa and as far inferior as a right inguinal hernia. Appearance of appendicitis varies but familiarity with the below findings will be helpful.
- Appearance of the appendix on CT scan:
  - The abnormal appendix diameter is typically >6 mm (although a normal appendix can exceed 6 mm) and may have wall thickening >3 mm. Enhancement of the wall indicates edema and hyperemia.
  - Arrowhead sign (see Figure 52.3): If oral contrast is given, cecal edema with wall thickening may be present with oral contrast in the cecum coming to a point at the base of the nonfilling appendix.
  - Fat stranding or fluid around the appendix suggests acute inflammation.
  - Findings indicative of perforation include extraluminal air and abscess.
  - Focus of calcification within the appendix represents an appendicolith, which can be the source of obstruction leading to appendicitis.

TABLE 52.6: Appendicitis findings on CT scan

Dilated appendix (diameter >6 mm)
Appendix wall thickening >3 mm
Appendicolith (bright white calcification within lumen)
Fat stranding or fluid around appendix
Extraluminal air or abscess (perforation likely)

 TABLE 52.7: CT scan: appendicitis

IV contrast	Yes
PO contrast	Varies by institution; usually not necessary unless the patient is thin
Amount of radiation	14 mSv

Classic Images

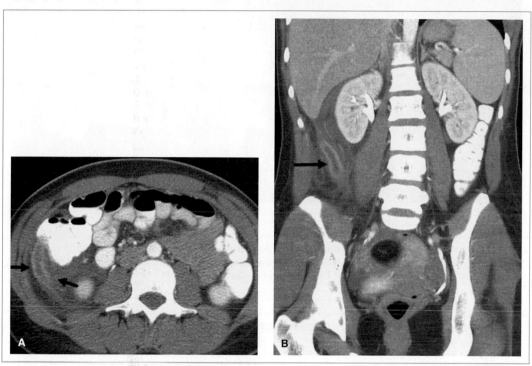

FIGURE 52.3: A 24-year-old female with right lower quadrant pain. Contrast-enhanced CT images of the abdomen and pelvis in axial (**A**) and coronal (**B**) planes demonstrate a dilated appendix in the right lower quadrant, measuring 11 mm in diameter, with a thick, enhancing, hyperemic wall. Oral contrast was administered and the appendix does not fill with contrast, further supporting the diagnosis of acute appendicitis. Adjacent haziness and fat stranding are consistent with periappendiceal inflammatory changes. (*Courtesy of Robin B. Levenson and Beth Israel Deaconess Medical Center, Department of Radiology, Boston, MA.*)

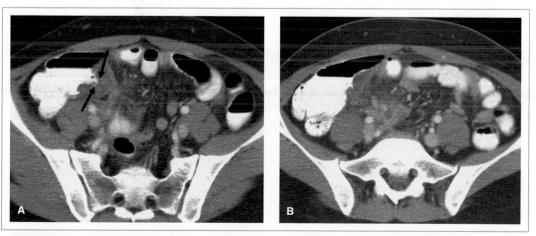

FIGURE 52.4: A 35-year-old female presenting with right lower quadrant pain due to acute appendicitis. Contrast-enhanced CT image of the abdomen and pelvis demonstrates the "arrowhead" sign (*black arrows*). Focal thickening of the cecal wall because of adjacent inflammatory changes from acute appendicitis leads to oral contrast collecting in the shape of an arrowhead. Appendix was not well defined on CT imaging because of extensive phlegmon (part B). (*Courtesy of Robin B. Levenson and Beth Israel Deaconess Medical Center, Department of Radiology, Boston, MA.*)

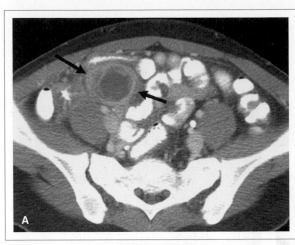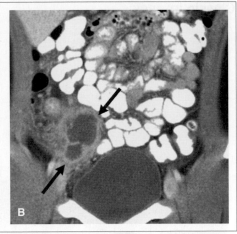

FIGURE 52.5: A 16-year-old female presenting with right lower quadrant pain. Axial (**A**) and coronal (**B**) images from contrast-enhanced CT of the abdomen and pelvis show a 5.6 × 3.9 × 3.8 cm fluid collection (*black arrows*) with thick rim enhancement, consistent with periappendiceal abscess and perforated appendicitis. Patient was initially treated with antibiotics and underwent CT-guided percutaneous drainage. (*Courtesy of Robin B. Levenson and Beth Israel Deaconess Medical Center, Department of Radiology, Boston, MA.*)

MRI

- MRI is particularly useful in the diagnosis of appendicitis in pregnant women after a nondiagnostic ultrasound.
- Not only does it spare radiation, but it can assess for other abdominopelvic pathology.
- Disadvantages include increased time to diagnosis when compared with CT scan.
- Availability of emergent MRI also varies by institution.
- Technique used for pregnant patient:
  - A 1.5 Tesla MRI scanner: Patient is placed in supine position and a body phased-array coil is used.
  - Oral contrast administration, using a 50/50 mixture of Gastromark (Mallinckrodt Medical, St. Louis, MO) and Readi-cat (E-Z-Em, Westbury, NY), creates negative contrast within the bowel lumen (lumen becomes dark/hypointense). Oral contrast should be given to the patient starting 1–1.5 hours prior to MRI.
  - Intravenous gadolinium administration is avoided as effects on the fetus are not well studied.
  - Magnetic resonance sequences obtained include triplanar single shot fast spin echo (SSFSE) T2-weighted images. Single shot imaging helps reduce motion artifact from the fetus. Fat-saturated axial SSFSE images help detect inflammation and edema, by darkening the adjacent intra-abdominal fat. Axial T1-weighted in- and opposed-phase gradient echo images can also be obtained to help identify hemorrhagic and fat-containing lesions.
- Appearance of the appendix on MRI:
  - Fluid-filled appendix >6 mm in diameter suggests acute appendicitis. Periappendiceal inflammation further supports the diagnosis. Periappendiceal edema can also be seen in early appendicitis before the appendix dilates, which helps make the diagnosis in cases in which the appendix has not yet dilated.
  - Walled-off fluid collection consistent with abscess may be seen in the region of the appendix.
  - An appendicolith, if present, is a dark focus on all sequences.

Classic Images

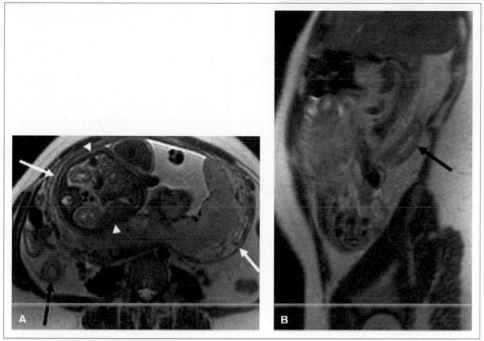

FIGURE 52.6: A 21-year-old woman, 31 weeks pregnant, presenting with right lower quadrant pain. T2-weighted axial (**A**) and sagittal (**B**) images through the abdomen and pelvis show a dilated (20 mm), thick-walled, retrocecal appendix (*black arrows*) with central T2 hyperintensity consistent with fluid within. Adjacent T2 iso- to hypointense stranding represents periappendiceal inflammation. Enlarged uterus (*white arrows*) with partially visualized fetus (*white arrowheads*) is also seen. (*Courtesy of Robin B. Levenson and Beth Israel Deaconess Medical Center, Department of Radiology, Boston, MA.*)

Basic Management
- Keep the patient NPO.
- Administer analgesia: The use of short-acting narcotics to relieve pain has not been shown to delay diagnosis or result in poor outcomes.
- If perforation is suspected, initiate antibiotic coverage.
- Early surgical consultation: If the patient is a male presenting with classic signs/symptoms of appendicitis, surgical consultation can preclude the use of imaging.
- Once appendicitis is confirmed, if noncomplicated, likely admit for definitive operative treatment. Percutaneous image-guided drainage may be performed before surgery in cases with drainable abscess formation and perforation.
- When appendicitis remains at the top of the differential diagnosis but has not been confirmed, admission for serial examinations is reasonable.

Summary

TABLE 52.8: Advantages and disadvantages of imaging modalities in appendicitis

Imaging modalities	Advantages	Disadvantages
Ultrasound	No radiation exposure Relative lower cost Available	Operator-dependent Patient body habitus limitations Often nonconclusive and may delay more definitive study
CT scan	High sensitivity/specificity Availability Detection of other pathology	Potential side effects of IV contrast Radiation exposure
MRI	Useful in pregnancy Identification of other abdominopelvic pathology	Expensive Not always available emergently Time-consuming

53

Acute Cholecystitis

Kaushal Shah

Background

It is estimated that gallstones are present in approximately 10–15% of Americans, and among people over the age of 40 years, more than 20% of women and over 8% of men have gallstones. Among patients with gallstones, it is estimated that new biliary pain will occur in 10% at 5 years, 15% at 10 years, and 18% at 15–20 years. Eighty percent of gallstones are predominantly composed of cholesterol and 20% are composed of calcium bilirubinate (pigment stones). There are 500,000 cholecystectomies performed each year and approximately 6,000–10,000 deaths associated with gallbladder (GB) disease annually in the United States.

TABLE 53.1: Classic history and physical

RUQ pain worse after fatty meal
4 F's: female, fat, forty, and fertile
RUQ tenderness
Murphy's sign: halting of inspiration when RUQ (suspected area of GB) is palpated

GB, gallbladder; RUQ, right upper quadrant.

TABLE 53.2: Potentially helpful laboratory tests

LFT: Often obtained but poor sensitivity and specificity; can be completely normal
Lipase: Elevated in cases of choledocholithiasis

LFT, liver function test.

Bedside Ultrasound

- Although the GB can be assessed well with ultrasound, it is one of the more difficult structures to locate; therefore, a methodological approach is recommended
- Use a 3.5–5.0 MHz ultrasound probe and scan the right upper quadrant of the abdomen in the longitudinal plane under the costal margin initially using the liver as an acoustic window to identify the GB
- If there is difficulty, ask the patient to take a slow deep breath because the GB moves significantly with respiration
- The probe can also be positioned in the intercostal space to avoid bowel gas and rib shadows
- Once the GB is identified, confirm that the structure is in fact the GB by identifying associated structures because the GB can easily be mistaken for a vessel (e.g., inferior vena cava), duct in the liver, or loop of intestine on cross section

TABLE 53.3: Helpful associated structures

Gallstones
Main lobar fissure of the liver
■ linear echogenic structure
■ points toward the GB neck and also connects the portal vein
Common bile duct
■ runs between the GB and the portal vein
■ usually seen when the probe is parallel to the subcostal margin

- Always visualize the GB in various planes (e.g., longitudinal and transverse) in order to see the entire extent of the structure
- If gallstones are suspected, change the position of the patient from lying flat to left lateral recumbent in order to see the stones shift position
- For diagnostic purposes, a sonographic Murphy's sign (halting of inspiration when the GB is compressed with the ultrasound probe) can be elicited
- Rarely, the GB can be scarred down on a large gallstone resulting in an atypical appearance of the GB; then there will be no standard "pear-shaped" GB and no lumen; there may only be a hyperechoic area with distal shadowing

Classic Images

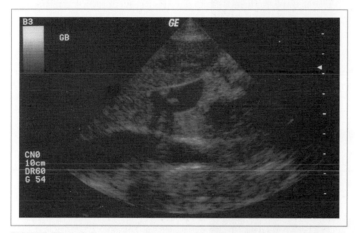

FIGURE 53.1: Gallstones in the gallbladder (GB) demonstrating acoustic shadowing.

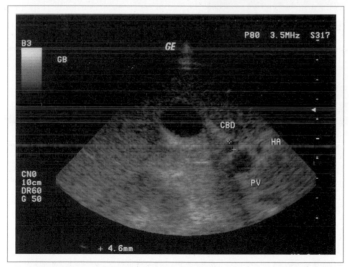

FIGURE 53.2: Mickey Mouse sign formed by portal vein (PV) in the center and the common bile duct (CBD) and hepatic artery (HA) adjacent to it.

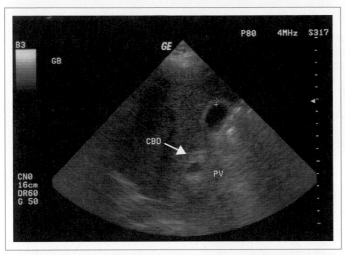

FIGURE 53.3: The common bile duct (CBD) is often found running between the GB and portal vein (PV).

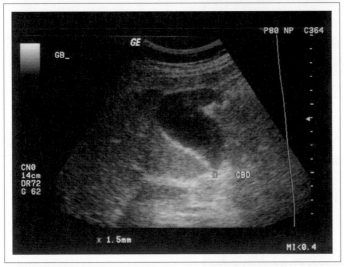

FIGURE 53.4: A pharygian cap is a normal variant of gallbladder appearance on ultrasonography.

Abdomen CT Scan

- A CT scan of the abdomen is not the gold standard or first-line imaging modality for suspected cholecystitis; however, it can be used if an ultrasound and HIDA scan are not available
- The sensitivity and specificity of a CT scan for diagnosis of cholecystitis has not been well studied
- Twenty percent of gallstones can me missed because they are of the same density as bile. Typically, cholesterol stones have low attenuation relative to bile; the best visualized are well-calcified stones
- A CT scan can demonstrate GB wall edema/thickening, pericholecystic stranding and fluid, and high-attenuation bile
- A CT scan provides significantly more information of the surrounding abdomen than an ultrasound or HIDA scan

 TABLE 53.4: CT scan: cholecystitis

IV contrast	Yes
PO contrast	No
Amount of radiation	14 mSv

Classic Images

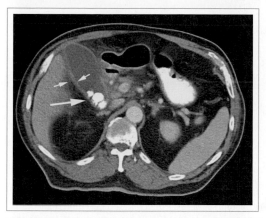

FIGURE 53.5: CT image showing the thickened GB wall (*small arrows*) and multiple stones (*large arrow*). (From Daffner RH. Clinical Radiology: The Essentials, 3rd ed. Philadelphia: Lippincott Williams & Wilkins, 2007.)

HIDA Scan
- HIDA and DISIDA scans are functional studies of the GB. Technetium-labeled analogues of iminodiacetic acid (IDA) or diisopropyl IDA-DISIDA are administered IV and secreted by hepatocytes into bile, enabling visualization of the liver and biliary tree
- Considered the gold standard for the diagnosis of cholecystitis
- HIDA scans have high sensitivity (94%) and specificity (65–85%) for acute cholecystitis
- The process of obtaining the scan requires a technician and injection of radionuclide particles
- Must wait for a radiologist to interpret study and determine results
  - Normal: visualization of the GB at 30 minutes
  - Abnormal/cholecystitis: nonvisualization of GB at 60 minutes
  - Rim sign: increased tracer adjacent to the GB at 60 minutes suggests gangrenous cholecystitis

 TABLE 53.5: HIDA Scan: cholecystitis

IV contrast	No
PO contrast	No
Amount of radiation	3 mSv

Classic Images

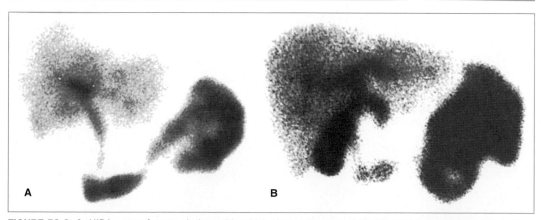

FIGURE 53.6: A: HIDA scan of acute cholecystitis which shows absence of GB filling and normal free-draining bile duct. **B:** HIDA scan showing normal filling of the GB and biliary tree with free flow into the duodenum and proximal bowel. (From Gorbach SL, Bartlett JG, and Blacklow NR. Infectious Diseases, 3rd ed. Philadelphia: Lippincott Williams & Wilkins, 2003.)

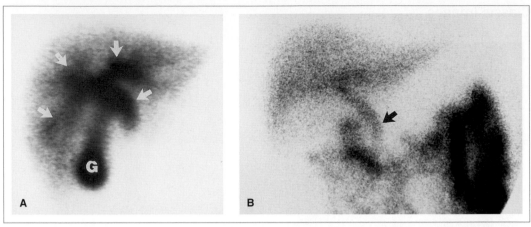

FIGURE 53.7: Abnormal technetium-99m-labeled mebrofenin biliary scans. **A:** Patient with a common duct stone. Ninety minutes after injection, the isotope is in the liver and gallbladder (G). There is no excretion into the duodenum, and the biliary tree is dilated (*arrows*). **B:** Patient with acute cholecystitis from cystic duct stone. No gallbladder filling occurs at 60 minutes. The isotope passes freely into the duodenum through the common bile duct (*arrow*). (From Daffner RH. Clinical Radiology: The Essentials, 3rd ed. Philadelphia: Lippincott Williams & Wilkins, 2007.)

Basic Management
- NPO and replace volume loss with normal saline followed by maintenance fluids
- Pain management
  - Both biliary colic and acute cholecystitis can be treated with opiate analgesia
  - Anti-inflammatory analgesia (i.e., ketorolac) is effective but the surgical consultation may not want antiplatelet activity preoperatively
- Antibiotics, especially for the elderly and immunocompromised
- Surgical consultation
- Admission for likely cholecystectomy

Summary

TABLE 53.6: Advantages and disadvantages of imaging modalities in cholecystitis

Imaging modalities	Advantages	Disadvantages
Ultrasound	Low cost Minimal patient discomfort No radiation Bedside availability Less time-consuming	Availability of official ultrasound Body habitus limitations
CT scan	Availability Other diagnoses also possible	IV contrast Radiation exposure
HIDA scan	Gold standard	Time–consuming

HIDA, hepatobiliary iminodiacetic acid.

54 Boerhaave's Syndrome

John Jesus and Leon D. Sanchez

Background

Esophageal perforation may occur from a variety of processes. Iatrogenic injury is the most frequent, accounting for approximately 75% of cases. Iatrogenic perforations generally occur in the cervical esophagus, are more indolent, and often respond to conservative treatment with antibiotics and IV hyperalimentation. Boerhaave's syndrome represents another 10–15% of perforations, and refers to a sudden, dramatic increase in intraluminal pressure causing spontaneous full thickness rupture of the esophageal tissue. Approximately 75% of cases are a result of forceful emesis, though spontaneous rupture has also been reported with coughing, seizures, childbirth, status asthmaticus, and weight lifting. Spontaneous ruptures usually occur at the left posterolateral border of the distal esophagus where there exists the least support from surrounding mediastinal structures. Alcohol binging is commonly associated with this pathology, and is seen more commonly in men. Unlike iatrogenic cervical perforations, spontaneous thoracic perforations generally require immediate surgical repair to prevent ensuing mediastinitis, sepsis, and death.

TABLE 54.1: Classic history and physical

Violent retching after an alcoholic binge and a large meal

Classic ("Mackler") triad: vomiting, lower thoracic chest pain, and subcutaneous emphysema

Sudden onset crushing substernal chest pain exacerbated by swallowing

Hamman's sign: mediastinal crunch or crackles that are associated with each heart beat rather than respiration

TABLE 54.2: Potentially helpful laboratory test

Pleural fluid analysis: pH < 6, amylase, and food particles within pleural fluid if a thoracentesis is performed (infrequently obtained due to available diagnostic imaging modalities)

Chest Radiograph

- Almost 75–90% of distal esophageal perforations are associated with a pleural effusion or hydropneumothorax, resulting from refluxed gastric contents, swallowed food, and a sympathetic reaction from irritation to the adjacent parietal pleura and pulmonary parenchyma
- Pneumomediastinum is often the earliest plain film finding and manifests as streaks of gas that track up the lateral border of the aortic arch and descending aorta or along the lateral border of the ascending aorta
- "V-sign" of Naclerio refers to the rare presentation of pneumomediastinum that tracks along diverging fascial planes of the mediastinal and diaphragmatic pleura adjacent to the distal esophagus
- The most common site of perforation abuts the parietal pleura on the left, resulting in *left*-sided hydropneumothoraces in 75% of cases
- Radiographs may be normal in as many as 12% of esophageal perforations

 TABLE 54.3: Chest x-ray (Portable AP): Boerhaave's syndrome

IV contrast	No
PO contrast	No
Amount of radiation	0.02 mSV

Classic Images

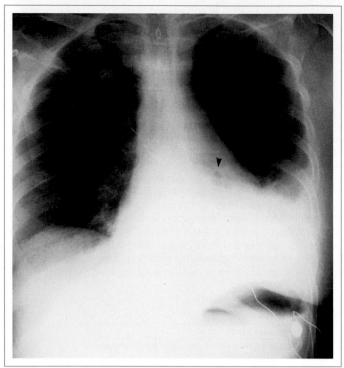

FIGURE 54.1: Pneumomediastinum (*black arrow*) and left-sided pleural effusion. (From Harris J and Harris W. The Radiology of Emergency Medicine, 4th ed. Philadelphia: Lippincott Williams & Wilkins, 2000.)

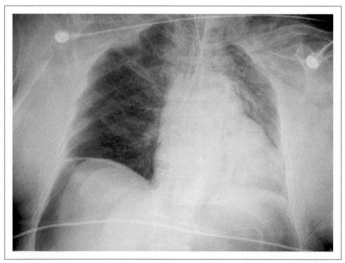

FIGURE 54.2: Pneumoperitoneum that reflects perforation of the distal esophagus below the diaphragm and subcutaneous air. (From Greenberg M. Greenberg's Text-Atlas of Emergency Medicine. Philadelphia: Lippincott Williams & Wilkins, 2005.)

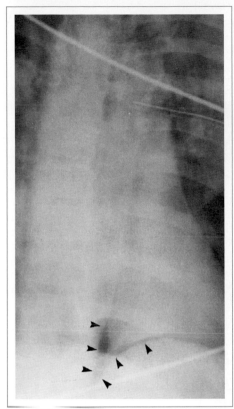

FIGURE 54.3: "V-sign" of Naclerio (*arrow heads*). (From Harris J and Harris W. The Radiology of Emergency Medicine, 4th ed. Philadelphia: Lippincott Williams & Wilkins, 2000.)

Esophagography

- Although esophagography is not as sensitive as a CT scan, it is a cheaper diagnostic modality that involves less patient exposure to radiation
- Esophagography is performed by having a patient slowly ingest water soluble Gastrografin or barium contrast while obtaining chest radiographs at various intervals
- Extravasation of contrast outside the esophagus is evidence of esophageal perforation
- Water soluble contrast is less radiopaque than barium and is unable to detect 15–25% of thoracic esophageal perforations (if the clinical presentation is concerning for perforation, however, the study should be repeated with barium contrast as the benefits of earlier diagnosis far outweigh the potential inflammatory fibrous reaction of extravasated barium contrast)

TABLE 54.4: Esophagography: Boerhaave's syndrome

IV contrast	No
PO contrast	Yes
Amount of radiation	6 mSV

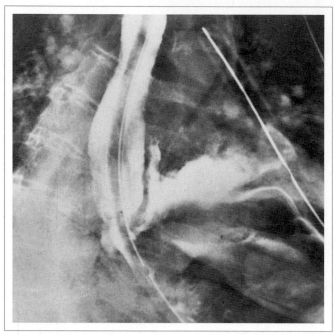

FIGURE 54.4: Esophagography demonstrating free extravasation of contrast outside the esophagus. (Eisenberg R. Gastrointestinal Radiology: A Pattern Approach, 4th ed. Philadelphia: Lippincott Williams & Wilkins, 2003.)

Chest CT

- Although CT studies expose patients to a significant amount of radiation, it is a far more sensitive diagnostic modality than esophagography or chest radiograph
- Findings without the use of contrast include esophageal thickening, pleural effusions, and mediastinal gas or fluid collections
- CT esophagography is performed by using a water-soluble contrast medium via a nasogastric tube or by rapid ingestion
- Contrast extravasation and paraesophageal air collections outside the gastrointestinal track are the principle findings of CT esophagography

■ Complications of esophageal perforation apparent on chest CT include streaky infiltration of mediastinal fat associated with mediastinitis, mediastinal widening or compression of mediastinal structures, and abscess formation

 TABLE 54.5: Chest CT scan: Boerhaave's syndrome

IV contrast	No
PO contrast	Yes
Amount of radiation	7–12 mSV

Classic Images

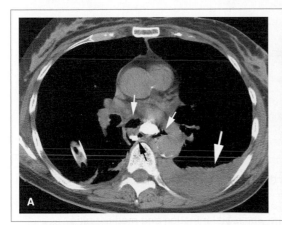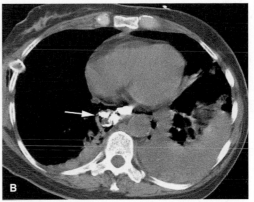

FIGURE 54.5: CT esophagography demonstrating contrast-enhanced esophagus with (**A**) contained extraluminal extravasation of contrast (*black arrow*), (**A** and **B**) paraesophageal air collections (*short white arrows*), and (**A**) left-sided effusion (*large white arrow*). (From Naidich D, Muller N, Krinsky G, et al. Computed Tomography and Magnetic Resonance of the Thorax. Philadelphia: Lippincott Williams & Wilkins, 2007.)

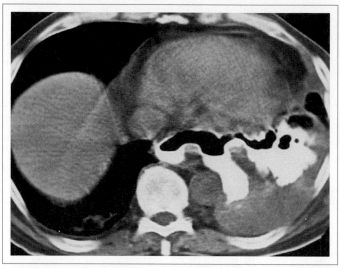

FIGURE 54.6: CT esophagography with extensive free extravasation of contrast with moderate left pleural fluid collection. (From Naidich D, Muller N, Krinsky G, et al. Computed Tomography and Magnetic Resonance of the Thorax. Philadelphia: Lippincott Williams & Wilkins, 2007.)

Basic Management
- Prevent the patient from eating or drinking and replace volume loss with normal saline followed by maintenance fluids
- Pain management
- Empiric broad spectrum antibiotics for likely polymicrobial infection and mediastinitis
- Emergent surgical consultation
- Admission for likely thoracotomy and perforation repair

TABLE 54.6: Advantages and disadvantages of imaging modalities for Boerhaave's syndrome

Imaging modality	Advantages	Disadvantages
Chest radiograph	Low cost Little radiation exposure Less time-consuming	Lowest sensitivity
Esophagography	Little radiation exposure More sensitive than chest radiograph	Lower sensitivity than CT Availability
CT esophagography	Most sensitive	IV contrast Increased radiation exposure Higher cost

55

Colitis

Kevin Nuttall and Michael Ganetsky

Background

Colitis can be divided into three broad categories: inflammatory bowel disease (IBD), infectious colitis, and ischemic colitis. IBD comprises ulcerative colitis (UC) and Crohn's disease. These have a bimodal age of onset, highest in the late teens and twenties, with a second smaller peak in the sixth to eighth decade. The pattern of affected bowel can help differentiate between UC and Crohn's disease. UC causes inflammation limited to the colon and almost always involves the rectum. Mucosa tends to be contiguously affected and involves a variable amount of colon. Conversely, Crohn's disease can affect the gastrointestinal (GI) tract anywhere from the mouth to the anus; patchy affected areas interspersed among normal bowel are common. Fifty percent have both small intestine and colon involvement and 20% have only colitis. The terminal ileum is the most commonly affected location.

Infectious colitis can be caused by viral, bacteria, fungal, or protozoal pathogens. Common invasive bacterial organisms that cause inflammatory diarrhea include Salmonella, Shigella, Campylobacter, Yersinia, *Escherichia coli* O157:H7, and *Clostridium difficile*. These are more likely to cause fever and bloody stool and elevate fecal leukocytes than the noninvasive bacterial pathogens such as enterotoxigenic *E. coli* and *Vibrio cholerae*. Viral pathogens such as rotavirus, Norwalk virus, and enteric adenoviruses also cause watery diarrhea and are very common, especially in the pediatric population.

Ischemic colitis is bowel infarction due to inadequate blood supply from the branches of the superior and inferior mesenteric arteries that supply the colon. The process is covered in detail in chapter 58 (Mesenteric Ischemia).

TABLE 55.1: Classic history and physical

Fever, chills, weight loss
Crampy abdominal pain
Diarrhea with variable amounts of bright red blood and mucous
Diarrhea which is watery and nonbloody
Tenesmus
Diffuse or localized abdominal tenderness
Extra-intestinal manifestations of inflammatory bowel disease: seronegative arthritis, episcleritis and iritis, erythema nodosum, pyoderma gangrenosum

TABLE 55.2: Potentially helpful laboratory tests

Fecal leukocytes: elevated in invasive infectious diarrhea
Stool culture and gram stain, stool ova, and parasites
Stool *Clostridium difficile* toxin A and B: classic EIA test is only moderately sensitive (79–80%), which necessitates repeat samples if negative; however, it is highly specific (98%)
CBC: leukocytosis seen in severe IBD and invasive infectious diarrhea; anemia if significant blood loss has occurred
ESR and CRP: very nonspecific but often elevated in IBD.

CBC, complete blood count; CRP, C-reactive protein; EIA, enzyme immunoassay; ESR, erythrocyte sedimentation rate; IBD, inflammatory bowel disease.

Abdominal X-ray

- Abdominal *plain films* may be useful in colitis when evaluating for complications such as toxic megacolon, ileus and obstruction, or free air.
- Nonspecific findings such as air-fluid levels in the colon and colonic distention of less than 6 cm in diameter may be seen in any type of colitis. Air within the rectum and the absence of free air under the diaphragm support an uncomplicated colitis.
- Radiographic findings suggestive of toxic megacolon include a measured diameter of the transverse colon greater than 6 cm, loss of haustra, and "thumbprinting" of the bowel wall because of inflammation and edema. When seen in the presence of signs of systemic toxicity, the diagnosis becomes likely.
- The *double contrast air-barium enema* abdominal x-ray allows for the evaluation of signs of IBD and is more sensitive than CT scan for the detection of the subtle colonic mucosal changes of early disease. It is also good at differentiating Crohn's disease from UC when only the colon is involved. In the emergency department setting, this study has largely been supplanted by abdominal CT.

 TABLE 55.3: Abdominal plain film: colitis

IV contrast	No
PO contrast	No, but may consider if looking for definitive signs of obstruction and CT scan not available
Recta contrast	No
Amount of radiation	0.7 mSv per view

Classic Images

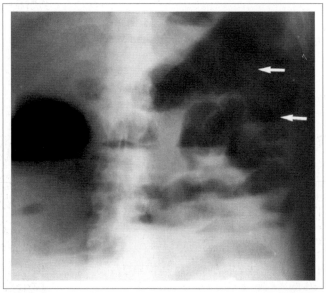

FIGURE 55.1: Plain upright abdominal radiograph of a patient with ileus. Air-fluid levels are present in the stomach and small intestine (*arrows*). Gas is seen in the colon. These findings are characteristic of, but not specific for, ileus. (From Mulholland MW, Lillemoe KD, Doherty GM, et al. Greenfield's Surgery Scientific Principles and Practice, 4th ed. Philadelphia: Lippincott Williams & Wilkins, 2006.)

Abdominal CT Scan

- CT scan allows visualization of the bowel wall as well as the surrounding tissues and structures.
- It is useful in the primary diagnosis of IBD as well as for evaluation of acute exacerbations.
- CT scan is also useful in excluding complications such as abscess, stricture, and fistula.
- Overall diagnostic sensitivity for IBD is about 84% and specificity 95% when PO and IV contrast used.

- Findings in IBD:
  - Bowel wall thickening:
    - ▶ Normal thickness: 1–4 mm
    - ▶ Crohn's disease: mean 11 mm
    - ▶ UC: mean 8 mm
  - Multiple wall densities indicative of edema, inflammation, and fatty infiltration
  - Pericolonic fat stranding (Crohn's disease due to *transmural* inflammation)
  - Lymphadenopathy
- Differentiating between UC and Crohn's disease can often be accomplished solely by examining the pattern of affected bowel. UC nearly always involves the rectum and spreads proximally to involve variable amounts of the colon contiguously. Crohn's disease has patchy involvement and can affect the small bowel or any part of the GI tract as well. Involvement of only the colon suggests UC, but Crohn's disease can mimic this pattern, thus making radiographic diagnosis difficult in this situation.
- CT scan should not be performed for the primary diagnosis of infectious colitis. However, if obtained for undifferentiated abdominal pain, the presence of pancolitis suggests an infectious process. CT findings are typically nonspecific, including circumferential wall thickening, air-fluid levels, and pericolonic fat stranding.
- Most infections manifest as pancolitis; however, Yersinia or amebiasis may be limited to proximal colon and gonorrhea or syphilis can be limited to the distal colon.
- *C. difficile* colitis tends to cause prominent colonic wall thickening (3–32 mm), "thumbprinting," and "accordion sign" indicative of contrast in-between thickened haustral folds. Ascites can occur in 35% of cases.

 TABLE 55.4: Abdominal CT scan: colitis

IV contrast	Yes
PO contrast	Yes
Amount of radiation	14 mSv

Classic Images

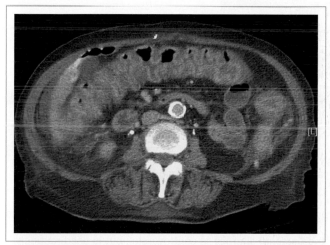

FIGURE 55.2: Thickened, edematous haustra of the transverse colon in a patient with *Clostridium difficile* pancolitis. (*Image courtesy of Beth Israel Deaconess Medical Center, Boston, MA.*)

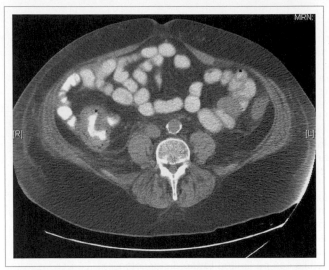

FIGURE 55.3: Crohn's disease affecting the ascending colon. Note the thickened bowel wall with oral contrast media within the lumen. (*Image courtesy of Beth Israel Deaconess Medical Center, Boston, MA.*)

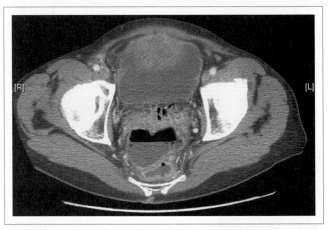

FIGURE 55.4: Abscess in ulcerative colitis. Note the fluid-and-air-filled collection compressing thickened sigmoid colon with surrounding fat stranding. (*Image courtesy of Beth Israel Deaconess Medical Center, Boston, MA.*)

Basic Management

- Analgesia, rehydration, and electrolyte repletion
- Complications such as toxic megacolon, abscess, obstruction, and perforation require urgent surgical consultation
- If treating infectious diarrhea:
  - Most cases of infectious diarrhea, especially with profuse watery stools, are noninvasive and do not require antibiotics
  - Empiric antibiotic use in suspected bacterial diarrhea is controversial, but is used routinely in patients with fever, heme- or leukocyte-positive stool, and traveler's diarrhea; currently, fluoroquinolones are recommended for 3–5 days
  - Persistent diarrhea for 2–4 weeks may be treated empirically with metronidazole to cover giardiasis
  - Antimotility agents such as loperamide have been shown to shorten duration of symptoms and number of diarrheal stools when given with an antibiotic
  - Outpatient referral to an infectious disease specialist may be indicated
- If treating IBD:
  - Relief of symptoms and treatment of complications are the principal goals

- For severe exacerbations, hospital admission for bowel rest, IV steroids, and broad-spectrum antibiotics is indicated
- If outpatient management is appropriate, consider oral steroids and antibiotics (e.g., ciprofloxacin and Flagyl), sulfasalazine, and bowel rest
- Discuss with the patient's primary physician or gastroenterologist and arrange for close follow-up.

Summary

TABLE 55.5: Advantages and disadvantages of imaging modalities in colitis

Imaging modalities	Advantages	Disadvantages
Abdominal x-ray	Fast Inexpensive Minimal radiation	Rarely a definitive study
CT scan	Gold standard for detection of complications of colitis	Expensive Time-consuming when used with oral contrast Higher radiation IV contrast

56

Diverticulitis

Amina Saghir and Marc A. Camacho

Background

Diverticulosis, multiple saccular outpouchings of the bowel, is a prerequisite condition for diverticulitis. The incidence of diverticulosis follows a clear geographic distribution, with greater prevalence in Western and urbanized countries, hypothesized to be caused by typical dietary habits low in fiber with a high intake of processed food. It can involve any part of the gastrointestinal tract, but most commonly the large bowel, more specifically the sigmoid colon. While diverticulosis may be seen in those younger than 30 years of age, the condition is more prevalent as people age, with 33–50% of those over 50 years of age afflicted. It is seen in >50% of those over 80 years of age.

Diverticulitis develops when one or more of these diverticula become impacted and locally inflamed with subsequent perforation. Ten to twenty-five percent of people with diverticulosis subsequently develop at least one acute episode of diverticulitis. A quarter of patients with diverticulitis will develop potentially life-threatening complications, including abscess, fistulae, obstruction, or stricture.

Plain films may demonstrate obstruction or free air but a CT scan is far more reliable for confirmation of the diagnosis.

TABLE 56.1: Classic history and physical

Colicky pain (LLQ in majority due to sigmoid involvement)
Vomiting
Dysuria and urinary frequency because of proximity of bladder
Tenderness
Palpable mass
Fever
Altered bowel habits

TABLE 56.2: Potentially helpful laboratory test

Elevated WBC count

Abdominal CT Scan

- Gold standard for diagnosis
- Findings include the presence of inflamed diverticula with pericolic infiltration, fat stranding (sensitivity 95%), fascial thickening, and free fluid
- Bowel wall thickening (sensitivity 96%), extensive inflammatory changes with or without a peridiverticular abscess
- Overall CT interpretation has a sensitivity of 99%, a specificity of 99%, a positive predictive value of 99%, a negative predictive value of 99%, and an overall accuracy of 99%
- Images demonstrate the spectrum of findings associated with diverticulitis

 TABLE 56.3: CT scan: diverticulitis

IV contrast	Yes
PO contrast	Yes
Rectal contrast	Yes, may be helpful as substitute for PO contrast
Amount of radiation	14 mSV

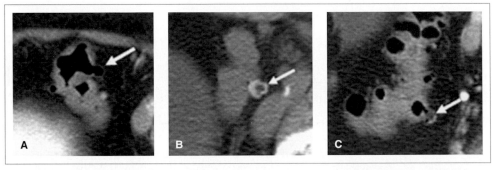

FIGURE 56.1: Sigmoid diverticulosis without diverticulitis. Axial contrast-enhanced CT images in three different patients. *Short white arrow* indicates: (**A**) air-filled diverticulum, (**B**) barium-filled diverticulum, and (**C**) stool-filled diverticulum. No thickening of the adjacent sigmoid colon wall is present and the adjacent fat demonstrates no inflammatory stranding.

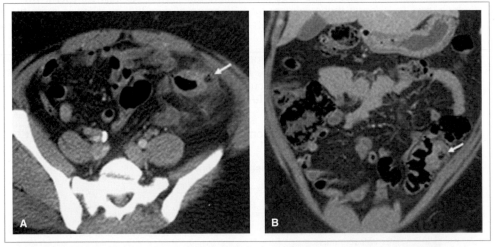

FIGURE 56.2: Uncomplicated sigmoid diverticulitis. **A:** Contrast-enhanced axial CT slice. **B:** Coronal reconstructed image at level of sigmoid colon. Marked inflammatory changes surrounding a segment of the sigmoid colon with eccentric wall thickening and an inflamed diverticulum (*white arrow*).

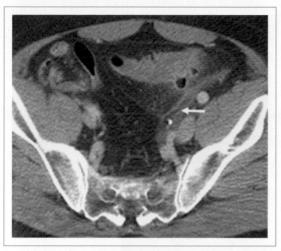

FIGURE 56.3: Early sigmoid diverticulitis. Contrast-enhanced axial CT slice through sigmoid colon. Minimal sigmoid wall thickening with minimal adjacent inflammatory stranding (*white arrow*).

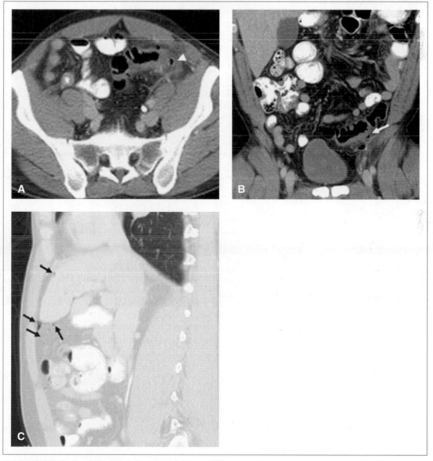

FIGURE 56.4: Complicated sigmoid diverticulitis with microperforation. **A:** Contrast-enhanced axial CT image at level of sigmoid colon. **B:** Coronal reconstruction demonstrating eccentric sigmoid colonic wall thickening, pericolonic inflammatory stranding, and an inflamed diverticulum (*arrowhead* in A, *white arrow* in B). **C:** Sagittal reconstructed images of upper abdomen in lung windows demonstrating multiple locules of extraluminal air indicating microperforation (*black arrows*).

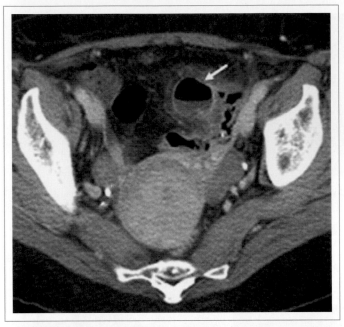

FIGURE 56.5: Complicated sigmoid diverticulitis. Contrast-enhanced axial CT image demonstrating an extraluminal air-fluid collection with thin enhancing rim consistent with abscess (*white arrow*) adjacent to sigmoid diverticulitis.

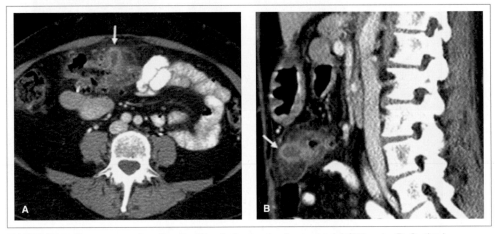

FIGURE 56.6: Transverse colon diverticulitis. **A:** Contrast-enhanced axial CT image. **B:** Sagittal reconstructed image demonstrating an inflamed diverticulum with surrounding inflammatory stranding in the transverse colon.

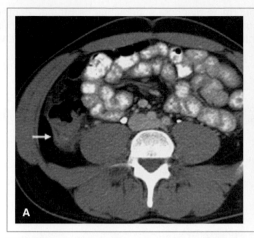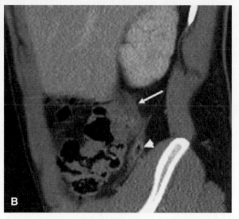

FIGURE 56.7: Ascending colon diverticulitis. **A:** Contrast-enhanced axial CT image through mid-abdomen. Inflamed diverticulum (*white arrow*) at posterior mid-ascending colon surrounded by marked inflammatory stranding. **B:** Sagittal reconstructed CT image. Proximity of appendiceal tip (*arrowhead*) to inflamed diverticulum (*white arrow*) explains initial clinical suspicion of appendicitis

Basic Management

- NPO
- Fluid replacement of volume loss with normal saline followed by maintenance fluids
- IV antibiotics
- Bowel rest
- Percutaneous drainage, if abscess present
- Emergent surgery, for perforation and peritonitis

Summary

TABLE 56.4: Advantages and disadvantages of CT scan in diverticulitis

Advantages	Disadvantages
Readily available	Contrast
Gold standard with overall accuracy of 99%	Radiation exposure
Easily identifies alternate diagnoses	

57

Abdominal Wall and Groin Hernias

Atif N. Khan and Marc A. Camacho

Background

The term hernia describes the protrusion of all or part of an organ, organs, or other anatomic structure through a defect in its surrounding support structure. While hernias can occur throughout the body and abdomen, those that occur in the abdominal wall and groin are the focus of this chapter. In the United States approximately 1.2 million abdominal hernia repairs are performed each year. Groin hernias account for 75% with the majority being inguinal (direct or indirect). Umbilical hernias are also common with 175,000 annual repairs but the majority do not require surgical repair. Incisional hernias account for approximately 10% of all repairs.

Radiologic examinations are useful for confirming diagnoses, depicting hernia sac contents for preoperative planning, and diagnosing complications such as obstruction and ischemia. The most common hernias seen in routine clinical practice include indirect inguinal, femoral, ventral, umbilical, and incisional.

TABLE 57.1: Subclassification of abdominal wall and groin hernias

Abdominal wall hernias	Umbilical
	Ventral (most, but not all, midline)
	Spigelian (at lateral edge of rectus abdominus muscle)
	Lumbar
	Incisional
Groin hernias	Inguinal (indirect, direct, and combined)
	Femoral
	Obturator
	Sciatica
	Perineal

Indirect inguinal hernias occur through a patent internal (deep) inguinal ring and into the inguinal canal. This is in contrast to direct inguinal hernias, which pass directly through fascial and muscular structures of the abdominal wall medial to the inferior epigastric vessels (in Hesselbach's triangle). Femoral hernias occur through a defect in the transversalis fascia inferior to the inguinal ligament. As the name implies, umbilical hernias occur through defects, again acquired or congenital, at the umbilicus. Ventral hernias describe other hernias through acquired or congenital disruptions in the anterior abdominal wall in other locations. Finally, incisional hernias intuitively occur at sites of acquired defects, most commonly postsurgical, although post-traumatic remains a diagnostic consideration.

Inguinal hernias have a male to female ratio of 9:1. In contrast, femoral hernias are more common in females by a 3:1 ratio. Approximately 10% of men during their lifetime will be diagnosed with an inguinal hernia.

TABLE 57.2: Classic history and physical (depends on size, location, and content of hernia)

Asymptomatic palpable mass, typically reducible and may enlarge with Valsalva
Crampy abdominal pain: intermittent, but progressively worse (possible obstruction)
Nausea with/without vomiting (indicates likely intestinal obstruction)
Pain, either focal at site or referred (e.g., scrotal pain in inguinal hernia)
Nonreducible palpable bulge (suggests incarceration)

TABLE 57.3: Potentially helpful laboratory tests

WBC: May be elevated in cases of peritonitis (insensitive and nonspecific)
Lactate: May be elevated in cases of ischemia (insensitive and nonspecific)

Plain Film Abdominal X-rays
- May reveal bowel gas over unusual site outside of typical peritoneal cavity (e.g., below obturator foramen, scrotum)
- Dilated loops of bowel with multiple air-fluid levels visible if obstruction present
- Free air: very rare; present only in cases of bowel perforation, presumably due to infarction
- Pneumatosis is a late manifestation of ischemia/infarction

 TABLE 57.4: Abdominal radiograph: hernia

IV contrast	No
PO contrast	No
Amount of radiation	0.7 mSv per view

Classic Images

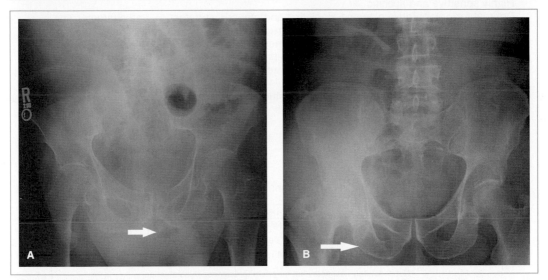

FIGURE 57.1: Abdominal radiography of indirect inguinal hernias in two different patients (**A** and **B**). Note the lucency (*white arrows*) in each case representing bowel gas within small bowel loops projecting below the superior pubic ramus (in the inguinal canal). Standard abdominal radiography is relatively insensitive, but more so for nearly all hernias except indirect inguinal hernias such as these.

Bedside Ultrasound
- Given variability in size and contents, ultrasound has limited utility with poor sensitivity and specificity
- Use of linear or curved array transducer depends on size of hernia
- May visualize homogenous fat or fat with bowel loops. May see bowel peristalsis and/or "dirty shadowing" of air in bowel lumen
- May detect defect in the anterior abdominal wall
- Contents of hernia sac may increase in size with Valsalva maneuver

Classic Images

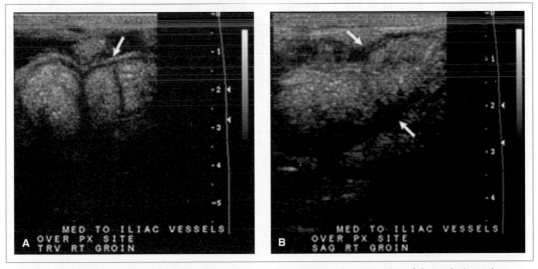

FIGURE 57.2: Transverse (**A**) and sagittal (**B**) images from an ultrasound examination of the groin (over the inguinal canal). Gray-scale images show loops of small bowel (white arrow at anterior wall in A between white arrows in B). In real-time imaging, peristalsis must be documented to confirm presence of bowel loops.

CT Scan

- Highly sensitive and specific
- Optimal for preoperative planning, depicting and measuring defect(s), and characterizing complications such as ischemia and/or obstruction
- Accurately depicts intraperitoneal contents (mesenteric fat, vessels and lymph nodes, and variable lengths of small and/or large bowel) protruding through variable-sized defects in peritoneum/abdominal wall musculature or internal ring of inguinal canal (in indirect inguinal hernias)
- If present, can accurately depict a focal transition in caliber at the hernia site with proximal bowel dilatation in bowel obstruction and/or bowel wall thickening and hernia sac fluid in ischemia
- If there is no bowel herniation (only fat and interstitium), fat may be infiltrated with stranding, which suggests fat infarction

 TABLE 57.5: CT scan: hernias

IV contrast	Yes, Useful*
PO contrast	No, Not necessary
Rectal contrast	May be helpful in equivocal cases
Amount of radiation	5–14 mSV

*Not absolutely necessary but may help to diagnose this condition in thin patients and to more accurately depict ischemia.

Classic Images

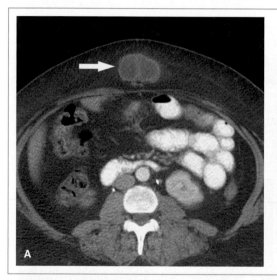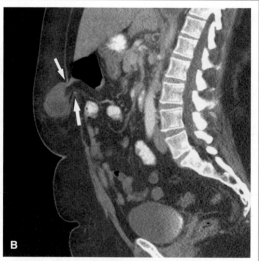

FIGURE 57.3: Axial (**A**) and sagittal (**B**) reconstructed images from a contrast-enhanced CT scan of the abdomen and pelvis. **A:** A "knuckle" of fluid-filled small bowel (*white arrow*) is seen within a small sac in the superficial abdominal wall fat. **B:** The cephalocaudal extent (the "neck") of the abdominal wall defect at the umbilicus is demonstrated (between white arrows).

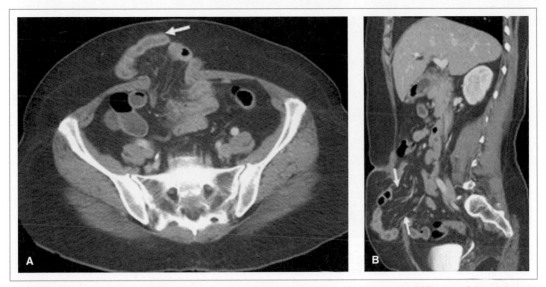

FIGURE 57.4: Axial (**A**) and sagittal (**B**) reconstructed images from a contrast-enhanced CT scan of the abdomen and pelvis. **A:** Numerous collapsed loops of small bowel and associated mesentery are present within a large hernia sac (*white arrow*) in the ventral abdominal wall right of midline at the site of a prior incision. **B:** The cephalocaudal extent (the "neck") of the incisional defect is demonstrated (between white arrows).

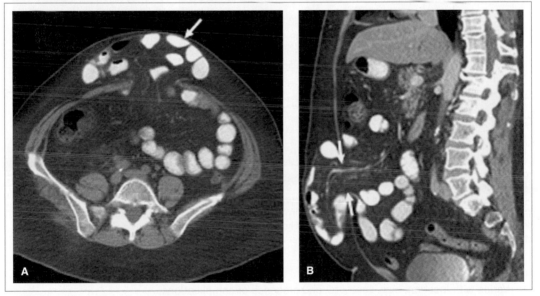

FIGURE 57.5: Axial (**A**) and sagittal (**B**) reconstructed images from a contrast-enhanced CT scan of the abdomen and pelvis. **A:** Numerous contrast-opacified loops of small bowel and associated mesentery are present within a large hernia sac in the ventral abdominal wall (*white arrow*). The presence of oral contrast in these involved loops and lack of dilatation of the more proximal loops are reassuring for the absence of obstruction. **B:** The cephalocaudal extent (the "neck") of the ventral abdominal wall defect is demonstrated (between white arrows).

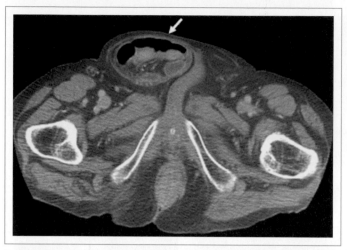

FIGURE 57.6: Axial reconstructed image from a contrast-enhanced CT scan of the abdomen and pelvis. Contrast-opacified small bowel loops and associated mesentery are present in a hernia sac in the right inguinal canal (*white arrow*).

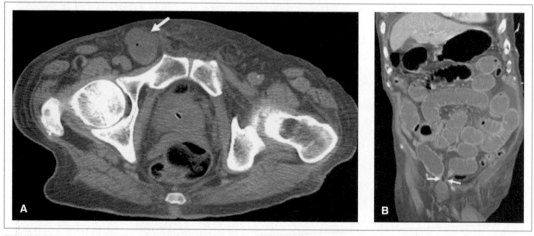

FIGURE 57.7: Axial (**A**) and coronal (**B**) reconstructed images from a contrast-enhanced CT scan of the abdomen and pelvis. **A:** Distended fluid-filled loops of small bowel and associated mesentery are present in a hernia sac in the right inguinal canal (*white arrow*). There is immediately adjacent free fluid by the small bowel within the hernia sac suggesting ischemia. **B:** Narrow neck of hernia (between white arrows) noted at right internal ring. Markedly dilated loops of more proximal small bowel are evident indicating obstruction.

Basic Management

- Varies with location, size, contents, and presence of complications
- Observe for passive reduction, may have to attempt manual reduction; if reducible, support and refer for surgical follow-up
- Pain management, opiate analgesia optimal
- If nonreducible, but no small bowel obstruction or signs of ischemia:
  - Conservative management
  - Surgical consult/referral
- If nonreducible and complicated by obstruction and/or ischemia:
  - Urgent surgical consult
  - NPO and replace volume loss with normal saline followed by maintenance fluids
  - NGT
  - Antibiotics for peritonitis and/or perforation
  - Admission for surgical repair

Summary

TABLE 57.6: Advantages and disadvantages of imaging modalities in hernia

Imaging modalities	Advantages	Disadvantages
Radiography	Low cost Fast, may quickly identify obstruction/ perforation	Insensitive and nonspecific Ionizing radiation
Ultrasound	Availability Nonionizing radiation	Cannot reliably exclude complications Poorly characterizes length and caliber of involved bowel
CT scan	Gold standard	Ionizing radiation IV contrast

58

Mesenteric Ischemia

Katherine Kroll, Peter Smulowitz, and Craig Sisson

Background

Mesenteric ischemia occurs when there is inadequate blood flow to the small intestine which results in inflammation and injury. This may occur as a result of mesenteric vein thrombosis, arterial embolism (majority from a cardiac source), nonocclusive low flow states (hypotension), arterial thrombosis (either slow progressive atherosclerosis with or without acute thrombus formation), vasospasm, or vasculitis. Mesenteric ischemia is relatively uncommon, accounting for just 0.1% of all hospital admissions and 1% of all patients with an acute abdomen; nonetheless, it may result in devastating consequences, including bowel infarction, sepsis, and death if early diagnosis and treatment are not achieved. While ischemia can be either acute or chronic, acute mesenteric ischemia (AMI) accounts for 60–70% of cases and has a mortality rate of greater than 60%. Despite advances in disease awareness and medical imaging, the mortality rate has not changed.

Risk factors for mesenteric ischemia include advanced age, a history of atherosclerosis, cardiac arrhythmias, valvular disease, recent myocardial infarction, intra-abdominal malignancy, congestive heart failure, hypercoagulability, and hypotension. Chronic mesenteric ischemia (CMI), also known as "intestinal angina," occurs in the setting of atherosclerotic disease of the mesenteric blood vessels, leading to intestinal hypoperfusion and ischemia during periods of increased demand (i.e., after eating).

TABLE 58.1: Classic history and physical

Acute mesenteric ischemia
  Rapid onset of symptoms
  Rapid clinical deterioration
  Abdominal pain out of proportion to physical examination findings
  Nausea, vomiting
  Late: confusion, tachycardia, tachypnea, circulatory collapse, hemoccult
  positive stools, abdominal distention
Chronic mesenteric ischemia
  Postprandial pain (intestinal angina)
  Nausea
  Fear of eating, weight loss

TABLE 58.2: Potentially helpful laboratory tests

Lactate: 77–100% sensitive but only 42% specific
WBC: Elevated in most cases, often markedly, but poor specificity
Amylase: Elevated in approximately 50% of cases, but poor specificity

Plain Abdominal X-rays

- Plain abdominal x-rays are nonspecific and, in a majority of cases, will be either normal or fail to suggest a specific pathologic process
- Most often, plain abdominal radiographs demonstrate a nonspecific ileus pattern with dilated, fluid-filled loops of bowel or, in 25% of cases, a normal abdomen
- While abdominal x-rays do not exclude mesenteric ischemia, they may help identify whether perforation has occurred with the presence of free air
- Findings on abdominal x-rays that are more specific for ischemia include thumbprinting (focal bowel wall thickening secondary to mucosal edema and hemorrhage), a picket-fence appearance of valvulae conniventes in the small bowel ("stacked coins"), separation of bowel loops due to mesenteric thickening, intramural gas, or mesenteric or portal venous gas; however, these are rare findings and usually indicate late-stage disease
- Mortality significantly increases with abnormal plain x-ray findings
- Primary role of x-ray is to exclude other causes of abdominal pain (i.e., perforation, small bowel obstruction, ileus, volvulus)

 TABLE 58.3: Abdominal radiograph: mesenteric ischemia

IV contrast	No
PO contrast	No
Amount of radiation	0.7 mSv per view

Classic Images

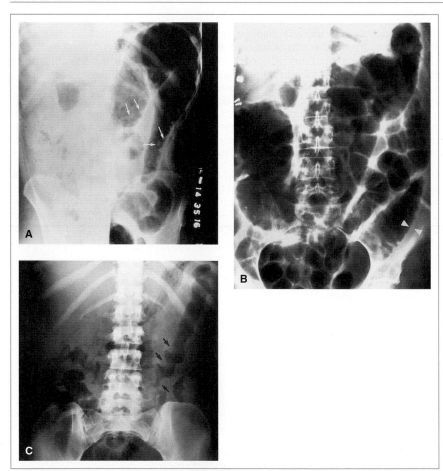

FIGURE 58.1: X-ray image showing (**A**) air in the bowel wall (*white arrows*) and (**C**) thumbprinting (*black arrows*). (**B**) The bowel wall appears thickened (*arrowheads*). (From Daffner RH. Clinical Radiology: The Essentials, 3rd ed. Philadelphia: Lippincott Williams & Wilkins, 2007.)

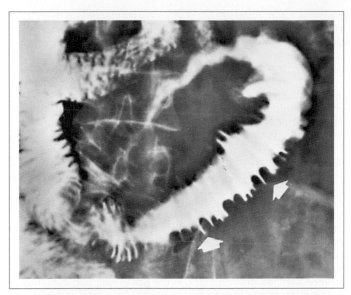

FIGURE 58.2: Small bowel ischemia producing a segmental picket-fence pattern of thickening of small bowel folds (*arrows*). (From Eisenberg RL. An Atlas of Differential Diagnosis, 4th ed. Philadelphia: Lippincott Williams & Wilkins, 2003.)

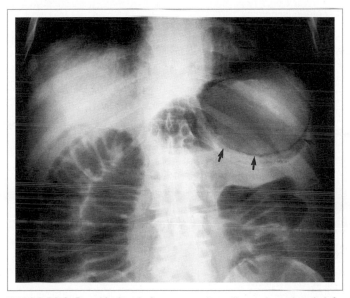

FIGURE 58.3: Bowel ischemia from a massive celiac and mesenteric infarction with pneumatosis in the stomach wall. (From Daffner RH. Clinical Radiology: The Essentials, 3rd ed. Philadelphia: Lippincott Williams & Wilkins, 2007.)

Abdominal CT Scan

- Although angiography was traditionally the gold standard for diagnosis of mesenteric ischemia, multidetector computer tomography (MDCT) has now become the examination of choice when mesenteric ischemia is suspected, because of its ability to image both the mesenteric blood vessels (with CT angiography) and the small intestine, as well as its capacity to evaluate the abdomen for other etiologies of abdominal pain

- CT evaluation for mesenteric ischemia is rapid, noninvasive, and widely available in a majority of medical centers. However, with the exception of acute mesenteric vein thrombosis, a normal CT scan of the abdomen cannot exclude the various causes of AMI
- Using MDCT technology, the sensitivity and specificity of abdominal CT scan for detecting mesenteric vein thrombosis exceeds 90%; the sensitivity for all-cause mesenteric ischemia is 65–80%
- Findings on CT suggestive of mesenteric ischemia include bowel wall thickening (the most common finding), bowel distention, intraperitoneal free fluid (ascites), "streaky" mesentery or mesenteric edema, intramural gas (pneumatosis intestinalis), portal vein gas, vascular occlusion or stenosis, a lack of bowel wall enhancement, as well as infarcts of liver, spleen, or kidney
- Findings on nonintravenous contrast-enhanced CT scan include hypoattenuated thickened bowel wall as a marker of bowel wall edema and hyperattenuated thickened bowel wall as a marker of bowel wall hemorrhage
- Findings on IV contrast-enhanced CT include areas of nonenhancing thickened bowel wall which has a 96% specificity for acute ischemia; other findings include hyperemia of thickened bowel as an indication of mesenteric venous outflow obstruction and hyperperfusion of thickened bowel as an indication of reperfusion after ischemia or a concomitant infectious process
- Mesenteric arterial and venous occlusions and stenosis can be shown on CT scan using timed IV contrast injections, which identify lack of enhancement or narrowing of the arteries and veins; however, these are less common findings than changes in the bowel wall and mesentery
- Limitations to abdominal CT scan still exist; in particular, early reversible mesenteric ischemia is difficult to identify on CT scan. Thus, angiography may play a role in cases where there is a very high clinical suspicion with unremarkable CT scan

 TABLE 58.4: CT scan: mesenteric ischemia

IV contrast	Yes, bowel wall enhancement indicates perfusion
PO contrast	Yes, to distend bowel for better assessment of bowel wall thickening
Amount of radiation	14 mSv

Classic Images

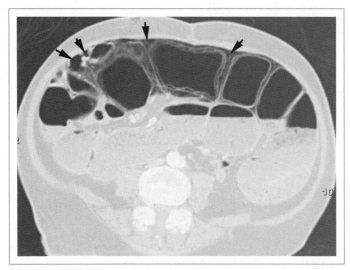

FIGURE 58.4: CT image showing dilated loops of bowel anteriorly with gas in the walls. Notice the pneumoperitoneum between the dilated loops. (From Daffner RH. Clinical Radiology: The Essentials, 3rd ed. Philadelphia: Lippincott Williams & Wilkins, 2007.)

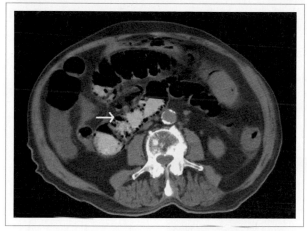

FIGURE 58.5: Pneumatosis of the small bowel (*arrow*). (*Courtesy of Turandot Saul, St. Luke's Roosevelt Hospital, New York, NY.*)

Abdominal MRI/MRA

- MRI should not be the initial diagnostic test for mesenteric ischemia because of the time necessary to obtain the examination
- Has been shown to have accurate imaging of the mesenteric vasculature; however, in the acute setting offers little over CT imaging
- May be used in planning surgical or endovascular repair

 TABLE 58.5: MRI/magnetic resonance angiography: mesenteric ischemia

IV contrast	Yes, to delineate vasculature
PO contrast	No
Amount of radiation	None

Classic Images

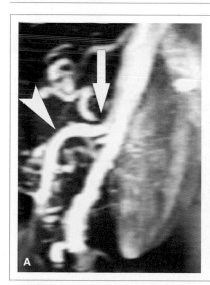
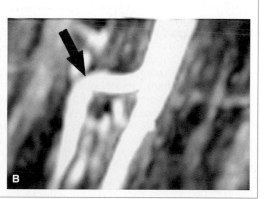

FIGURE 58.6: Mesenteric magnetic resonance angiography (MRA). **A:** Sagittal maximum intensity projection of data from three-dimensional gadolinium-enhanced MRA obtained in coronal plane clearly shows severe celiac artery stenosis (*arrow*) and widely patent superior mesenteric artery (SMA) (*arrowhead*). **B:** No signal is present in proximal celiac artery on phase contrast MRA due to severity of stenosis (*arrow* denotes SMA). (From Leyendecker JR and Brown JJ. Practical Guide to Abdominal and Pelvic MRI. Philadelphia: Lippincott Williams & Wilkins, 2004.)

Doppler Ultrasonography

- Sensitivity is 70–89% and specificity is 92–100% for identification of severe or complete proximal splanchnic vessel occlusion
- Cannot diagnose emboli beyond proximal main vessel and cannot diagnose nonocclusive mesenteric ischemia
- Arterial stenosis alone does not establish a diagnosis of mesenteric ischemia, as significant stenosis can be present in asymptomatic patients secondary to increased collateral blood flow

Classic Images

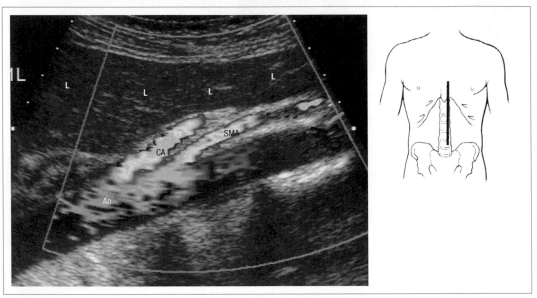

FIGURE 58.7: Doppler ultrasound of the abdomen at level of aorta, celiac artery superior mesenteric artery. Small image at right indicates level of scan (line D). AO, aorta; CA, celiac artery; SMA, superior mesenteric artery (*Courtesy of Dr. J. Lai, University of Toronto, Toronto, Ontario, Canada.*) (From Agur A and Dalley A, eds. Grant's Atlas of Anatomy, 12th ed. Philadelphia: Lippincott Williams & Wilkins, 2008.)

Angiography

- Angiography can identify the location of vascular occlusion (important for surgical planning) and can also evaluate the mesenteric vasculature for atherosclerosis; as noted above, it may also be more sensitive for early, reversible ischemia
- Gold standard for the diagnosis of AMI (excluding ischemic colitis), including nonocclusive mesenteric ischemia, *prior* to the onset of acute peritonitis (bowel necrosis); angiography is very sensitive (74–100%) and specific (100%) for identifying arterial occlusion
- Angiography can be therapeutic as well as diagnostic; selected vasodilators (e.g., papaverine or prostaglandin E1) or thrombolytic agents may be infused into affected vessels
- Angiography must be biplanar; branches are best visualized with anterior-posterior fluoroscopic views and the origins of major vessels are best seen on lateral fluoroscopic views
- Arterial thrombosis occurs most commonly at the origin of the superior mesenteric artery (SMA)
- Mesenteric venous thrombosis shows vessel-specific increased arterial filling times and corresponding lack of mesenteric venous and portal venous opacification
- Nonocclusive mesenteric ischemia shows diffuse increased arterial filling times with normal venous drainage; narrowing in multiple areas in the SMA distribution leading to the "string of sausages" sign may also be seen
- Although highly sensitive and specific, angiography is also an invasive, time-consuming, potentially nephrotoxic, and costly procedure; angiography is most likely to cause complications in the very patient population in which intestinal ischemia is most common, that is, elderly patients with atherosclerosis; it may not be available in every hospital on a consistent basis, as angiography requires an endovascular specialist to be available

TABLE 58.6: Angiography: mesenteric ischemia

IV contrast	Yes, to visualize vasculature
PO contrast	No
Amount of radiation	12 mSv

Classic Images

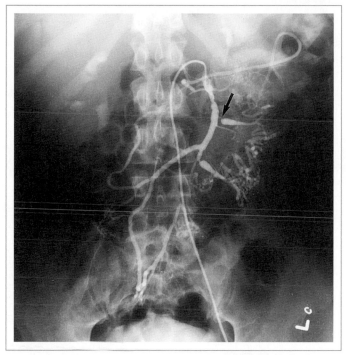

FIGURE 58.8: Stenosis of a jejunal branch (*arrow*) of the superior mesenteric artery. (*Courtesy of Dr. Ernest Ring.*) (From Koopman WJ and Moreland LW. Arthritis and Allied Conditions: A Textbook of Rheumatology, 15th ed. Philadelphia: Lippincott Williams & Wilkins, 2004.)

Basic Management

- AMI is a true emergency, requiring rapid initiation of volume resuscitation and aggressive monitoring of hemodynamic status, as hypotension may result from third-spacing of fluid into the ischemic bowel, further worsening bowel ischemia
- Empiric, broad-spectrum antibiotics (such as imipenem) should be used early, as bowel ischemia can lead to translocation of bacteria through the intestinal wall
- A nasogastric tube should be placed for gastric decompression
- Surgical revascularization is indicated for mesenteric artery thrombosis
- Vasodilators such as papaverine hydrochloride may be used for nonocclusive mesenteric ischemia
- In cases of mesenteric artery embolism, treatment choices include surgical embolectomy, thrombolytic agents, and anticoagulants
- Anticoagulation, usually an unfractionated heparin drip, is useful to prevent clot propagation in the setting of an embolism or thrombus; a heparin drip can be titrated quickly and turned off, should surgery be required
- When vasopressors are needed, dopamine, a β-adrenergic agonist, is preferred in order to avoid aggravation of intestinal ischemia
- Early surgical consultation is imperative, and is also associated with decreased morbidity and mortality; admission to a surgical service is likely
- Pain management is generally with parenteral opiate analgesics
- Treatment of patients with chronic mesenteric ischemic is generally less acute, and is surgical or endovascular in nature

Summary

TABLE 58.7: Advantages and disadvantages of imaging modalities in mesenteric ischemia

Imaging modalities	Advantages	Disadvantages
Abdominal x-ray	Fast Noninvasive Low dose of radiation Low cost Widely available	Neither sensitive nor specific Pathologic findings occur late in disease
CT scan	Fast Noninvasive Other diagnoses can be made Widely available Sensitive and specific	IV and PO contrast Radiation exposure Nephrotoxic contrast
MRI	Accurate assessment of vasculature Surgical planning	Time-consuming Less monitored setting
Ultrasound	Sensitivity 70–89% for *proximal* splanchnic vessel occlusion	Cannot exclude occlusion in distal vessels Arterial stenosis alone is nondiagnostic
Angiography	Gold standard Possibly therapeutic May reveal early reversible ischemia Sensitive and specific	Time-consuming Invasive Radiation exposure Question of availability Nephrotoxic contrast Costly

59

Small Bowel Obstruction

Erin Horn and Jason Imperato

Background

Small bowel obstruction (SBO) causes nontraumatic, acute abdominal pain in 4% of patients presenting to the emergency department and it accounts for approximately 20% of all surgical admissions. The most common etiologies of SBO include postoperative adhesions, which accounts for 50–60%, as well as inflammatory bowel disease, especially Crohn's disease, hernias, neoplasms, and strictures. Surgeries most closely associated with adhesions leading to SBO are appendectomy, colorectal surgery, gynecologic procedures, and upper gastrointestinal procedures.

SBO occurs when the flow of normal luminal contents, which includes the 8–10 L of fluid secreted by the stomach, small bowel, biliary tract, and pancreas, is interrupted. Usually, this volume is reabsorbed in the large bowel, but in cases of SBO, the fluid accumulates in the small bowel proximal to the obstruction. Swallowed air and gas from bacterial fermentation adds to the distention. As the process continues, the bowel wall becomes edematous, leading to transudative fluid loss into the peritoneal cavity. The final common pathway, regardless of the cause of the SBO, is dehydration with electrolyte abnormalities.

SBO can be partial or complete, simple or strangulated—although strangulation usually occurs in the setting of complete obstruction. Strangulation occurs when there is decreased blood flow to the bowel wall. Hypoperfusion and the resulting ischemia is usually caused by one of two distinct mechanisms: (i) increasing edema and elevated intraluminal pressure and (ii) when there is mesenteric twisting around a fixed point such as an adhesive band. Strangulation ultimately leads to necrosis, perforation, and increased morbidity and mortality.

A specific type of SBO is a closed loop obstruction, which occurs when a segment of intestine is blocked at two locations such that there is no proximal or distal outlet.

TABLE 59.1: Classic history and physical

Abdominal pain and distention
Nausea/vomiting
Inability to pass flatus (variable especially early in course)
Fever, tachycardia, and hypotension (a late finding in strangulation)
Hyperactive bowel sounds (early)
Hypoactive bowel sounds (late)

TABLE 59.2: Potentially helpful laboratory tests

Standard metabolic panel: not diagnostic but may suggest dehydration
Metabolic alkalosis: early sign (vomiting)
Metabolic acidosis: late sign (strangulation)
CBC: elevated WBC

CBC, complete blood count; WBC, white blood cell.

Plain Radiography

- Obtain plain radiographs first if SBO is suspected; they are widely available and relatively inexpensive when compared to other radiographic studies
- At least two views are required, supine/flat and upright (a decubitus film may be performed if the patient is unable to stand or sit)
- Plain radiographs can reveal a spectrum of small bowel gas patterns
  - **Normal:** either absence of gas or small amounts of gas in up to four nondistended (less than 25 mm) loops of small bowel and a normal distribution of colonic air and stool
  - **Abnormal but nonspecific:** at least one loop of mildly distended small bowel (25–30 mm) with three or more air-fluid levels on upright x-ray; the colonic gas and stool distribution is either normal or slightly decreased, which indicates very early or low-grade obstruction, ileus, or hypoperistalsis
  - **Probable SBO:** multiple gas- or fluid-filled loops of dilated small bowel but with colonic gas and stool, which indicates early complete obstruction, partial obstruction, or ileus
  - **Definite SBO:** dilated gas- or fluid-filled loops of small bowel with air-fluid levels and a gasless colon
- Upright films with air-fluid levels in the same loop of bowel and with a mean air-fluid level width greater than 25 mm are more likely to be indicative of a high-grade obstruction
- May also see "small bowel fecalization," although more commonly seen on CT scan
  - Occurs when the solid material in the dilated segment of bowel contains gas bubbles resembling feces
  - Feces should usually only be seen in the large bowel (this sign is associated with SBO in 82% of patients)
- Plain films are diagnostic in 50–60%, equivocal in 20–30% and normal, nonspecific, or misleading in 10–20% of cases
- Supine x ray:
  - the air-fluid interface is parallel to the x-ray plate, showing the entire width of gas- or fluid-filled loops of bowel
  - allows an estimation of the degree of distention
- Upright x-ray:
  - the air-fluid interface is perpendicular to the x-ray plate, showing the characteristic air-fluid levels

 TABLE 59.3: Abdominal radiograph: small bowel obstruction

IV contrast	No
PO contrast	No
Amount of radiation	0.7 mSv per view

Classic Images

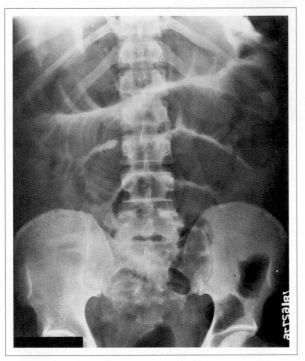

FIGURE 59.1: Supine film showing multiple dilated small bowel loops. (From Daffner RH. Clinical Radiology: The Essentials, 3rd ed. Philadelphia: Lippincott Williams & Wilkins, 2007.)

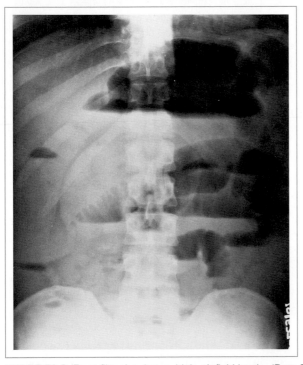

FIGURE 59.2: Erect film showing multiple air-fluid levels. (From Daffner RH. Clinical Radiology: The Essentials, 3rd ed. Philadelphia: Lippincott Williams & Wilkins, 2007.)

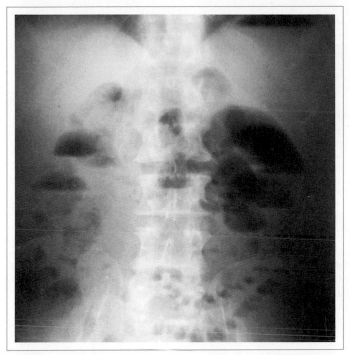

FIGURE 59.3: Stepladder pattern of air-fluid levels on upright view in a patient with small bowel obstruction. (From Harwood-Nuss A, Wolfson AB, et al. The Clinical Practice of Emergency Medicine, 3rd ed. Philadelphia: Lippincott Williams & Wilkins, 2001.)

Abdominal CT Scan
- About 90% sensitive and specific in detecting SBO
- Has several advantages over plain films, as a CT scan can:
  - identify the cause of the obstruction
  - differentiate between ileus and SBO
  - provide information regarding the presence of either strangulation or a closed loop obstruction
- Does not require PO contrast for diagnosis because the intraluminal fluid serves as a natural contrast agent
- Diagnostic if the small-bowel loop is dilated greater than 25 mm in diameter proximal to a distinct transition zone of collapsed bowel less than 10 mm in diameter
- Signs of strangulation can include:
  - bowel wall thickening
  - increased mural attenuation
  - portal venous gas
  - the double halo or target sign, which arises from submucosal edema
  - intestinal pneumatosis and hemorrhagic mesenteric changes can be seen in advanced ischemia
- Closed-loop obstruction can be signified by:
  - distended, fluid-filled, sometimes C-shaped or U-shaped loop of bowel
  - prominent mesenteric vessels converging on the point of torsion or incarceration
  - proximal loops are dilated and filled with gas and fluid

 TABLE 59.4: CT scan: small bowel obstruction

IV contrast	Yes
PO contrast	No, this can obscure the etiology of the obstruction and enhancement of the mucosal bowel lumen
Amount of radiation	14 mSV

Classic Images

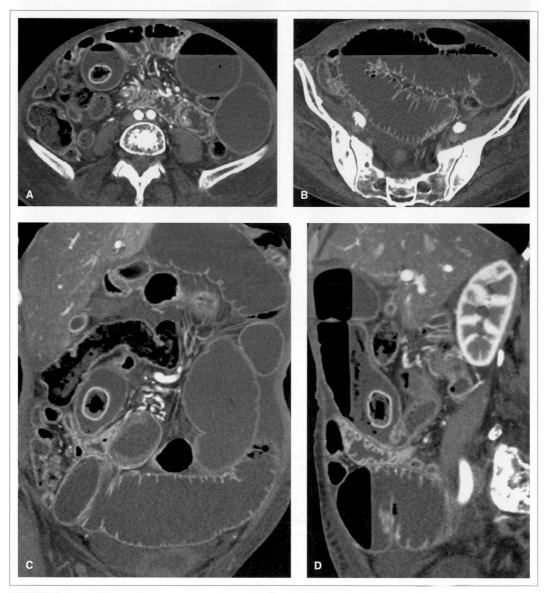

FIGURE 59.4: Axial (**A** and **B**) and coronal reformatted (**C** and **D**) Contrast enhanced CT scan images demonstrate multiple dilated loops of small bowel (up to 6 cm), with an acute transition point at the level of the proximal ileum. (Reproduced with permission from Ros PR and Mortele K. CT and MRI of the Abdomen and Pelvis, 2nd edition: Philadelphia, Lippincott Williams & Wilkins, 2007.)

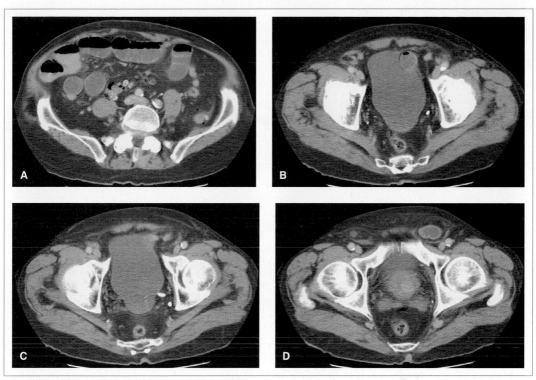

FIGURE 59.5: Axial contrast enhanced CT scan images demonstrate multiple dilated loops of small bowel (**A**) which can be followed into the left groin (**B**, **C**, and **D**), anteromedially to the femoral vessels (**D**). (Reproduced with permission from Ros PR and Mortele K. CT and MRI of the Abdomen and Pelvis, 2nd ed. Philadelphia, Lippincott Williams & Wilkins, 2007.)

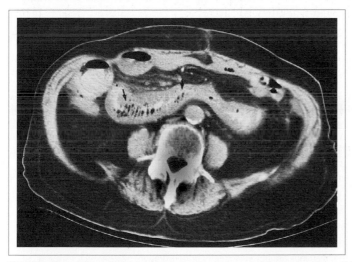

FIGURE 59.6: CT section shows pneumatosis (*arrows*) in a loop of small bowel. (From Daffner RH. Clinical Radiology: The Essentials, 3rd ed. Philadelphia: Lippincott Williams & Wilkins, 2007.)

Basic Management

- Bowel decompression with nasogastric tube for suctioning of gastrointestinal contents
- Aggressive fluid resuscitation
- Pain control and antiemetics

- Antibiotics
- Surgical consultation
- Admission for operative repair or serial abdominal examinations

Summary

TABLE 59.5: Advantages and disadvantages of imaging modalities in small bowel obstruction

Imaging modality	Advantages	Disadvantages
Plain radiographs	Low cost Minimal radiation Not time-consuming May give immediate diagnosis	Nonspecific results Does not identify cause of obstruction
CT scan	Identifies complications and etiology of SBO	Radiation exposure Time-consuming

60

Large Bowel Obstruction

Daniel Henning and Sejal Shah

Background

The majority of large bowel obstructions (LBOs) in adults are caused by neoplasms (60%), most commonly colon carcinoma. Volvulus accounts for another 10–17%; of these, 76% involve the sigmoid colon and 22% involve the cecum. Strictures from chronic diverticulitis cause another 10–12%. Other less common causes of LBO include fecal impaction, acute diverticulitis, inflammatory bowel disease, hernia, intussusception, and colonic infections. These percentage values reflect LBOs that required surgery, and may not accurately reflect the patient population presenting acutely with LBO to the emergency department.

The radiologic findings of LBO are related to its pathophysiology. Mechanical obstruction leads to dilation of the proximal segments of bowel secondary to increased intraluminal pressure. This pressure can result in decreased blood flow to the bowel. Ischemia may ensue, which can manifest as bowel wall thickening (edema) and free fluid (transudation of fluid) on CT. Ultimately, necrosis of the bowel wall can cause bowel perforation, resulting in free intraperitoneal air, and air within the bowel wall (pneumatosis). Specific to volvulus, two pathologic mechanisms occur: gas created within the closed loop cannot escape resulting in massive dilation of the loop, and twisting of the vascular pedicle results in bowel wall ischemia.

TABLE 60.1: Classic history and physical

Abdominal pain and distention, may be sudden onset or progressive
Obstipation or constipation
Nausea and vomiting typically occur later, and may be feculent
Abdominal distension with peritoneal signs on examination

TABLE 60.2: Potentially helpful laboratory tests

CBC: Elevated WBC may suggest infection/inflammation
Lactate: If elevated, may indicate bowel ischemia or dehydration

CBC, complete blood count.

Abdominal Radiographs

- Sensitivity and specificity for LBO 84% and 72% respectively
- Abnormally dilated bowel (3,6,9 rule)
  - Small bowel >3 cm
  - Large bowel >6 cm
  - Cecum >9 cm

- Differentiate small from large bowel
  - Large bowel is characterized by haustral folds and fecal content
  - Small bowel is characterized by circumferential folds (valvulae conniventes), most abundant in the jejunum
- Obstruction with perforation is suggested by free air beneath the diaphragm on upright/decubitus film or air outlining bowel wall both internally and externally on supine film
- Disease-specific findings:
  - Sigmoid volvulus (more common in elderly)
    - ▶ Bent inner tube sign or coffee bean sign
    - ▶ Colon distends proximal to twist
  - Cecal volvulus (more common in young adults)
    - ▶ Dilated loop in the mid upper abdomen
    - ▶ Decompressed distal large bowel

 TABLE 60.3: Abdominal radiograph: large bowel obstruction

IV contrast	No
PO contrast	No
Amount of radiation	0.7 mSv per view

Classic Images

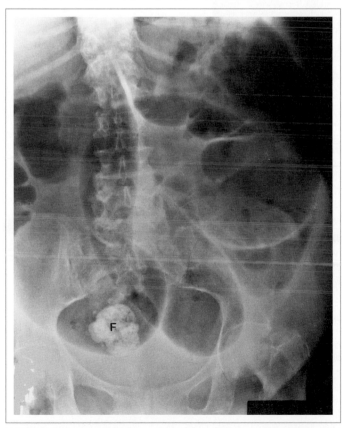

FIGURE 60.1: Sigmoid volvulus. Note distended proximal large bowel and coffee bean appearance of volvulus loop. The F denotes an incidental fibroid, and is not related to the volvulus. (From Daffner RH. Clinical Radiology: The Essentials, 3rd ed. Philadelphia: Lippincott Williams & Wilkins, 2007.)

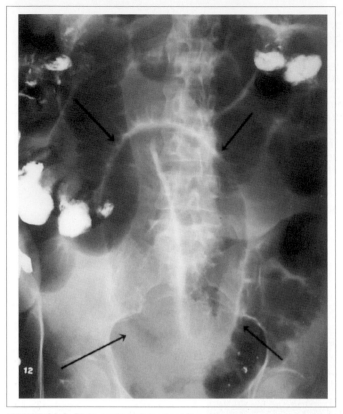

FIGURE 60.2: Plain supine abdominal film of a patient with sigmoid volvulus. The centrally located sigmoid loop is outlined by trapped air. Notice the coffee bean appearance. The proximal small intestine is dilated as well, suggesting that the volvulus has been present for sufficient time to cause accumulation of air and fluid proximally. (*Courtesy of John Braver, Department of Radiology, Brigham and Women's Hospital, Harvard Medical School, Boston, MA.*) (From Mulholland M, Lillemoe K, Doherty G, et al. Greenfield's Surgery: Scientific Principles and Practice, 4th ed. Philadelphia: Lippincott Williams & Wilkins, 2006.)

Abdominal CT Scan
- Both sensitivity and specificity of 90% in diagnosing LBO
- With 64 slice and multiplanar reformatting, the need for PO contrast to identify bowel obstruction is limited to patients with surgical changes to abdominal anatomy and patients with minimal intra-abdominal fat (generally less than 120 lb)
- CT scan is indicated for any patient with strong clinical suspicion of LBO, with or without evidence of LBO on KUB
- Value of CT for LBO
  - Clearly identify point of obstruction
  - Assess bowel wall for signs of edema/necrosis
  - Assess for free air, pneumatosis
  - Assess for other causes of abdominal pain such as appendicitis or inflammatory bowel disease

- Disease-specific findings:
  - Colorectal cancer
    - ▶ Mass visible within bowel lumen
    - ▶ Bowel wall thickening causing luminal compromise
  - Sigmoid volvulus
    - ▶ Dilated, U-shaped loop of large bowel
    - ▶ Twisted mesentery and blood vessels at point of volvulus make "whirl" sign
  - Cecal volvulus
    - ▶ Cecal pole appears in left upper quadrant of the abdomen
    - ▶ Extreme dilation of the cecum

 TABLE 60.4: CT scan: large bowel obstruction

IV contrast	Yes
PO contrast	Yes, Helpful
Amount of radiation	14 mSv

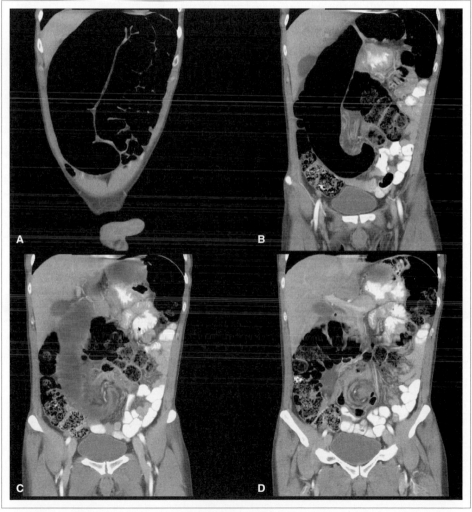

FIGURE 60.3: Sigmoid volvulus. Image **A** through **D** in sequential order anterior to posterior. Note in image A the distended, large U-shaped bowel loop, with proximal bowel dilation. Moving posterior, the vascular pedicle is seen as the whirl emerging in the middle of the image. (*Courtesy of Beth Israel Deaconess Medical Center, Boston, MA.*)

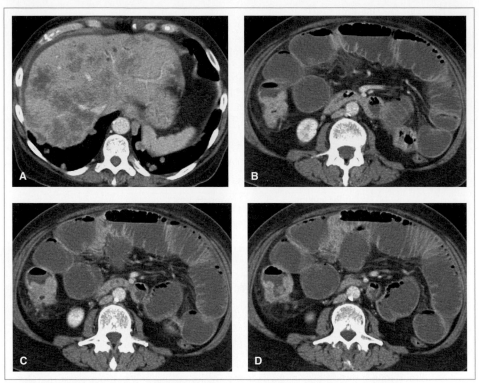

FIGURE 60.4: Colon cancer with bowel obstruction. (**A**) CT scan demonstrates pulmonary nodules and low attenuation masses in the liver. (**B–D**) Mid-abdomen images reveal a constricting lesion of the ascending colon and associated bowel obstruction. (From Ros PR and Mortelle KJ. CT and MRI of the Abdomen and Pelvis: A Teaching File, 2nd ed. Philadelphia: Lippincott Williams & Wilkins, 2007.)

Basic Management
- NPO and replace volume loss with normal saline followed by maintenance fluids
- Pain management
- Antibiotics, especially for the elderly and/or immunocompromised
- Fecal disimpaction if necessary
- Surgical consultation
- Gastrointestinal (GI) tract decompression
  - Place a nasogastric tube to decompress the upper GI tract, if necessary
  - Sigmoid volvulus may resolve with placement of rectal tube for decompression
  - Cecal volvulus typically requires surgical correction
- Admission for bowel decompression and likely resection

Summary

TABLE 60.5: Advantages and disadvantages of imaging modalities in large bowel obstruction

Imaging modalities	Advantages	Disadvantages
Abdominal radiograph	Low cost Low radiation Less time-consuming	Decreased sensitivity and specificity Will likely require further imaging regardless of findings
CT scan	Higher sensitivity and specificity Other pathology discerned Easy availability	IV contrast Radiation exposure

TABLE 60.6: Sensitivity and specificity of imaging modalities in large bowel obstruction

Imaging modalities	Sensitivity	Specificity
Abdominal radiograph	84%	72%
CT scan	90%	90%

61

Acute Pancreatitis

Kathryn Volz and Todd Seigel

Background

More than 220,000 patients with acute pancreatitis are admitted to hospitals each year. Alcohol abuse and gallstones represent the most common etiologies of acute pancreatitis (60–70%). Almost 70–80% cases of acute pancreatitis are self-limited, with the remainder developing severe complications or progressing to fulminant pancreatitis.

TABLE 61.1: Etiologies of pancreatitis

Alcohol abuse
Biliary stone disease
Hypertriglyceridemia
Hypercalcemia
ERCP procedure
Drugs*
Viral infections, e.g., mumps, CMV, EBV, Coxsackie
Trauma
Scorpion bites

CMV, cytomegalovirus; EBS, Epstein barr virus.
*Drugs: estrogen-containing oral contraceptives, corticosteroids, sulfonamides, thiazide diuretics, furosemides, nonsteroidal anti-inflammatory drugs (NSAIDs) and tetracyclines.

TABLE 61.2: Classic history and physical

Mid to upper abdominal pain radiating to the back
Nausea and vomiting
Restlessness and agitation
Relief on bending forward
SOB (may be from reactive pleural effusion, ARDS, or depressed myocardial function)
Grey Turner sign (ecchymosis of the flanks) and Cullen sign (ecchymosis of the periumbilical area) caused by hemorrhagic pancreatitis

ARDS, acute respiratory distress syndrome; SOB, shortness of breath

TABLE 61.3: Potentially helpful laboratory tests

Lipase, elevation above two times the normal value is the hallmark of pancreatitis; may be elevated or normal in chronic pancreatitis
Amylase,* less specific than lipase
Calcium, hypocalcemia may be present, but is a very nonspecific marker
LFTs, elevation is suggestive of gallstone pancreatitis

*Lipase has been shown to be more accurate and specific than amylase in the evaluation of acute pancreatitis. Amylase plus lipase adds no diagnostic accuracy over lipase alone and therefore lipase alone can safely be used in screening for pancreatitis.

Abdominal CT Scan
- The pancreas can be identified in the midabdomen, caudad from the gallbladder, draped over the aorta, and in the same plane as the adrenal glands
- A normal pancreas will evenly enhance with IV contrast
- IV contrast-enhanced CT scan is the gold standard imaging modality in the diagnosis of acute pancreatitis

■ CT can confirm the diagnosis of pancreatitis, rule out other etiologies of patient's pain, and may identify the underlying cause of disease

TABLE 61.4: Indications for CT scan in suspected pancreatitis

Clinical diagnosis in doubt
Hyperlipasemia and severe clinical pancreatitis, abdominal distension, tenderness to palpation, fever >102°F, or leukocytosis
Ranson score > 3 or APACHE score > 8
No clinical improvement within 72 hr
Acute change in clinical status including fever, pain, inability to take PO, hypotension, and drop in hematocrit

■ CT is useful to grade severity of disease and identify complications including necrosis, and late complications such as abscess and pseudocyst
  ● Necrosis, resulting from enzymatic destruction of the parenchyma, is seen as an area of low-attenuation or gas bubbles within the pancreatic bed; it is one of the most concerning findings because infected necrotizing pancreatitis is associated with a high mortality rate

TABLE 61.5: CT severity index (Balthazar classification)

Grade A	Normal
Grade B	Focal or diffuse enlargement of pancreatitis with contour irregularities
Grade C	Grade B plus peripancreatic inflammation
Grade D	Grade C plus one fluid collection or phlegmon
Grade E	Grade D plus two or more fluid collections or gas in the pancreas or retroperitoneum

TABLE 61.6: Complications of pancreatitis seen on CT scan

Acute peripancreatic fluid collection	Collection of fluid not enclosed by a wall that occurs within hours in 30–50% of patients Usually self-resolving but may progress to pseudocyst or abscess
Acute pseudocyst	Collection of fluid (low attenuation) with well-circumscribed wall seen >4 wk from onset of symptoms
Pancreatic abscess	Collection of purulent fluid with a thick, irregular wall seen > 4 wk from onset of symptoms
Pancreatic necrosis	Nonviable pancreatic tissue (fat necrosis and nonenhancing tissue), may be infectious or noninfectious

■ Notably, CT is not necessary in cases of clinically diagnosed mild pancreatitis and may be negative in 14–28% of these patients
■ Contrast CT may be contraindicated in patients with an elevated creatinine
■ Noncontrast CT scan is unable to evaluate pancreatic necrosis as is and therefore is less useful clinically, but may still be useful to see fluid collections, retroperitoneal air, or inflammation in patients with contraindications to IV contrast

 TABLE 61.7: Abdomen CT scan: pancreatitis

IV contrast	Yes
PO contrast	No
Amount of radiation	8 mSV

Classic Images

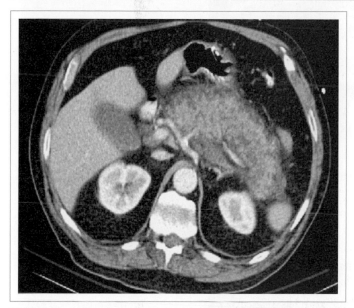

FIGURE 61.1: CT scan demonstrating acute interstitial pancreatitis. (From Mulholland MW, Maier RV, et al. Greenfield's Surgery: Scientific Principles and Practice, 4th ed. Philadelphia: Lippincott Williams & Wilkins, 2006.)

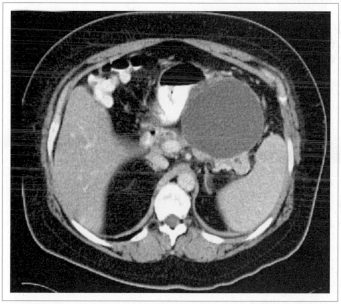

FIGURE 61.2: CT scan demonstrating pancreatic pseudocyst. (From Mulholland MW, Maier RV, et al. Greenfield's Surgery: Scientific Principles and Practice, 4th ed. Philadelphia: Lippincott Williams & Wilkins, 2006.)

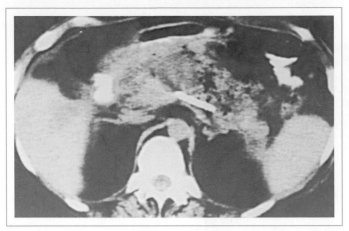

FIGURE 61.3: CT scan demonstrating pancreatic abscess. (From Gorbach SL, Bartlett JG, and Blacklow NR. Infectious Diseases, 3rd ed. Philadelphia: Lippincott Williams & Wilkins, 2003.)

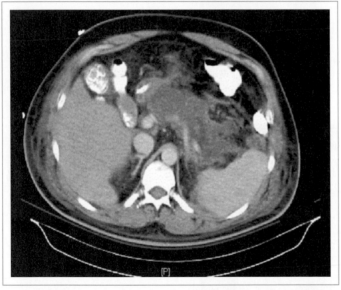

FIGURE 61.4: CT scan demonstrating pancreatic necrosis. (From Mulholland MW, Maier RV, et al. Greenfield's Surgery: Scientific Principles and Practice, 4th ed. Philadelphia: Lippincott Williams & Wilkins, 2006.)

Abdominal Ultrasound
- Ultrasound of the abdomen provides poor visualization of the pancreas and is essentially unhelpful in diagnosing acute pancreatitis
- Ultrasound more reliably identifies biliary pathology, and therefore may be most helpful in either confirming biliary disease as an alternative diagnosis or identifying gallstones as a likely etiology for gallstone pancreatitis
- Ultrasound in the nonacute phase may identify pseudocyst formation or visualize calcifications

Classic Images

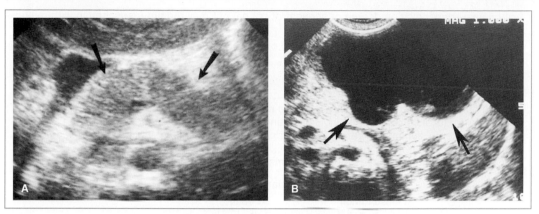

FIGURE 61.5: A: Acute pancreatitis: ultrasonographic findings. Note the enlarged and slightly hypoechoic pancreas (*arrows*). **B:** Pseudocyst: ultrasonographic findings. Note the anechoic, lobulated pancreatic pseudocyst (*arrows*). (From: Swischik LE. Emergency Imaging of the Acutely Ill or Injured Child, 4th ed. Philadelphia: Lippincott Williams & Wilkins, 2000.)

MRI
- As sensitive as CT in identifying pancreatitis, but more effective in characterizing the consistency of pancreatic fluid collections
- Less sensitive than CT in identifying pancreatic necrosis
- Magnetic resonance cholangiopancreatography (MRCP) is useful in diagnosing choledocholithiasis and gallstone pancreatitis
- Less available, more time consuming
- Useful in patients with renal failure unable to undergo contrast-enhanced CT imaging

TABLE 61.8: MRI: pancreatitis

IV contrast	No*
PO contrast	Yes
Amount of Radiation	None

*Gadolinium is helpful

Classic Images

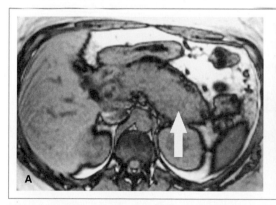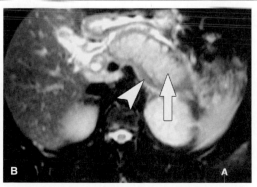

FIGURE 61.6: Pancreatitis as seen on MRI. (**A**) T1-weighted gradient echo and (**B**) fat-suppressed T2-weighted images of the abdomen show diffuse enlargement of the pancreas (*arrows*) with low-signal intensity rim (*arrowhead*) on T2-weighted image. (From Leyendecker JR and Brown JJ. Practical Guide to Abdominal and Pelvic MRI. Philadelphia: Lippincott Williams & Wilkins, 2004.)

Basic Management

- NPO
- IV fluids—depending on degree of sequestration, patient may require resuscitation with multiple liters of normal saline or lactated ringers
- Pain management
  - Opiate analgesia
  - Anti-inflammatory analgesia
- Antiemetics
- Consider surgical consultation in severe acute pancreatitis and when there is evidence of a large fluid collection, abscess, or pancreatic necrosis
- Monitor for local complications (including pancreatic necrosis and abscess formation) and systemic complications indicating fulminant pancreatitis (including shock, sepsis, pulmonary insufficiency, and renal failure)
- ICU admission is often necessary for patients with fulminant pancreatitis

TABLE 61.9: Ranson criteria

At presentation	At 48 hr
Glucose > 200 mg/dL	Calcium < 8 mg/dL
Age > 55 yr	Hct drop > 10%
LDH > 350 IU/L	PO$_2$ < 60 mm Hg
AST > 250 IU/L	BUN rise > 5 mg/dL
WBC > 16,000/mm^3	Base deficit > 4 mEq/L
	Fluid sequestration > 6 L

AST, aspartate aminotransferase; BUN, blood urea nitrogen; Hct, hematocrit; LDH, lactate dehydrogenase; PO, partial pressure of oxygen; WBC, white blood cell count.

TABLE 61.10: Predicted Mortality at 48 Hours

Number of Ranson criteria	Mortality
3–4	20%
5–6	40%
≥7	100%

Summary

TABLE 61.11: Advantages and disadvantages of imaging modalities in pancreatitis

Imaging modality	Advantages	Disadvantages
CT scan	Gold standard Availability Other diagnoses possible	IV contrast Radiation exposure Poor biliary system visualization
Ultrasound	Assessment of gallstone disease	Poor pancreas visualization
MRI	Useful when IV contrast is contraindicated	Time-consuming Poor availability

62

Gastrointestinal Foreign Body

Shannon Straszewski and Daniel McGillicuddy

Background

An estimated 1,500 deaths annually occur from gastrointestinal (GI) foreign bodies. Of all foreign body ingestions, children comprise 80% of those seeking emergency care, predominately between 6 months and 6 years of age. In the adult population, prisoners, psychiatric patients, and edentulous adults comprise the majority of individuals seeking care. The majority of objects will pass uneventfully through the GI tract. However, objects greater than 6 cm long or 2.5 cm wide or sharp objects are more likely to require extraction. The main anatomical sites for a foreign body to become trapped include the esophagus and rarely the pylorus and ileocecal valve.

TABLE 62.1: Classic history and physical

Foreign body sensation in throat
Palpable rectal foreign body
Drooling, vomiting
Chest or abdominal pain
Children are often asymptomatic (up to 35%)
Peritonitis or signs of GI bleeding indicating perforation

GI, gastrointestinal.

TABLE 62.2: Potentially helpful laboratory tests

Coagulation panel: Obtained for preoperative planning purposes
CBC: With concern for GI bleeding

CBC, complete blood count; GI, gastrointestinal.

Neck/Chest X-ray

- Orthogonal views of the chest and neck allow detection of mediastinal, peritoneal, or subcutaneous air
- The lateral image confirms foreign body is in esophagus and aids in detection of multiple foreign bodies
- Esophageal edema is an indication for emergent endoscopy
- Oral contrast should not be used routinely as it risks aspiration and makes retrieval more difficult
- A negative study does not exclude presence of foreign body

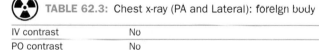 **TABLE 62.3:** Chest x-ray (PA and Lateral): foreign body

IV contrast	No
PO contrast	No
Amount of radiation	0.1 mSv

Classic Images

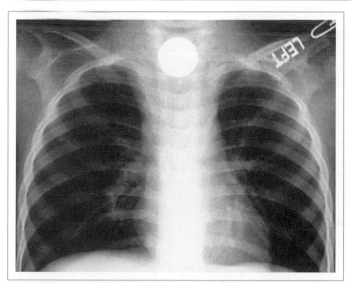

FIGURE 62.1: Esophageal coin located at the thoracic inlet on chest radiograph. (From Fleisher GR, Ludwig S, and Baskin MN. Atlas of Pediatric Emergency Medicine. Philadelphia: Lippincott Williams & Wilkins, 2004.)

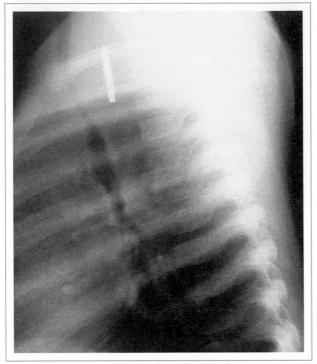

FIGURE 62.2: Lateral chest radiograph of ingested coin. (From Fleisher GR, Ludwig S, and Baskin MN. Atlas of Pediatric Emergency Medicine. Philadelphia: Lippincott Williams & Wilkins, 2004.)

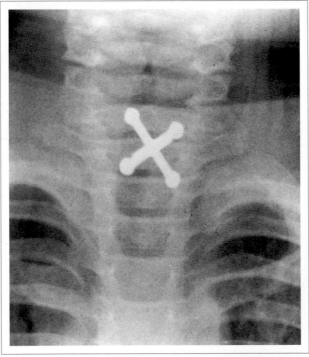

FIGURE 62.3: Esophageal foreign body. (From Daffner RH. Clinical Radiology: The Essentials, 3rd ed. Philadelphia: Lippincott Williams & Wilkins, 2007.)

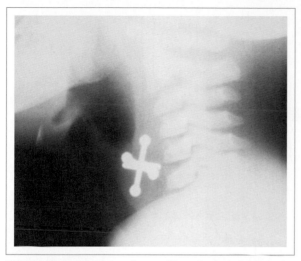

FIGURE 62.4: Jack in esophagus. (From Stedman's Medical Dictionary, 28th ed. Baltimore: Lippincott Williams & Wilkins, 2006.)

Abdominal X-ray
- Allows imaging to ensure an object has passed the esophagus
- Outlines object shape, indicating if passage unlikely
- Allows identification of free air if perforation has occurred
- Allows for identification of rectal foreign bodies, and is recommended prior to digital rectal examination if object in question may have sharp edges so as to prevent injury to the examiner
- Can have characteristic findings for drug packers, aiding in the diagnosis and deciphering type of material inserted

TABLE 62.4: Abdominal x-ray: foreign body

IV contrast	No
PO contrast	No
Amount of radiation	0.7 mSv per view

Classic Images

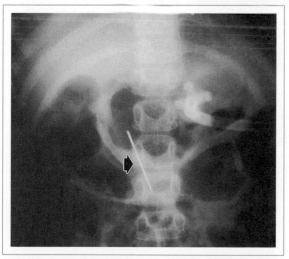

FIGURE 62.5: Ingested strait pin in gastric antrum on abdominal x-ray. (From Fleisher GR, Ludwig S, and Baskin MN. Atlas of Pediatric Emergency Medicine. Philadelphia: Lippincott Williams & Wilkins, 2004.)

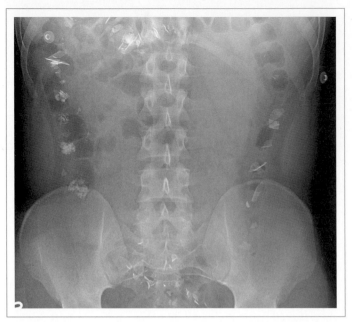

FIGURE 62.6: Abdominal x-ray of a 22-year-old male who swallowed a light bulb with shards of glass located throughout intestinal tract. No evidence of perforation identified. (*Courtesy of BIDMC Department of Radiology, Boston, MA.*)

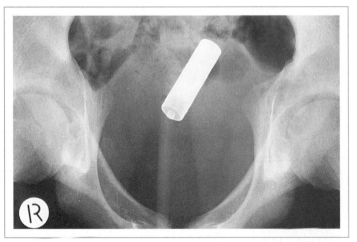

FIGURE 62.7: Rectal battery. Anteroposterior pelvis x-ray. This metallic artifact represents a flashlight battery within the rectum. (*Courtesy of David P. Thomas, MD, Melbourne, Australia.*) (From Yochum TR and Rowe LJ. Yochum and Rowe's Essentials of Skeletal Radiology, 3rd ed. Philadelphia: Lippincott Williams & Wilkins, 2004.)

CT Scan

- Highly accurate with sensitivity of up to 100%, but depends on material ingested
- Recommended if perforation is suspected
- Recommended for nonradiopaque foreign bodies that have not passed esophagus, or in cases where patient is symptomatic and other imaging modalities have failed
- In the case of children, many experts recommend proceeding directly to endoscopy to save the radiation exposure

TABLE 62.5: CT scan: foreign body

IV contrast	No
PO contrast	Possibly, not necessary to simply identify free air
Amount of radiation	Neck: 3 mSv
	Abdomen: 8 mSv
	Pelvis: 6 mSv

Classic Images

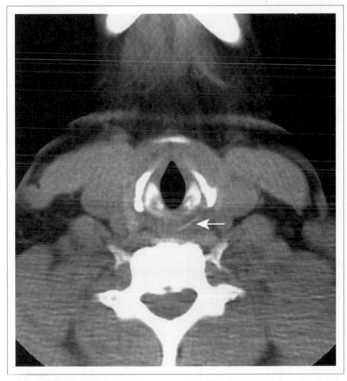

FIGURE 62.8: An axial image of the neck of a 43-year-old female who felt a foreign body sensation in her throat after eating fish. The CT scan shows a slender radiolucent foreign body located in the left side of the esophagus. (*Courtesy of BIDMC Department of Radiology, Boston, MA.*)

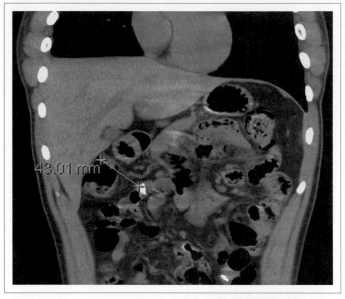

FIGURE 62.9: Two discrete foreign bodies resembling razorblade fragments identified in loops of small bowel in the right upper quadrant and left lower quadrant. There is no evidence of esophageal or bowel injury. (*Courtesy of BIDMC Department of Radiology, Boston, MA.*)

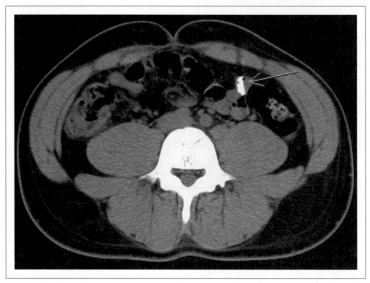

FIGURE 62.10: An axial CT image from a 26-year-old man who ingested a razorblade. No evidence of bowel injury or perforation is identified. (*Courtesy of BIDMC Department of Radiology, Boston, MA.*)

Basic Management

- Make patient NPO and replace volume loss with normal saline followed by maintenance fluids
- Pain management
- Administer antibiotics if perforation is suspected
- For esophageal foreign bodies consider use of glucagon or nitroglycerin if object has potential to pass and has not been impacted for more than a few hours
- GI consultation for therapeutic endoscopy or diagnostic use if mucosal tear is suspected
- Surgical consultation if unable to extract rectal foreign body or perforation suspected anywhere in GI tract
- Admission if patient warrants endoscopy or surgical extraction

Summary

TABLE 62.6: Advantages and disadvantages of imaging modalities in gastrointestinal foreign body

Imaging modalities	Advantages	Disadvantages
Chest x-ray	Low cost Minimal patient discomfort	Unable to detect radiolucent material
Abdominal x-ray	Low cost Minimal patient discomfort	Unable to detect radiolucent material
CT scan	Detects images not seen on plain film Potential to avoid endoscopy	Costly Radiation exposure

Section Editor: Arun Nagdev

63   Abdominal Aortic Aneurysm
Sachita Shah

Background

Abdominal aortic aneurysm (AAA) can be a life-threatening condition which may be difficult to diagnose in the emergency department because of its commonly atypical presentation. As the 13th leading cause of death in the United States, ruptured AAA is a relatively common surgical emergency. The incidence of AAA is 2–4% in the adult population, and elderly white males have the highest incidence. The most common misdiagnosis for AAA is renal colic, as aortic pathology involving the renal artery may cause hematuria with flank pain.

AAA arises when the media layer of the aortic wall degenerates, allowing steady dilation of the vessel lumen and weakening of the vessel wall. While the exact etiology of the disease remains unclear, association with atherosclerotic disease and collagen-vascular disorders such as Marfan's disease or Ehlers-Danlos syndrome has been established. An average of 65% of patients with ruptured AAA die prior to arrival at a hospital, and most patients with ruptured AAA were unaware of their disease.

TABLE 63.1: Classic history and physical

Severe sudden back, flank, groin, or abdominal pain
Ruptured AAA may present with syncope, shock
Family history of AAA increases risk
Pulsatile mass on abdominal examination
Hematuria

AAA, abdominal aortic aneurysm.

TABLE 63.2: Potentially helpful laboratory tests

Hematocrit: Decreasing hematocrit suggests leakage of an AAA
Type and screen, coagulation panel: In case emergent operative intervention is necessary
Urinalysis: Hematuria with renal artery involvement

AAA, abdominal aortic aneurysm.

Aortic Ultrasound

- In a hemodynamically unstable patient, bedside ultrasound is the optimal tool in the timely diagnosis of AAA.
- It is extremely important to visualize the entire abdominal aorta, from the superior mesenteric artery to the bifurcation of the aorta into the iliac arteries, when attempting to rule out the presence of AAA.
- Retroperitoneal hemorrhage secondary to a rupturing AAA cannot be detected by bedside ultrasound, but must be assumed with a patient with severe pain and unstable vital signs.

323

- Intraperitoneal rupture of AAA is often immediately fatal and rarely amenable to resuscitative efforts by emergency services in the field. Thus, AAA with intraperitoneal rupture is rarely diagnosed in the emergency department setting. In these cases, fluid accumulates in the usual recesses (i.e., Morison's pouch).
- Place a 3.5–5 MHz ultrasound probe in a transverse position on the abdomen with the probe marker pointed to the patient's right side. Begin in the subxiphoid region (using the liver as a window) and apply gentle, steady pressure with your hand, or the probe, to displace bowel gas. Scan the aorta in a transverse plane to visualize the proximal (level of the superior mesenteric artery), mid, and distal aorta to the bifurcation.
- Landmarks seen on ultrasound include the vertebral body shadow, appearing as a hyperechoic curved rim with hypoechoic shadow posteriorly. The aorta and inferior vena cava (IVC) should be seen in the transverse plane as a round (aorta) structure on the left of the screen and an oblong (IVC) hypoechoic structure on the right of the screen just anterior to the vertebral body.
- Once the aorta is identified, be sure to measure the aortic diameter, anterior to posterior, from the outer wall to the outer wall using the calipers on the ultrasound machine. Measure the aorta in the proximal, mid, and distal areas.
- The aorta is measured outer wall to outer wall as there may be intraluminal clot making the lumen smaller than the actual aorta diameter.
- The normal caliber of the abdominal aorta is <3 cm, and the normal iliac arteries are <1.5 cm.
- In cases where bowel gas obstructs visualization of the abdominal aorta, gentle/steady pressure with the palm of your hand or the ultrasound probe may displace peristaltic small bowel.
- Placing the patient in a left lateral decubitus position may also displace bowel gas.
- False positives can result from pancreatic cysts, and para-aortic lymphadenopathy (both noncontiguous structures) with absent to minimal flow on color Doppler.
- False negatives can result from failure to visualize the entire aorta, measurement of aortic luminal diameter without including the associated aortic wall thrombus, and improper long-axis aortic measurement lateral to the true midline.

TABLE 63.3: Common abdominal aortic aneurysm ultrasonographic errors

False positive	False negative
Pancreatic cyst	Not visualizing entire aorta
Para-aortic lymphadenopathy	Measuring lumen size without including thrombus
	Non-midline long-axis measurement

- Always visualize the aorta in various planes (e.g., longitudinal and transverse) in order to visualize the entire extent of the structure to avoid missing an AAA.
- When evaluating the aorta longitudinally, scan through the aorta in its entirety in this plane to avoid missing a saccular aneurysm.
- If you note an AAA, note the presence of free fluid surrounding the aorta, or free fluid in Morison's pouch (hepatorenal space) if you suspect leakage into the abdomen.

TABLE 63.4: Helpful associated structures

Vertebral body shadow
The inferior vena cava is the oblong, hypoechoic vascular structure to the right of the aorta on the screen, generally thinner walled and not pulsatile
The proximal aorta is identified by visualizing either the liver or the superior mesenteric artery on the screen

Classic Images

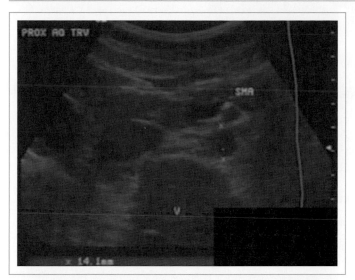

FIGURE 63.1: Ultrasound image of normal aortic anatomy including superior mesenteric artery, aorta, inferior vena cava, and vertebral body. (*Courtesy of the Division of Emergency Ultrasound, St. Luke's Roosevelt Hospital Center, New York, NY.*)

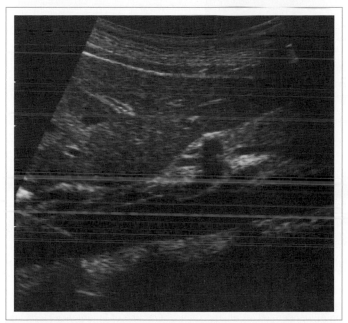

FIGURE 63.2: A longitudinal view of the aorta on ultrasound. Probe marker positioned toward the patient's head. The celiac trunk and the superior mesenteric artery are seen arising from the proximal aorta in this image. (From Moore KL and Agur A. Essential Clinical Anatomy, 2nd ed. Philadelphia: Lippincott Williams & Wilkins, 2002.)

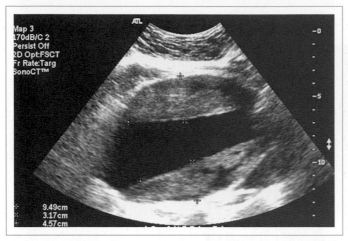

FIGURE 63.3: Gray-scale longitudinal duplex ultrasound image of a large abdominal aortic aneurysm. The maximal diameter of the abdominal aortic aneurysm is 9.49 cm. There is extensive thrombus formation within the aneurysm. (From Topol EJ, Califf RM, Prystowsky EN, et al. Textbook of Cardiovascular Medicine, 3rd ed. Philadelphia: Lippencott Williams & Wilkins, 2006.)

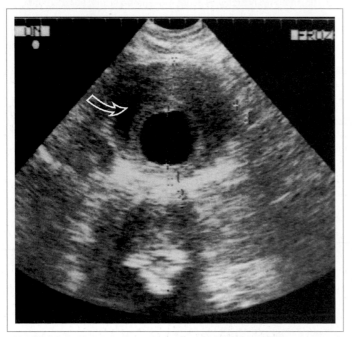

FIGURE 63.4: Abdominal aortic aneurysm. This is a transverse image of a large abdominal aortic aneurysm with mural thrombus (*arrow*). Intraluminal clot makes the lumen appear smaller than the actual aortic diameter. (From Harwood-Nuss A, Wolfson AB, Linden CH, et al. The Clinical Practice of Emergency Medicine, 3rd ed. Philadelphia: Lippincott Williams & Wilkins, 2001.)

Abdominal CT Scan

- CT scan of the abdomen is the current gold standard for rapid detection of AAA, and is helpful in determining retroperitoneal rupture not well visualized with ultrasound
- Using CT, it is possible to view the extent of the AAA and involvement of renal arteries, which can help in surgical planning
- CT scan quality is not limited by patient body habitus or intestinal gas
- The sensitivity and specificity of CT scan for diagnosis of AAA is nearly 100%
- Major disadvantages to CT imaging in patients with suspected AAA include additional time to diagnosis, movement of a potentially unstable patient from the emergency department, IV contrast, and reliance on a radiologic interpretation

 TABLE 63.5: CT scan: abdominal aortic aneurysm

IV contrast	Yes, to visualize vascular structures
PO contrast	No, bowel not organ of interest
Amount of radiation	8 mSv

Classic Image

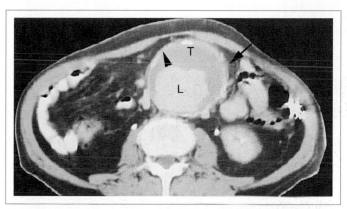

FIGURE 63.5: Abdominal aortic aneurysm. Soft tissue window CT, axial abdomen. Note the pronounced aneurysmal dilatation of the abdominal aorta (*arrow*). Observe the atherosclerotic plaquing in the wall of the aneurysm (*arrowhead*). T, thrombus; L, lumen of the abdominal aorta. (*Courtesy of Department of Radiology, Wood River Memorial Township Hospital, Wood River, IL.*) (From Yochum TR and Rowe LJ. Yochum and Rowe's Essentials of Skeletal Radiology, 3rd ed. Philadelphia: Lippincott Williams & Wilkins, 2004.)

Magnetic Resonance Imaging/Magnetic Resonance Angiography

- MRI may be useful in patients with severe allergy to IV contrast used for CT scanning
- Patients must be hemodynamically stable to undergo an MRI with contrast for imaging of the abdominal aorta because it is a lengthy examination
- Provides excellent details for preoperative evaluation

 TABLE 63.6: MRI/magnetic resonance angiography: abdominal aortic aneurysm

IV contrast	Yes, to visualize vascular structures
PO contrast	No, bowel not organ of interest
Amount of radiation	None

Classic Image

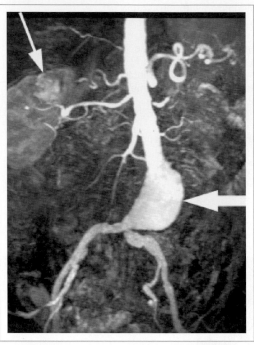

FIGURE 63.6: Abdominal aortic aneurysm. Maximum intensity projection image of three-dimensional gadolinium-enhanced magnetic resonance angiography of infrarenal abdominal aortic aneurysm (*arrow*) that extends to bifurcation. Note incidentally discovered renal cell carcinoma in right kidney (*thin arrow*). (From Leyendecker JR and Brown JJ. Practical Guide to Abdominal and Pelvic MRI. Philadelphia: Lippincott Williams & Wilkins, 2004.)

Aortogram

- Previously used extensively in the preoperative evaluation of AAA; however, it has been replaced with less invasive technologies
- More recently, used more selectively in patients with possible stenosis of other nearby vessels that may alter plans for surgical repair
- May also be used for the placement of endovascular stent grafts
- Can underestimate aortic size if intraluminal clot is present

 TABLE 63.7: Aortogram: abdominal aortic aneurysm

IV contrast	Yes, to visualize vascular structures
PO contrast	No, bowel not organ of interest
Amount of radiation	12 mSv, more if used for stent placement

Classic Images

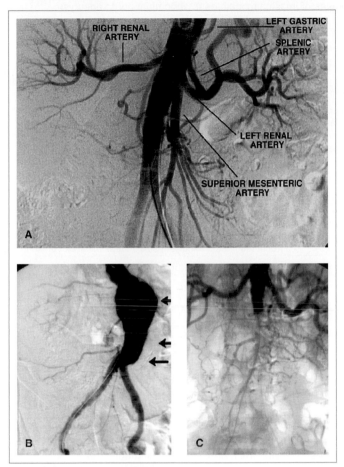

FIGURE 63.7: A: Normal abdominal aortogram in anteroposterior projection. **B:** Aortogram demonstrating an intrarenal abdominal aortic aneurysm (4.7 cm) that underestimates the accurate size owing to the presence of mural thrombus (*arrows*). **C:** Distal aortic occlusion below the renal arteries. (From Baim DS. Grossman's Cardiac Catheterization, Angiography, and Intervention, 7th ed. Philadelphia: Lippincott Williams & Wilkins, 2005.)

Basic Management

- Unruptured, asymptomatic AAA found incidentally may be managed conservatively based on the size of the aorta and recommendations of surgical consultation
- Ruptured and symptomatic aneurysms should be treated emergently with:
  - Pain management
  - Preoperative laboratory work-up
  - Correction of coagulopathies, anemia, and thrombocytopenia as needed with blood products and medications
  - Large-bore peripheral access or central venous access for fluid resuscitation
  - Emergent consultation with a vascular surgeon
  - Admission to the surgical intensive care unit after the planned intervention

Summary

TABLE 63.8: Advantages and disadvantages of imaging modalities in abdominal aortic aneurysm

Imaging modalities	Advantages	Disadvantages
Ultrasound	Low cost Minimal patient discomfort No radiation Bedside availability Less time-consuming	Body habitus limitations Bowel gas limitations Operator-dependent
CT scan	Availability Other diagnoses also possible Modality of choice to determine if ruptured	IV contrast Radiation exposure Transfer of patient to a less monitored setting Moderately time-consuming
MRI	For use in presence of dye allergy No radiation	Time-consuming Expensive Lack of monitoring equipment during the examination Availability Transfer of patient to less monitored setting
Aortogram	Can also evaluate nearby vessel pathology	Invasive Expensive Large amounts of IV contrast Underestimates aneurysm size if intraluminal clot present

64

Aortic Dissection

Jolene Nakao and Turandot Saul

Background

Aortic dissection is an uncommon but potentially life-threatening condition. Overall in-hospital mortality is estimated at 27% and varies depending on the type of dissection, age of patient, presence of comorbid conditions, and the modality chosen for treatment. The incidence is esti-mated at 5–30 cases per million people per year. Aortic dissection has a 2:1 male predominance with greatest incidence in the seventh decade of life. The approximate mortality rate in acute dissection is 1–2% per hour for the first 24–48 hours. A history of hypertension is present in more than 70% of cases.

Classification of aortic dissection guides treatment and informs prognosis. In the Stanford classi-fication, type A (proximal) dissection involves the ascending aorta, while type B (distal) dissection does not. Type A dissections are more often lethal and require a surgical treatment approach.

The pathognomonic finding to diagnose aortic dissection on imaging is the intimal flap that sepa-rates the true and false aortic lumen. The goals of imaging are to determine:
- presence, location, and extent of dissection
- involvement of arteries and arteries involved
- associated complications, including aortic rupture, valvular involvement, and pericardial effusion
- presence of intramural hematoma or penetrating ulcer

TABLE 64.1: Classic history and physical

Sudden onset severe chest and/or back pain; maximal at onset; sharp, tearing, or ripping in character
Chest pain with syncope or neurologic symptoms should increase suspicion
Risk factors include hypertension, advanced age, and connective tissue disorders such as Ehlers-Danlos and Marfan syndromes
Diastolic murmur of aortic insufficiency
Differential pulsations and/or blood pressure between the two upper extremities

TABLE 64.2: Potentially helpful laboratory tests

Hematocrit: Decreasing hematocrit suggests hemorrhage from an aortic dissection
BUN/creatinine: May be elevated with renal artery involvement
Troponin/CK: May be elevated if the dissection extends to the aortic root with compromise of the coronary arteries
Type and screen, coagulation panel: In case of the need for emergent operative intervention
Urinalysis: Hematuria with renal artery involvement
D-dimer, soluble elastin fragments, and myosin heavy-chain concentrations: May prove useful pending clinical trials

BUN, blood urea nitrogen; CK, creatine kinase.

X-ray

- Chest x-ray is often abnormal in aortic dissections, especially when the dissection involves the ascending aorta
- Most common abnormal finding is a widened mediastinum:
  - A widened mediastinum is difficult to determine on anteroposterior radiographs; if the patient is stable, a PA radiograph is preferred
  - A mediastinal width of greater than 8 cm on anteroposterior radiograph is considered abnormal
- With a calcified aortic arch, the external contour of the tunica media and adventitia of the aorta lay within a few millimeters of the calcification; during aortic dissection, this wall may be thickened away from the calcified plaque (>5 mm between calcification and edge of wall is abnormal)
- More subtle findings include a hemothorax, left apical cap (blood accumulation at the left lung apex from blood leaking from a ruptured aorta), tracheal deviation, depression of the left main stem bronchus, esophageal deviation, or loss of the paratracheal stripe (indicating adjacent pathology)
- There is no single finding to look for but rather a combination of findings to make this diagnosis
- A normal chest x-ray is inadequate to rule out dissection

 TABLE 64.3: Chest X-ray (PA and lateral): Aortic dissection

IV contrast	No
PO contrast	No
Amount of radiation	0.10 mSv

Classic Images

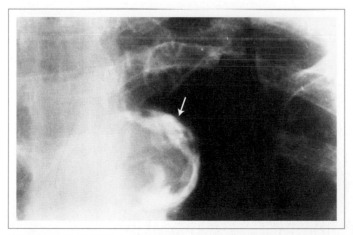

FIGURE 64.1: Aortic arch calcification. Note that the external contour of the tunica media and adventitia of the aorta lay within a few millimeters of the calcification. During aortic dissection, thickening of this wall away from the calcified plaque may sometimes be seen on a chest radiograph. (From Yochum TR and Rowe LJ. Yochum and Rowe's Essentials of Skeletal Radiology, 3rd ed. Philadelphia: Lippincott Williams & Wilkins, 2004.)

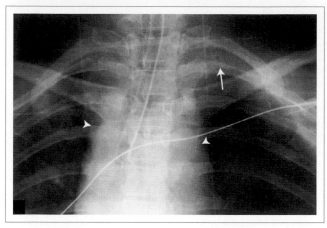

FIGURE 64.2: The mediastinum is widened (*arrowheads*), the aortic contour is absent, and there is an apical pleural cap (*arrow*). (From Yochum TR and Rowe LJ. Yochum and Rowe's Essentials of Skeletal Radiology, 3rd ed. Philadelphia: Lippincott Williams & Wilkins, 2004.)

CT Scan

- The sensitivity of CT for aortic dissection ranges from 83%–94%, with a specificity of 87–100%
- IV contrast aids in visualizing the intimal flap (seen within the lumen of the aorta)
- CT provides information about the location and the extent of the dissection
- The true and false lumens and any associated vessel involvement (i.e., renal arteries) are easily assessed to aid in presurgical planning
- CT is helpful in determining retroperitoneal rupture
- Major disadvantages of CT in patients with suspected aortic dissection include additional time to diagnosis, movement of a potentially unstable patient from the emergency department, IV contrast, and reliance on a radiologic interpretation

 TABLE 64.4: CT scan: aortic dissection

IV contrast	Yes, to visualize vascular structures
PO contrast	No
Amount of radiation	23 mSv (chest + abdomen)

Classic Images

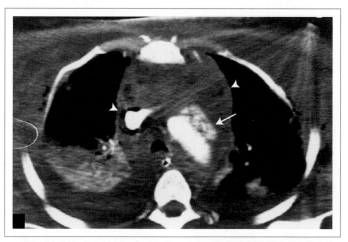

FIGURE 64.3: Contrast-enhanced CT (axial chest). At the level of the aortic arch, note the contrast extravasation beyond the vessel wall (*arrow*). Accumulated blood distends the mediastinum (*arrowheads*). (From Yochum TR and Rowe LJ. Yochum and Rowe's Essentials of Skeletal Radiology, 3rd ed. Philadelphia: Lippincott Williams & Wilkins, 2004.)

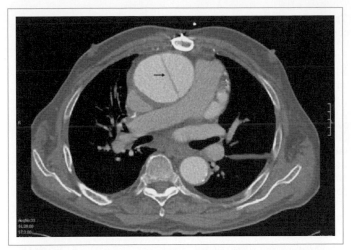

FIGURE 64.4: Type A aortic dissection. The CT slice demonstrates a dissection flap (*black arrow*) with two separate lumens in the aneurysmal ascending thoracic aorta. (From Topol EJ, Califf RM, et al. Textbook of Cardiovascular Medicine, 3rd ed. Philadelphia: Lippincott Williams & Wilkins, 2006.)

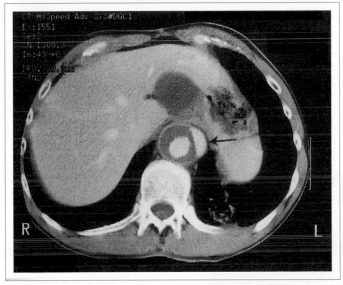

FIGURE 64.5: CT (midthorax). Observe the aortic dissection with rupture (*arrow*). (*Courtesy of Robert Heigans, MD, Department of Radiology, University Hospital, Denver, CO.*) (From Yochum TR and Rowe LJ. Yochum and Rowe's Essentials of Skeletal Radiology, 3rd ed. Philadelphia: Lippincott Williams & Wilkins, 2004.)

Transthoracic Echocardiogram/Transabdominal Aortic Ultrasound

- Retroperitoneal hemorrhage secondary to a ruptured aortic dissection cannot be detected by bedside ultrasound
- Transthoracic echocardiogram (TTE) is most useful in diagnosing ascending aortic dissections involving the aortic root, within a few centimeters of the aortic valve
- TTE can also diagnose cardiac tamponade, involvement of the coronary arteries, and aortic insufficiency
- TTE has a sensitivity of 80% and a specificity of 90%
- TTE is limited in its ability to accurately visualize the aorta beyond the root
- In the abdomen, landmarks include the vertebral body shadow, appearing as a hyperechoic, curved rim with a hypoechoic shadow posteriorly
- The aorta and inferior vena cava should be seen in transverse plane as a round (aorta) structure on the left of the screen and oblong (inferior vena cava) hypoechoic structure on the right of the screen just anterior to the vertebral body
- The aorta is measured outer wall to outer wall as there may be intraluminal clot making the lumen smaller than the actual aorta diameter
- The normal diameter of the abdominal aorta is <3 cm, and the normal diameter of each iliac artery is <1.5 cm
- An aortic dissection appears as a floating membrane dividing the aorta in two
- In the abdomen, the aorta may be scanned proximally and distally observing the flap in an attempt to define the extent of the dissection
- Color flow Doppler on each side of the flap may give information regarding the false versus true lumen
- Imaging quality and diagnostic ability is limited by patient body habitus and operator experience

TABLE 64.5: Helpful associated structures

Abdominal aorta	Vertebral body shadow
	Inferior vena cava: the oblong, hypoechoic vascular structure to the right of the aorta on the screen—generally thinner walled and not pulsatile
Thoracic aorta	Aortic valve
	Cardiac chambers

Classic Images

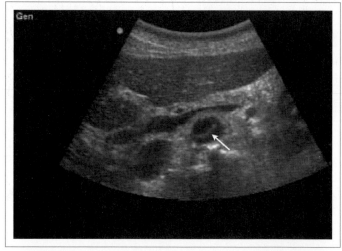

FIGURE 64.6: Abdominal aortic dissection demonstrating an intimal flap (arrow). (*Courtesy of the Division of Emergency Ultrasound, St. Luke's Roosevelt Hospital Center, New York, NY.*)

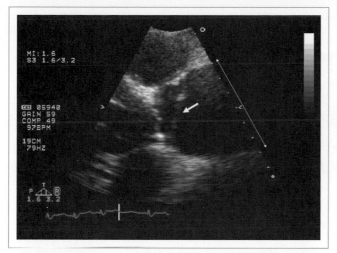

FIGURE 64.7: Type A aortic dissection. Transthoracic echo, parasternal long-axis view. A dissection flap (*white arrow*) is visualized within the proximal aorta above the aortic valve leaflets. The tubular ascending aorta is 6.2 cm in diameter, consistent with prior thoracic aortic aneurysm. (From Topol EJ, Califf RM, et al. Textbook of Cardiovascular Medicine, 3rd ed. Philadelphia: Lippincott Williams & Wilkins, 2006.)

Transesophageal Echocardiogram Ultrasonography

- Transesophageal echocardiogram (TEE) is most useful in assessing ascending aortic dissections involving the aortic root
- It can also diagnose cardiac tamponade, involvement of the coronary arteries, and aortic insufficiency—all potential complications of aortic dissection
- TEE has a sensitivity of 97–99% and a specificity of 97–100% with an experienced operator
- Disadvantages of TEE are its dependence on the operator's experience and the potential to increase blood pressure and aggravate the dissection
- TEE can miss localized dissection of the upper ascending aorta and proximal aortic arch
- TEE cannot be performed in patients with esophageal varices or stenosis

Classic Images

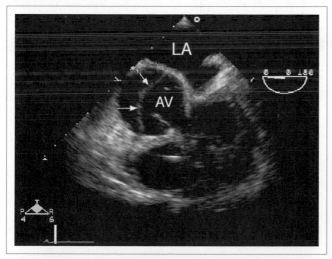

FIGURE 64.8: A transesophageal echocardiogram at the base of the heart is shown from a patient with an aortic dissection involving the proximal aorta. The aortic valve (AV) is seen in an off-axis plane. The arrows point to the dissection flap within the aortic root. The location of the dissection flap affected the ability of the valve to close in diastole, thereby causing aortic regurgitation. LA, left atrium. (From Feigenbaum H, Armstrong WF, and Ryan T. Feigenbaum's Echocardiography, 6th ed. Philadelphia: Lippincott Williams & Wilkins, 2005.)

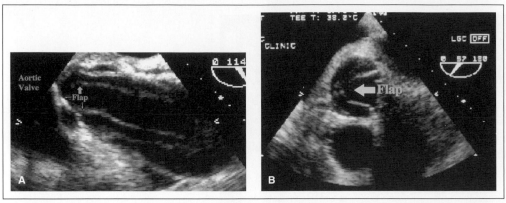

FIGURE 64.9: Aortic dissection with a flap in the ascending aorta. **A:** Long axis. **B:** Short axis. (From Topol EJ, Califf RM, et al. Textbook of Cardiovascular Medicine, 3rd ed. Philadelphia: Lippincott Williams & Wilkins, 2006.)

MRI/MRA

- MRI may be useful in patients with severe allergy to IV contrast used for CT scanning and who require aortic imaging
- MRI/MRA provides excellent details for preoperative evaluation
- MRI/MRA is useful in imaging chronic dissections and patients after endovascular or open repair
- The sensitivity of MRI/MRA is >90% and the specificity is >95%
- Patients must be hemodynamically stable to undergo an MRI with contrast

 TABLE 64.6: MRI/MRA: aortic dissection

IV contrast	Yes, to visualize vascular structures
PO contrast	No
Amount of radiation	None

Classic Images

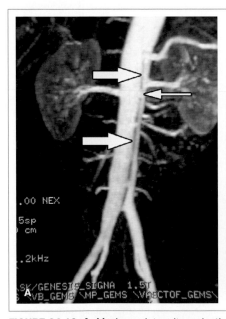
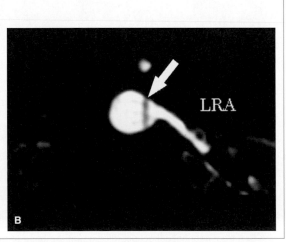

FIGURE 64.10: A: Maximum intensity projection image from three-dimensional gadolinium-enhanced MR angiograph of abdominal aorta shows dissection flap (*arrows*) and fenestrations. **B:** Flap (*arrow*) is clearly demonstrated on axial reformation at the level of the left renal artery (LRA). (From Leyendecker JR and Brown JJ. Practical Guide to Abdominal and Pelvic MRI. Philadelphia: Lippincott Williams & Wilkins, 2004.)

Aortogram

- Aortogram is still considered the gold standard
- The sensitivity is 88% and the specificity is 94%
- Aortogram aids the surgeon in preoperative planning because the aortic arch and vessels are easily assessed
- False-negative results can occur in the cases of thrombosed false lumens and intramural hematomas (intramural hemorrhages)
- Disadvantages include the invasive and time-consuming nature, necessity of transport to a less monitored setting, the use of IV contrast, and cost

TABLE 64.7: Aortogram: aortic dissection

IV contrast	Yes, to visualize vascular structures
PO contrast	No
Amount of radiation	7–12 mSv, depending on area visualized

Classic Images

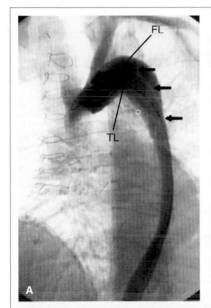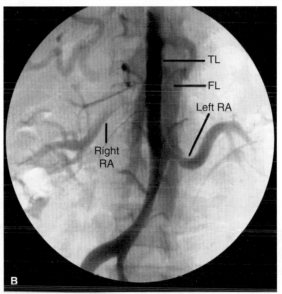

FIGURE 64.11: A: Stanford type A aortic dissection following aortic valve replacement. The intimal dissection flap (*arrows*) separates the contrast-filled true lumen (TL) from the false lumen (FL) that compromises the TL as it proceeds distally. **B:** The dissection extending into the abdominal aorta with origination of the left renal artery (RA) from the FL and TL supplying the right (RA). (From Baim DS. Grossman's Cardiac Catheterization, Angiography, and Intervention, 7th ed. Philadelphia: Lippincott Williams & Wilkins, 2005.)

Basic Management

- Immediately place two large bore IVs oxygen and cardiac monitor, and obtain emergent surgical consultation
- Patients hypotensive secondary to aortic rupture or pericardial tamponade should be resuscitated with IV fluids and immediately transported to the operating room
- Heart rate and blood pressure should be aggressively managed, with a target heart rate of less than 60 beats per minute and systolic blood pressure of 100–120 mm Hg
- Pain should be adequately managed
- A preoperative laboratory work-up should be sent
- Coagulopathies, anemia, and thrombocytopenia should be corrected as needed with blood products and medications
- Type A dissections involving the ascending aorta will require surgery, and type B dissections involving only the descending aorta may be medically or surgically managed on a case-by-case basis

Summary

TABLE 64.8: Advantages and disadvantages of imaging modalities in aortic dissection

Imaging modality	Advantages	Disadvantages
X-ray	Low cost Rapid No exposure to IV contrast Minimal radiation exposure	May be normal No one specific finding confirms diagnosis
CT scan	Widely available Can assess for other pathology Defines extent of dissection Procedure of choice for suspected rupture	Exposure to IV contrast Radiation exposure Need to transfer patient to a less-monitored setting Moderately time-consuming
Ultrasound	Low cost Rapid Available at bedside; portable No exposure to IV dye No radiation exposure	TTE/transabdominal: body habitus and bowel gas limitations TEE: contraindicated with esophageal varices or stenosis May increase blood pressure and aggravate dissection Operator-dependent Does not provide complete information Does not detect rupture
MRI	No exposure to IV dye No radiation exposure Useful in chronic dissection and postoperative patients	Time-consuming Expensive Not widely available Need to transfer patient to a less-monitored setting
Aortogram	Can also evaluate nearby vessel pathology	Invasive Expensive Time-consuming Large amount of IV contrast needed May not detect false lumen if thrombosed or intramural hemorrhages

65

Deep Vein Thrombosis

Jason W.J. Fischer

Background

The true incidence of deep vein thrombosis (DVT) is unknown. It is estimated that first-time venous thromboembolism (VTE) occurs in approximately 100 per 100,000 persons per year of which approximately one third of cases are pulmonary embolism (PE) and two thirds of cases are DVT. Thrombi from deeper and more proximal vessels are believed to be of greater risk for embolization. The formation of a thrombus is associated with the classic triad of factors described by Rudolf Virchow: stasis, endothelial injury, and hypercoagulable state.

TABLE 65.1: Classic history and physical

Pain in the calf or thigh

Unilateral leg edema, warmth, and tenderness

Risk factors: history of venous thromboembolism, major surgery, trauma, immobility, cancer, increased estrogen state, indwelling central venous catheter, smoking, age >45 years, obesity, inherited coagulopathy, and medical comorbidity

TABLE 65.2: Potentially helpful laboratory test

D-dimer—For low probability patients, the moderately sensitive latex agglutination assay has a sensitivity of 86% and a specificity of 78% and the highly sensitive ELISA has a sensitivity of 95% and a specificity of 58%; values below 500 ng/mL have a high negative predictive value in low- and intermediate-risk patients

Limited Compression Ultrasound

- Ultrasound is used to diagnose DVT by performing a compressibility study
- A normal vein will compress with minimal pressure without neighboring arterial collapse, while the inability to compress a vein is an indication that it is filled with a thrombus or clot
- Intraluminal clot may vary in appearance from hypo- to hyperechoic depending on age, and therefore the visualization of a clot is not necessary for the diagnosis of DVT nor is its absence an indication of vessel patency
- The deep femoral vein travels deep in Hunter's (adductor) canal making it difficult to image in the thigh; it is easily imaged in the popliteal fossa
- Distal to the popliteal fossa, the popliteal vein trifurcates into the anterior and posterior tibial veins and the peroneal vein; ultrasound cannot adequately evaluate these smaller veins, but the risk of embolization is low if clot is present
- The concern for calf vein DVT is if thrombosis propagates proximally into the popliteal vein; for this reason, repeat ultrasound should be performed within 7 days
- The common femoral vein is best visualized when the patient is in reverse Trendelenburg position (to aid in venous pooling), with the leg externally rotated and the knee slightly flexed
- A 5–12 MHz linear high-resolution probe should be used in the transverse plane, just distal to the inguinal ligament to visualize the common femoral artery and common femoral vein
- The vein should compress with both walls touching completely
- The popliteal vein requires less pressure to compress and is best visualized when the patient is in the supine position, with the knee slightly flexed and externally rotated
- The probe should then be positioned in the transverse plane in the popliteal fossa to visualize the popliteal artery and popliteal vein
- After DVT diagnosis and treatment, it may take many months for the clot to organize and dissolve completely; for this reason, compressibility studies cannot diagnose acute DVT in a patient with previous DVT unless a normal compressibility study was documented prior to the onset of new symptoms

TABLE 65.3: Helpful associated structures

Common femoral artery—thick walled, pulsatile, noncompressible, typically lateral to common femoral vein
Great saphenous vein—arises from the proximal common femoral vein
Superficial and deep femoral veins—arise from the bifurcation of the common femoral vein in the thigh
Femoral lymph nodes—round and noncompressible; similar in appearance to a DVT and a common cause of false-positive interpretation (when the probe is tilted back and forth, edges can be seen differentiating them from vessels)
Popliteal artery—thick walled, pulsatile, noncompressible, typically deep to the popliteal vein

DVT, deep vein thrombosis.

Classic Images

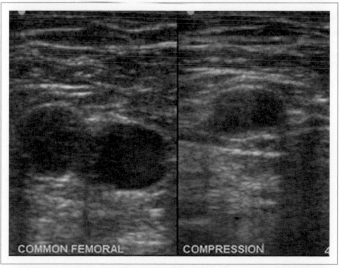

FIGURE 65.1: Limited compression ultrasound of common femoral vein (*arrows*). Vein collapses with compression indicating no deep vein thrombosis (*right*). (*Courtesy of Turandot Saul, St. Luke's Roosevelt Hospital, New York.*)

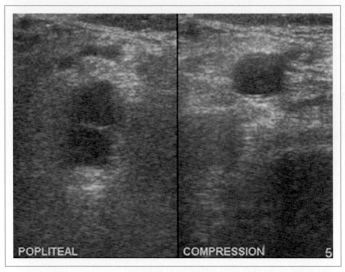

FIGURE 65.2: Limited compression ultrasound of popliteal vein (*arrows*). Vein collapses with compression indicating no deep vein thrombosis (*right*). (*Courtesy of Turandot Saul, St. Luke's Roosevelt Hospital, New York.*)

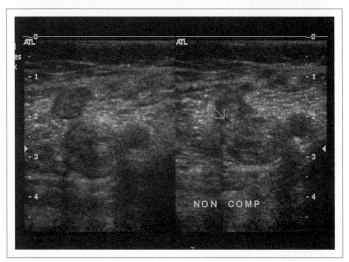

FIGURE 65.3: Ultrasound demonstrating a noncompressible femoral vein indicating venous thrombosis. (Courtesy of Dr. Marie Gerhard-Herman, Brigham and Women's Hospital, Boston Massachusetts) (From Baim DS. Grossman's Cardiac Catheterization, Angiography, and Intervention, 7th ed. Philadelphia: Lippincott Williams & Wilkins, 2005.)

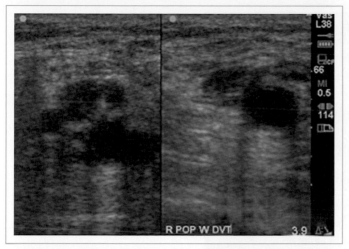

FIGURE 65.4: Limited compression ultrasound of popliteal vein (*arrows*). Vein does not collapse with compression indicating deep vein thrombosis (*right*). (*Courtesy of Turandot Saul, St. Luke's Roosevelt Hospital, New York.*)

Duplex Ultrasound

- Duplex ultrasound adds spectral and color flow Doppler to compression B-mode ultrasonography
- It is 95–100% sensitive and 91–100% specific for proximal vein DVT
- Looks for normal flow patterns within the vessel as markers of patency; compressibility is still the major criterion used to exclude DVT
- An increase in the size of the vein during Valsalva maneuver or with compression of the leg distally can be used as another indicator of vessel patency

Classic Images

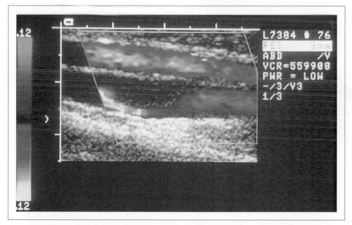

FIGURE 65.5: Color flow Doppler showing femoral vein thrombus. (*Courtesy of Acuson Computed Sonography Corporation, Mountain View, CA.*) (From Stedman's Medical Dictionary, 28th ed. Baltimore: Lippincott Williams & Wilkins, 2006.)

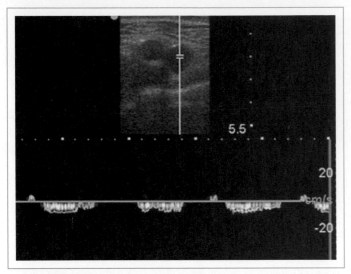

FIGURE 65.6: Normal spectral Doppler venous flow in the common femoral vein. Venous flow varies with respiration. (*Image courtesy of Turandot Saul, Department of Emergency Medicine, St. Luke's Roosevelt Hospital Center, New York.*)

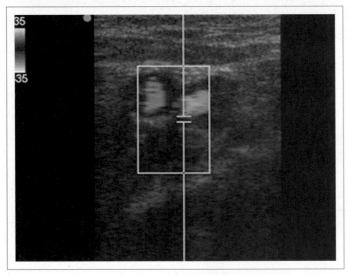

FIGURE 65.7: Normal color Doppler venous flow in the common femoral vessels. (*Image courtesy of Turandot Saul, Department of Emergency Medicine, St. Luke's Roosevelt Hospital Center, New York.*)

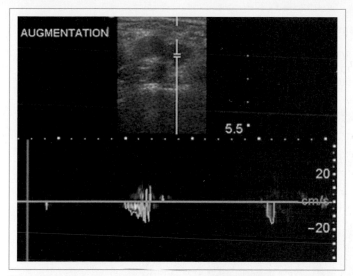

FIGURE 65.8: Augmentation: increase in size of the common femoral vein with distal compression of the leg. (*Image courtesy of Turandot Saul, Department of Emergency Medicine, St. Luke's Roosevelt Hospital Center, New York.*)

CT Venography

- CT venography (CTV) has equivalent sensitivity and specificity to limited compression ultrasound for proximal DVT but can also diagnose pelvic and calf DVT
- Intravenous contrast is administered usually via an antecubital vein
- Identification of a filling defect in a deep vein is indicative of DVT

 TABLE 65.4: CT venography

IV contrast	Yes, to visualize venous system
PO contrast	No
Amount of radiation	10 mSv

Classic Images

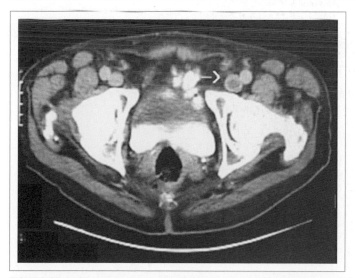

FIGURE 65.9: Contrast-enhanced CT reveals a large thrombosis in the left femoral vein. Acute pulmonary embolism was also visualized in this patient. (From Topol EJ, Califf RM, Isner, J, et al. Textbook of Cardiovascular Medicine, 3rd ed. Philadelphia: Lippincott Williams & Wilkins, 2006.)

MR Venography

- MR venography (MRV) has a sensitivity of 100% and a specificity of 99% for pelvic vein and proximal vein DVT
- MRV is less sensitive for calf DVT (68%) but may provide alternative diagnoses
- Performed in a similar fashion to CTV
- May be able to differentiate acute versus chronic DVT

 TABLE 65.5: MR venography

IV contrast	Yes, to visualize venous system
PO contrast	No
Amount of radiation	None

Classic Images

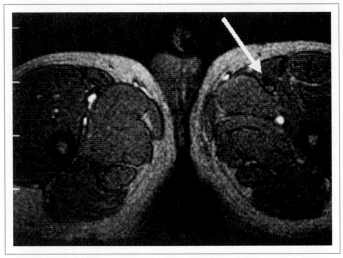

FIGURE 65.10: Magnetic resonance venography showing left superficial femoral venous thrombosis *(arrow)*. Note dilatation of ipsilateral deep femoral vein. (From Bucholz RW and Heckman JD. Rockwood and Green's Fractures in Adults, 5th ed. Philadelphia: Lippincott, Williams & Wilkins, 2001.)

Contrast Venography

- Gold standard with 99–100% sensitivity and specificity
- Contrast is administered intravenously via a foot vein IV, and then a series of x-rays are performed
- Invasive test with 2% chance of inducing DVT
- Contrast venography is resource heavy and rarely performed

 TABLE 65.6: Contrast venography

IV contrast	Yes, to visualize venous system
PO contrast	No
Amount of radiation	Variable, multiple x-rays of extremity, 0.01 mSv each

Classic Images

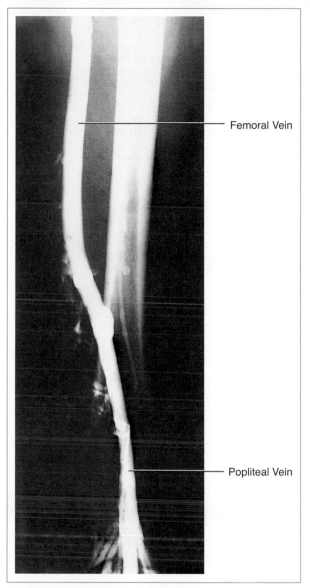

Femoral Vein

Popliteal Vein

FIGURE 65.11: Venogram of the deep venous system of the left lower extremity showing the popliteal and femoral veins. From Uflacker R. Atlas of Vascular Anatomy: An Angiographic Approach, 2nd ed. Philadelphia: Lippincott Williams & Wilkins, 2006.)

Basic Management
- Anticoagulation with low-molecular-weight heparin is the outpatient treatment of choice because of easy dosing and no need for serial laboratory testing
- The appropriate treatment of calf vein thrombosis remains unclear
- Pain management
- Patients should be encouraged to elevate the affected extremity to decrease swelling
- Patients with suspected calf vein DVT with a normal ultrasound compressibility study should have repeat imaging done in 7 days for confirmation and to ensure there is no proximal propagation of a missed DVT

Summary

TABLE 65.7: Advantages and disadvantages of imaging modalities in deep vein thrombosis

Imaging modalities	Advantages	Disadvantages
Limited compression ultrasound	Low cost No radiation Bedside availability Less time-consuming	Less sensitive for calf DVT May require repeat ultrasound in 7 days Limited by body habitus Unable to differentiate acute vs. chronic DVT
Duplex ultrasound	Increased sensitivity for calf DVT No radiation	Time–consuming Expensive Limited by body habitus Unable to differentiate acute vs. chronic DVT
CT venography	Evaluate both DVT and PE Diagnose pelvic and calf DVT	Radiation exposure IV contrast Time-consuming Expensive
MR venography	Provides alternative nonthrombotic diagnoses No radiation	Less sensitive for calf DVT Availability Time-consuming Expensive
Contrast venography	Gold standard	May induce DVT Time-consuming Expensive

DVT, deep vein thrombosis; PE, pulmonary embolism.

Section Editor: Daniel J. Egan

66

Renal Calculi

Jonathan Ilgen and Lalena Yarris

Background

Acute flank pain is a frequent complaint of patients seen in the emergency department. It is estimated that up to 12% of the population will have a urinary stone during their lifetime, and after the primary event, there is a 50% probability of having a recurrent stone within 5–7 years. A family history of kidney stones substantially increases an individual's risk of developing nephrolithiasis, tripling the rate of incident stone formation among men in one large population survey. Other risk factors for developing kidney stones include history of prior nephrolithiasis, history of surgical procedures that may enhance enteric oxalate absorption (e.g., gastric bypass or bariatric surgery), frequent urinary tract infections, and dehydration. Kidney stones are most commonly composed of calcium salts, though also form from uric acid, magnesium ammonium phosphate (struvite), and cysteine. Drug-induced urolithiasis is an infrequent etiology of kidney stones overall, but should be considered in certain patient populations. Of note, Indinavir, a protease inhibitor used in the treatment of HIV, may cause stone formation in up to 50% of patients.

TABLE 66.1: Classic history and physical

Colicky flank pain radiating to the groin
Nausea and vomiting
Patient writhing in distress, unable to find a comfortable position
Possible urinary frequency, urgency, and dysuria

TABLE 66.2: Potentially helpful laboratory test

Urinalysis: Gross or microscopic hematuria very common, though absent in 10% of patients with urinary stones; also helpful in identifying infection

X-ray

- Calcium-containing stones are radiopaque and appear as distinct structures in the kidneys, ureters, or bladder on a KUB x-ray
- Ten to fifteen percent of kidney stones do not have enough calcium content to be visible on x-ray
- Serial films may be used in following the passage of a previously documented radio-opaque stone
- Does not give information about degree of obstructive uropathy

 TABLE 66.3: X-ray: renal calculi

IV contrast	No
PO contrast	No
Amount of radiation	0.70 mSv per view

Classic Images

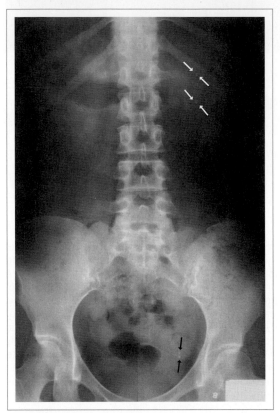

FIGURE 66.1: Kidney stones (*arrows*) in ureter and bladder. (From Moore KL and Dalley AF II. Clinical Oriented Anatomy, 4th ed. Baltimore: Lippincott Williams & Wilkins, 1999.)

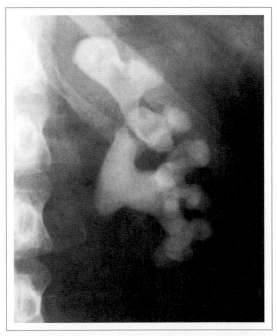

FIGURE 66.2: Large complete left staghorn calculus. (From Harwood-Nuss A, Wolfson AB, Linden CH, et al. The Clinical Practice of Emergency Medicine, 3rd ed. Philadelphia: Lippincott Williams & Wilkins, 2001.)

Abdominal-Pelvic CT Scan

- Unenhanced CT scan is the preferred modality because the intravenous contrast appears bright white and may obscure small stones.
- CT scan has the best test characteristics to confirm the presence of urinary stone: sensitivity of 94–100%, specificity of 92–99%, positive predictive value (PPV) 93–98%, negative predictive value (NPV) 83–97%.
- It is able to directly identify all types of stones except those formed by pure Indinavir precipitates.
- It allows the clinician to directly assess the location of the stone, its size, and the presence of additional stones.
- It can show indirect signs of urolithiasis, such as ureteral dilatation, perinephric and periureteral stranding, renal enlargement, renal sinus fat blurring, or the "rim sign" (circumferential soft tissue attenuation surrounding a stone).
- CT scan is able to detect non-stone-related urinary problems, as well as extra-urinary conditions that manifest as acute flank pain such as those that affect the intestinal tract (appendicitis, Crohn's disease, intussusceptions, hernia, volvulus), vascular system (abdominal aortic aneurysm, renal vein thrombosis), liver and biliary tree, and adnexa (ovarian pathology, hydrosalpinx, endometriosis).
- Radiation exposure is inherent in all CT scans, and given the frequent recurrence of renal calculi, clinicians must consider the cumulative effect of multiple CT studies. In one study, the average cumulative dose over a 6-year period for patients presenting with flank pain ranged from 8.5 to 17.0 mSv for multidetector CT examinations. However, 4% of patients who presented during that period had three or more examinations, with estimated radiation exposure from 19.5 to 153.7 mSv.
- Low-dose protocols for the identification of urinary stones have been developed to address the concern of radiation exposure, achieving doses as low as 1.5 mSv per study, with similar test characteristics to traditional protocols.

TABLE 66.4: CT scan: renal calculi

IV contrast	No, may obscure small stones
PO contrast	No, bowel not organ of interest
Amount of radiation	14 mSv

Classic Images

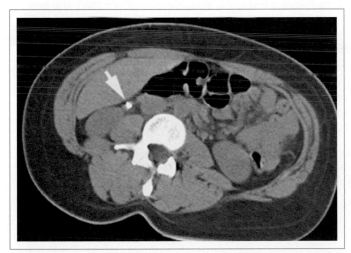

FIGURE 66.3: CT image shows a stone in the ureter *(arrow)*. (From Daffner RH. Clinical Radiology: The Essentials, 3rd ed. Philadelphia: Lippincott Williams & Wilkins, 2007.)

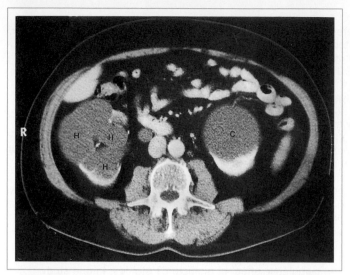

FIGURE 66.4: CT image shows the hydronephrotic collecting system (H) on the right. The mass on the left is a renal cyst (C). (From Daffner RH. Clinical Radiology: The Essentials, 3rd ed. Philadelphia: Lippincott Williams & Wilkins, 2007.)

Renal Ultrasound

- Traditionally, diagnosis of renal calculi was based on indirect anatomic changes such as dilatation of the pelvicalyceal system and ureter proximal to the stone.
- The accuracy of ultrasound is limited by its ability to visualize the ureters. Reported sensitivities and specificities are in the range of 11–93% and 95–100%, respectively.
- Use a 3.5–5.0 MHz ultrasound probe and scan through both long-axis and transverse views of the kidney with the patient supine.
- Having the patient take a deep breath will displace the kidney inferiorly and may bring it out from behind rib shadows.
- In the right upper quadrant, the liver acts as an acoustic window. The probe may be placed in the anterior, mid, or posterior axillary line.
- In the left upper quadrant, images can be more difficult to obtain. Positioning the patient in the right lateral decubitus position and placing the probe along the posterior axillary line may improve the views.
- Doppler sonographic data of intrarenal arterial perfusion can provide secondary evidence of ureteral obstruction. The resistive index (RI) is calculated by subtracting the peak diastolic velocity from the peak systolic velocity, and then dividing it by the latter. RI is designated to be abnormal if it is greater than 0.70, with an inter-renal difference in RI (ΔRI) greater than 0.08. Both the RI and ΔRI can improve the sensitivity and specificity of ultrasonography for renal calculi.
- Ultrasonography should be considered in pregnant women and patients with chronic renal stones, given the teratogenic risk and potential risk of malignancy inherent in multiple CT scans, respectively.
- The combination of ultrasonography and abdominal radiography may be considered in patients with known chronic stones. This combined approach reduces the radiation exposure by an order of magnitude, with improved test characteristics: sensitivity 77–100%, specificity 85–96%, PPV 95%, and NPV 68%.
- Ultrasound has some ability to detect other pathologies that cause acute flank pain but not nearly as reliably as CT scan.

Classic Images

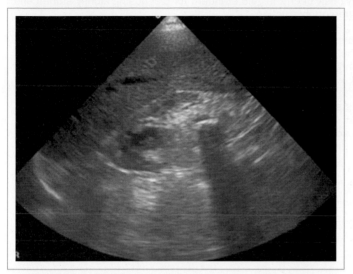

FIGURE 66.5: Intrarenal stone. The calcified stone appears bright white with posterior shadowing. (*Courtesy of Resa Lewiss, St. Luke's Roosevelt Hospital Center, New York, NY.*)

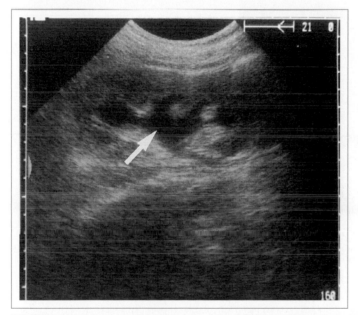

FIGURE 66.6: This is a longitudinal view of the right kidney. There is moderate hydronephrosis, which is seen as separation of the pelvic calyces by fluid (*arrow*). (From Harwood-Nuss A, Wolfson AB, Linden CH, et al. The Clinical Practice of Emergency Medicine, 3rd ed. Philadelphia: Lippincott Williams & Wilkins, 2001.)

Intravenous Urography

- Intravenous pyelogram had previously been the gold standard for diagnosing kidney stones and identifying the location and degree of obstruction
- Intravenous urography (IVU) has a higher sensitivity and specificity than plain radiograph for detecting renal calculi; it also provides structural and functional information about the kidneys, ureters, and bladder, and may help identify congenital anomalies
- Drawbacks include need for contrast, which may cause adverse reactions, and length of time needed to obtain optimal study, which can be quite long if bowel preparation was used for another study
- IVU may be helpful in identifying stones not readily seen on CT scans (stones of protease inhibitors or cold matrix stones)
- Because of the availability and advantages of CT scan, IVU is rarely used in most emergency departments today

 TABLE 66.5: IVU: renal calculi

IV contrast	Yes, shows renal collecting system as contrast is filtered through the renal cortex
PO contrast	No, bowel not organ of interest
Amount of radiation	3 mSv

Classic Image

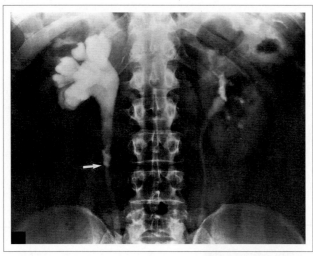

FIGURE 66.7: IVU demonstrates partial obstruction on the right secondary to the ureteral stone (*arrow*). The left kidney is not obstructed. (From Daffner RH. Clinical Radiology: The Essentials, 3rd ed. Philadelphia: Lippincott Williams & Wilkins, 2007.)

Magnetic Resonance Urography

- MRI may offer potential advantages in patients who are pregnant, or have other strong contraindications to ionizing radiation
- Like CT urography, MR urography has the potential to provide a detailed assessment of the urinary tract structures, kidneys, and the surrounding structures
- The cost and the lack of availability of MRI currently limit its practical utility for this diagnosis

 TABLE 66.6: MR urography: renal calculi

IV contrast	Yes, visualization of the collecting system
PO contrast	No, bowel not organ of interest
Amount of radiation	None

Classic Images

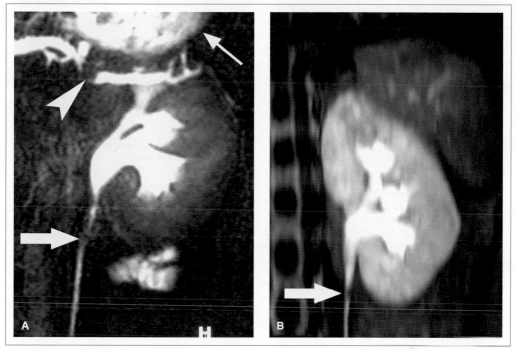

FIGURE 66.8: A: Coronal static MR urogram in patient with tiny proximal left ureter stone (*arrow*) demonstrates multiple overlapping fluid-filled structures such as stomach (*thin arrow*) and pancreatic duct (with intraductal stone) (*arrowhead*). **B:** Excretory urogram performed with 20 mL intravenous gadolinium is not limited by overlying fluid and demonstrates nonobstructing nature of ureteral stone (*arrow*). (From Leyendecker JR and Brown JJ. Practical Guide to Abdominal and Pelvic MRI. Philadelphia: Lippincott Williams & Wilkins, 2004.)

Basic Management
- Intravenous fluids may be helpful in patients with dehydration
- Pain management
  - Nonsteroidal anti-inflammatory drugs (NSAIDs) have been shown to be as effective as opiates
- Facilitating stone passage
  - Most stones will pass without intervention
  - Stones > 4mm in diameter are at higher risk for failure to pass
  - Alpha$_1$ blockade therapy may help facilitate stone passage as compared to conservative therapy alone
- Urologic consultation and admission should be considered in patients with concomitant urinary tract infection or urosepsis, acute renal failure, anuria, or uncontrolled pain despite conservative measures

Summary

TABLE 66.7: Advantages and disadvantages of imaging modalities in renal calculi

Imaging modalities	Advantages	Disadvantages
X-ray	Fast Low radiation Low cost	Not all stones visualized No information about degree of obstruction
CT urography	Gold standard Can identify direct and indirect signs of urinary calculi Can identify other causes of flank pain Rapidly obtained and interpreted	Radiation, especially in cumulative doses
Ultrasonography	Low cost Minimal patient discomfort No radiation Useful in pregnancy Bedside availability	Inferior sensitivity/specificity, though improved when used with KUB
Intravenous urogram	Prior gold standard Lower radiation dose Higher sensitivity than plain film Provides information about location and obstruction	Time-consuming Inferior sensitivity/specificity Limited availability Cannot identify extra-urinary pathology
MR urography	No radiation Can identify other causes of flank pain	Cannot visualize calcification, only filling defects Underestimates stone size and renal caliceal stone burden High cost Limited availability

67

Renal Infarct

Kriti Bhatia

Background

Renal infarct can be an elusive diagnosis. There can be many presentations of this rare entity and symptoms can mimic other more common conditions. The major causes are thromboemboli usually originating from the heart or aorta and primary thrombosis of the renal artery, which is less common. Standard initial imaging for the work-up of flank pain may not detect renal infarction, and therefore the clinician must have a high enough suspicion to order the appropriate diagnostic imaging.

TABLE 67.1: Classic history and physical

Acute onset flank pain or generalized abdominal pain
Nausea, vomiting
Low grade fever
Risk factors for atherosclerotic and thromboembolic disease

TABLE 67.2: Potential helpful laboratory tests

Urinalysis: Hematuria, gross or microscopic
Lactate Dehydrogenase (LDH): Elevated (low sensitivity, high specificity)

X-ray—Nephrotomogram
- A series of x-rays of the kidneys taken from varying angles showing the kidneys clearly without the shadows of overlying organs
- IV contrast is administered to improve visualization of the renal parenchyma

 TABLE 67.3: Nephrotomogram: renal infarct

IV contrast	Yes, to evaluate renal parenchyma
PO contrast	No, bowel is not area of interest
Amount of radiation	0.7 mSv per view

Classic Image

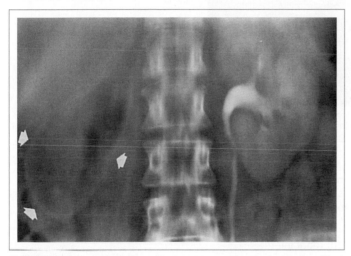

FIGURE 67.1: Renal infarction due to acute renal artery occlusion. Nephrotomogram demonstrating a thin cortical rim surrounding the right kidney (*arrows*), reflecting viable renal cortex perfused by perforating collateral vessels from the renal capsule. (From Eisenberg RL. An Atlas of Differential Diagnosis, 4th ed. Philadelphia: Lippincott Williams & Wilkins, 2003.)

Abdominal CT Scan
- CT scan without contrast is the preferred initial test for the work-up of flank pain
- It allows for diagnosis of intrarenal pathology and ureteral stones which occur much more frequently than renal infarction
- An IV contrast-enhanced CT scan is necessary for diagnosis of renal infarction
- The classic finding is a wedge-shaped perfusion defect
- There is often a high-attenuation cortical rim peripheral to the lesion

 TABLE 67.4: CT scan: renal infarct

IV contrast	Yes, to evaluate vasculature and parenchyma
PO contrast	No, bowel is not area of interest
Amount of radiation	8 mSV

Classic Image

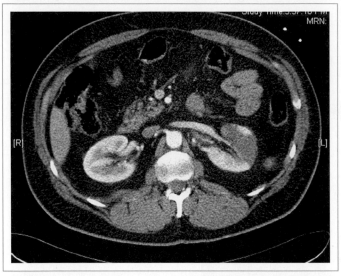

FIGURE 67.2: CT scan with IV contrast demonstrating a renal infarct of the left kidney. (Image courtesy of Daniel J. Egan, Brigham and Women's Hospital, Boston, MA.)

Magnetic Resonance Imaging

- This modality can be helpful for patients with IV contrast allergy or renal failure
- This modality demonstrates low signal intensity of the lesion on both T1- and T2-weighted images
- If there is a hemorrhagic component of the infarct, the signal intensity may be high

 TABLE 67.5: MRI: renal infarct

IV contrast	Yes, to evaluate the renal vasculature and parenchyma
PO contrast	No, bowel is not area of interest
Amount of radiation	None

Classic Image

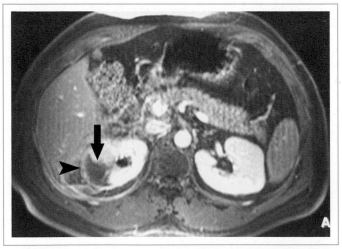

FIGURE 67.3: Fat-suppressed, gadolinium-enhanced T1-weighted gradient echo image demonstrating wedge-shaped, nonenhancing area (*arrow*) involving lateral right kidney. Capsular enhancement is present (*arrowhead*). (From Leyendecker JR and Brown JJ. Practical Guide to Abdominal and Pelvic MRI. Philadelphia: Lippincott Williams & Wilkins, 2004.)

Ultrasound

- Findings of renal parenchymal diseases are nonspecific
- Spectral Doppler ultrasound can be helpful to evaluate renal blood flow
- Color Doppler ultrasound can demonstrate increase or decrease in renal blood flow
- This modality has relatively low sensitivity

Classic Images

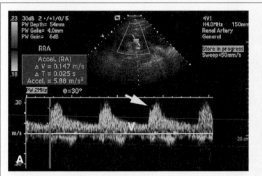
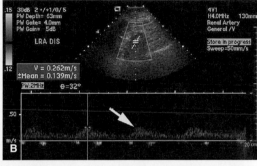

FIGURE 67.4: Renal artery Doppler examinations. **A:** Normal Doppler waveform of an arcuate branch of the right renal artery. The slope (*arrow*) of the systolic upstroke is normal (>300 cm/sec^2). Velocities (V) in the normal right renal artery are less than 180 cm/sec, consistent with no significant renal artery stenosis. **B:** Doppler waveform of an arcuate branch of the left renal artery in the same patient shows slow systolic upstroke and delay to peak (parvus tardus morphology, *arrow*) distal to a significant stenosis. Right renal artery (RRA); left renal artery (LRA); distal (DIS). (*Courtesy of H. Scott Beasley, Department of Radiology, Western Pennsylvania Hospital.*)

Abdominal Angiography

- In the setting of inconclusive CT or MRI, angiography may be useful; this modality is invasive, time-consuming, and requires contrast and specialized personnel, and therefore it is not recommended in the initial diagnostic evaluation
- A wedge-shaped cortical defect is diagnostic of infarct

 TABLE 67.6: Angiography: renal infarct

IV contrast	Yes, to evaluate the renal vasculature and parenchyma
PO contrast	No, bowel is not area of interest
Amount of radiation	12 mSv

Classic Image

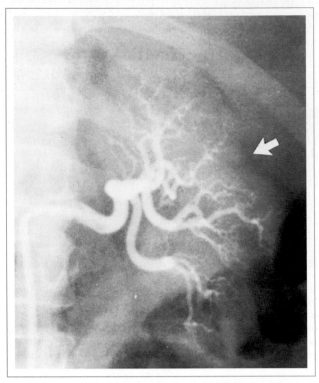

FIGURE 67.5: Renal infarction. Selective left renal arteriogram shows a wide-based cortical depression (*arrow*) reflecting an infarct scar. Note the tortuosity and rapid tapering of interlobar arteries and their branches that is characteristic of arteriolar nephrosclerosis. (From Eisenberg RL. An Atlas of Differential Diagnosis, 4th ed. Philadelphia: Lippincott Williams & Wilkins, 2003.)

Basic Management
- Conservative management is usually preferred
- Anticoagulation, thrombolysis, or embolectomy may minimize loss of renal function
- Pain management
- In-patient admission for further evaluation of underlying problem (e.g., hematologic evaluation for coagulopathy may be useful to identify patients at high risk for further thromboembolic events).

Summary

TABLE 67.7: Advantages and disadvantages of imaging modalities in renal infarct

Imaging modalities	Advantages	Disadvantages
X-ray—nephrotomogram	Fast Low radiation	IV contrast
CT scan	Fast High sensitivity	IV contrast Radiation exposure
MRI	No radiation exposure	Time to obtain and interpret
Ultrasound	Portable No radiation exposure Noninvasive	Operator-dependent Low sensitivity Body habitus limitations
Abdominal angiography	Definitive diagnosis	Invasive Special personnel required Radiation exposure

68

Renal Cell Carcinoma

Jarone Lee

Background

Renal cell carcinoma (RCC) accounts for about 2% of all cancers. Approximately 54,000 people are diagnosed with and 13,000 people die from RCC annually in the United States. RCC is responsible for approximately 80% of all primary renal cancers; however, metastatic cancers are still the most common cause of renal neoplasms. Epidemiologically, RCC is a disease primarily in North America and Scandinavia, with a very low incidence in Africa. Recent studies show that over the past 30 years, the incidence of RCC is increasing. The increasing use of noninvasive imaging has led to many diagnoses early in disease. Approximately 60% of RCCs are discovered incidentally now, compared to 10% in 1970.

TABLE 68.1: Renal cell carcinoma risk factors

Smoking
Occupational exposure (cadmium, asbestos, petroleum)
Obesity
Acquired renal cystic disease
Analgesic abuse nephropathy
Cytotoxic chemotherapy
Alcohol use
Unopposed estrogen use
Prior radiation therapy
Sickle cell anemia
Genetic and family history (e.g., Von Hippel-Lindau disease)

TABLE 68.2: Classic history and physical*

Flank pain
Hematuria
Palpable abdominal mass

*This classic triad is found in only 9% of cases. More commonly, patients are asymptomatic and diagnosis is discovered based on renal or abdominal imaging for another indication. RCC can also present atypically or late in the disease with anemia, hepatic dysfunction (Stauffer's syndrome), fevers, hypercalcemia, thrombocytosis, polymyalgia rheumatica, or paraneoplastic symptoms.

TABLE 68.3: Potentially helpful laboratory tests

Urinalysis: Hematuria
CBC: Anemia of chronic disease; thrombocytosis in late disease. Both associated with a poor prognosis
LFT: Transaminitis in the absence of metastatic disease (Stauffer's syndrome). Resolves with nephrectomy. Associated with poor prognosis
Calcium: Hypercalcemia in 15% of patients

CBC, complete blood count; LFT, liver function test.

Renal Ultrasound

- Sensitivity 56–91%, specificity 86–99%
- Consider contrast-enhanced renal ultrasound to increase sensitivity and specificity (sensitivity 96.6%, specificity 100%, PPV 100%, NPV 95.8%)

- Use a 3.5–5.0 MHz ultrasound probe and scan the right upper quadrant (RUQ) and the left upper quadrant (LUQ) of the abdomen. Scan through both kidneys in two planes (longitudinal and transverse). Also image the bladder in two planes in the suprapubic area.
- Having the patient take a deep breath will displace the kidney inferiorly and may bring it out from behind rib shadows
- In the RUQ, the liver acts as an acoustic window. The probe may be placed in the anterior, mid, or posterior axillary line.
- In the LUQ, images can be more difficult to obtain. Positioning the patient in the right lateral decubitus position and placing the probe along the posterior axillary line may improve the views.
- RCC appearance is typically different from the following simple cyst criteria:
  - Round and well demarcated, smooth edges
  - Anechoic interior and no solid elements
  - Strong posterior wall acoustic enhancement
  - Well-defined interface between cyst and renal parenchyma
  - Peripheral location
- Simple renal cysts do have a small chance of associated malignancy. Appropriate follow-up should be arranged.

Classic Image

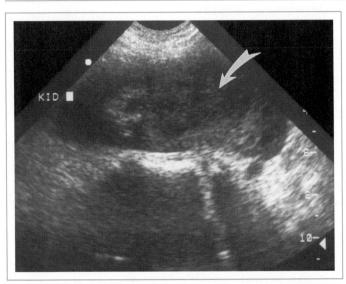

FIGURE 68.1: Renal cell carcinoma. Solid hypoechoic mass (*arrow*) in the inferior half of the kidney (KID) that disrupts the collecting system and distorts the renal outline. (From Eisenberg RL. An Atlas of Differential Diagnosis, 4th ed. Philadelphia: Lippincott Williams & Wilkins, 2003.)

Abdominal CT Scan
- Sensitivity 83–100%, specificity 79–100%
- Increasingly, renal masses are being found when a CT is ordered for another indication; approximately % of RCCs are now diagnosed incidentally
- CT is the diagnostic modality of choice to image for RCC and also to stage metastatic disease
- Patients with renal cysts that do not fit the ultrasound criteria for simple cysts should undergo both an unenhanced and IV contrast-enhanced CT of the abdomen
- The renal mass is suspicious for malignancy if it has thickened and irregular walls or enhancement after IV contrast

 TABLE 68.4: CT scan: renal cell carcinoma

IV contrast	Yes, contrast enhancement is marker for malignancy
PO contrast	No, bowel not area of interest
Amount of radiation	8 mSv

Classic Images

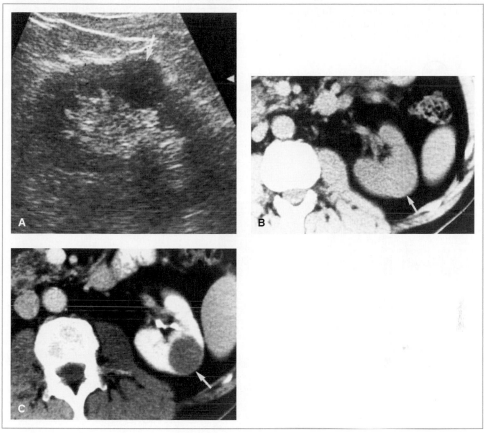

FIGURE 68.2: Renal cell carcinoma. **A:** Longitudinal ultrasound image of the left kidney demonstrates a 3-cm hypoechoic mass with no distal acoustic enhancement (*white arrow*). **B:** Unenhanced CT image through the mid left kidney demonstrates no visible mass (*white arrow*). **C:** Contrast-enhanced CT image at the same level demonstrates a well-defined mass with minimal enhancement (*white arrow*). The CT appearance could be confused with a cystic mass, but the ultrasound shows that this is a solid tumor. (From Kawashima A, Goldman SM, and Sandler CM. The Indeterminate Renal Mass. Radiol Clin North Am 1996;34:997–1015. Used with permission.)

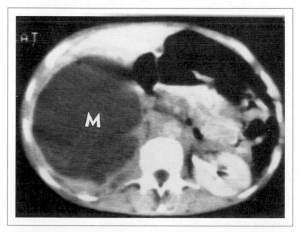

FIGURE 68.3: Necrotic renal cell carcinoma. The huge nonenhancing, cyst-like mass (M) has irregular margins (especially on its medial and posterior aspects). (From Eisenberg RL. An Atlas of Differential Diagnosis, 4th ed. Philadelphia: Lippincott Williams & Wilkins, 2003.)

Abdominal MRI

- Imaging study of choice if ultrasound and CT are nondiagnostic
- Similar to CT, it can be used for staging; studies report that MRI is excellent at detecting lymph node involvement with a sensitivity of 100%
- Again, a renal mass can be found when imaging is ordered for another indication

 TABLE 68.5: MRI: renal cell carcinoma

IV contrast	Yes, not necessary to visualize mass but may be used for further general evaluation
PO contrast	No, bowel not area of interest
Amount of radiation	None

Classic Image

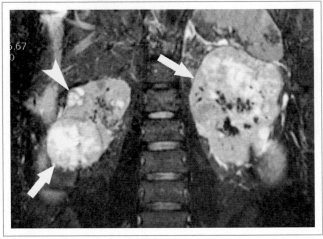

FIGURE 68.4: Coronal fat-suppressed T2-weighted image of the kidneys shows bilateral clear cell carcinomas (*arrows*) and right upper pole papillary renal cell carcinoma (*arrowhead*). (From Leyendecker JR and Brown JJ. Practical Guide to Abdominal and Pelvic MRI. Philadelphia: Lippincott Williams & Wilkins, 2004.)

Basic Management

- If the patient has reliable medical follow-up, consider outpatient management with the primary care physician and oncologic referral
- Consider in-patient admission for sick, debilitated patients, and patients with poor follow-up and social support
- Pain management

Summary

TABLE 68.6: Advantages and disadvantages of imaging modalities in renal cell carcinoma

Imaging modalities	Advantages	Disadvantages
Ultrasound	Low cost Minimal patient discomfort No radiation Availability Less time-consuming	Availability (off hours) Body habitus limitations
CT scan	Availability Diagnosis of other diseases also possible Lymph node staging	IV contrast Radiation exposure
MRI	Diagnosis of other diseases also possible No radiation Lymph node staging	IV contrast Availability Time-consuming Expensive

69

Polycystic Kidney Disease

Daniel J. Egan

Background

Polycystic kidney disease (PKD) is the most common genetic cause of renal failure in adults. Typically the disease is passed on in an autosomal dominant fashion affecting somewhere between 1 in every 400–1,000 births annually. There are several possible genetic mutations that are essentially clinically indistinguishable. The disease is progressive with development of cystic lesions in the parenchyma of the kidney ultimately leading to renal failure. Other organ systems may develop cystic lesions as well, including the liver, spleen, cerebral vascular system (berry aneurysms), and the vasculature of the heart. As mentioned above, the disease is progressive with children rarely developing renal failure as a result of PKD. Most patients begin to develop cysts in the first decade of life, but clinical manifestations usually are not apparent until the fourth or fifth decade. The average age at which patients require hemodialysis is 53.

TABLE 69.1: Classic history and physical

Pain in the flank or back is the most common complaint
Abdominal pain may be present directly from the enlarged kidneys or because of other organ involvement
Patients may develop hematuria
Peripheral edema may be present because of worsening renal function
Palpable bilateral flank masses
Hepatosplenomegaly may be present if these organs are involved
Generalized findings of renal failure (mental status changes from uremia, edema, skin changes)

TABLE 69.2: Potentially helpful laboratory tests

BUN and creatinine: Evaluation of renal function
Urinalysis: Evaluates for presence of infection. Other markers such as degree of proteinuria may also be helpful

BUN, blood urea nitrogen.

Renal Ultrasound

- Ultrasound is the preferred modality for imaging the kidneys in a patient with suspected PKD. It is valuable as a screening test for patients at risk.
- Ultrasound should detect cysts 1 cm in size or greater.
- The 3.5-MHz probe is typically used to scan patients. Images in both the longitudinal and transverse planes should be obtained.
- Having the patient take a deep breath will displace the kidney inferiorly and may bring it out from behind rib shadows.
- In the right upper quadrant, the liver acts as an acoustic window. The probe may be placed in the anterior, mid, or posterior axillary line.
- In the left upper quadrant, images can be more difficult to obtain. Positioning the patient in the right lateral decubitus position and placing the probe along the posterior axillary line may improve the views.
- Renal cysts should fit the following criteria:
  - Round and well demarcated, smooth edges
  - Anechoic interior and no solid elements
  - Strong posterior wall acoustic enhancement
  - Well-defined interface between cyst and renal parenchyma
  - Peripheral location
- The cysts typically are spread throughout the cortex of the kidney.

- Normal renal parenchyma is usually visualized between the cysts.
- Over time, repeat examinations will show an increase in both the number and overall size of the cysts.
- Cysts are at risk for both hemorrhage and infection, which show a change in echogenicity inside the cyst if present.
- As a screening modality, if no cysts are present by the end of the second decade of life, patients are unlikely to develop PKD.

Classic Image

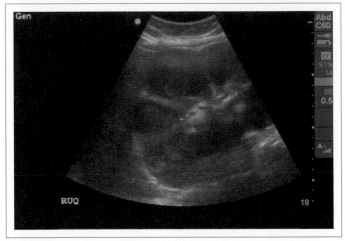

FIGURE 69.1: Renal ultrasound demonstrating multiple cysts. RUQ, right upper quadrant. (*Image courtesy of the Division of Emergency Ultrasound, Massachusetts General Hospital, Boston, MA.*)

Abdominal CT Scan

- CT scan has the same sensitivity as ultrasound in identifying cysts
- On CT imaging, cysts appear as well-defined low-attenuation masses that do not enhance with the administration of IV contrast
- CT allows for identification of complications such as cyst rupture into the retroperitoneum, or the development of blood or pus within a cyst

 TABLE 69.3: CT scan: polycystic kidney disease

IV contrast	Yes, cysts do not enhance with contrast; however, abscesses do
PO contrast	No, bowel not organ of interest
Amount of radiation	8 mSv

Classic Image

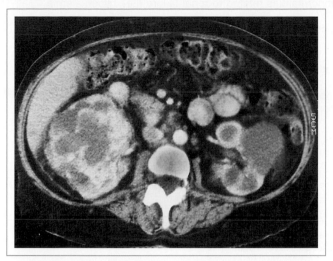

FIGURE 69.2: CT image through the kidneys in an adult patient showing multiple renal cysts. Notice the enhancement of the surrounding renal parenchyma after IV contrast administration. (From Daffner RH. Clinical Radiology: The Essentials, 3rd ed. Philadelphia: Lippincott Williams & Wilkins, 2007.)

Magnetic Resonance Imaging

- MRI is indicated only for further evaluation of documented PKD; additionally, it can be used to further clarify cysts or structures that are not clear on ultrasound or CT scan
- On T1 imaging, cysts have a low to intermediate signal intensity
- On T2-weighted images, the cysts appear with high signal intensity

 TABLE 69.4: MRI: polycystic kidney disease

IV contrast	Yes, changes signal intensity of cysts for evaluation
PO contrast	No, bowel not area of interest
Amount of radiation	None

Classic Image

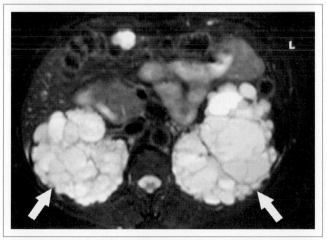

FIGURE 69.3: Autosomal dominant polycystic kidney disease. Fat-suppressed T2-weighted image demonstrating extensive bilateral renal involvement with cysts (*arrows*). (From Leyendecker JR and Brown JJ. Practical Guide to Abdominal and Pelvic MRI. Philadelphia: Lippincott Williams & Wilkins, 2004.)

Basic Management

- Check renal function and correct abnormalities related to renal failure (i.e., hyperkalemia, hypocalcemia, acidosis)
- Treat urinary tract infection if present
- Control blood pressure
- Pain control
- Admission to hospital recommended if renal failure is present
- Surgical or interventional radiologic consultation for drainage of infected cysts
- Nephrology follow-up if admission not required
- Advise patient to keep away from contact sports to avoid traumatic cyst rupture

Summary

TABLE 69.5: Advantages and disadvantages of imaging modalities in polycystic kidney disease

Imaging modalities	Advantages	Disadvantages
Ultrasound	Minimal patient discomfort No radiation Availability	Difficulty identifying complications of PKD
CT scan	Availability Diagnosis of other diseases also possible Ability to identify associated lesions in other organs	IV contrast Radiation exposure
MRI	Excellent identification of kidneys and other parenchyma Evaluation of lesions not clearly identifiable with other modalities	Expensive Time-consuming IV contrast

PKD, polycystic kidney disease.

70   Perinephric Abscess

Kathleen Wittels

Background

A perinephric abscess is a rare but serious infection located in the space between the renal capsule and Gerota's fascia. It most commonly occurs as a complication of an ascending urinary tract infection, but it can also develop by hematogenous spread of another infection (often from the skin). *Escherichia coli* and other gram-negative bacteria are the most common pathogens, but other species such as Staph aureus may be present (particularly when hematogenous spread is the etiology). Most patients have an underlying urinary tract abnormality, and up to one third of patients with a perinephric abscess have diabetes.

TABLE 70.1: Classic history and physical

Flank pain and/or tenderness
Persistent fever despite >72 hr of antibiotics
Insidious onset of symptoms (often >5 d)
Palpable abdominal or flank mass (~50% of the time)

TABLE 70.2: Potentially helpful laboratory tests

CBC: Leukocytosis
Urinalysis: Pyuria (although urinalysis may be normal)
Creatinine: Elevated
Urine and blood cultures: Often negative

CBC, complete blood count.

X-ray

- X-ray is not the diagnostic modality of choice for perinephric abscess
- Perinephric abscess may be seen on x-ray if gas is present

 TABLE 70.3: X-ray: perinephric abscess

IV contrast	No
PO contrast	No
Amount of radiation	0.7 mSv per view

Classic Image

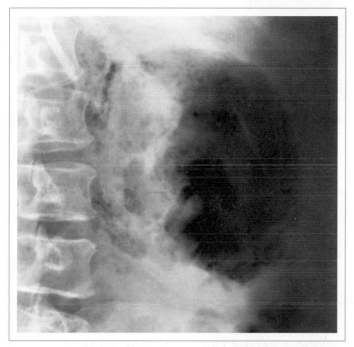

FIGURE 70.1: Renal abscess. Large amounts of extraluminal gas in and around the left kidney. (From Eisenberg RL. An Atlas of Differential Diagnosis, 4th ed. Philadelphia: Lippincott Williams & Wilkins, 2003.)

Renal Ultrasound

- The kidney is an easily identifiable organ on ultrasound, which makes it a good initial test if there is a suspicion of perinephric abscess.
- Use a 3.5–5.0 MHz ultrasound probe and scan through both long-axis and transverse views of the kidney with the patient supine.
- Having the patient take a deep breath will displace the kidney inferiorly and may bring it out from behind rib shadows.
- In the right upper quadrant, the liver acts as an acoustic window. The probe may be placed in the anterior, mid, or posterior axillary line.
- In the left upper quadrant, images can be more difficult to obtain. Positioning the patient in the right lateral decubitus position and placing the probe along the posterior axillary line may improve the views.
- The perinephric abscess may appear as either a hypo- or hyperechoic mass.
- The use of Doppler can be helpful to distinguish between an abscess (avascular) and a malignancy (vascular).

Classic Images

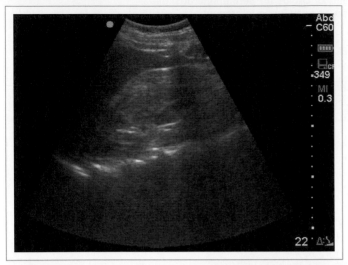

FIGURE 70.2: Ultrasound image demonstrating pyelonephritis before the development of an abscess. Notice the increased echogenicity of the renal parenchyma when compared to the liver suggesting infection. (*Courtesy of the Division of Emergency Ultrasound, Massachusetts General Hospital, Boston, MA.*)

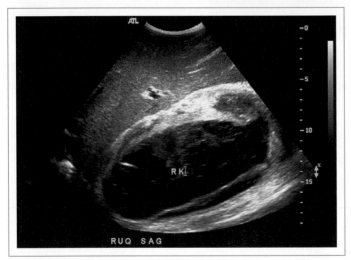

FIGURE 70.3: Ultrasound image demonstrating a perinephric abscess. (*Courtesy of the Division of Emergency Ultrasound, Mount Sinai Department of Emergency Medicine, New York, NY.*)

Abdominal CT Scan
- CT scan of the abdomen is the imaging modality of choice
- A perinephric abscess will appear as a low-attenuation mass that enhances with IV contrast
- Thickening of Gerota's fascia is often present
- CT will also define the extension of the abscess and possible spread of infection to adjacent tissues (i.e., psoas muscle)

 TABLE 70.4: CT scan: perinephric abscess

IV contrast	Yes, abscess enhances with contrast
PO contrast	No, bowel not area of interest
Amount of radiation	8 mSv

Classic Image

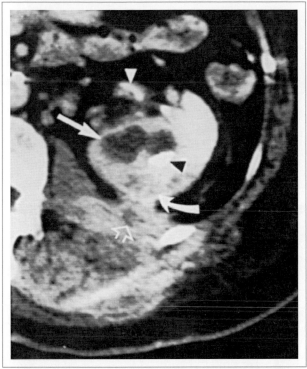

FIGURE 70.4: CT scan of the left kidney after IV injection of contrast material shows calculi (*arrowheads*), hydronephrosis (*straight white arrow*), parenchymal suppuration with liquefaction (*curved white arrow*), and extension of the process through the renal capsule into the perinephric space forming a perinephric abscess (*short open arrow*). (From Gorbach SL, Bartlett JG, Blacklow NR, et al. Infectious Diseases. Philadelphia: Lippincott Williams & Wilkins, 2004.)

Magnetic Resonance Imaging
- Similar sensitivity to CT scan in identifying a perinephric abscess
- MRI is an alternative to consider in patients with iodinated contrast allergy or contraindication to radiation

 TABLE 70.5: MRI: perinephric abscess

IV contrast	Yes, changes signal intensity of abscess
PO contrast	No
Amount of radiation	None

Classic Images

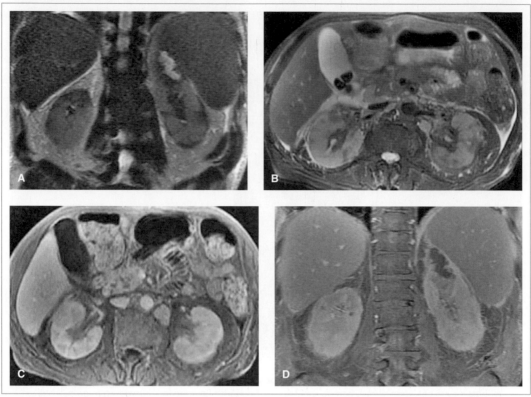

FIGURE 70.5: Coronal T2-weighted imaging (WI) (**A**) demonstrates a 2.8 × 4.8 × 3.4 cm, exophytic, left upper pole, hyperintense, thick-walled lesion. Fat-suppressed axial T2-WI (**B**) shows wedge-shaped areas of decreased signal intensity. Gadolinium-enhanced, fat-suppressed axial (**C**) and coronal (**D**) T1-WI show enhancement of the irregular wall of the left upper pole cystic lesion and wedge-shaped areas of decreased enhancement of the renal parenchyma. Note left interpolar renal scarring, cholelithiasis, and para-aortic lymph node. (From Ros PR, Mortele KJ, Lee S, et al. CT and MRI of the Abdomen and Pelvis: A Teaching File, 2nd ed. Philadelphia: Lippincott Williams & Wilkins, 2007.)

Basic Management

- Small abscesses (less than 3 cm) may be treated with antibiotics alone, but most abscesses require drainage
- Depending on the location and size of the abscess, percutaneous drainage may be performed with ultrasound or CT guidance
- Severe cases may require open surgical drainage and rarely partial or complete nephrectomy is necessary

Summary

TABLE 70.6: Advantages and disadvantages of imaging modalities in perinephric abscess

Imaging modalities	Advantages	Disadvantages
X-ray	Availability Low radiation	May only see abscess if gas is present
Ultrasound	Availability No radiation	Operator-dependent Less sensitive than CT scan
CT scan	High sensitivity Evaluates extent of infection	Radiation exposure IV contrast
MRI	No radiation High sensitivity	Less accessible Expensive IV contrast

71

Scrotal Pain

Sanjay Shewakramani

Background

Because of the emergent nature of testicular torsion, it is necessary to expedite the evaluation in patients presenting with acute onset scrotal pain and swelling. While testicular torsion is most common in males between 10 and 20 years of age, it can occur at any age. After the age of 20, epididymitis is the most common cause of testicular pain. Other differential diagnoses to consider include torsion of the testicular appendage, orchitis, hydrocele, varicocele, trauma, hernia, and Henoch-Schönlein purpura. The evaluation and management for testicular torsion and epididymitis will be outlined below.

Testicular Torsion

Testicular torsion occurs in approximately 1 in 4,000 males, peaking in incidence at 13 years of age, and comprises 16% of all patients presenting to the emergency department with an acute scrotum. It occurs secondary to a congenital defect in testicular suspension (bell-clapper deformity, found in 12% of males), resulting in twisting (180–720 degrees) of the spermatic cord, ischemia, and eventual necrosis. Testicular salvage is likely if detorsion occurs within 6 hours, but if left untreated for greater than 24 hours, testicular necrosis is almost certain.

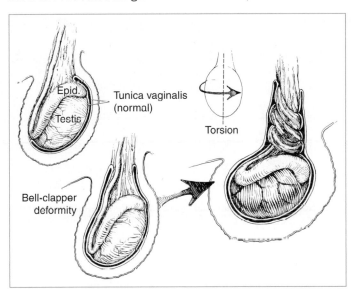

FIGURE 71.1: Torsion testis. Abnormality of testicular fixation—bell-clapper deformity—permits torsion of spermatic vessels with subsequent infarction of the gonad. (From Fleisher GR, Ludwig S, and Henretig FM. Textbook of Pediatric Emergency Medicine, 5th ed. Philadelphia: Lippincott Williams & Wilkins, 2005.)

TABLE 71.1: Classic history and physical for torsion

Sudden onset of pain and swelling, typically unilateral
Trauma or vigorous activity may have been the inciting event
May have had prior episodes of similar, milder symptoms (torsion/detorsion)
Classic examination reveals a swollen, tender, high-riding testis in a horizontal lie
Absent cremasteric reflex

TABLE 71.2: Potentially helpful laboratory test for torsion

Urinalysis: Can evaluate for other causes of testicular pain if etiology unclear

Ultrasound

- A linear probe should be used to scan the entire scrotum, identifying traverse and longitudinal views of both testes, epididymal heads and tails, and spermatic cords.
- High-frequency (7.5–10.0 MHz) color Doppler imaging should always be used in evaluating torsion to determine whether there is flow within the intratesticular arteries, which can be missed using a 5 MHz probe.
- The straddle view can be used to ultrasound both testicles at once and compare the affected and unaffected sides.
- Blood supply to the testicle is via the testicular artery. Blood supply to the scrotal skin is via the internal pudendal artery. Care must be taken to visualize Doppler flow within the testicle itself as visualizing arterial flow to the surrounding scrotal skin can result in a false negative for torsion.
- In prepubertal children with small testicular volumes, power Doppler may be necessary to evaluate for intratesticular blood flow and avoid a false positive for torsion.
- Sensitivity of ultrasound ranges from 86% to 98%; specificity approaches 100%.
- Signs of torsion include:
  - Enlarged testicle
  - Hypoechoic testicle
  - Complete lack of blood flow within the testicle
  - Edema/hydrocele (nonspecific)
- After detorsion, the testicle can have increased Doppler flow, potentially leading to a false diagnosis of epididymitis.

Classic Images

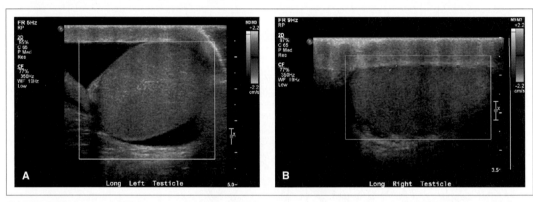

FIGURE 71.2: Images of bilateral testes. Note the enlargement and surrounding edema within the torsed left testicle (**A**) compared to the right testicle (**B**). (*Courtesy of Department of Emergency Medicine, Georgetown University Hospital, Washington, D.C.*)

Nuclear Scintigraphy

- It has fallen out of favor as the test of choice for testicular torsion, but is still occasionally used when ultrasound findings are inconclusive
- Technetium-99m is used to demonstrate perfusion of the testicles, as well as the surrounding structures
- Sensitivity and specificity are comparable to ultrasound
- Risks include radiation and potential delay in obtaining imaging
- Sensitivity of nuclear imaging decreases significantly 4 hours after the onset of symptoms
- After manual detorsion, repeat injection of technetium is often not needed, and imaging can be repeated to demonstrate successful return of blood flow

 TABLE 71.3: Nuclear scintigraphy: testicular torsion

IV contrast	No
PO contrast	No
Amount of radiation	2–3 mSv

Classic Image

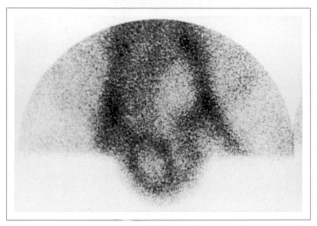

FIGURE 71.3: The "doughnut" sign: Lack of blood flow within the right testicle, with a rim of peripheral hyperemia. (From Fleisher GR, Ludwig S, and Baskin MN. Atlas of Pediatric Emergency Medicine. Philadelphia: Lippincott Williams & Wilkins, 2004.)

Management
- Due to the time-sensitive nature of the disease, if torsion is clinically evident, surgical management should not be delayed to obtain imaging
- With high clinical suspicion, even without imaging, manual detorsion should be attempted by twisting the affected testicle using an "open-book" technique; turning the testicle outward is the correct direction in two thirds of cases
- Urology consultation should be obtained immediately
- If manual detorsion is unsuccessful, detorsion must be performed in the operating room
- Even if manual detorsion is successful, orchiopexy is often performed to prevent future occurrences
- Bilateral orchiopexy is preferred, as the bell-clapper deformity tends to occur bilaterally
- Spontaneous detorsion can occur prior to evaluation; if the clinical presentation is concerning, the patient can be admitted for observation to monitor for recurrence

Epididymitis

Epididymitis is the most common cause of the acute scrotum encountered in the emergency department, with an incidence of approximately 1:1,000 per year. Inflammation is most often caused by infection, resulting in pain. Causative organisms often reach the epididymis via the urethra, but blood-borne infections can occur as well. In patients 35 years and younger, *Chlamydia trachomatis* and *Neisseria gonorrhoeae* are the most frequently encountered microbes, whereas *Escherichia coli* is the most commonly encountered microbe in men over the age of 35.

TABLE 71.4: Classic history and physical for epididymitis

Gradual onset of pain, peaking after 24 hr
Associated urinary symptoms—dysuria, frequency, urgency, or retention
Fever and flank pain can occur
Ten percent of cases are bilateral
Tender, warm, and edematous epididymis (posterior aspect of the testicle)
Cremasteric reflex should be present
Prehn sign: elevation of the scrotum relieves pain (not reliable for ruling out torsion)

TABLE 71.5: Potentially helpful laboratory tests for epididymitis

Urinalysis: 50% will be abnormal
Urethral swab for Gonorrhea/Chlamydia

Ultrasound

- A linear probe (as in cases of suspected torsion) should be used with color Doppler flow
- Hyperemia of the enlarged and inflamed epididymis is diagnostic in the absence of torsion
- Reactive hydroceles may form
- Increased Doppler flow within the testis in addition to the epididymis indicates epididymo-orchitis
- Sensitivity and specificity approach 100% with ultrasound
- The epididymis can become hyperemic and enlarged in some cases of testicular torsion, and intratesticular blood flow should always be evaluated

Classic Image

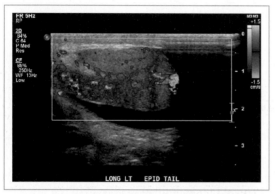

FIGURE 71.4: Doppler ultrasound reveals epididymitis of the left testicle evidenced by hyperemia and enlargement of the epididymis as well as a reactive hydrocele. Note the presence of blood flow within the testicle, ruling out torsion. (*Courtesy of Department of Emergency Medicine, Georgetown University Hospital, Washington, D.C.*)

Nuclear Scintigraphy

- As with torsion, this test has fallen out of favor in place of ultrasonography
- Technetium-99 injection reveals increased perfusion of the epididymis
- Sensitivity and specificity are both less in comparison to ultrasound
- Late complications of epididymitis, such as abscess or hydrocele, can lead to a hypervascular rim with a photopenic center, which could potentially mimic torsion

 TABLE 71.6: Nuclear scintigraphy: epididymitis

IV contrast	No
PO contrast	No
Amount of radiation	2–3 mSv

Classic Image

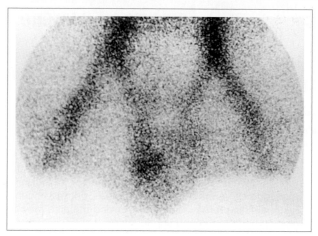

FIGURE 71.5: Epididymitis of the right testicle. Note the increased uptake indicating hyperemia. (From Fleisher GR, Ludwig S, and Baskin MN. Atlas of Pediatric Emergency Medicine. Philadelphia: Lippincott Williams & Wilkins, 2004.)

Basic Management
- Antibiotics should be tailored to treat the most likely causative agents
- Postpubertal men under the age of 35 should receive treatment for *N. gonorrhoeae* and *C. trachomatis*
- Prepubertal males and men over the age of 35 should receive treatment for enteric organisms
- Supportive care including scrotal elevation and analgesia

Summary

TABLE 71.7: Advantages and disadvantages of imaging modalities in testicular torsion/epididymitis

Imaging modalities	Advantages	Disadvantages
Ultrasound	Fast and readily available No radiation Bedside availability Patient discomfort	Operator-dependent
Nuclear scintigraphy	Not operator-dependent	Radiation exposure Time-consuming Transport to radiology suite Less accurate

72

Fournier's Gangrene

Emily L. Senecal

Background

Fournier's gangrene is a life-threatening soft tissue infection of the perineum which occurs most commonly in men. Patients with diabetes and those that abuse alcohol are at high risk. Initial symptoms often involve perineal itching or irritation after a break in the skin, followed by diffuse edema, erythema, and tenderness of the soft tissue as polymicrobial bacteria invade the underlying soft tissues and fascial planes. Crepitus develops when *Clostridium* or other gas-forming bacteria are present. The perineum, scrotum, and penis are most often involved, but the abdominal wall may become affected as well. Systemic symptoms including fever and malaise may be present, and patients are at risk for developing bacteremia and septic shock.

Although Fournier's gangrene is often suspected based on history and examination findings, soft tissue CT scan is the definitive diagnostic test. Prompt diagnosis is critical, as bacterial destruction of fascial planes can be as fast as 2–3 cm/hour. Mortality, which is high in this disease process at 7–33%, increases up to 75% with delay in diagnosis.

TABLE 72.1: Classic history and physical

Initial break in skin allowing bacteria to invade the soft tissues and fascial planes
Increased risk in diabetes; men affected 10 times more than women
Erythema, edema, tenderness of perineum or scrotum
Crepitus when gas-forming organisms present
Bacteremia and septic shock may develop

TABLE 72.2: Potentially helpful laboratory tests

CBC: Leukocytosis
BMP: To assess for dehydration, acidosis, and potential hyper- or hypoglycemia
Lactate, coagulation profile, and DIC panel: Evidence of severe sepsis
Blood, urine, wound cultures
ABG: To assess for acid/base disturbance

ABG, arterial blood gas; BMP, basic metabolic panel; CBC, complete blood count; DIC, disseminated intravascular coagulation.

Pelvic Radiograph

- May demonstrate air in soft tissues
- Absence of air on plain films does not rule out Fournier's gangrene

TABLE 72.3: Pelvis x-ray: Fournier's gangrene

IV contrast	No
PO contrast	No
Amount of radiation	0.6 mSv per view

Classic Image

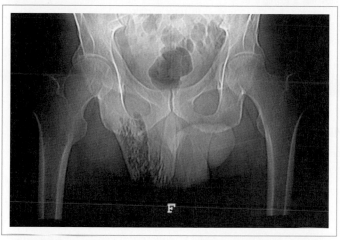

FIGURE 72.1: Air in the soft tissues of the scrotum and perineal area in a patient with Fournier's gangrene. (*Courtesy of Dr. Jose Medina Polo, Department of Urology, Hospital Universitario 12 de Octubre, Madrid, Spain.*)

Scrotal Ultrasound
- Bedside ultrasound aids in rapidly confirming this life-threatening diagnosis
- Air in the scrotal wall is diagnostic
- Subcutaneous air appears as numerous discrete, hyperechoic foci
- Testes and epididymis appear normal
- Alternate causes of acute testicular pain and swelling may be identified (e.g., testicular torsion, epididymitis, inguinal hernia)

Classic Image

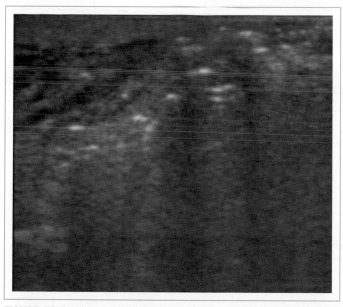

FIGURE 72.2: Ultrasound image of the perineal soft tissue demonstrating inflammatory changes consistent with subcutaneous edema and hyperechoic areas consistent with subcutaneous air. (*Courtesy of Eitan Dickman, Division of Emergency Ultrasound, Maimonides Medical Center, Brooklyn, NY.*)

Abdominal-Pelvic CT Scan

- Gold standard for diagnosis of Fournier's gangrene
- CT findings include soft tissue thickening, fat stranding, soft tissue gas
- Classic finding is gas dissecting along fascial planes
- CT determines the extent of disease and assists in operative planning
- CT may identify an underlying etiology of Fournier's gangrene (e.g., abdominal or pelvic abscess, incarcerated hernia, perianal fistula or abscess)
- IV contrast assists with visualization of soft tissue stranding and extent of tissue necrosis; however, soft tissue gas is visible without IV contrast

 TABLE 72.4: CT scan: Fournier's gangrene

IV contrast	Yes, enables visualization of soft tissue stranding and extent of tissue necrosis
PO contrast	No, bowel wall typically not involved
Amount of radiation	14 mSv

Classic Image

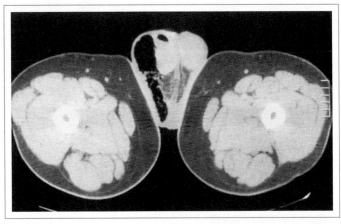

FIGURE 72.3: Uninfused CT image of the upper scrotum demonstrating scrotal thickening with subcutaneous gas. (From Pope TL. Aunt Minnie's Atlas and Imaging-Specific Diagnosis, 3rd ed. Philadelphia: Lippincott Williams & Wilkins, 2009.)

Basic Management

- Immediate urologic consultation for debridement
- Aggressive fluid resuscitation
- Early broad-spectrum antibiotics
- Tetanus prophylaxis if skin breakdown is present

Summary

TABLE 72.5: Advantages and disadvantages of imaging modalities in Fournier's gangrene

Imaging modalities	Advantages	Disadvantages
Plain film	Low radiation	Cannot rule out diagnosis
Ultrasound	No radiation Bedside availability Gas in scrotal wall is diagnostic; can rule in other causes of acute testicular pain (torsion, epididymitis)	Second line diagnostic test unless credentialed ultrasonographer immediately available May be painful for patient
CT scan	Gold standard for diagnosis Reveals extent of disease and pathway of spread Assists with operative planning Often identifies etiology (i.e., underlying abscess)	Radiation exposure IV contrast exposure

73

Acute Urinary Retention

Sonya Seccurro

Background

Acute urinary retention is the most common urologic emergency. It is most common in men and the incidence increases with age. In most cases, it is due to urethral obstruction, secondary to a nonprimary urethral process like BPH (benign prostatic hypertrophy) in men or a displaced cystocele or rectocele in women. Other nonobstructive causes include neurologic disorders, medication side effects, and infection.

Acute urinary retention is much less common in women than men. It is most likely due to distorted anatomy of the bladder outlet because of fibroids, malignant tumors, postpartum vulvar edema, or labial fusion/imperforate hymen. The work-up includes an evaluation of an anatomic cause and if no clear etiology is found, then urodynamic studies should be performed.

TABLE 73.1: Classic history and physical

Abrupt inability to pass urine
Abdominal or suprapubic pain
Fullness on palpation of the lower abdomen and suprapubic region
Rectal examination in men may suggest prostate fullness
Pelvic examination in women may show uterine prolapse, bladder prolapse, or masses
In straightforward urinary retention, neurologic examination of the motor and sensory system of the extremities as well as rectal tone should be normal
Use of recent pharmacologic agents that could lead to acute urinary retention (e.g., antihistamines, anticholinergics)

TABLE 73.2: Potentially helpful laboratory tests

Urinalysis: To evaluate for infection
BUN and creatinine: Limited utility if acute process; may be useful if history suggests chronic retention
Urine pregnancy test

BUN, blood urea nitrogen.

Renal Ultrasound

- Urinary catheterization was historically the diagnostic and therapeutic modality of choice and easily quantified the amount of urine retained
- However, as it is invasive, uncomfortable, and introduces the possibility of infection, ultrasound can be used to make a diagnosis prior to catheterization
- Use a 3.5–5.0 MHz ultrasound probe and scan through the bladder in both sagittal and transverse planes; place the probe just superior to the pubic symphysis and tip down into the pelvis to bring the bladder into view
- Using ultrasound, a markedly distended bladder can be easily recognized
- For chronic or acute urinary retention, the bladder volume (mL) can be estimated by $0.7 \times$ the width (cm) $\times$ the height (cm) $\times$ the depth (cm).
- A post-void residual can be performed by having the patient urinate and then repeating the volume measurement; if it is greater than 100 mL, chronic urinary retention should be suspected
- If retention is severe, the kidneys may show signs of hydronephrosis; the medulla of the kidney will appear hypoechoic from fluid within the dilated collecting system
- If the obstruction is acute, the hydronephrosis should resolve upon relief of the obstruction

Classic Images

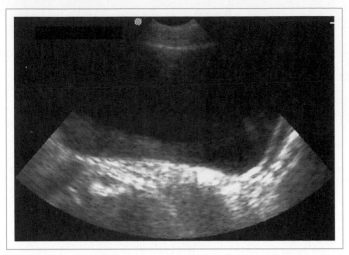

FIGURE 73.1: Sagittal view of the bladder. The hyperechoic area in the inferior portion of the bladder represents clotted blood which caused the retention. (*Courtesy of Kamal Medlej, St. Luke's Roosevelt Hospital Center, New York, NY.*)

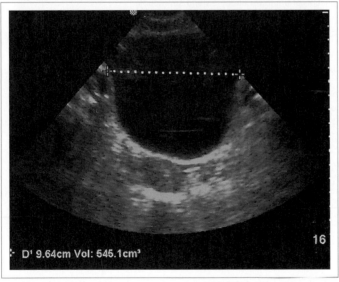

FIGURE 73.2: The use of bedside ultrasound estimating bladder volume. (*Division of Emergency Ultrasound, St. Luke's Roosevelt Hospital Center, New York, NY.*)

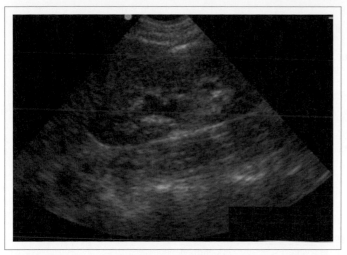

FIGURE 73.3: Mild hydronephrosis of the right kidney. The hypoechoic area in the renal medulla illustrates the dilated collecting system. (*Courtesy of Turandot Saul, St. Luke's Roosevelt Hospital Center, New York, NY.*)

Abdominal-Pelvic CT Scan
- CT scan is not the imaging modality of choice for the diagnosis of acute urinary retention
- A markedly distended bladder or hydronephrosis may be seen incidentally on CT scan, prompting the physician to investigate further

 TABLE 73.3: Abdomen-Pelvis CT scan: Acute urinary retention

IV contrast	No, may obscure urolithiasis
PO contrast	No, bowel is not area of interest
Amount of radiation	14 mSv

Classic Image

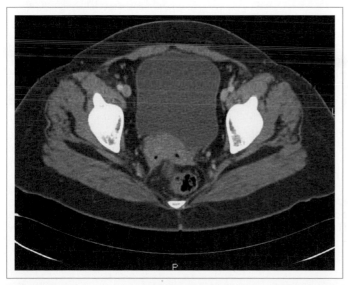

FIGURE 73.4: CT scan demonstrating a markedly distended bladder in this patient undergoing CT scan for right lower quadrant (RLQ) pain. (*Courtesy of St. Luke's Roosevelt Hospital Center Department of Emergency Medicine, New York, NY.*)

Basic Management

- Definitive treatment of acute or chronic urinary retention is bladder decompression with a Foley catheter
- A 14- to 18-French Foley catheter is used unless there is concern for a narrow lumen (e.g., a recent TURP, urethral stricture) in which a smaller catheter may pass easier and with less urethral trauma
- If an enlarged prostate is suspected or difficulty is encountered during passage, a larger catheter or a firm coudé tip may be needed
- Suprapubic needle aspiration is sometimes necessary in cases of severe patient distress and the inability to place a Foley catheter
- Urologic consultation may provide cystoscopic guidance prior to suprapubic catheterization

Summary

TABLE 73.4: Advantages and disadvantages of imaging modalities for acute urinary retention

Imaging modalities	Advantages	Disadvantages
Ultrasound	No radiation exposure Noninvasive Bladder is easily identifiable Kidneys may be evaluated as well	Operator-dependent Availability
CT scan	Can image the entire urinary system	Radiation exposure

74

Urethral Injury

Jonathan Kirschner

Background

Genitourinary trauma typically does not take first priority in the multiple trauma patient; however, it may have significant morbidity. Early identification of a partial urethral injury is important because manipulation can convert a partial tear to a complete tear. Urethral injury is present in 10% of major pelvic fractures with a higher risk of urethral injury in Malgaigne fractures and straddle fractures.

Urethral injury can be classified by anatomic location. Anterior urethral injury occurs distal to the urogenital diaphragm and is often caused by straddle injuries, falls, direct blows, or penetrating trauma. Posterior urethral injury occurs proximal to the urogenital diaphragm and is primarily caused by pelvic fractures. The membranous and prostatic urethras are fixed by the puboprostatic ligaments. Fracture of the pelvis and subsequent displacement of the pubic symphysis creates shearing forces that lacerate or avulse the fixed urethra. Urethral injuries in females are less common due to the mobility of the female urethra. In the setting of pelvic fracture, the "Classic history and physical" findings necessitate further evaluation prior to Foley catheter placement.

TABLE 74.1: Classic history and physical

Major pelvic fracture
Inability to void
Gross hematuria
Blood at penile meatus
Elevation of the prostate on rectal examination (sensitivity 2%)
Perineal swelling and hematoma

Retrograde Urethrogram

- Retrograde urethrogram is the diagnostic procedure of choice in all cases of suspected urethral injury. Occasionally, preliminary CT scan may identify signs of urethral injury such as prostatic apex elevation or extravasation of contrast above or below the urogenital diaphragm.
- Classically, urethrography is performed with the patient in the oblique position. However, in the setting of significant pelvic fracture and hematoma, the supine position is preferred with the penis stretched obliquely over the thigh.
- The procedure is performed by placing a Toomey syringe with Cooke adapter snugly in the urethral meatus and gently injecting 30–60 mL of diluted contrast (1:10 with saline). A radiograph is shot during the final 10 mL of contrast injection. Some sources suggest using a Foley catheter in the fossa navicularis with 2 mL of water in the balloon for contrast injection.
- A normal study shows retrograde flow into the bladder without extravasation of contrast indicating no urethral tear or disruption.
- Extravasation of contrast material outside of the urethra with concomitant filling of the bladder indicates a partial tear.
- The location of contrast extravasation helps identify the anatomic location of the injury and allows classification of injury.

TABLE 74.2: Urethral injury classification (Goldman and Sandler)

Type 1	Stretched posterior urethra, no tear
Type 2	Partial or complete urethral tear above an intact urogenital diaphragm
Type 3	Partial or complete urethral tear of combined anterior/posterior urethra with torn urogenital diaphragm
Type 4	Bladder neck injury with extension to the urethra
Type 5	Isolated anterior urethral injury

- In anterior urethral injury, contrast leakage may be limited to the corporal bodies or may spread throughout the scrotum and perineum if Buck's fascia is disrupted.
- If a partial urethral tear is suspected after successful placement of a Foley catheter, a modified retrograde urethrogram may be performed by placing a small feeding tube alongside the Foley catheter and injecting contrast through the feeding tube. The successfully placed Foley catheter is not removed so that a standard retrograde urethrogram may be performed.

 TABLE 74.3: Retrograde urethrogram: urethral injury

IV contrast	No
PO contrast	No
Amount of radiation	0.6 mSv per view

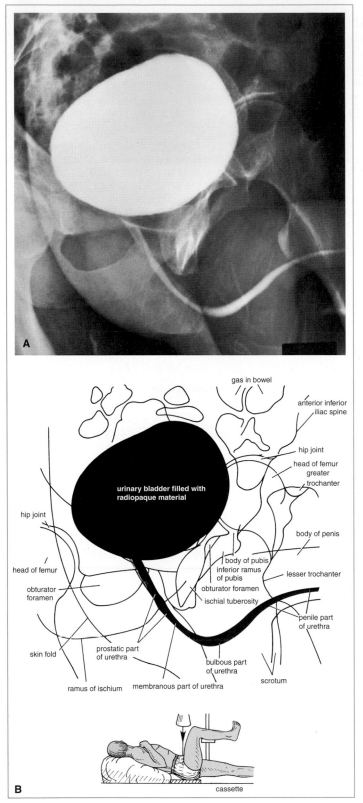

FIGURE 74.1: A: Demonstration of a retrograde urethrogram. **B:** The main features seen in the previous retrograde urethrogram. (From Snell RS. Clinical Anatomy by Regions, 8th ed. Philadelphia: Lippincott Williams & Wilkins, 2008.)

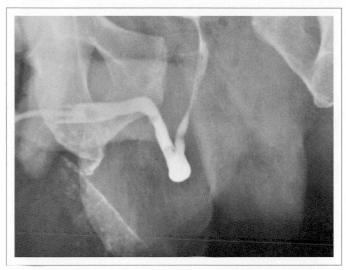

FIGURE 74.2: Type I urethral injury. Retrograde urethrogram shows a stretched but intact urethra with elevation of the bladder base. Marked diastsis of the pubic symphysis is evident. (From Mirvis SE, Dunham CM 1992 Abdominal-pelvic trauma. In: Mirvis SE, Young JWR Eds. Imaging in trauma and critical care. Lippincott Williams & Wilkins. P 230).

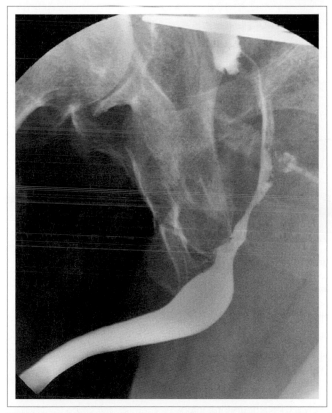

FIGURE 74.3: Type II urethral injury. Retrograde urethrogram with partial tear of membranous urethra. (From Harwood-Nuss A, Wolfson AB, eds. The Clinical Practice of Emergency Medicine, 3rd ed. Philadelphia: Lippincott Williams & Wilkins, 2001.)

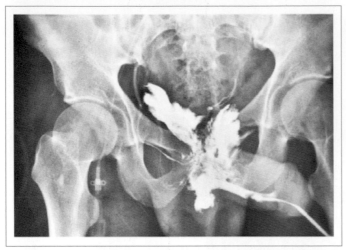

FIGURE 74.4: Type III urethral injury. Retrograde urethrogram reveals extravasaition of contrast material from the posterior urethra extending above and below the level of the urogenital diaphragm. (From Mirvis SE, Dunham CM 1992 Abdominal-pelvic trauma. In: Mirvis SE, Young JWR Eds. Imaging in trauma and critical care. Lippincott Williams & Wilkins. P 230).

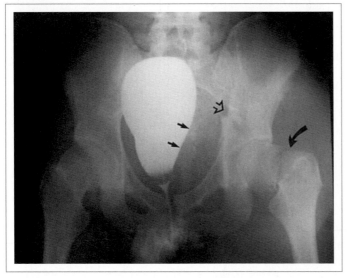

FIGURE 74.5: Pelvic fractures. Frontal radiograph shows fractures involving the left acetabulum (*open arrow*) and left femoral neck (*curved arrow*). A large pelvic hematoma compresses and displaces the contrast-filled bladder to the right (*small arrows*). There is extravasated contrast just below the pubic symphysis as a result of a urethral injury. The floor of the bladder is elevated as another manifestation of this injury. (From Daffner RH. Clinical Radiology: The Essentials, 3rd ed. Philadelphia: Lippincott Williams & Wilkins, 2007.)

Pelvic CT Scan

- CT scan may identify signs of urethral injury such as prostatic apex elevation or extravasation of contrast above or below the urogenital diaphragm

 TABLE 74.4: Pelvis CT scan: urethral injury

IV contrast	Yes, as part of trauma protocol
PO contrast	Yes/No, only if needed as part of trauma protocol
Amount of radiation	6 mSv

Classic Image

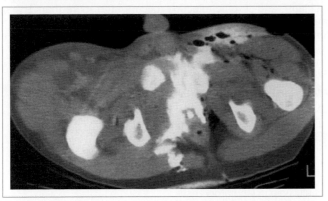

FIGURE 74.6: Posterior urethral disruption and pelvic fracture. CT scan of pelvis shows extravasation of contrast from posterior urethra into the surrounding tissues. (From Fleisher GR, Ludwig S, and Henretig FM. Textbook of Pediatric Emergency Medicine, 5th ed. Philadelphia: Lippincott Williams & Wilkins, 2005.)

Basic Management

- Partial tears may be treated with one careful attempt at catheterization with a 12- or 14-French Foley catheter
- Complete disruption necessitates urology consultation for primary or delayed surgical repair and placement of a suprapubic catheter for urinary drainage
- Experimental studies suggest bedside retrograde urethrocystoscopy may identify urethral injury while aiding in simultaneous catheter placement

Summary

TABLE 74.5: Advantages and disadvantages of imaging modalities in urethral injury

Imaging modalities	Advantages	Disadvantages
Retrograde urethrogram	Low cost Less time-consuming Less radiation	Requires technical experience to inject contrast
CT scan	Often performed in setting of pelvic fracture/other trauma Relatively good specificity	IV contrast Radiation exposure Poor sensitivity

75

Renal Transplant Imaging
Megan Fix

Background

Renal transplantation has become the preferred treatment for end-stage renal disease and there are currently more than 200,000 living renal transplant recipients. Renal transplants account for the majority of solid organ transplants in the United States, with more than 14,000 per year. The majority of these transplants are from cadaveric donors (60%) and the rest from living donors, either related or unrelated. Recipients of cadaveric kidneys typically experience higher rejection rates. The graft survival rate from living donors is 95% at 1 year and 76% at 5 years; while the graft survival rate from cadaveric donors is 89% at 1 year and 61% at 5 years. The major complications of kidney transplantation include infection, graft failure, hypertension, hyperlipidemia, cardiovascular disease, diabetes mellitus, osteoporosis, and malignant neoplasm. Rejection can be divided into hyperacute rejection (occurs in the operating room), acute rejection (occurs within the first 6 months after transplant), and chronic rejection (occurs after more than 1 year of transplantation). Other complications that can lead to graft failure include renal artery or vein stenosis, thrombosis, or obstruction.

TABLE 75.1: Classic history and physical

Hypertension
Decreased urine output
Fever
Bruit over graft site
Pain over graft site

TABLE 75.2: Potentially helpful laboratory tests

Urinalysis: red blood cells are a marker of glomerulonephritis and white blood cells are a marker of infection or obstruction
Creatinine: the best marker of renal dysfunction   In a renal transplant patient, acute renal failure is defined as a 20% rise (as opposed to a 50% rise in the general population)
Cultures: blood and urine if febrile
Immunosuppressive drug levels: cyclosporine levels >300 ng/mL are associated with nephrotoxicity

Renal Ultrasound

- The transplanted kidney is usually in the pelvis and more often on the patient's right
- Ultrasound is the preferred method to identify obstruction (hydronephrosis) and peritransplant fluid collections
- Color Doppler of the renal artery and vein are necessary to evaluate stenosis or thrombosis, as grayscale 2D images cannot
- Acute rejection will manifest as an increase in renal volume from edema
- Chronic rejection will manifest as:
  - small atrophic appearance of the kidney with a thin cortex
  - diminished number of intrarenal vessels
  - mild hydronephrosis
- Obstruction can be seen in the form of:
  - ureteral obstruction
  - urine extravasation
  - fluid collection (hematoma, urinoma, abscess, and lymphocele)

TABLE 75.3: Helpful associated structures

Variable site of transplanted kidney: incision and palpable mass can guide probe placement

Classic Images

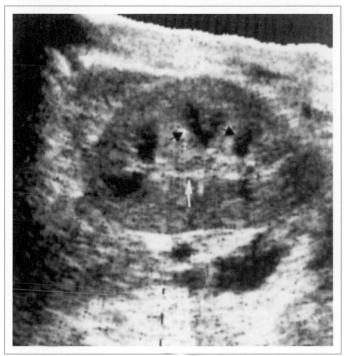

FIGURE 75.1: Renal transplant rejection. Sagittal supine sonogram shows enlargement of the renal transplant with increased sonolucency of the medullary pyramids (*black arrows*) and thinning of the central echogenic hilar structures (*white arrow*). (From Eisenberg RL. An Atlas of Differential Diagnosis, 4th ed. Philadelphia: Lippincott Williams & Wilkins, 2003.)

Renal Ultrasound with Color and Spectral Doppler
- Color Doppler can visualize long segments of vessels, but cannot quantify flow disturbances.
- Duplex Doppler can identify flow disturbances using waveforms. Important values are the peak flow rates and the resistive index. These are calculated by the radiologist. The peak flow rate in systole and diastole are important in the diagnosis of renal artery stenosis. The resistive index is a marker of resistance to renal blood flow and is elevated in transplant rejection. It is calculated by subtracting the peak diastolic velocity from the peak systolic velocity, then dividing it by the latter. Normal resistive index is <0.7, indicating lower resistance to flow.
- Markers of acute rejection include:
  - increase in the resistive index >0.8 (a resistive index of >0.9 has a 100% positive predictive value for rejection).
  - reversal of diastolic flow
- Drug nephrotoxicity usually does not show a change in the resistive index.
- Renal artery stenosis demonstrates an increased peak systolic velocity and dampened signals distal to the stenosis. Peak systolic velocity of 190–250 cm/second has a sensitivity of 90–100% for renal artery stenosis with greater than 50% luminal narrowing.
- Renal artery thrombosis will manifest as an absence of intrarenal arterial and venous flow, cortical thickening, and areas of infarction.
- Pseudoaneurysm will manifest as an extra- or intrarenal area of disorganized flow.
- Arteriovenous fistula will manifest as high-velocity, low-resistance flow in the feeding artery with a pulsatile "arterialized" waveform in the draining vein.
- Renal vein thrombosis will manifest as an enlarged hypoechoic transplant with diminished cortical perfusion and absent venous flow.

Classic Image

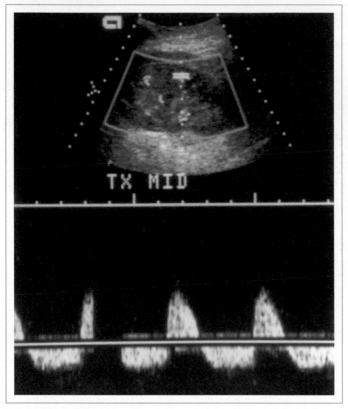

FIGURE 75.2: Duplex Doppler ultrasound obtained from an interlobar vessel of the midportion of the renal allograft demonstrates reversed end diastolic arterial flow. No flow is identified in the renal vein. (From Provenzale JM and Nelson RC. Duke Radiology Case Review: Imaging, Differential Diagnosis, and Discussion. Philadelphia: Lippincott Williams & Wilkins, 1998.)

Abdominal CT Scan
- CT scan of the abdomen is not the gold standard or first-line imaging modality for suspected renal transplant rejection; however, it can be utilized if ultrasound is not available to diagnose fluid collections or obstruction
- Contrast-enhanced CT scanning can give limited information on the vascular flow of the renal transplant
- CT is generally not used in transplant patients with elevated creatinine because of concern for IV contrast further compromising renal function

 TABLE 75.4: Abdomen CT scan: renal transplant

IV contrast	Yes, can evaluate vasculature and parenchyma
PO contrast	No, bowel is not area of interest
Amount of radiation	8 mSv

Classic Image

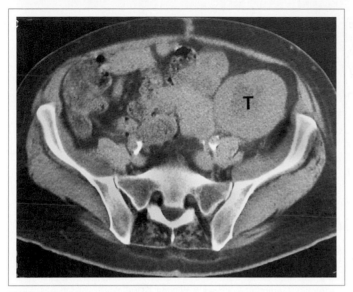

FIGURE 75.3: Polycystic kidney disease with renal failure. CT image through the pelvis shows a transplanted kidney (T). (From Daffner RH. Clinical Radiology: The Essentials, 3rd ed. Philadelphia: Lippincott Williams & Wilkins, 2007.)

Renal Scintlgraphy

- Renal scintigraphy is a nuclear imaging test that assesses vascular perfusion, parenchymal extraction, and excretion
- Process of obtaining scan requires a technician and the injection of radionuclide particles
- Scintigraphy can be interpreted as:
  - normal uptake
  - impaired uptake (consistent with obstruction or hyperacute rejection)
  - decreased uptake (consistent with chronic rejection)
- Scintigraphy has limited utility because an abnormal uptake can be seen with renal artery stenosis, graft rejection, or cyclosporine toxicity, and these cannot be distinguished using this method

 TABLE 75.5: Renal scintigraphy: renal transplant

IV contrast	No, but roquires radionuclide particle IV injection
PO contrast	No, bowel is not area of interest
Amount of radiation	2.6 mSv

Classic Images

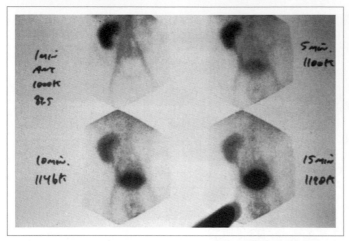

FIGURE 75.4: Renal scintigraphy of a transplanted kidney. The images demonstrate normal flow of radiotracer to the renal transplant and clearance into the bladder in the subsequent 15 minutes. A failing transplant would demonstrate a photopenic region (no uptake) in the area of the transplanted kidney. (From Schrier RW. Diseases of the Kidney and Urinary Tract, 8th ed. Philadelphia: Lippincott Williams & Wilkins, 2006.)

Abdominal Angiography

- Gold standard for the diagnosis of renal artery stenosis and arteriovenous fistulas
- It also allows for potential treatment of the above
- Angiography is rarely performed because it is invasive, uses nephrotoxic contrast agents, and cannot be used in those with contrast allergy
- Complications include hemorrhage and AV fistula

 TABLE 75.6: Angiography: renal transplant

IV contrast	Yes, to evaluate perfusion of parenchyma
PO contrast	No, bowel is not area of interest
Amount of radiation	12 mSv

Classic Images

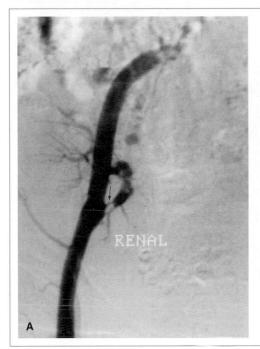
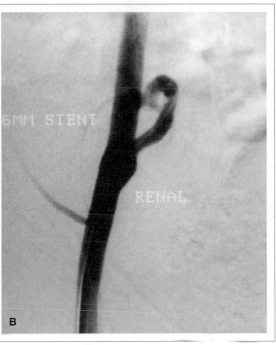

FIGURE 75.5: Renal artery stenosis in a transplanted kidney. **A:** Digital subtraction angiogram shows stenosis of the transplanted renal artery (*arrow*). **B:** After placement of a stent, the lumen of the transplanted artery is restored. (From Daffner RH. Clinical Radiology: The Essentials, 3rd ed. Philadelphia: Lippincott Williams & Wilkins, 2007.)

Management

- Fluid replacement if the patient is hypovolemic
- Consultation with transplant physician
- Surgical consultation if a vascular complication is present
- An ultrasound-guided biopsy may be obtained to evaluate degree of rejection
- Antibiotics if UTI or other infection is present
- Hospital admission is recommended for signs of infection, acute renal failure (defined as serum creatinine rise of 20% from baseline), rejection, perinephric fluid collection, obstruction, or immunosuppressive toxicity

Summary

TABLE 75.7: Advantages and disadvantages of imaging modalities in renal transplant rejection

Imaging modality	Advantages	Disadvantages
Ultrasound with color/ spectral Doppler	Minimal patient discomfort No radiation Screens for most major complications	Availability of official ultrasound Difficult to distinguish between causes of parenchymal failure
CT scan	Availability Other diagnoses possible	IV contrast: nephrotoxic Radiation exposure
Renal scintigraphy	None	Time-consuming Availability Cannot distinguish between rejection, cyclosporine toxicity, and renal artery stenosis
Angiography	Gold standard for diagnosing renal artery stenosis and other vascular complications Therapeutic for some vascular complications	Availability IV contrast: nephrotoxic Invasive

Section Editor: Gregory Press

76

Normal Pregnancy

Christopher Freeman

Background

There were approximately 4.2 million live births in the United States in the year 2008. While most women deliver without complications, emergency departments (EDs) see about 500,000 annual visits for bleeding in the first trimester of pregnancy. Identification of a normal intrauterine pregnancy (IUP) is the primary decision point in the ED management of these patients. In patients without reproductive assistance, the presence of an IUP effectively rules out ectopic pregnancy given the very low rates of heterotopic pregnancy. ED physicians can rapidly diagnose an IUP allowing for prompt, appropriate management of complaints in the first trimester of pregnancy.

TABLE 76.1: Classic history and physical

Absent menses
Irregular menses or vaginal spotting
Nausea or vomiting
Breast tenderness
Generalized malaise

TABLE 76.2: Potentially helpful laboratory tests

Urine β-human chorionic gonadotrophin (β hCG)	Can detect pregnancy at levels of 20–25 mIU/ml or 99% sensitive at first missed menses May have false negative with dilute urine in early pregnancy
Quantitative serum β-hCG	Dependent on assay but capable of detecting β-hCG at levels of 5 mIU/mL Expected to double every 48 hr in the first 7–10 wk
Complete blood count (CBC)	Assess for blood loss
Blood type	Assess Rh status and potential need for Rhogam when bleeding

Pelvic Ultrasound

- Ultrasound is the modality of choice for evaluating pregnancy.
- At some institutions, ultrasound evaluation for IUP is performed in the ED at the bedside, while at others, all ultrasounds are performed in the department of radiology. Practitioners should follow the guidelines in place at their institution.
- Imaging of the pelvis in pregnancy can be obtained by both a transvaginal and transabdominal approach.

- Transvaginal ultrasound (TVUS) allows for earlier diagnosis of IUP but can be limited in evaluation of structures outside of the pelvis, such as free fluid in the right upper quadrant or advanced pregnancy.
  - For TVUS evaluation of the pelvis, a high-frequency microconvex endocavitary probe should be used with a conducting medium applied both inside and outside a latex or vinyl sheath cover.
  - An empty bladder is optimal for TVUS scanning, as it is more comfortable for the patient, and a full bladder distorts the anatomy making it more difficult to visualize the structures of interest.
  - For TVUS, the patient should be placed in the lithotomy position as for a pelvic examination.
  - For TVUS, the uterus should be scanned through in sagittal (probe indicator pointed anteriorly toward the pubic bone) and coronal (probe indicator pointed to the patient's right) planes, and evaluation of both adnexae should be performed. An anteverted uterus will lie just posterior to the bladder.
- Transabdominal ultrasound (TAUS) is less invasive and allows for a larger field of view for structures inside and outside the pelvis. However, it is also less sensitive for the identification of early IUP.
  - For TAUS evaluation of the pelvis, a low-frequency curved array transducer should be placed just superior to the pubic bone.
  - A full bladder is optimal for TAUS and can be used as an acoustic window to identify the uterus.
  - The uterus should be scanned through in sagittal (probe indicator pointed cephalad) and transverse (probe indicator pointed to the patient's right) planes, and both ovaries evaluated. Nonpathologic adnexa will be difficult to visualize during a TAUS.
- To visualize a normal pregnancy, the uterus, a thick-walled pear-shaped structure of medium echogenicity, should be identified adjacent to the bladder.
- The entire uterus should be scanned through to identify structures inside the uterus.
- A complete evaluation of the pregnant patient includes assessing both adnexa and the periuterine pouches for free fluid.
- The ovaries are best visualized with TVUS. The ovaries are typically located lateral to the fundus of the uterus and anteromedial to the iliac vessels.
- The ovaries appear as ovoid heterogeneous structures with multiple cystic (anechoic) areas. It may be difficult to visualize the fallopian tubes in the area between the ovaries and uterus in a normal patient. A corpus luteal cyst, the remnant of the ovulated follicle, is visualized as an anechoic dominant cyst. If there is bleeding into the cyst, it can appear as a complex or echogenic material.
- Fluid may also be visualized in the area of the adnexa. A small amount of simple fluid can be normal. A large amount of fluid or fluid that appears complex is abnormal. Heterogeneous or echogenic fluid may represent blood or pus.
- In a normal IUP, gestational age is the most helpful predictor of what structures can be seen by ultrasound. However, gestational age by last menstruation may be inaccurate.
- The β-hCG level at which early pregnancy may be first visualized is termed the "discriminatory zone." The discriminatory zone for TVUS is 1000–2000 mIU/mL, and for TAUS it is approximately 6500 mIU/mL.
- The gestational sac is the first structure visualized in pregnancy. In normal pregnancy, it appears as a small anechoic pocket surrounded by an echogenic rim centrally located in the uterus. The pseudogestational sac of ectopic pregnancy is a simple fluid collection within the uterus and can mimic a gestational sac.
- The double decidual sign consists of two concentric echogenic rings around the central anechoic sac. Its value in excluding ectopic pregnancy is limited because of the subjective nature of this finding on ultrasound and its variable sensitivity (60–99%) in confirming IUP. For this reason, this finding should not be used in the ED setting to rule out ectopic pregnancy.
- The yolk sac, a thin circular hyperechoic structure, is the first definitive sign of an IUP. The yolk sac appears as a bright white ring located within the anechoic gestational sac. It is first visualized at about 5 weeks gestation.
- The next structure visualized in normal pregnancy is a fetal pole adjacent to the yolk sac. The fetal pole appears as a small echogenic mass of tissue, often described as peanut-shaped.
- At approximately 6 weeks from the last menstrual period, cardiac activity may be visualized by TVUS. Early cardiac activity appears as flickering within the torso of the fetus.

TABLE 76.3: Expected ultrasound findings based on gestational age and β-hCG level

Approximate gestational age	Serum β-hCG	Transvaginal ultrasound	Transabdominal ultrasound
4–5 wk	500–1000	Gestational sac	+/− Gestational sac
5 wk	1000–7000	Yolk sac +/− fetal pole	Gestational sac +/− yolk sac
6 wk	5000–20,000	Fetal pole with cardiac activity	Yolk sac +/− fetal pole

- Cardiac activity in early pregnancy is best measured by M-mode as it transmits less output to the fetus than Doppler measurements of fetal heart rate.
- A normal heart rate for an embryo less than 5 mm (or 6.2 weeks) should be greater than 100 beats per minute (bpm) and greater than 120 bpm for an embryo greater than 5 mm. Slow fetal heart rates correspond with a higher incidence of intrauterine demise.
- Estimation of fetal age is most accurate in the first trimester and is determined by mean gestational sac diameter, crown rump length, or biparietal diameter later in the first trimester.
- Crown rump length is measured as the maximal length of the embryo excluding yolk sac and limb buds.
- Biparietal diameter is the transverse diameter of the skull at the level of the thalamus measured from leading edge of the skull to leading edge of the skull.

TABLE 76.4: Helpful associated structures

Iliac vessels: The adnexae lies just medial and anterior of these vessels.
Bladder: The uterus lies just posterior to the bladder in TAUS transverse view and TVUS coronal view. It appears on the right when looking at the screen in TAUS sagittal view but on the left when looking at the screen in TVUS sagittal view. It should be emptied prior to a TVUS examination to avoid the full bladder displacing the uterus posteriorly.
Posterior cul-de-sac: Fluid may accumulate here in pathologic states; however, a small amount may be physiologic.

TAUS, transabdominal ultrasound; TVUS, transvaginal ultrasound.

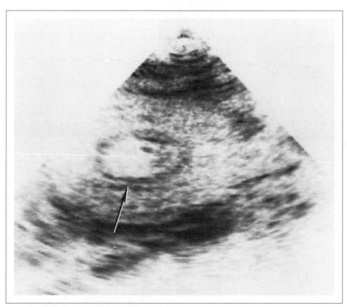

FIGURE 76.1: Double decidual sign. Transverse sonogram shows a second line (*arrow*) parallel to a portion of the decidual sac. (From Eisenberg RL. An Atlas of Differential Diagnosis, 4th ed. Philadelphia: Lippincott Williams & Wilkins, 2003.)

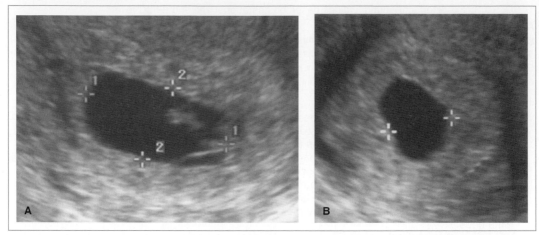

FIGURE 76.2: Measurement of the mean sac diameter (MSD). The distances measured by the calipers in the longitudinal axis (**A,** number one) and the depth (**A,** number two) and the transverse diameter measured in (**B**) are added together and divided by three to produce the MSD. Some use only the sum of the longitudinal and depth measurements divided by two. (From Gibbs RS, Karlan BY, Haney AF, et al. Danforth's Obstetrics and Gynecology, 10th ed. Philadelphia: Lippincott Williams & Wilkins, 2008.)

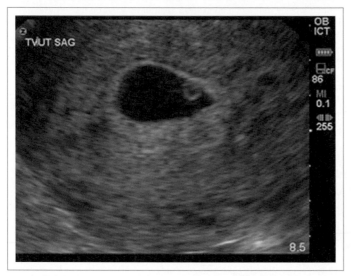

FIGURE 76.3: A yolk sac (*arrows*) is visualized inside the intrauterine gestation sac (*arrowheads*) confirming an intrauterine pregnancy. (*Courtesy of Turandot Saul, MD. St. Luke's Roosevelt Hospital Center, New York, NY.*)

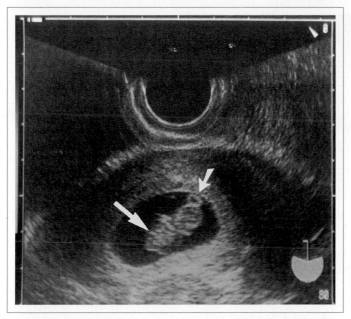

FIGURE 76.4: Intrauterine pregnancy with yolk sac and fetal pole. This is a transvaginal view of an intrauterine gestational sac with fetal pole (*large arrow*) and yolk sac (*small arrow*). (From Harwood-Nuss A, Wolfson AB, ct al. The Clinical Practice of Emergency Medicine, 3rd ed. Philadelphia: Lippincott Williams & Wilkins, 2001.)

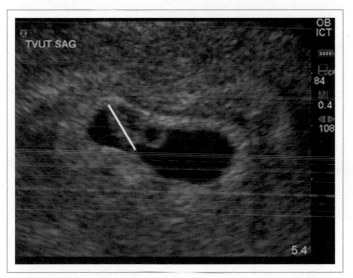

FIGURE 76.5: Measurement of crown rump length. Crown rump length (calipers) is measured in a 7-week pregnancy. The yolk sac (*arrow*) should not be included in the measurement. Transvaginal ultrasound of the uterus in the sagittal plane (TVUT SAG). (*Courtesy of Turandot Saul, MD. St. Luke's Roosevelt Hospital Center, New York, NY.*)

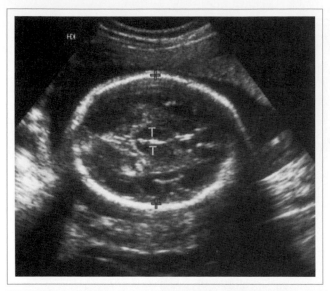

FIGURE 76.6: Fetal biparietal diameter (BPD). Axial scan of the head at the standardized level for BPD measurement shows the thalami. (From MacDonald MG, Seshia MMK, et al. Avery's Neonatology Pathophysiology & Management of the Newborn, 6th ed. Philadelphia: Lippincott Williams & Wilkins, 2005.)

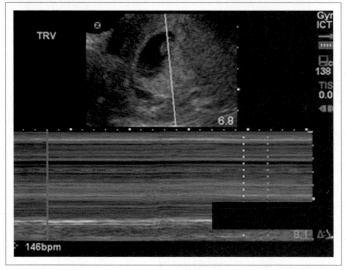

FIGURE 76.7: Measurement of the fetal heart rate by M-mode. The M-mode vertical marker is placed over the visualized fetal heart, and the heart rate is measured over the distance of one cardiac cycle. Transvaginal ultrasound of the uterus in the transverse plane (TRV). (*Courtesy of Turandot Saul, MD. St. Luke's Roosevelt Hospital Center, New York, NY.*)

MRI

- There is currently no indication for MRI in the evaluation of the fetus in the first trimester of pregnancy.
- While there is still concern about the safety of MRI, especially in the first trimester, it may be a safer method of evaluation of other maternal structures in the abdomen and pelvis, such as the appendix, than CT imaging.
- MRI may have utility in later pregnancy in assessment of fetal central nervous system and thoracic abnormalities.
- Ultrasound is the imaging modality of choice in pregnancy, for both mother and fetus, for all structures that can be accurately evaluated via ultrasound.

TABLE 76.5: MRI: pregnancy

IV contrast	Yes/No, depending on primary indication for study
PO contrast	Yes/No, depending on primary indication for study
Amount of radiation	None

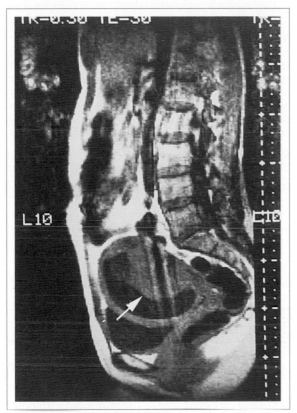

FIGURE 76.8: MRI was performed in the 14th week of pregnancy due to neurologic compromise from a disk herniation. T1-weighted MRI, sagittal lumbar spine. Observe the fetus in utero (*arrow*). (*Courtesy of Marsha I. Carry, MS, DC, Manhattan Beach, CA.*) From Yochum TR and Rowe LJ. Yochum and Rowe's Essentials of Skeletal Radiology, 3rd ed. Philadelphia: Lippincott Williams & Wilkins, 2004.

Basic Management
- Prenatal vitamins
- Complete ultrasound in department of radiology if bedside ultrasound performed
- Rhogam if vaginal spotting
- Obstetric follow-up

Summary

TABLE 76.6: Advantages and disadvantages of imaging modalities in pregnancy

Imaging modality	Advantages	Disadvantages
Ultrasound	Low cost Bedside availability No ionizing radiation Safe for the fetus	Body habitus limitations Operator-dependent
MRI	Safer than CT in the evaluation of other abdominal pathology Can be used to evaluate the fetus in later stages of pregnancy	Safety concerns

77 Ectopic Pregnancy

Turandot Saul

Background

The incidence of ectopic pregnancy in women presenting to the emergency department with vaginal bleeding or pain in the first trimester has been estimated at approximately 10%, and it remains the leading cause of maternal death in the first trimester. The increasing incidence of ectopic pregnancy is due to a number of factors including treatments for infertility, pelvic inflammatory disease, tubal surgery, and the use of intrauterine devices. An ectopic pregnancy can be located in the fallopian tube, the ovary, the cervix, or the peritoneum. The emergency physician evaluating a patient who is pregnant with complaints concerning for an ectopic pregnancy should consider related diagnoses such as a cornual ectopic or a heterotopic pregnancy.

TABLE 77.1: Classic history and physical

Amenorrhea
Positive pregnancy test
Vaginal bleeding
Hypotension or tachycardia
Abdominal pain or tenderness
Adnexal mass or tenderness

TABLE 77.2: Potentially helpful laboratory tests

Quantitative serum β-hCG	Can be abnormally low for pregnancy dates May rise slower or plateau as compared to a normal pregnancy Can be followed every 2 d for doubling as a marker for normal development High levels of β-hCG may be seen in molar pregnancies and multiple gestations
Complete blood count (CBC)	May be used to assess degree of bleeding or anemia
Blood type	Bleeding pregnant patients who are Rh (−) will require Rho-GAM

TABLE 77.3: Expected ultrasound findings based on gestational age and β-hCG level

Approximate gestational age	Serum β-hCG (mIU/ml)	Transvaginal ultrasound	Transabdominal ultrasound
4–5 wks	500–1000	Gestational sac	+/− Gestational sac
5 wks	1000–7000	Yolk sac +/− fetal pole	Gestational sac +/− yolk sac
6 wks	5000–20,000	Fetal pole with cardiac activity	Yolk sac +/− fetal pole

Bedside Pelvic Ultrasound

- In the emergency department, bedside ultrasound can be used to identify the presence of an intrauterine pregnancy. At many institutions, however, this evaluation takes place in the department of radiology or by the gynecologic consultant. Practitioners should follow the guidelines in place at their institution.
- Transabdominal ultrasound using a low-frequency probe should be performed first to examine the pelvic structures and also Morison's pouch (hepatorenal interface) for free fluid. If present, significant hemorrhage is likely present.
- A high-frequency endocavitary probe should then be used to evaluate early pregnancy. The patient should be given the opportunity to void. A full bladder during the examination will posteriorly displace the uterus and can be uncomfortable for the patient.
- Always visualize the uterus in two planes (e.g., sagittal and coronal) in order to see the entire extent of the structure. The bladder should appear on the left side when looking at the screen in sagittal scanning.
- Adjust the depth of the image to evaluate the posterior cul-de sac for free fluid. A small amount of fluid may be normal.

- If an intrauterine gestation (yolk sac, fetal pole, fetal pole with cardiac activity) is not visualized, a high index of suspicion must be maintained for ectopic pregnancy.
- Measure the endomyometrial mantle (edge of the gestational sac to outer edge of the uterine myometrium) at the thinnest area; if <7 mm, be concerned for a cornual (in a bicornuate uterus) or interstitial ectopic pregnancy.
- Perform careful evaluation of the adnexa by scanning up toward the uterine fundus, then move the probe in a plane parallel to this level toward the lateral fornix on each side. Following the cornual region laterally will bring the fallopian tube and ovary into view.
- Ninety-five percent of ectopic pregnancies occur in the fallopian tube and ultrasound evaluation may reveal an adnexal mass external to the uterus with a yolk sac or fetus.
- Independent movement of the mass and ovary when gently probed with the ultrasound transducer is highly suggestive of ectopic pregnancy and can differentiate it from an ovarian cyst.
- Heterotopic pregnancies have increased in frequency up to 1 in 100 in patients undergoing assisted reproductive techniques. In these high-risk patients, careful evaluation of the adnexa should take place despite the presence of an intrauterine pregnancy and obstetric/gynecologic consultation is advised in all cases.
- Vascular flow around an ectopic pregnancy is related to the amount to trophoblastic tissue present. This classically presents as a "ring of fire" on color Doppler ultrasound.

TABLE 77.4: Helpful associated structures

Iliac vessels: The adnexa lies just medial and anterior to these vessels
Uterus in the coronal plan

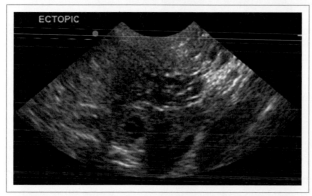

FIGURE 77.1: Ectopic pregnancy in the posterior cul-de-sac with formed yolk sac. A portion of the empty uterus can be seen on the left. (*Courtesy of Turandot Saul, MD. St. Luke's Roosevelt Hospital Center, New York, NY.*)

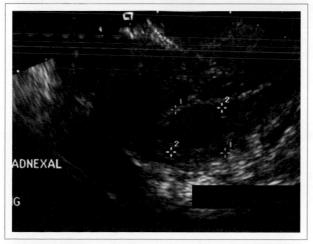

FIGURE 77.2: Ectopic pregnancy in the area of the right adnexa. (*Courtesy of Turandot Saul, MD. St. Luke's Roosevelt Hospital Center, New York, NY.*)

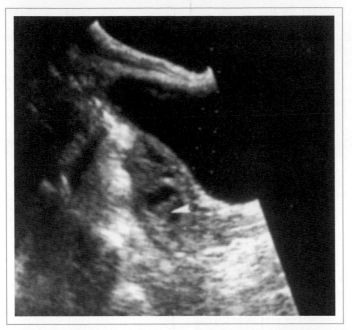

FIGURE 77.3: Ectopic pregnancy. Sagittal sonogram of the left adnexa identifies the gestational sac and the fetal pole (arrowhead). (From Eisenberg RL. An Atlas of Differential Diagnosis, 4th ed. Philadelphia: Lippincott Williams & Wilkins, 2003.)

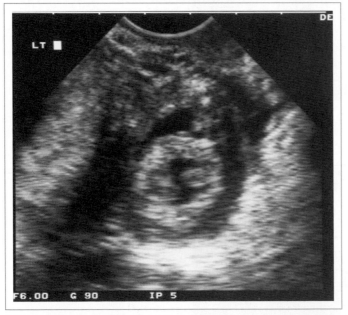

FIGURE 77.4: Ectopic pregnancy. Unruptured ectopic pregnancy appearing as a "tubal ring" in the left adnexa. (From Gibbs RS, Karlan BY, Haney AF, et al. Danforth's Obstetrics and Gynecology, 10th ed. Philadelphia: Lippincott Williams & Wilkins, 2008.)

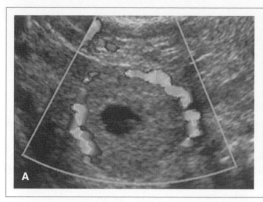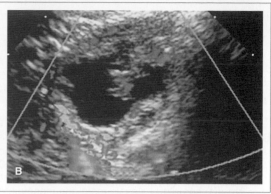

FIGURE 77.5: Rings of fire. A corpus luteum (**A**) can be confused with an ectopic pregnancy (**B**). (From Gibbs RS, Karlan BY, Haney AF, et al. Danforth's Obstetrics and Gynecology, 10th ed. Philadelphia: Lippincott Williams & Wilkins, 2008.)

Basic Management

- Emergent obstetric/gynecologic consultation if there is a positive beta-hCG and no visualized intrauterine pregnancy, a visualized or suspected ectopic pregnancy, a thin endomyometrial mantle or risk factors for heterotopic pregnancy
- Pain control
- Volume replacement if rupture present/hypotension
- Type and screen for RhoGAM administration if necessary
- Preoperative workup
- Methotrexate may be used at the discretion of the gynecologic consult
- In patients who do not meet criteria for methotrexate, laparoscopy with salpingostomy, or in some cases salpingectomy, is necessary.

Summary

TABLE 77.5: Advantages and disadvantages of ultrasound for ectopic pregnancy

Advantages	Disadvantages
Low cost	Operator dependent
No ionizing radiation	Body habitus limitations
Bedside availability	
Serial examinations easily done	
No risk to fetus	

Background

Hydatidiform mole, commonly referred to as molar pregnancy, is a type of gestational trophoblastic disease that affects approximately 1 in 1,000 pregnancies in the United States. On the basis of genetic karyotype, morphology, and histopathology, molar pregnancy is divided into two main groups: complete/classic mole and incomplete/partial mole.

Complete moles occur when an ovum devoid of genetic material is fertilized either by two unique sperms or by a single sperm that subsequently duplicates its genetic material such that the resulting entity contains a diploid karyotype with genetic material exclusively of paternal origin. Histologically, the aberrant changes in the placenta of a complete mole consist of generalized edema of chorionic villi and diffuse trophoblastic hyperplasia. Grossly, these changes give the villi a cluster-like vesicular appearance similar to a "bunch of grapes." Of note, fetal tissue is absent. Rarely, however, a complete mole may coexist with a normal pregnancy in which a healthy fetus and placenta are identified separate from the molar pregnancy.

Incomplete or partial moles are the result of dispermic fertilization of a single ovum resulting in a triploid karyotype, with two sets of chromosomes of paternal origin while one set is maternally derived. Histologically, partial moles have focal swelling of chorionic villi and only mild trophoblastic hyperplasia. Although fetal tissue is present, the fetus is generally growth-retarded and nonviable.

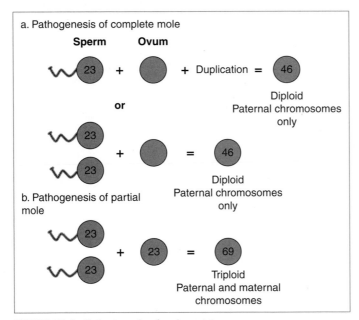

FIGURE 78.1: Pathogenesis of molar pregnancy

As a result of the greater extent of trophoblastic proliferation in complete versus incomplete moles, the former secrete comparatively higher levels of beta human chorionic gonadotropin (β-hCG) and may result in uterine size that is out of proportion to gestational age as well as the formation of large theca lutein cysts. The first clinical clue is usually the presence of vaginal bleeding and β-hCG hormone levels exceeding those expected during a normal pregnancy of similar gestational age.

TABLE 78.1: Classic history and physical

Extremes of reproductive age or history of molar pregnancy
Higher incidence rates have been noted in Asian populations
Uterine size large (complete mole) for gestational age
Uterine size normal (partial mole) for gestational age
Vaginal bleeding
Hyperemesis gravidarum
Pre-eclampsia
Pain from ruptured or torsion of enlarged theca lutein cysts
Hyperthyroidism
Symptoms of invasive disease 15–20% (complete mole), 0.5–2.0% (partial mole) (pulmonary, central nervous system)

TABLE 78.2: Potentially helpful laboratory tests

β-hCG	Markedly elevated (complete mole) or elevated (partial mole) compared with gestational age
p57Kip2 immunostain	Negative (complete mole), p57Kip2 immunostain positive (partial mole)
TSH	Depressed

Pelvic Ultrasound

- Radiological investigations of choice
- Appearance varies greatly depending on the timing of imaging and on its classification of complete versus partial mole
- During the first trimester, complete moles have relatively small villi resulting in an overall homogenous echogenic endometrial mass within a normal or enlarged uterus
- As the pregnancy progresses and the placenta enlarges, villi become grossly swollen and appear as multiple small anechoic areas, 3–10 mm in diameter, giving a "snow storm" appearance
- No fetal tissue is identified on ultrasound of a complete hydatidiform mole
- Rarely a living fetus is associated with a complete molar pregnancy
- The presence of a thickened placenta with cystic degeneration and a coexisting fetus raises the suspicion of a partial mole
- An accurate assessment of uterine volume should be obtained on ultrasound (uterine size may correlate with extrauterine tumor burden)
- Intraoperative ultrasound during suction curettage is sometimes employed to confirm adequate uterine evacuation
- Theca lutein ovarian cysts, resulting from overstimulation of lutein cells by excessively high levels of β-hCG during complete molar pregnancy appear multiseptated bilaterally

Role of Doppler

- Doppler evaluation of the uterine arteries further confirms and assesses for invasive disease
- During the first trimester of a normal pregnancy, Doppler of the intrauterine arterial system shows high impedance waveforms with low diastolic velocities; as pregnancy progresses, physiologic arterial invasion by trophoblastic tissue occurs which reduces the vascular impedance such that by the third trimester, high-velocity low-impedance flow patterns are expected
- Abnormal trophoblastic proliferation accelerates uterine arterial invasion such that Doppler studies may reveal high-velocity, low-impedance flow as early as the first trimester (typically seen in the third trimester)
- Once trophoblastic tissue invades maternal circulation, it can be carried to extrauterine locations including the lung, liver, and brain

Classic Images

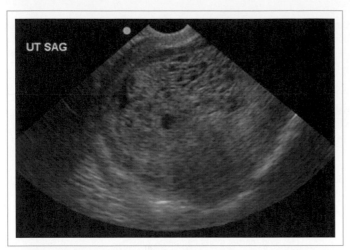

FIGURE 78.2: "Snowstorm" appearance of complete mole on ultrasound examination. (*Courtesy of Turandot Saul, St. Luke's Roosevelt Emergency Ultrasound Division, New York.*)

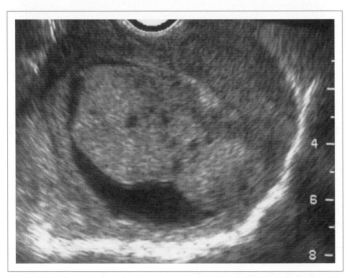

FIGURE 78.3: Partial mole. The placenta appears cystic and enlarged for gestation. No fetal heartbeat was noted and, although fetal tissue was found at pathology, no chromosome studies were obtained. (From Gibbs RS, Karlan BY, Haney AF, et al. Danforth's Obstetrics and Gynecology, 10th ed. Philadelphia: Lippincott Williams & Wilkins, 2008.)

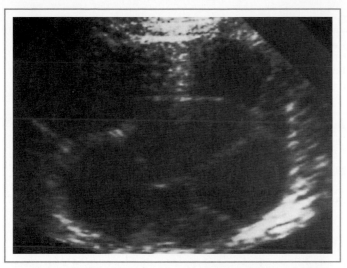

FIGURE 78.4: Theca lutein cyst. Multiseptated structure in the adnexal region. (From Eisenberg RL. An Atlas of Differential Diagnosis, 4th ed. Philadelphia: Lippincott Williams & Wilkins, 2003.)

MRI

- On T2-weighted MRI, a hydatidiform mole appears as a heterogenous mass of high signal intensity that distends the endometrial cavity; numerous cystic spaces may be present in the mass giving a classic "cluster of grapes" appearance
- Particularly helpful in the assessment of brain and spinal cord metastases

 TABLE 78.3: MRI: molar pregnancy

IV contrast	No
PO contrast	No
Amount of radiation	None

Classic Images

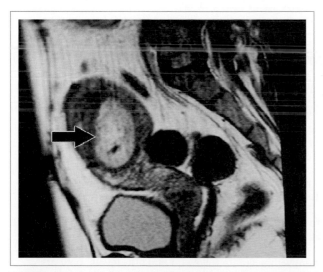

FIGURE 78.5: Gestational trophoblastic disease. Sagittal T2-weighted fast spin echo image through uterus in patient with abnormally elevated human chorionic gonadotropin level and abnormal transvaginal ultrasound. Nonspecific thickening of the endometrium is seen (*arrow*) without evidence of fetal development or gestational sac. Dilatation and curettage revealed complete molar pregnancy. (From Leyendecker JR and Brown JJ. Practical Guide to Abdominal and Pelvic MRI. Philadelphia: Lippincott Williams & Wilkins, 2004.)

Other Imaging Modalities

- CT scans of hydatidiform moles may demonstrate a normal-sized uterus with areas of low attenuation, an enlarged uterus with a central area of low attenuation, or hypoattenuating foci surrounded by highly enhanced areas in the myometrium
- Chest x-ray may demonstrate metastatic disease

Classic Images

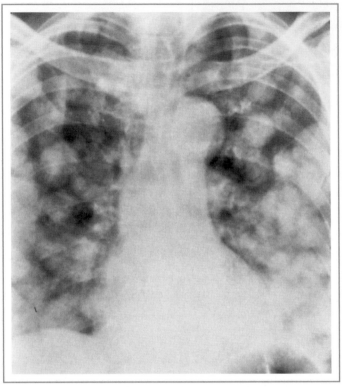

FIGURE 78.6: Cannonball metastases in a patient with gestational trophoblastic neoplasia. Fuzzy margins around the nodular opacities may represent hemorrhage given the marked vascularity of these lesions. (From Eisenberg RL. An Atlas of Differential Diagnosis, 4th ed. Philadelphia: Lippincott Williams & Wilkins, 2003.)

Basic Management

- Urine and serum hCG measurement
- Ultrasound evaluation
- Ob-gyn consultation
- Initial management of molar pregnancy involves uterine evacuation by suction curettage
- Close follow-up of the β-hCG level is required to ensure return to undetectable levels, which is evidence of complete disease resolution
- Persistent elevation of β-hCG levels is indicative of ongoing disease caused by invasion of abnormal trophoblast cells into the uterine wall; distant organ metastases can also occur, particularly to the lung
- It is believed that 15–20% of complete moles and 0.5–2.0% of partial moles lead to the development of gestational trophoblastic neoplasia, including locally invasive moles and malignant choriocarcinoma
- Because a new pregnancy would interfere with accurate follow up of β-hCG levels, patients treated for molar pregnancy are advised to use contraception during the interval of hormone level monitoring
- Women with a malignant form of gestational trophoblastic disease require further treatment with chemotherapy; with appropriate treatment and follow-up, trophoblast tumors are highly curable

- Given increased risk of recurrent hydatidiform moles, women with a prior history of gestational trophoblastic disease are advised to undergo first trimester ultrasound examination during subsequent pregnancies

Summary

TABLE 78.4: Advantages and disadvantages of imaging modalities in hydatidiform mole

Imaging modalities	Advantages	Disadvantages
Ultrasound	Low cost No ionizing radiation Safe for the fetus	Body habitus limitations Operator-dependent
MRI	Useful to identify presence and extent of invasive disease	Time-consuming More costly

79 Select Etiologies of Third Trimester Hemorrhage: Placenta Previa, Placental Abruption, and Uterine Rupture

Sara Miller

Background

Placenta previa presents with vaginal bleeding in the second and third trimesters of pregnancy and refers to the implantation of the placenta over or near the internal os of the cervix. This occurs in 5 of 1,000 deliveries and has a mortality rate of 0.03%. In complete placenta previa, the placenta completely obscures the internal os. In marginal placenta previa, implantation occurs within 2 cm of the internal os. The diagnosis should be confirmed in the third trimester, as the placenta may be further removed from the internal os since the lower uterine segment grows during this time.

Placental abruption occurs when the normally located placenta separates from the uterine wall after 20 weeks of gestation and prior to birth. Hematoma formation continues the separation, resulting in compromise of the fetal blood supply. Bleeding may be visible and draining from the cervix, most often with incomplete abruption. If the hemorrhage is concealed, the hematoma is contained within the uterus, often with complete abruption and an increased incidence of coagulopathy.

Uterine rupture occurs with complete transection of the uterine wall and overlying serosa. This occurs in both the scarred and unscarred uterus, and can precipitate preterm labor or occur during the course of labor.

TABLE 79.1: Classic history and physical

	Placenta previa	Placental abruption	Uterine rupture
Vaginal bleeding	Spotting in first and second trimester Sudden, painless, profuse, bright red in third trimester	Bleeding with abdominal pain (80%) Concealed (20%)	Small amounts to massive hemorrhage
Uterus	Soft and nontender	Firm, tender, and irritable	Sudden loss of contractions and recession of presenting part
Fetal distress	None (fetal heart tracing most often normal)	Dependent on severity of abruption	Severe
Maternal symptoms	Cramping (10%) No shock	Severe low abdominal pain and DIC	Low abdominal pain with "tearing" sensation and DIC

DIC, disseminated intravascular coagulopathy.

TABLE 79.2: Potentially helpful laboratory tests

CBC: to assess anemia
Coagulation profile, fibrinogen, and fibrin split products: preoperative testing and DIC assessment
Kleihauer-Betke test: if Rh negative, to assess degree of fetal-maternal transfusion
Type and crossmatch: preoperative testing and for Rh status

Pelvic Ultrasound
- Bedside ultrasound by emergency physicians is not the standard of care for these disease entities
- Studies should be performed by the department of radiology or the obstetrical consult
- For a transabdominal ultrasound, the patient should ideally have a full bladder
- For transvaginal ultrasound, the bladder should be empty

Placenta Previa
- The accuracy of diagnosis of placenta previa with ultrasound is 93–98%
- Placenta previa can be ruled out if the internal cervical os is visualized without overlying placental tissue
- The lowest-lying portion of the placenta should be visualized and the distance between this portion and the internal os should be measured (greater than 2 cm excludes the diagnosis)
- Uterine contraction may also contribute to a false-positive diagnosis of placenta previa, as the wall of the uterus thickens and may look like placental tissue
- A repeated ultrasound in the absence of contraction can exclude the diagnosis

Placental Abruption
- Hyperechoic or isoechoic foci posterior to the placenta may be seen in acute hemorrhage
- Hypoechoic foci are more suggestive of a formed clot, usually within a week of hemorrhage
- Ultrasound has a low sensitivity for detecting placental abruption (25–50%), and fetal monitoring should be initiated in patients with suspected abruption. More recent reports that take into account advances in ultrasound technology have found the sensitivity of ultrasound to be as high as 80%.

Uterine Rupture
- Hemoperitoneum may be seen on ultrasound
- Fetal parts may be seen adjacent to a small contracted uterus

TABLE 79.3: Helpful associated structures

Uterus scanned in two planes: sagittal and transverse
Bladder: anterior to the uterus
Posterior cul-de-sac: free fluid will likely accumulate here first when there is intraperitoneal pelvic pathology

Classic Images

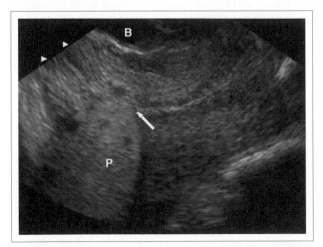

FIGURE 79.1: A transvaginal ultrasound image of a complete placenta previa. The arrow points to the internal os. P, placenta; B, bladder. (From Gibbs RS, Karlan BY, Haney AF, et al. Danforth's Obstetrics and Gynecology, 10th ed. Philadelphia: Lippincott Williams & Wilkins, 2008.)

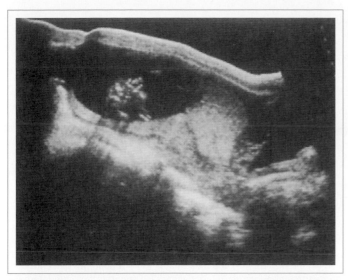

FIGURE 79.2: Posterior placenta previa shown on transabdominal ultrasound. (From Beckmann CRB, Frank W, et al. Obstetrics and Gynecology, 5th ed. Philadelphia: Lippincott Williams & Wilkins, 2006.)

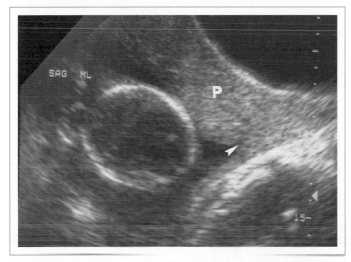

FIGURE 79.3: Partial placenta previa. Sagittal sonogram shows the placenta (P) partially covering the cervical os (*arrowhead*). (From Eisenberg RL. An Atlas of Differential Diagnosis, 4th ed. Philadelphia: Lippincott Williams & Wilkins, 2003.)

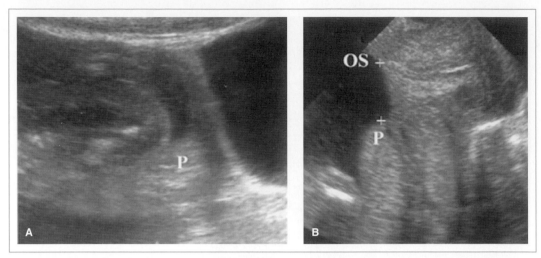

FIGURE 79.4: Low-lying posterior placenta. In (**A**) the placenta (P) could be mistaken for a posterior placenta previa. Transvaginal ultrasound (**B**) demonstrates the lower border of the placenta (P) separate from the internal os (OS) by the distance indicated between the plus signs. (From Gibbs RS, Karlan BY, Haney AF, et al. Danforth's Obstetrics and Gynecology, 10th ed. Philadelphia: Lippincott Williams & Wilkins, 2008.)

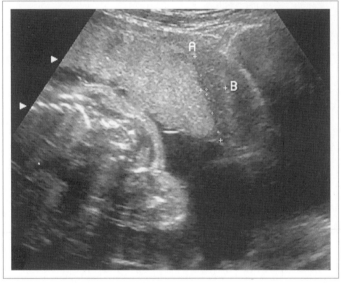

FIGURE 79.5: Transvaginal ultrasound image of a retroplacental abruption. The markers indicate the size of the clot. (From Gibbs RS, Karlan BY, Haney AF, et al. Danforth's Obstetrics and Gynecology, 10th ed. Philadelphia: Lippincott Williams & Wilkins, 2008.)

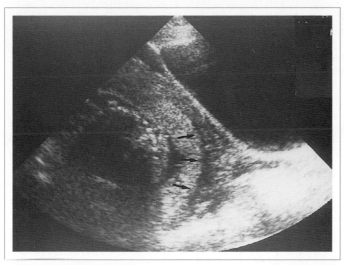

FIGURE 79.6: Abruptio placentae. Longitudinal scan shows separation of the placenta from the uterine wall (*arrows*). (From Daffner RH. Clinical Radiology: The Essentials, 3rd ed. Philadelphia: Lippincott Williams & Wilkins, 2007.)

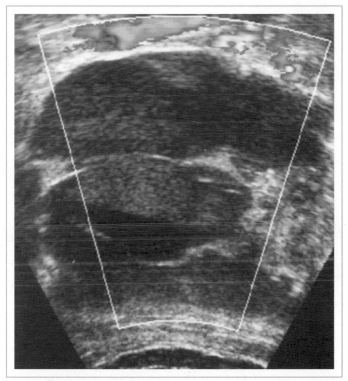

FIGURE 79.7: Uterine rupture: transverse image of pelvis shows complex hematoma. (Reprinted with permission from Kaakaji Y, Nnghiem HV, Nodell C, Winter TC. Sonography of obstetric and gynecologic emergencies. Part 1, obstetric emergencies. Am J Roentgenol. 174: 2000; 641–649. Figure 11B.)

Pelvic MRI

- Utility is limited by potential maternal hemorrhage during the time required to complete the study
- On T1-weighted images, the signal intensity of the placenta is low, whereas on T2-weighted images, the signal intensity of the placenta is high and can be clearly differentiated from surrounding structures
- There may be excessive motion artifact due to fetal movement and maternal breathing

 TABLE 79.4: Pelvic MRI: placental previa, placental abruption, and uterine rupture

IV contrast	No, not necessary to view pathology
PO contrast	No, bowel not organ of interest
Amount of radiation	None

Classic Images

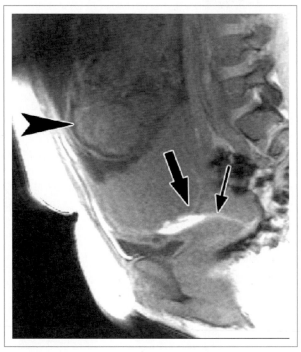

FIGURE 79.8: Central placenta previa. Sagittal T1-weighted gradient echo image shows placenta completely covering internal cervical os *(arrow)* in a patient with vaginal bleeding. Fetal head notated by *arrowhead*. High signal intensity within cervical canal *(thin arrow)* represents hemorrhage. (From Leyendecker JR and Brown JJ. Practical Guide to Abdominal and Pelvic MRI. Philadelphia: Lippincott Williams & Wilkins, 2004.)

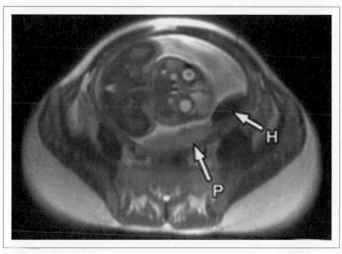

FIGURE 79.9: Placental Hematoma. Axial T2-weighted SSFSE MR image shows a low–signal-intensity mass (H) along the margin of the placenta (P). (*Courtesy of Khaled M. Elsayes, MD. Department of Radiology, University of Michigan, Ann Arbor, MI.*)

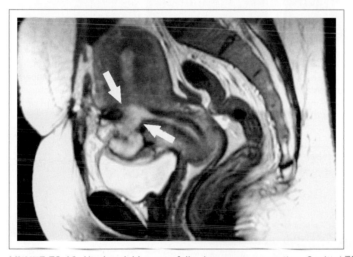

FIGURE 79.10. Uterine dehiscence following cesarean section. Sagittal T2-weighted Image of uterus in patient with pain and bleeding after cesarean section. Note disruption of myometrium at the incision site (*arrows*). (From Leyendecker JR and Brown JJ. Practical Guide to Abdominal and Pelvic MRI. Philadelphia: Lippincott Williams & Wilkins, 2004.)

Pelvic CT Scan
- CT is used most often in the setting of trauma to evaluate a hemodynamically stable mother
- Uterine rupture and placental abruption may be diagnosed with CT
- Placenta previa may be incidentally identified, but because of ionizing radiation, CT should not be utilized for the purpose of diagnosing this condition

Placental Abruption
- Best viewed when IV contrast administered for primary indication
- Normal placental perfusion can be distinguished from areas of hypoperfusion and/or hemorrhage

Uterine Rupture
- Hemoperitoneum and fetal parts outside of the uterus may be identified
- This imaging modality has limited use in the diagnosis of uterine rupture, as the likelihood of maternal hemodynamic instability is high

TABLE 79.5: Pelvic CT scan: placental previa, placental abruption, and uterine rupture

IV contrast	Yes, to evaluate placental perfusion
PO contrast	Not necessary but may be given
Amount of radiation	6 mSv

Classic Images

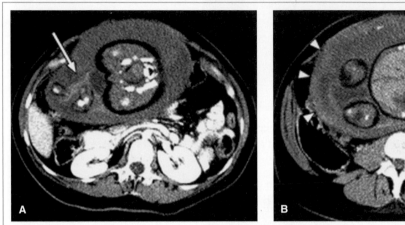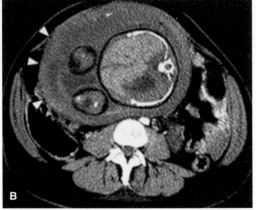

FIGURE 79.11: CT images show placental abruption after a motor vehicle collision at 40 weeks of gestation. The amniotic fluid is high in attenuation because of hemorrhage (*arrow* in **A**), making the devascularized placenta difficult to identify. Careful inspection reveals an anterior and right lateral placenta (*arrowheads* in **B**), which has only slightly higher attenuation than the amniotic fluid. (*Courtesy of Khaled M. Elsayes, MD. Department of Radiology, University of Michigan, Ann Arbor, MI.*)

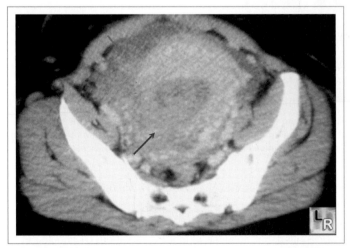

FIGURE 79.12: Uterine rupture in a postpartum woman. Contrast-enhanced CT scan demonstrates a large discontinuity in the right posterolateral wall (*blue arrow*). There is a moderate amount of blood in the pelvis (*red arrow*). The pelvic veins are dilated from the recent pregnancy. (Reprinted with permission from LearningRadiology.com.)

Basic Management
- Emergent obstetric consultation
- The method and timing of delivery is dependent on evidence of maternal or fetal distress

- Steroids should be considered in stable patients to promote lung maturity for a fetus of 24–34 weeks of gestation
- Monitor for the presence of life-threatening complications such as hypovolemic shock, DIC, and amniotic fluid embolism

Placental Previa
- In stable patients with bleeding from placenta previa, hemorrhage can be managed with transfusion, tocolytics, bedrest, and expectant management
- If significant hemorrhage is present or there is concern for fetal well-being, emergent delivery may be indicated

Placental Abruption and Uterine Rupture
- Continuous monitoring of the fetus and uterine contractions are ultimately the best indicator of clinically significant placental abruption or uterine rupture
- In the case of rupture, there is loss of contractions and potential loss of fetal heart tones as the fetus looses amnionic fluid and shifts position into the peritoneum
- Because placental abruption is a difficult radiologic diagnosis, fetal monitoring and clinical judgment should direct management decisions

Summary

TABLE 79.6: Advantages and disadvantages of imaging modalities in placenta previa, placental abruption, and uterine rupture

Imaging modality	Advantages	Disadvantages
Ultrasound	Low cost No ionizing radiation Bedside availability Safe for fetus	Body habitus limitations Operator-dependent Cannot exclude diagnosis of abruption or rupture
MRI	No ionizing radiation Extremely accurate	Time-consuming Requires a stable patient
CT scan	Availability Evaluates other intra-abdominal structures (especially in the setting of trauma)	IV contrast Radiation (to mother and fetus) Requires a stable patient

80

Ovarian Cysts and Polycystic Ovarian Syndrome

Katrin Takenaka

Background

Ovarian cysts most commonly occur in women during their childbearing years. Follicular cysts, the most common type, develop during the first half of the menstrual cycle when physiologic follicles fail to rupture. They are often multiple and are considered pathologic if greater than 2.5 cm in diameter. Corpus luteum cysts arise following ovulation if the physiologic corpus luteum becomes greater than 3 cm in diameter. Theca-lutein cysts are least common and develop due to excessive stimulation by or a hypersensitivity to β-hCG (e.g., polycystic ovarian syndrome, clomiphene therapy, gestational trophoblastic disease). These cysts are usually bilateral and can cause moderate to massive ovarian enlargement. Potential complications of cysts, if ruptured, include hemorrhagic hypovolemia and, if large, ovarian torsion.

Polycystic ovarian syndrome (PCOS) is estimated to occur in 3–7% of women in their reproductive years. This syndrome is characterized by abnormal gonadotrophin release and increased circulating androgen levels. The diagnosis depends on the presence of at least two of the following findings: biochemical or clinical evidence of hyperandrogenism (e.g., acne, male pattern hair loss, hirsutism), anovulation or irregular menses, and polycystic ovaries on ultrasound. Patients with PCOS are often overweight, have some degree of insulin resistance, and suffer from infertility. Long-term complications may include diabetes mellitus, hypertension, dyslipidemia, ovarian cancer, endometrial hyperplasia, and nonalcoholic fatty liver.

TABLE 80.1: Classic history and physical

Follicular cyst	Usually asymptomatic
	May present with vague heaviness in pelvis if large
	May rupture, but rarely associated with hemorrhage
	Occasionally associated with abnormal uterine bleeding
Corpus luteum cyst	May be asymptomatic
	Often causes dull, unilateral lower abdominal and pelvic pain
	Frequently associated with significant hemorrhage (causing sudden, severe lower abdominal pain)
	May be associated with amenorrhea or delayed menstruation
Theca-lutein cyst	Usually asymptomatic
	May present with sensation of pelvic pressure if large
	Rarely associated with hemorrhage
	May be associated with ascites
	Ovarian torsion rare
All cysts	Tenderness on the affected side on pelvic examination with associated mass
	Acute pelvic pain after vaginal intercourse
PCOS	Obese, hirsute with acne and/or alopecia, and irregular menses

PCOS, polycystic ovarian syndrome.

TABLE 80.2: Potentially helpful laboratory tests

Urinalysis	Evaluate for infection
hCG	Evaluate for pregnancy
CBC, coagulation profile, type, and screen	Evaluate for anemia due to hemorrhage Preoperative planning

CBC, complete blood count; hCG, human chorionic gonadotropin.

Pelvic Ultrasound

- Bedside ultrasound may be performed by the emergency physician but note that this is not the standard of care for cyst evaluation
- Ultrasound is the preferred initial imaging modality to assess for ovarian pathology
- Both transabdominal (sagittal and transverse views) and transvaginal (sagittal and coronal views) approaches should be used
- The transabdominal approach is useful to assess for the presence of free fluid in the pelvis and potential spaces such as Morison's pouch and to visualize large pelvic masses
- Normal ovaries "may be" difficult to visualize with transabdominal scanning
- The transvaginal approach allows for a more detailed view of the ovary itself
- The ovary is usually found anterior and medial to the internal iliac vessels
- Functional cysts are round, thin-walled, anechoic, and unilocular
- Hemorrhage into a cyst may result in a heterogeneous echogenic pattern
- Although ultrasound cannot definitively differentiate between benign and malignant ovarian masses, findings concerning for malignancy include solid elements, internal septations or echoes, thickened walls, or a large amount of free fluid
- Findings consistent with PCOS include enlarged ovaries (>10 cm) with a dense central stroma and 10 or more peripheral cysts (2–8 mm each)
- Vascular flow to the ovary should be evaluated and documented using spectral color and/or power flow Doppler mode with concern for ovarian torsion

TABLE 80.3: Helpful associated structures

Iliac vessels: The adnexa lies just medial and anterior to these vessels
Uterus in the coronal plan: Scan the uterine fundus until you visualize a uterine endometrial stripe; move the probe in a plane parallel to this level toward the lateral fornix of each side; follow the cornua laterally to bring the fallopian tube and ovary into view

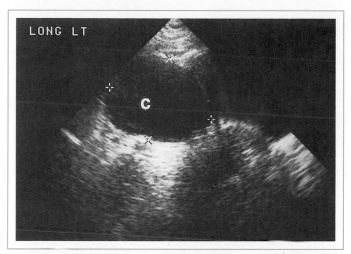

FIGURE 80.1: Ovarian cyst (C): anechoic, unilocular, and devoid of internal echoes. (From Daffner RH. Clinical Radiology: The Essentials, 3rd ed. Philadelphia: Lippincott Williams & Wilkins, 2007.)

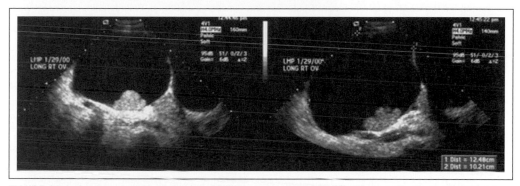

FIGURE 80.2: Ovarian cyst with internal solid elements concerning for malignancy. The final pathology of this cyst was clear cell adenocarcinoma. (From Gibbs RS, Karlan BY, Haney AF, et al. Danforth's Obstetrics and Gynecology, 10th ed. Philadelphia: Lippincott Williams & Wilkins, 2008.)

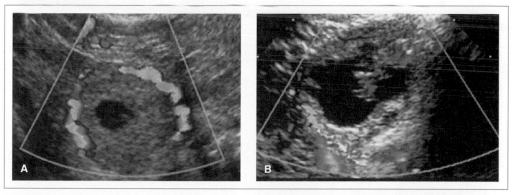

FIGURE 80.3: Rings of fire. A corpus luteum (**A**) can be confused with an ectopic pregnancy (**B**). The arrow indicates blood flow in the embryo (**B**). (From Gibbs RS, Karlan BY, Haney AF, et al. Danforth's Obstetrics and Gynecology, 10th ed. Philadelphia: Lippincott Williams & Wilkins, 2008.)

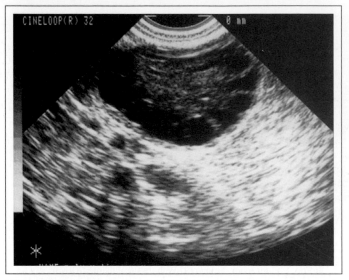

FIGURE 80.4: Polycystic ovary with a string of subcapsular cysts and dense central stroma. (From Gibbs RS, Karlan BY, Haney AF, et al. Danforth's Obstetrics and Gynecology, 10th ed. Philadelphia: Lippincott Williams & Wilkins, 2008.)

Pelvic CT Scan

- CT and all verb tenses to singular are not the imaging modality of choice for identifying ovarian cysts although they may be helpful in patients with pelvic pain in order to rule out other disease processes such as appendicitis or renal colic
- CT scans may identify large adnexal lesions or complications of ovarian cysts better than ultrasound

 TABLE 80.4: CT scan: ovarian cyst

IV contrast	Not necessary but may be given
PO contrast	Not necessary but may be given
Amount of radiation	6 mSv

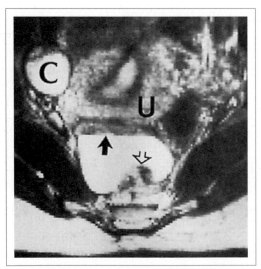

FIGURE 80.5: Ovarian cyst (C) and uterus (U). (From Eisenberg RL. An Atlas of Differential Diagnosis, 4th ed. Philadelphia: Lippincott Williams & Wilkins, 2003.)

MRI

- Although MRI is not the preferred initial imaging for ovarian cysts, they can provide more detailed information than CT scan
- Simple functional cysts demonstrate a low T1-weighted signal intensity and high T2-weighted intensity
- Internal hemorrhage of cysts results in high-signal intensity on T1-weighted MRI

 TABLE 80.5: MRI: ovarian cyst

IV contrast	No, but may have been used for primary indication for study
PO contrast	No, bowel is not area of interest
Amount of radiation	None

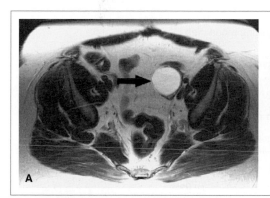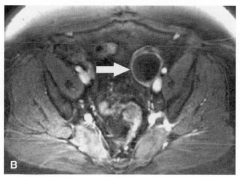

FIGURE 80.6: A: Left ovarian cyst (*arrow*) seen on axial T2-weighted image. **B:** Same cyst (*arrow*) seen on T1-weighted image. (From Leyendecker JR and Brown JJ. Practical Guide to Abdominal and Pelvic MRI. Philadelphia: Lippincott Williams & Wilkins, 2004.)

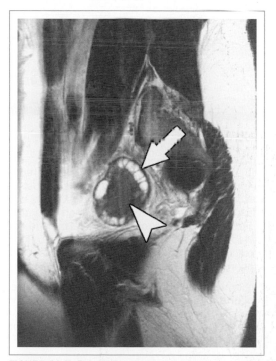

FIGURE 80.7: Polycystic ovary (*arrow*) seen on sagittal T2-weighted image. Prominent low-signal intensity ovarian stroma (*arrowhead*) is also present. (From Leyendecker JR and Brown JJ. Practical Guide to Abdominal and Pelvic MRI. Philadelphia: Lippincott Williams & Wilkins, 2004.)

Basic Management

- Analgesia
- Hemodynamic monitoring and serial hematocrit with concern for ongoing bleeding
- Most uncomplicated cysts will resolve spontaneously; therefore, observation with adequate analgesia and serial ultrasound exam is a common initial therapeutic approach
- Emergent gynecology consultation in cases of ovarian torsion or hemodynamic compromise from a hemorrhagic cyst
- Consider gynecology consultation in cases of persistent cysts (lasting longer than 12 weeks) and those that increase in size
- Ruptured corpus luteum cysts may require cystectomy
- Outpatient gynecology follow-up in patients with PCOS who require a combination of lifestyle interventions, hormonal therapy, androgen blockade, metformin, cosmetic treatments, and infertility therapy

Summary

TABLE 80.6: Advantages and disadvantages of imaging modalities in ovarian cysts

Imaging modality	Advantages	Disadvantages
Ultrasound	Detailed evaluation of ovarian pathology Low cost No ionizing radiation Bedside availability Easily repeatable Safe in pregnancy	Operator dependent Body habitus limitations Unable to evaluate large ovarian masses well
CT scan	Can rule out other abdominal pathology Can identify complications of ovarian cysts Availability	Can be difficult to differentiate ovarian pathology from other pelvic structures IV contrast Radiation Cost
MRI	No ionizing radiation Can provide detailed information regarding ovarian pathology	Availability Cost

81 Ovarian Torsion

Lisa Freeman Grossheim

Ovarian torsion is a gynecologic emergency with a reported incidence of 3%. Women of reproductive age are the most commonly affected, although torsion can present at any age. Most cases of ovarian torsion (50–80%) in adults are associated with adnexal pathology such as ovarian tumors or cysts. In contrast to adults, the affected ovary in children with torsion is more likely to be normal. Approximately 15% of cases of torsion occur in neonatal, prepubertal, and adolescent girls. Torsion in children has been attributed to excessive mobility of the adnexa. Potential mechanisms for torsion in children include tortuosity and elongation of the fallopian tube or mesosalpingeal vessels, congenitally long supportive ligaments or tubal spasm.

The ovary has a dual blood supply. The primary vascular supply is from the ovarian artery, a branch of the hypogastric artery, but additional arterial flow is provided by the ovarian branches of the uterine artery. Torsion is caused by rotation of the adnexal vascular pedicle on its axis, resulting in arterial, venous, and lymphatic compromise. Initially, the obstruction of the lymphatic drainage leads to edema and ovarian enlargement, followed by venous obstruction. The final step is interruption of the arterial blood supply and hemorrhagic infarction. The length of time from onset of pain to nonreversible ovarian loss is reported to be highly variable due to the extent of torsion and dual blood supply.

TABLE 81.1: Pathology that mimics ovarian torsion

Ovarian cyst rupture
Ectopic pregnancy
Pelvic inflammatory disease
Appendicitis
Kidney stone
Biliary colic

TABLE 81.2: Risk factors for ovarian torsion

Unilateral ovarian cysts or tumors
Hormone induction/hyperstimulation syndrome
Pregnancy

TABLE 81.3: Classic history and physical

Lower quadrant abdominal pain
Colicky or constant pain, but usually intense and progressive
Pain out of proportion to other findings
The pain may be intermittent with periods of spontaneous resolution of symptoms
Associated fever and nausea and/or vomiting
Tenderness on the affected side on pelvic examination, and an adnexal mass may be appreciated

TABLE 81.4: Potentially helpful laboratory tests

Urinalysis: To evaluate for infection
CBC: Leukocytosis may be present, preoperative planning
HCG: To evaluate for pregnancy
Coagulation profile, type, and screen: Preoperative planning

Pelvic Ultrasound

- Transvaginal ultrasound is the preferred imaging modality to diagnose ovarian torsion, as it provides characterization of the internal architecture of the uterus, ovary, and vascular anatomy
- The standard of care is to have this examination performed in the department of radiology, as most emergency departments do not have the proper equipment or skilled staff to perform an adequately sensitive exam for this gynecologic emergency
- The most common sonographic gray-scale finding of ovarian torsion is an enlarged ovary or ovarian tubal complex with prominent heterogeneous central stroma and small peripheral follicles
- Although the lack of intraovarian arterial or venous flow is highly indicative of adnexal torsion, Doppler flow, either pathologic or normal, can be recorded in a significant percentage of patients who have surgically proven torsion; reasons for this include intermittent, incomplete or early torsion, and dual blood supply
- Doppler flow patterns in torsion are variable, depending on the degree of torsion and its chronicity
- Complete absence of arterial and venous flow in a morphologically abnormal ovary is diagnostic of ovarian torsion; however, the presence of blood flow does not exclude ovarian torsion
- A complete absence of flow appears to be a late finding of ovarian torsion and an insensitive but highly specific criterion
- When evaluating with Doppler, the flow-pattern distribution probably has greater diagnostic significance than the presence or absence of flow; incomplete torsion can be associated with apparently normal adnexal flow
- Venous thrombosis may cause symptoms before the development of arterial occlusion, resulting in early absence of venous Doppler signals

- The sonographic appearance of the adnexa is related to the duration and degree of torsion and to the presence of associated masses or hemorrhage
- In patients with torsion and no pathological adnexal mass or cyst, the affected ovary is typically enlarged at baseline
- It is always important to interrogate the opposite ovary because torsion is usually unilateral and flow in the contralateral ovary is usually detectable
- Torsed adnexa are usually medial to the normal expected location, often at midline, positioned cranial to the uterine fundus
- A variable amount of free pelvic fluid may be present
- The echo texture of the ovary can be variable, depending on the extent of necrotic changes
- Hemorrhage usually produces hypoechoic areas that are either homogenous or contain punctate echogenicities
- Extensively necrotic ovaries present with cystic, solid, or mixed echogenicity
- The normal fallopian tube is not usually seen on ultrasound; however, an ischemic tube can occasionally be identified as a thickened elongated structure, either void or fluid-filled, in patients with torsion
- On cross section, the enlarged tube and twisted vascular pedicle are identified as an extraovarian echogenic mass that may have a concentric or "target-like" appearance with alternating hypoechoic and echogenic bands; the hypoechoic bands are believed to represent twisted vessels in the adnexal pedicle and can best be seen with color Doppler imaging (whirlpool sign)
- Scanning parameters must be adjusted for detection of low-velocity flows and color Doppler gain should be turned just below the noise threshold
- In patients with hemorrhagic or leaking cysts, it may be incorrectly assumed that the cyst pathology is the cause of the patient's acute pelvic pain and the associated torsion may be overlooked

TABLE 81.5: Helpful associated structures

Iliac vessels: The adnexa lies just medial and anterior of these vessels
Uterus in the coronal plan: Scan up toward the uterine fundus, until the uterine stripe is visible; move the probe in a plane parallel to this level toward either lateral fornix; follow the cornua laterally to bring the fallopian tube and ovary into view; evaluated the ovary in two planes

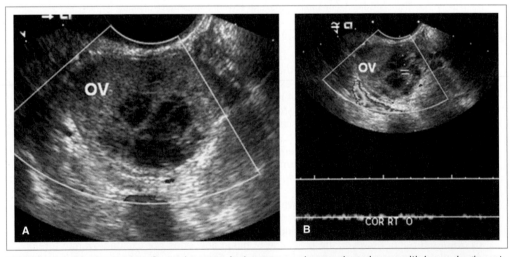

FIGURE 81.1: Ovarian torsion. Coronal transvaginal sonogram shows enlarged ovary with hemorrhagic cyst demonstrating (**A**) no color flow and (**B**) no flow on duplex Doppler examination because of ovarian torsion. (Reproduced with permission from Jain KA. Gynecologic causes of acute pelvic pain: ultrasound imaging. *Ultrasound Clin* 3: 2008; 1–12.)

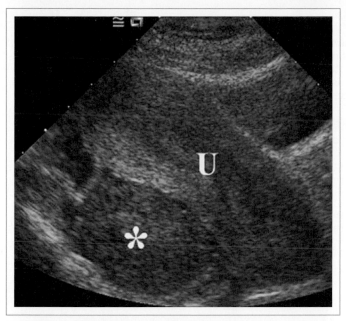

FIGURE 81.2: Right adnexal torsion in a 32-year-old woman. The right ovary (*asterisk*) is enlarged and has slightly increased echogenicity. No peripheral follicular cysts are recognized. U, uterus. (Reproduced with permission from Bertolotto M, Serafini G, Toma P, et al. Adnexal torsion. *Ultrasound Clin* 3: 2008; 109–119.)

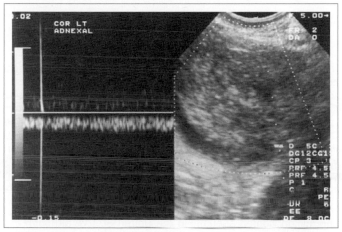

FIGURE 81.3: Doppler sonogram of enlarged left ovary containing venous flow. This finding suggests potential viability of this partial ovarian torsion. (From Gibbs RS, Karlan BY, Haney AF, et al. Danforth's Obstetrics and Gynecology, 10th ed. Philadelphia: Lippincott Williams & Wilkins, 2008.)

Basic Management

- Pain control
- Emergent gynecologic consultation
- Preoperative laboratory testing
- To maximize reproductive potential, laparoscopic adnexal detorsion with surgical aspiration and removal of cysts and other associated adnexal masses is preferred
- If adnexal necrosis has occurred, an oophorectomy must be performed

Summary

TABLE 81.6: Advantages and disadvantages of ultrasound in ovarian torsion

Advantages	Disadvantages
Low cost	Body habitus limitations
Bedside availability	Operator dependent
No ionizing radiation	
Can be performed in the pregnant patient	
Provides information about the structure of the ovary as well as vascular anatomy	

82

Imaging of PID and TOA

Joanne L. Oakes

Background

Primary pelvic inflammatory disease (PID) is a spectrum of ascending pelvic infection and inflammation that typically progresses from the lower genital tract to the upper genital tract. The progression of PID consists of the following inflammatory/infectious conditions: cervicitis, endometritis, salpingitis, salpingo-oophoritis, pyosalpinx and/or hydrosalpinx, tubo-ovarian complex, tubo-ovarian abscess (TOA), pelvic peritonitis, ascending peritonitis, and perihepatitis. Perihepatitis, known as the Fitz-Hugh-Curtis syndrome, affects 1–30% of the women with PID and presents with right upper quadrant pain that may mimic gallbladder disease or hepatitis. Inflammation and adhesion formation between the anterior liver capsule and the anterior abdominal wall is seen as "violin strings" when visualized surgically. Secondary PID (not related to sexually transmitted disease) may present in postpartum patients, postabortion patients, or after ruptured appendicitis or diverticulitis.

PID affects approximately one million women annually in the United States, although the disease prevalence is probably underestimated. PID is associated with greater than $1 billion annual health care costs. Approximately 300,000 women per year are hospitalized for PID-associated conditions. TOA is present in an estimated 33% of women hospitalized for PID. The rate of TOA rupture may reach 15% and is associated with mortality rates as high as 9%. PID may result in significant lifetime morbidity such as infertility, ectopic pregnancy, pelvic adhesions, recurrent pelvic infections, and/or chronic pelvic pain. Laparoscopic surgical evaluation is generally considered the gold standard for diagnosis, but it is invasive and not routinely performed.

TABLE 82.1: Classic history and physical

No single symptom, physical findings, serologic test, or imaging study is sensitive and specific for the diagnosis of PID.
Vague or nonspecific findings or symptoms with acute, subacute, or subclinical presentations.
Young, sexually active, reproductive age women (14–40 years old), with highest prevalence in the 15- to 19-year-old age group.
Definite risk factors for PID: young age, multiple sexual partners, prior history of PID, history of gonorrhea or chlamydia, and not using barrier contraceptives
Additional possible risk factors: low socioeconomic status, race, unmarried, urban living, high frequency of sexual intercourse, coitus during menses, use of intrauterine device, recent uterine instrumentation, douching, smoking, and substance abuse
Abdominal pain (90–100%), fevers (50–65%), nausea (25–30%), vaginal discharge (19–30%), or abnormal bleeding (19–21%)
Acute symptoms may worsen with menstruation, worsen over 2–3 days, and persist for <3 wk
Cervical motion tenderness and/or purulent discharge from cervical os
A palpable adnexal mass or adnexal fullness on physical examination is not common

TABLE 82.2: Potentially helpful laboratory test results

CBC: Leukocytosis is nonspecific and elevated in only 44–75% of patients
Elevated erythrocyte sedimentation rate or elevated C-reactive protein have a sensitivity of 74–93% and specificity of 25–90%
Vaginal wet smear: 87–91% sensitive for upper tract infection if ≥ 3WBC/high powered field; absence of WBCs on wet smear has a 94.5% negative predictive value for upper tract infection
HCG: To evaluate for pregnancy
CA-125 levels may be elevated in PID, but are inconsistent and not helpful in the diagnosis

Pelvic Ultrasound

- Bedside ultrasound in the emergency department may be performed, but is not considered standard of care or sufficient to completely evaluate all pelvic structures
- Transabdominal ultrasound should be combined with transvaginal ultrasound to obtain the best possible images.
- Imaging should include scanning in two planes through the uterus: adnexae and cul-de-sac.
- Endometritis, salpingitis, and oophoritis may appear with uterine enlargement or indistinctness, endometrial thickening with possible endometrial fluid, larger than normal ovarian volumes, or complex free fluid with internal echoes
- For the diagnosis of TOA, a thick-walled, tubular adnexal mass with or without intrapelvic free fluid has a sensitivity of 85% and specificity of 100%
- Fallopian tubes are normally less than 4 mm in diameter and not visible on imaging unless filled with fluid, thickened due to inflammation, or surrounded by fluid
- Dilated fallopian tubes may appear as tubular, ovoid, or pear-shaped configurations with wall thickening >5 mm and anechoic or layering echogenic fluid with debris
- Pathologic fallopian tubes may have a "cogwheel" appearance due to thickened endosalpingeal folds and demonstrate increased flow with color Doppler ultrasound
- Dilated fallopian tubes are the most striking and specific sonographic finding for diagnosis
- A tubo-ovarian complex is visualized when an ovary is adherent to an inflamed tube but maintains its architecture and is still visible as a separate structure from the fallopian tube.
- A TOA is visualized when there is destruction of the usual distinct ovarian architecture into a solid and/or cystic adnexal mass involving the fallopian tube and ovary
- Speckled fluid in the abdomen or cul-de-sac correlates with purulent material

TABLE 82.3: Helpful associated structures

Iliac vessels: The adnexa lies just medial and anterior of these vessels
Uterus in the coronal plan: Scan up toward the uterine fundus, until the uterine stripe is visible; move the probe in a plane parallel to this level toward either lateral fornix; follow the cornua laterally to bring the fallopian tube and ovary into view; evaluated the ovary in two planes
Bladder: anterior to the uterus (coronal plane)
Posterior cul-de-sac: Free fluid will likely accumulate here first when there is pelvic pathology

Classic Images

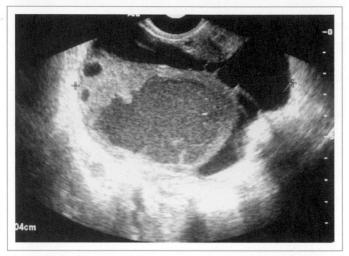

FIGURE 82.1: Ultrasound of pyosalpinx. (From Sweet RL, Gibbs RS. Atlas of Infectious Diseases of the Female Genital Tract. Philadelphia: Lippincott Williams & Wilkins, 2005.)

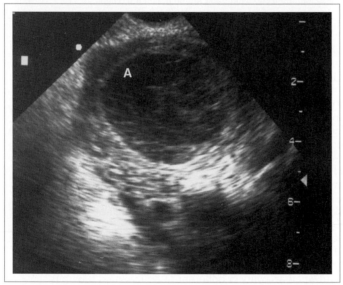

FIGURE 82.2: Pelvic inflammatory disease. Endovaginal scan shows an abscess (A) that contains low-level echoes and is surrounded by a well-defined wall. (From Eisenberg RL. An Atlas of Differential Diagnosis, 4th ed. Philadelphia: Lippincott Williams & Wilkins, 2003.)

Abdominal/Pelvic CT Scan
- Pelvic CT images may reveal enlarged and abnormally enhancing ovaries when involved, occasionally with a polycystic appearance
- The endocervical and/or endometrial cavities may contain hypodense fluid contents or a fluid/debris level
- Pyosalpinx presents as an enhancing serpiginous or dilated tubular structure with thick enhancing walls and mural nodules corresponding to thickened endosalpingeal folds
- Tubo-ovarian complex presents with regular margins, thick walls, an adnexal mass with an associated serpiginous structure (hydro- or pyosalpinx) that may be better visualized in coronal or sagittal planes

- TOA presents as a complex fluid collection or mass in unilateral or bilateral adnexa with loss of normal ovarian architecture, thickened walls, an enhancing rim, internal septations, and/or a fluid-debris level
- CT may reveal a connection of the TOA cystic mass to a dilated tubular structure (hydro- or pyosalpinx)
- The presence of gas is an infrequent but specific finding for TOA
- Other possible findings for PID on CT include a thickened round or uterosacral ligament, fat stranding or loss of normal fat planes, lymphadenopathy, pelvic free fluid, or right upper quadrant enhancement in Fitz-Hugh-Curtis syndrome

 TABLE 82.4: Pelvic CT scan: PID and TOA

IV contrast	Yes, enhancement in abscesses and other inflamed structures
PO contrast	Yes, to differentiate gynecologic anatomy from adjacent bowel
Amount of radiation	6 mSv

Classic Images

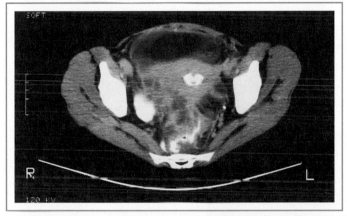

FIGURE 82.3: CT scan of tubo-ovarian abscess. (From Sweet RL, Gibbs RS. Atlas of Infectious Diseases of the Female Genital Tract. Philadelphia: Lippincott Williams & Wilkins, 2005.)

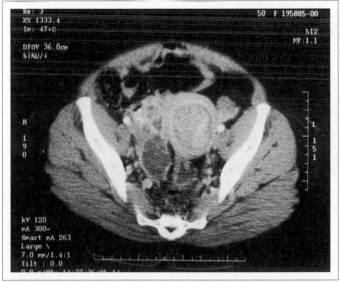

FIGURE 82.4: CT scan of a tubo-ovarian abscess. (From Sweet RL, Gibbs RS. Atlas of Infectious Diseases of the Female Genital Tract. Philadelphia: Lippincott Williams & Wilkins, 2005.)

Pelvic MRI

- MRI is considered a second-line "problem-solving" imaging modality after CT or ultrasound
- MRI is approved by the Food and Drug Administration Guidelines for safety in pregnancy and so should be used if ultrasound is indeterminate or equivocal and CT imaging is undesirable due to radiation risk for the fetus
- T2-weighted fat-saturated images depict parametrial signal hyperintensity due to adnexal edema and inflammation
- Hydrosalpinx may be confirmed as a dilated tubular structure arising from the upper lateral margin of the uterine fundus and separate from the ipsilateral ovary
- A dilated fallopian tube folds upon itself to form a sausage-like "C"- or "S"-shaped cystic mass; hydrosalpinges are well visualized on MR
- Pyosalpinx presents as a dilated tortuous fallopian tube with thickened walls with variable or heterogeneous signal intensity, well visualized on T2-weighted images
- TOA is seen as a multilocular round adnexal mass, predominantly dark on T1-weighted images and heterogeneously bright on T2-weighted images with intense enhancement of the thick irregular surrounding wall, internal debris, and adjacent soft tissue inflammation

TABLE 82.5: MRI: PID and TOA

IV contrast	Yes, to further delineate structures of interest
PO contrast	No, bowel not organ of interest
Amount of radiation	None

Classic Images

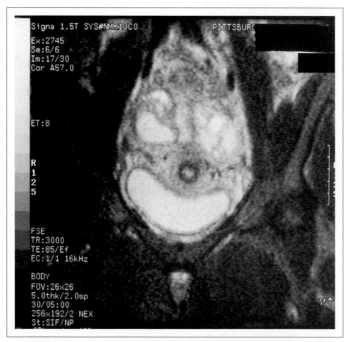

FIGURE 82.5: MRI of a tubo-ovarian abscess. (From Sweet RL, Gibbs RS. Atlas of Infectious Diseases of the Female Genital Tract. Philadelphia: Lippincott Williams & Wilkins, 2005.)

Nuclear Medicine

- Radionuclide scintigraphy has been demonstrated to diagnose sites of bacterial infection and PID (gallium-67 and indium-111)
- Single photon emission CT (SPECT) images of technetium 99 m ciprofloxacin imaging may correlate with areas of clinical symptoms

 TABLE 82.6: Nuclear medicine: PID and TOA

IV contrast	Yes, uptake of radioactive nucleotide in structures of interest
PO contrast	No, bowel not organ of interest
Amount of radiation	6–7 mSv

Classic Images

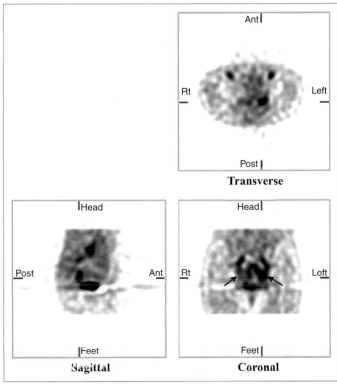

FIGURE 82.6: Scintigraphy images. Single photon emission CT scintigraphic images are shown. A 31-year-old patient met diagnostic criteria for PID. The ultrasound revealed a 3.5 cm right adnexal cystic mass. The patient had a twisted right ovarian cyst that was confirmed by surgical operation. There is an area of increased uptake in the right ovary with remarkably decreased uptake in the center. Right arrow in the coronal section indicates the ovarian cyst, and the left arrow in the coronal section indicates an area of adhesion between the cyst and the rectum. Culture of the adhesion area grew Pseudomonas aeruginosa. (Reproduced with permission from Im MW, et al., Pelvic inflammatory disease with ciprofloxacin Tc-99m imaging. *J. Obstet. Gynaecol. Res.* 34(4, part II): 2008; 754–758.)

Basic Management

- Analgesia
- Mild to moderate PID may be managed with outpatient antibiotic therapy
- Cervical culture sample for chlamydia/gonorrhea
- Assess HIV status and perform testing if status is unknown
- Indications for hospitalization and intravenous antibiotics include insufficient response to oral therapy, severe illness, persistent nausea and vomiting, high fever, or presence of TOA
- Gynecologic consult for TOA
- Operative intervention may be required

Summary

TABLE 82.7: Advantages and disadvantages of imaging modalities in PID and TOA

Imaging modality	Advantages	Disadvantages
Ultrasound	First-line imaging modality of choice Low cost Bedside availability May follow treatment response May use to guide abscess drainage Safe for pregnant patients	Availability Body habitus limitations May be normal in early disease Operator dependent
CT scan	Evaluates other diagnoses Early or mild inflammation better seen than with ultrasound Higher sensitivity than ultrasound Multiplanar reconstruction useful for visualizing TOA and pyosalpinx	IV contrast Radiation exposure Higher cost than ultrasound
MRI	Superior contrast resolution of pathologic tissue or fluid Multiplanar images helpful for visualization	Higher cost than CT or ultrasound IV contrast Patient claustrophobia Time-consuming Incompatibility with monitoring equipment/ internal metallic devices
Nuclear medicine scintigraphy	Localizes abscesses	Very time intensive Technically difficult Not widely used High cost Frequent false-positive studies due to tracer affinity for any inflammation Radioactive substance injected

83 Fibroid Uterus and Degenerative Fibroids

Iman Hassan

Background

Uterine leiomyomas, more commonly referred to as fibroids, are benign tumors that develop from uterine smooth muscle. Fibroids occur in up to 70% of women, most of whom experience no symptoms. They can occur as solitary lesions, but more often present as multiple lesions of varying size and location. The pathogenesis of uterine leiomyoma growth is thought to be hormone related, with evidence showing that high estrogen states can cause an increase in fibroid size, while low estrogen states such as menopause cause a decrease in their size. Generally, the presence of symptoms has been associated with larger fibroid size and a submucosal location. As fibroids outgrow their blood supply, they undergo degeneration that can exacerbate symptoms. The various types of degeneration include hyaline, cystic, myxoid, and red degeneration. Symptomatic fibroids are the most common indication for hysterectomy. Other treatment options for fibroids include myomectomy, uterine artery embolization, thermo-ablation, and hormone therapy directed toward halting ovulation.

TABLE 83.1: Common risk factors for the development of fibroids

Age > 30 years through menopause
Nulliparous
Childbirth later in life
Early age at menarche
Family history
African American
Obesity

TABLE 83.2: Classification of uterine fibroids

Submucosal: Grow immediately below the inner surface of the uterine cavity
Least common type but most likely to be symptomatic as they protrude into endometrial cavity
May be pedunculated

Intramural: Grow within the wall of the uterus
Most common type, but usually asymptomatic

Subserosal: Grow beneath the outer layer of the uterus and can project into the abdomen and pelvis
May be pedunculated

TABLE 83.3: Classic history and physical

Heavy menstrual bleeding (menorrhagia) and associated anemia
Increased pain with menstruation (dysmenorrhea)
Pain during sexual intercourse (dyspareunia)
Infertility
Miscarriage
Increased abdominal/pelvic girth and compression of surrounding tissues, which may result in hydronephrosis, urinary frequency, constipation, bloating, varicose veins, and back or pelvic pain
Acute pain, fever, and leukocytosis can occur with fibroid degeneration and torsion of a pedunculated fibroid

TABLE 83.4: Potentially helpful laboratory tests

Urinalysis: To evaluate for infection
HCG: To evaluate for pregnancy
CBC: To evaluate for anemia from vaginal bleeding or leukocytosis from fibroid degeneration
Metabolic panel: To evaluate renal function if fibroid mass causes obstructive uropathy

Pelvis X-Ray

Fibroids are usually not seen on plain radiographs unless they are heavily calcified or large enough to displace other structures such as bowel.

 TABLE 83.5: Pelvis x-ray: uterine fibroids

IV contrast	No
PO contrast	No
Amount of radiation	0.6 mSv

Classic Images

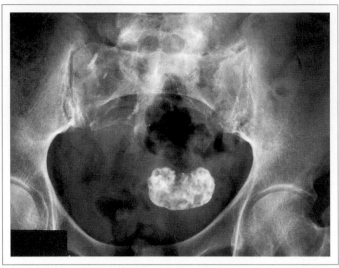

FIGURE 83.1: Pelvic radiograph shows a calcified mass to the left of midline. (From Daffner RH. Clinical Radiology: The Essentials, 3rd ed. Philadelphia: Lippincott Williams & Wilkins, 2007.)

Ultrasound

- Ultrasound is usually the first imaging modality used to investigate the female pelvis
- Although bedside ultrasound in the ED is not the gold standard, it may be performed but should not be considered the definitive imaging examination
- Both transabdominal and transvaginal approaches can be used
- Although obesity may limit the use of the transabdominal scan, an enlarged bulky uterus may be well visualized with this approach
- A transabdominal scan may be performed first, then prior to initiation of the transvaginal scan, the patient should be asked to empty her bladder allowing for improved patient comfort and visualization, as a full bladder will distort the ability to fully visualize the uterus
- Transvaginal ultrasounds are more sensitive than transabdominal scans for detecting small fibroids, and, in the hands of a skilled operator, fibroids as small as 5 mm can be seen on transvaginal ultrasound
- The uterus should be visualized in both sagittal and transverse planes (sagittal and coronal planes on transvaginal view) and scanned through its entirety
- The fibroid uterus may appear bulky or have an irregular contour
- Fibroids generally appear as well-circumscribed, solid masses with a whorled appearance
- Fibroids have variable patterns of echogenicity; although fibroids usually have echogenicity similar to surrounding myometrium, degenerating fibroids are more heterogeneous and often have hypoechoic and anechoic areas corresponding to cystic changes
- Calcified fibroids are hyperechoic and may cast an acoustic shadow
- Doppler ultrasonography typically shows circumferential vascularity
- Degenerate fibroids that are necrotic or have undergone torsion will have an absence of blood flow on Doppler ultrasonography
- Sonohysterography entails instillation of sterile saline into the uterine cavity via a transcervical catheter while performing a transvaginal ultrasound
- Sonohysterography allows better visualization of the endometrium and has been shown to increase the sensitivity for detection of submucosal fibroids
- Because fibroids have many sonographic appearances, ultrasound may be unable to reliably distinguish leiomyomas from other pelvic pathology

Classic Images

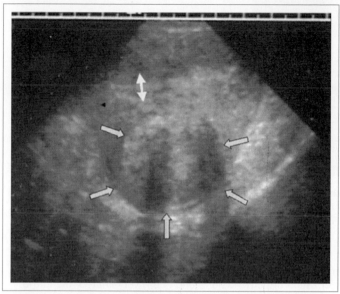

FIGURE 83.2: Ultrasound of uterine leiomyoma. This is a transvaginal ultrasound in a woman who has an intramural myoma (*arrows*). The myoma clearly does not impinge on the endometrial cavity with intervening myometrium. The endometrial stripe is defined by a double arrow. (From Gibbs RS, Karlan BY, Haney AF, et al. Danforth's Obstetrics and Gynecology, 10th ed. Philadelphia: Lippincott Williams & Wilkins, 2008.)

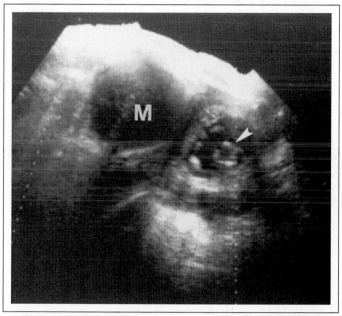

FIGURE 83.3: Coexisting *leiomyoma*. Longitudinal sonogram demonstrates the pregnant uterus (arrowhead) and the hypoechoic mass (M). (From Eisenberg RL. An Atlas of Differential Diagnosis, 4th ed. Philadelphia: Lippincott Williams & Wilkins, 2003.)

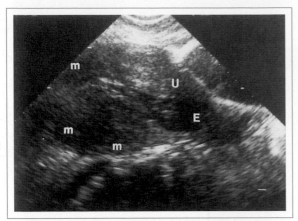

FIGURE 83.4: Uterine fibroids. Sagittal sonogram of the uterus (U) shows multiple hypoechoic masses (m) within the uterus. The dilated endometrial cavity (E) contains low-level echoes representing blood. (From Eisenberg RL. An Atlas of Differential Diagnosis, 4th ed. Philadelphia: Lippincott Williams & Wilkins, 2003.)

Pelvic CT Scan

- Although CT scan of the abdomen may incidentally show uterine fibroids, it is not the imaging modality of choice for the characterization of pelvic lesions and has a very limited role in the work up of fibroids
- Findings may include uterine enlargement, abnormal uterine contour, and fibroid calcifications
- On contrast-enhanced scans, fibroids are usually of lower attenuation relative to the normal myometrium, although they may be of the same or higher attenuation
- Degenerative fibroids with cystic changes and necrosis may demonstrate areas of fluid attenuation, while acute fibroid torsion may demonstrate peripheral rim enhancement corresponding to obstructed peripheral veins

 TABLE 83.6: Pelvis CT scan: uterine fibroids

IV contrast	No, not necessary to visualize fibroids
PO contrast	No, bowel is not area of interest
Amount of radiation	6 mSv

Classic Images

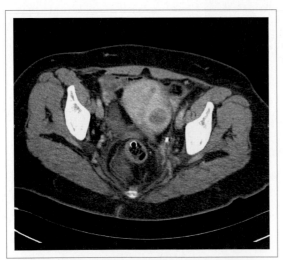

FIGURE 83.5: CT image of a uterine fibroid. (From http://commons.wikimedia.org/wiki/File:Uterine_fibroid_CT.JPG, per the *GNU Free Documentation License*, *Version 1.2 or later*.)

MRI

- MRI is the most accurate imaging modality to visualize, characterize, and localize uterine fibroids
- T2-weighted (T2W) sequences offer the best contrast resolution for delineation of pelvic anatomy and identification of fibroids
- On normal T2W images, the endometrium is of high-signal intensity, while the surrounding myometrium is of low to intermediate signal
- Nondegenerate fibroids are typically well-defined masses with low-signal intensity relative to normal myometrium on T2W images and isointense to the myometrium on T1-weighted (T1W) images
- T2W images show a clear demarcation between lower intensity fibroids and higher intensity normal surrounding myometrium
- Thirty percent of fibroids will have a hyperintense rim on T2W images that is thought to correspond to edema, dilated veins, and dilated lymphatics
- Calcifications associated with fibroids can appear as signal voids on MRI
- In contrast to the characteristic MRI appearance of nondegenerate myomas, degenerating fibroids have a variable and heterogeneous appearance
- Areas of hemorrhage have varying signal depending on the age of the blood; recent hemorrhage has high-signal intensity on both T1W and T2W images
- MRI characteristics of fibroids can help predict response to uterine artery embolization
- MRI is also helpful in differentiating fibroids from other pelvic pathology such as leiomyosarcomas, adenomyosis, and fibrothecomas

TABLE 83.7: Pelvis MRI: uterine fibroids

IV contrast	Yes/no, not necessary to visualize fibroids but will improve visualization
PO contrast	No, bowel is not area of interest
Amount of radiation	None

Classic Images

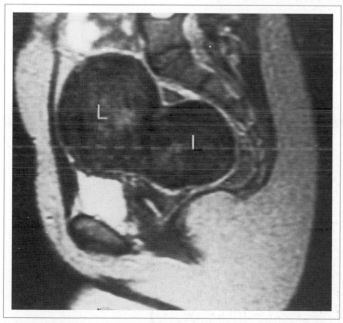

FIGURE 83.6: Subserosal leiomyomas of the uterus. Sagittal T2-weighted image shows two large subserosal leiomyomas (L), which appear as well-defined hypointense lesions along the superior surface of the uterus. (From Eisenberg RL. An Atlas of Differential Diagnosis, 4th ed. Philadelphia: Lippincott Williams & Wilkins, 2003.)

Hysterosalpingography

- Hysterosalpingography (HSG) is typically a test performed for the evaluation of infertility and allows visualization of the uterine cavity as well as patency of fallopian tubes
- It is useful for the evaluation of submucosal fibroids, as these will appear as filling defects
- Neither intramural nor subserosal fibroids can be visualized with this modality

TABLE 83.8: Hysterosalpingogram: uterine fibroids

IV contrast	No, contrast is injected transcervically
PO contrast	No, bowel is not area of interest
Amount of radiation	0.7 mSv

Classic Images

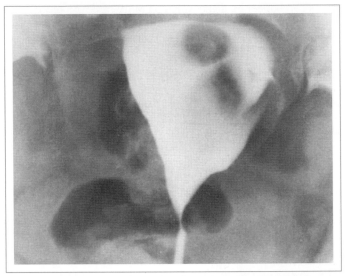

FIGURE 83.7: Hysterosalpingogram of a patient with submucosal myoma and recurrent abortion. (From Baggish MS, Valle RF, and Guedj H. Hysteroscopy: Visual Perspectives of Uterine Anatomy, Physiology and Pathology. Philadelphia: Lippincott Williams & Wilkins, 2007.)

Basic Management

- Treatment is not indicated unless fibroids become symptomatic
- Type of therapy is guided by fibroid size and location as well as patient's age and desire for future fertility
- Gynecology consultation in cases of hemodynamic instability, intractable pain, or tumor bulk preventing urine output or pelvic congestion
- Outpatient gynecology referral

SUMMARY

TABLE 83.9: Advantages and disadvantages of imaging modalities

Imaging modality	Advantages	Disadvantages
X-ray	Fast Low radiation	Visualizes only calcified fibroids
Ultrasound	Low cost Bedside possible No ionizing radiation Improved endovaginal visualization with sonohysterography Can be performed in the pregnant patient	Body habitus limitations Decreased sensitivity in larger uteri that extend out of visual field Decreased sensitivity with increasing number of fibroids and acoustic shadows Operator dependent
CT scan	Availability Allows for evaluation for other pathology	Radiation Cannot reliably distinguish fibroids from other uterine masses
MRI	No ionizing radiation Most accurate for fibroid visualization, localization, and characterization Increased anatomic detail and spatial resolution can better help target therapy Helpful in distinguishing fibroids from other pelvic pathology	Expensive Availability IV contrast
HSG	Other etiologies of infertility can be investigated concurrently	Does not visualize intramural or subserosal fibroids

HSG, hysterosalpingography.

Section Editors: Bret Nelson and Phillip Andrus

84 Peritonsillar Abscess

Matthew Constantine

Background

Peritonsillar abscess is considered the most common infection of the head and neck. Although this infection may occur at any age, it is most common in young adults (20–40 years old) with peak incidence in the late fall and winter months. The exact pathophysiology of this infection is not exactly known; however, it appears to be associated with episodes of exudative pharyngitis and tonsillitis. The abscess forms in the area between the palatine tonsil and its capsule. Additionally, there may be involvement of the Weber glands (salivary glands located just superior to the tonsil in the soft palate), which may trap necrotic tissue secondary to the inflammatory changes of the tonsil. These abscesses are generally found superior to the tonsil extending into the soft palate. Infection can occasionally spread into the deep tissues of neck leading to mediastinal involvement, airway compromise, or carotid sheath involvement leading to life-threatening hemorrhage. The patient is at risk for aspiration and sequelae of streptococcus infection.

TABLE 84.1: Classic history and physical

Severe sore throat (worse on affected side), dysphagia, fever, malaise, and ipsilateral ear pain, worsening over a 2- to 3-day period
Trismus, "hot-potato" or muffled voice and drooling
Unilateral soft palate tense swelling, enlarged tonsils, uvular deviation to the contralateral side, cervical lymphadenopathy, and fetid breath

TABLE 84.2: Potentially helpful laboratory tests

CBC: Nonspecific; may show inflammatory/infectious pattern
Rapid Strep testing: Sensitivity ranges greatly and negative testing does not exclude diagnosis
Throat cultures: Generally not available at the time of diagnosis; although streptococcal involvement is common, most abscesses are polymicrobial
Abscess cultures: Important to obtain at time of diagnosis; may guide later antibiotic therapy

CBC, complete blood count.

Plain Radiographs

- Findings will be only nonspecific or normal
- Subcutaneous air and/or significant neck swelling may be present; however, these findings are not specific to peritonsillar pathology
- May help identify other possible diagnoses such as foreign bodies or retropharyngeal abscess (with prevertebral space widening)
- Unable to show extension of abscess or assist in drainage guidance

- Chest x-ray may help to show any extending of infection into mediastinum or concomitant pneumonia

 TABLE 84.3: X-ray: peritonsillar abscess

IV contrast	No
PO contrast	No
Amount of radiation	0.20 mSv per view

Classic Images

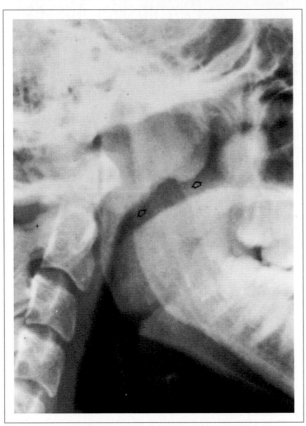

FIGURE 84.1: Enlarged tonsils and adenoids. Marked impressions (*arrows*) on the upper airway. (From Eisenberg RL. An Atlas of Differential Diagnosis, 4th ed. Philadelphia: Lippincott Williams & Wilkins, 2003.)

Bedside Ultrasound

- Both intraoral and transcutaneous approaches have been described, with intraoral generally accepted as more reliable
- Use a high-frequency endocavitary probe (5–10 MHz) with probe cover
- Preprocedural treatment with topical anesthetic or oral/IV pain medication is recommended
- Scan directly over the area of swelling (central landmark) or on the soft palate between the uvula medially and the peripharyngeal arch laterally
- Scan both axially and longitudinally through the soft palate area superior and medial to the tonsil and peripharyngeal arch
- Scan for a hypoechoic cystic structure generally just below the surface of the tissue

- May be used real-time to guide drainage or needle aspiration of abscess
- Sensitivity ranges from 89% to 92% and specificity ranges from 80% to 100%

TABLE 84.4: Helpful associated structures

Carotid artery
Internal jugular vein

Classic Images

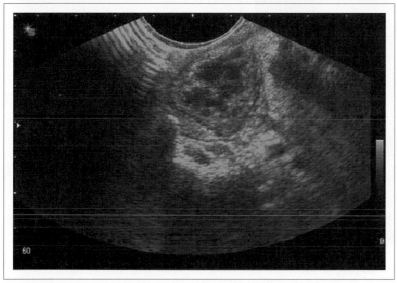

FIGURE 84.2: Ultrasound image demonstrating hypoechoic collection consistent with peritonsillar abscess. (*Courtesy of Danny Duque, MD, The Elmhurst Hospital Center, New York, NY.*)

Neck CT Scan

- Allows for identification of abscess, differentiating it from peritonsillar cellulitis, and also the extent of soft tissue involvement or encroachment into contiguous spaces
- Will differentiate between areas of soft tissue induration versus areas of fluid collection to assist with drainage efforts
- Generally regarded as more sensitive and more specific than intraoral ultrasound or clinical examination alone with sensitivities nearing 100%; however, specificity may be as low as 75%
- More expensive and time-consuming than clinical evaluation or ultrasound
- Exposes patient to ionizing radiation as well as IV contrast
- Cannot be used for real time guidance

 TABLE 84.5: CT scan: peritonsillar abscess

IV contrast	Yes, to evaluate vasculature and soft tissue inflammation
PO contrast	No, bowel not organ of interest
Amount of radiation	6 mSv

Classic Images

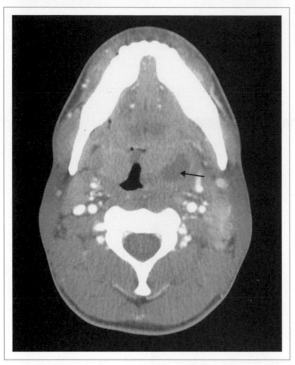

FIGURE 84.3: Axial view of neck CT with IV contrast demonstrating a peritonsillar abscess. (*Courtesy of The Department of Emergency Medicine, The Mount Sinai Hospital, New York, NY.*)

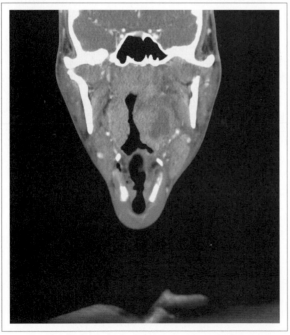

FIGURE 84.4: Sagittal view of neck CT with IV contrast demonstrating peritonsillar abscess. (*Courtesy of The Department of Emergency Medicine, The Mount Sinai Hospital, New York, NY.*)

Basic Management
- Drainage of the abscess is the definitive treatment
- Antibiotics generally are also accepted as adjunctive therapy; although most abscesses are polymicrobial, penicillins remain the most commonly used medications
- Steroids may provide additional symptomatic relief and more rapid resolution of inflammation
- Supportive care including antipyretics, analgesics, and correction of dehydration

Summary

TABLE 84.6: Advantages and disadvantages of imaging modalities in peritonsillar abscess

Imaging modality	Advantages	Disadvantages
X-ray	Lateral neck x-ray can evaluate for other etiologies Chest x-ray may show mediastinal involvement	Unable to visualize abscess
Ultrasound	Less expensive No radiation Bedside availability Real-time drainage guidance	Operator dependent Less reliable visualization of other involved structures
CT scan	Availability Defines extent of abscess as well as involvement of adjacent structures	IV contrast Radiation exposure Outside of emergency department Longer to perform than other modalities

85

Epiglottitis

Jennifer Galjour

Background
As most children in the United States have completed vaccination regimens including *Haemophilus influenzae*, epiglottitis has become a disease of adults rather than children. Although the most common pathogens are *H. influenzae*, *Streptococcus* species, and *Staphylococcus* species, viruses and fungi have also been identified as causes of epiglottitis. With all imaging, care must be taken in children as precipitation of crying during radiologic examinations can lead to rapid inspiration past the swollen epiglottis and closure of the airway.

TABLE 85.1: Classic history and physical

1–2 d of worsening dysphagia, dyspnea, odynophagia

Incomplete vaccination schedule (in children) or middle-aged adults

Symptoms worsen when patient is supine

Patient may assume a "tripod" position to assist breathing

Lateral Cervical Soft Tissue Films
- Structural changes in epiglottitis include elimination of the vallecula, aryepiglottic swelling, "ballooning" of the hypopharynx, soft tissue swelling (prevertebral, retropharyngeal), and the "thumbprint" sign
- In patients with epiglottitis, the vallecula (which normally extends almost to the hyoid bone) will appear diminished and shallower due to swelling
- "Ballooning" of the hypopharynx refers to widening of the airway superior to the epiglottis; the subglottic airway will appear unchanged in diameter

- The "thumbprint" sign refers to the swollen, edematous appearance of the epiglottis
- Diagnostic accuracy is limited if patient is unable to hyperextend the neck due to irritability

TABLE 85.2: Helpful associated structures

Vallecula
Hyoid bone

 TABLE 85.3: Neck x-ray: epiglottitis

IV contrast	No
PO contrast	No
Amount of radiation	0.2 mSv per view

Classic Images

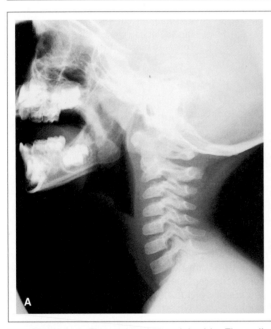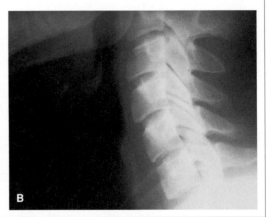

FIGURE 85.1: A: The patient has epiglottitis. The radiograph demonstrates a swollen epiglottis at the level of the hyoid bone, which is convex on both sides and appears in the shape of a thumbprint. Edema anterior to the epiglottis has obliterated the vallecula, which usually appears as an elongated black shadow. Note the marked swelling of the aryepiglottic folds, projecting inferiorly and posteriorly from the epiglottis, and the arytenoid cartilages at the base of the folds. **B:** For comparison, a normal epiglottis is shown, which is thin and fine with a concave surface posteriorly and the appearance of a slightly bent finger. (From Fleisher GR, Ludwig W, and Baskin MN. Atlas of Pediatric Emergency Medicine. Philadelphia: Lippincott Williams & Wilkins, 2004.)

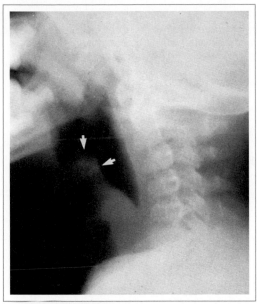

FIGURE 85.2: Epiglottitis. There is blunting and thickening of the epiglottis (*arrows*). This has severely narrowed the airway immediately below. Note the dilated hypopharynx. (From Daffner RH. Clinical Radiology: The Essentials, 3rd ed. Philadelphia: Lippincott Williams & Wilkins, 2007.)

Laryngoscopy
- All patients with suspected or confirmed epiglottitis should be evaluated by an otolaryngologist, who may perform direct or fiberoptic laryngoscopy
- Because of the potential for rapid airway compromise, care should be taken when performing either direct or fiberoptic laryngoscopy and the physician should be prepared to establish a definitive airway

Classic Images

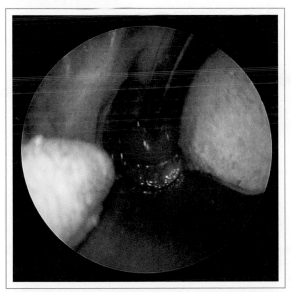

FIGURE 85.3: Epiglottis. A swollen, cherry-red epiglottis with an endotracheal tube passing posteriorly. (From Fleisher GR, Ludwig W, and Baskin MN. Atlas of Pediatric Emergency Medicine. Philadelphia: Lippincott Williams & Wilkins, 2004.)

Neck CT Scan

- Although the diagnosis of epiglottitis can typically be made with history, examination, and lateral cervical soft tissue radiographs, cervical CT scan can be used when the diagnosis is unclear
- Findings include swelling of the supraglottic structures, thickening of the platysma, and soft tissue swelling (prevertebral, retropharyngeal)
- Cervical CT scan should be considered only in patients with a stable airway as many patients with epiglottitis report worsening of symptoms in the supine position
- CT scan can afford better visualization of abscesses and other complications of epiglottitis, but should never delay management and treatment

TABLE 85.4: CT scan: epiglottitis

IV contrast	Yes/no, not necessary, but may increase yield of study for alternate diagnoses
PO contrast	No
Amount of radiation	6 mSv

Classic Images

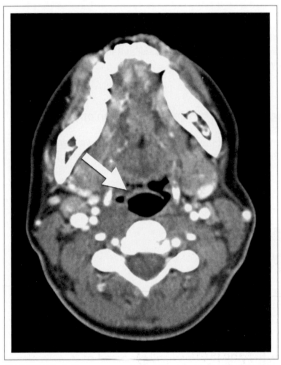

FIGURE 85.4: Transverse plane CT scan through epiglottis demonstrating thickening at the base (*arrow*). (*Courtesy of Mt. Sinai Department of Emergency Medicine, New York, NY.*)

MRI

- Although MRI findings in patients with epiglottitis have been described, MRI should be performed with even more caution than CT, as airway intervention can be even more difficult given the physical constraints of MRI scanning, the length of the examination, and the general lack of proximity to the emergency department or operating room
- Findings on MRI are similar to those on CT

Basic Management

- Urgent/emergent otolaryngologist consultation
- Oxygen should be humidified, as it reduces the crusting of secretions that can precipitate airway blockage

- Heliox may be useful in decreasing airway resistance
- Antibiotics
- Cardiac monitoring and pulse oximetry
- Definitive airway preparation, including cricothyrotomy (adults) and needle cricothyrotomy (children)
- Steroids are often administered to reduce swelling and inflammation in the airway

Summary

TABLE 85.5: Advantages and disadvantages of imaging modalities in epiglottitis

Imaging modality	Advantages	Disadvantages
X-ray	Rapid Low radiation risk Findings frequently diagnostic	Limited diagnostic accuracy if patient cannot hyperextend neck
Laryngoscopy	Low cost Defines airway anatomy Rapid	Best performed in operating room setting Manipulation of epiglottis will worsen swelling
CT Scan	Availability Other diagnoses also possible	IV contrast Radiation exposure Patient stability
MRI	Noninvasive Other diagnoses also possible	Time-consuming Patient stability

86

Subcutaneous Abscesses

Jasmine Koita

Background

Subcutaneous abscesses are collections of pus located in the dermis or deeper skin tissues. Furuncles are infections of the hair follicle that extend deeper and cause small abscesses in the subcutaneous tissues. These can coalesce into carbuncles. Furuncles and carbuncles are usually seen in areas of friction and perspiration such as the axilla or buttocks.

Initially, the tissue becomes infected and inflamed through either a break in the skin or hematogenous spread of bacteria. The tissue is then walled off with vascular fibrous tissue and the infected tissue liquefies. Abscesses are usually polymicrobial, containing normal skin flora. Notably, methicillin-resistant *Staphylococcus aureus* (MRSA) is increasingly noted as a pathogen in abscesses.

Diagnosis of an abscess is usually a clinical diagnosis but imaging modalities such as x-ray, ultrasound, or CT can be helpful in unclear clinical pictures.

TABLE 86.1: Classic history and physical

Presents initially as a painful bump or erythematous patch of skin
Systemic symptoms such as fever
Erythematous fluctuant nodule
Pain to palpation
Central pustule surrounded by a rim of erythema
Spontaneously draining pustule

TABLE 86.2: Potentially helpful laboratory tests

CBC: Leukocytosis is nonspecific, but may provide support for active infection
Blood cultures: May be helpful in patients with systemic symptoms, but generally does not guide acute management

CBC, complete blood count.

Plain Radiographs

- Not a reliable imaging modality for abscess
- Often will be normal in spite of significant soft tissue abscesses
- Secondary signs may be seen such as an air-fluid level, periosteal reaction, reactive joint effusion, obliterated facial plane, or dystrophic calcification in a chronic abscess

 TABLE 86.3: X-ray: subcutaneous abscess

IV contrast	No
PO contrast	No
Amount of radiation	0.01 mSv (extremity)

Classic Images

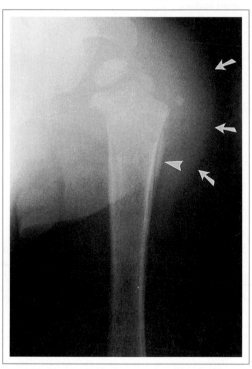

FIGURE 86.1: An abscess may not be visualized on x-ray; however, secondary signs such as soft tissue swelling (*arrows*) and lifting of the periosteum as a result of the infectious process (*arrowhead*) may be noted. (From Yochum TR and Rowe LJ. Yochum and Rowe's Essentials of Skeletal Radiology, 3rd ed. Philadelphia: Lippincott Williams & Wilkins, 2004.)

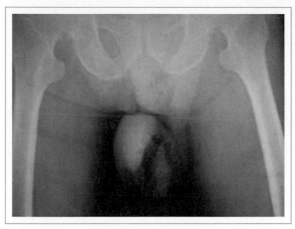

FIGURE 86.2: Pelvic x-ray of a left scrotal abscess with subcutaneous emphysema. (Reproduced with permission from Dr. El Fortia Mohamed, Department of Radiology, Misurata, Libya.)

Ultrasound

- In the emergency department, ultrasound can be the quickest and easiest imaging modality to visualize abscesses
- Ultrasound can be the most useful in differentiating between cellulitis and progression of the infection to an abscess
- A high-frequency linear probe (5–10 MHz) should be initially used but a low-frequency probe may be needed for deeper abscesses
- The probe should be positioned to scan over the area of greatest fluctuance
- The classic findings of abscess on ultrasound include an anechoic/hypoechoic fluid collection with irregular borders; septations may be seen inside the abscess cavity.
- An abscess is usually compressible, with swirling inside the abscess cavity when pressure is applied
- Posterior acoustic enhancement may be seen
- The sensitivity and specificity of clinical examination plus ultrasound for an abscess are 98% and 88%, respectively, with a positive-predictive value and negative-predictive value of 93% and 97%, respectively
- Color and power Doppler can assist with imaging, as the abscess wall may be vascular; proximity to vessels is also important when planning incision and drainage procedures
- Ultrasound can be used for real time guidance of incision and drainage
- The contralateral unaffected side can be evaluated to determine normal anatomy

Classic Images

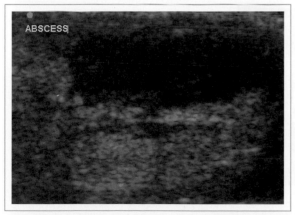

FIGURE 86.3: Ultrasound image demonstrating hypoechoic collection typical of abscess. (*Courtesy of Bret P. Nelson, MD, The Mount Sinai School of Medicine, New York, NY.*)

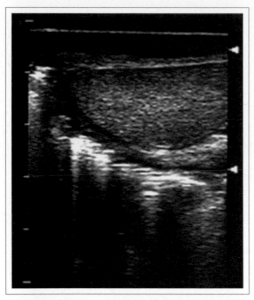

FIGURE 86.4: Left scrotal abscess with subcutaneous emphysema. Artifacts arise from air present within the soft tissues. (Reproduced with permission from Dr. El Fortia Mohamed, Department of Radiology, Misurata, Libya.)

CT Scan

- CT scanning is the most helpful in the evaluation of deep abscesses or those where borders are unclear
- IV contrast will improve the evaluation of inflamed tissue as well as vascular structures
- An abscess on CT scan will have a low-density center surrounded by a ring of higher density; the surrounding ring is made of granulation tissue and fibrosis and will enhance on contrast studies; septations within the abscess cavity may also enhance
- Tissue inflammation or cellulitis surrounding the abscess may be visible

 TABLE 86.4: CT scan: subcutaneous abscess

IV contrast	Yes, to evaluate abscess as well as nearby vascular structures
PO contrast	No, bowel not organ of interest
Amount of radiation	Variable depending on area of interest

Classic Images

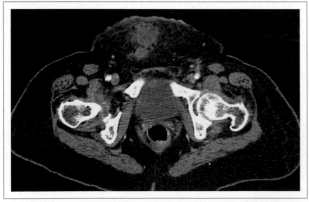

FIGURE 86.5: Contrast-enhanced CT scan of the abdomen demonstrating subcutaneous abscess and overlying cellulitis. (From Heiken JP, Menias CO, Elsayes K. Abdominal wall and peritoneal cavity. In: Lee JKT et al., ed. Computed Body Tomography with MRI Correlation. New York: Lippincott Williams & Wilkins, 2006, 1106.)

Basic Management

- Small furuncles can be treated with warm compresses and antibiotics
- The definitive management of abscesses and carbuncles is incision and drainage
- The cavity should be probed to open any loculations
- Antibiotics are not usually necessary except in cases with multiple lesions, cutaneous gangrene, impaired host defenses, extensive cellulitis, or systemic symptoms such as fever
- Ensure that tetanus is up to date

Summary

TABLE 86.5: Advantages and disadvantages of imaging modalities in subcutaneous abscesses

Imaging modality	Advantages	Disadvantages
X-ray	Quick and available Minimal radiation	Very poor test characteristics for abscess detection
Ultrasound	Bedside availability No radiation Excellent imaging Can guide procedures	Operator dependent Difficult to image deeper structures Body habitus limitations
CT	Availability Excellent imaging Can guide procedures	IV contrast Radiation

87

Cellulitis

Christopher Tainter

Background

Cellulitis is a bacterial infection of the deep dermal layer of skin and underlying subcutaneous tissue. It differs from erysipelas, which involves only the superficial dermis, and fasciitis or myositis, which involve the underlying fascial or muscle layers, respectively. It may occur on any part of the body, but most often affects the lower extremities. Gram-positive bacteria are implicated in about 80% of cases of cellulitis, most commonly beta-hemolytic streptococci, followed by staphylococcal species, and then gram negative organisms.

TABLE 87.1: Classic history and physical

Warm, erythematous with distinct borders
Fever may or may not be present
Often with associated vesicles, bullae, ecchymoses, petechiae
Edematous, may cause "peau d'orange" hair follicle dimpling
Look for inciting source (break in skin, venous insufficiency, onychomycosis, or toe web intertrigo)

TABLE 87.2: Potentially helpful laboratory tests

CBC: Nonspecific but leukocytosis may provide support for infection
Blood cultures: Not helpful, <5% sensitivity; may help direct antibiotic therapy for toxic patients

CBC, complete blood count.

Plain Radiograph
- Cellulitis is not apparent on plain radiography
- In some cases, it may be helpful to determine underlying pathology such as subcutaneous emphysema (gas-gangrene), osteomyelitis, or foreign body

 TABLE 87.3: X-ray: cellulitis

IV contrast	No
PO contrast	No
Amount of radiation	0.01 mSv

Classic Images

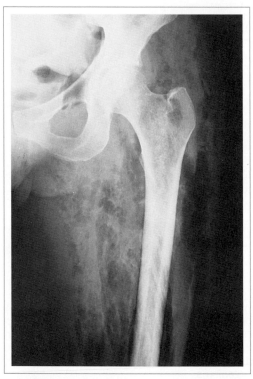

FIGURE 87.1: Gas gangrene, thigh. Observe the extensive radiographic presentation of subcutaneous emphysema (gas) scattered throughout the myofascial planes of the entire visualized portion of the hip and thigh. (*Courtesy of Bryan Hartley, MD, Melbourne, Australia.*) From Yochum TR and Rowe LJ. Yochum And Rowe's Essentials of Skeletal Radiology, 3rd ed. Philadelphia: Lippincott Williams & Wilkins, 2004.

CT Scan
- Cellulitis traditionally has the appearance of edema, stranding, and skin thickening; when IV contrast is used, hyperemic areas may enhance.
- It may be useful to evaluate for underlying foreign body, abscess, or DVT, especially in the limbs
- May help to distinguish cellulitis from other pathology, like myositis or fasciitis, though CT alone will not exclude these diagnoses

 TABLE 87.4: CT scan: cellulitis

IV contrast	Yes, helps to delineate vasculature and hyperemic areas may enhance
PO contrast	No, bowel not organ of interest
Amount of radiation	Variable depending on site

Classic Images

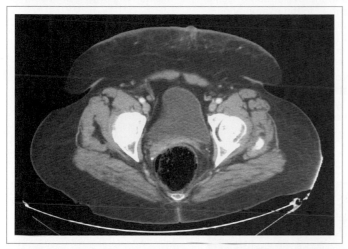

FIGURE 87.2: Abdominal CT image demonstrating abdominal wall cellulitis, with edema, stranding, and superficial skin thickening. (*Courtesy of The Department of Emergency Medicine, The Mount Sinai Hospital, New York, NY.*)

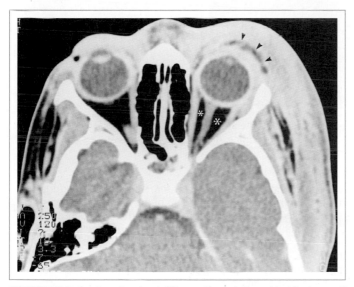

FIGURE 87.3: Axial postcontrast CT scan through the midorbits in a patient with a spider bite on the lower eyelid. CT shows extensive preseptal soft tissue swelling with extension over the left temporal scalp. There is reticulation of the subcutaneous fat and edema within the eyelid (*arrowheads*). The retro-orbital fat (*asterisks*) is of normal density. (From Harris JH, Jr., and Harris WH. The Radiology of Emergency Medicine, 4th ed. Philadelphia: Lippincott Williams & Wilkins, 2000.)

Bedside Ultrasound

- Bedside ultrasound can be used in the evaluation of cellulitis to exclude underlying abscess, which may not be readily apparent on initial examination
- Able to visualize many foreign bodies
- Use a high-frequency transducer (7.5 MHz or higher)
- May need lower frequency transducer to evaluate deep abscesses
- May see classical features of interstitial edema, including increased echogenicity (seen early) and cobblestoning (separation from hyperechoic fat lobules and hypoechoic interstitial fluid)
- Comparing the contralateral unaffected side may be useful in determining anatomy
- A stand-off pad or water bath may be used to visualize very superficial structures; it may also be more comfortable for the patient as there is less probe contact with the affected area

Classic Images

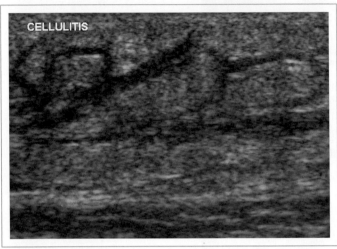

FIGURE 87.4: Ultrasound image of cellulitis, demonstrating interstitial edema causing "cobblestoning" effect. (*Courtesy of Bret P. Nelson, MD, The Mount Sinai School of Medicine, New York, NY.*)

Basic Management

- Evaluation of patients with cellulitis should include evaluation for more concerning underlying pathology such as fasciitis or myositis, foreign body, abscess, and deep venous thrombosis
- Assess patient for comorbidities or complicating factors that may direct therapy such as diabetes, immunocompromised state, lymphatic or venous insufficiency, or bite or marine animal injuries
- In almost every case, antibiotic therapy is indicated
- In toxic-appearing patients, IV antibiotic treatment and surgical consult should be initiated immediately; these patients generally require admission
- Laboratory test results are generally not helpful, but blood cultures may help guide antibiotic therapy in patients with systemic toxicity
- Pain management and elevation of the affected area when applicable
- Nonsteroidal anti-inflammatory medications help reduce inflammation and may improve symptoms as well.
- Ensure that tetanus immunization status is up-to-date

Summary

TABLE 87.5: Advantages and disadvantages of imaging modalities in cellulitis

Imaging modality	Advantages	Disadvantages
X-ray	Low cost, readily available May help diagnose osteomyelitis, gas gangrene, or foreign body	Unable to visualize soft tissues Poor sensitivity
CT scan	May visualize myositis, fasciitis, abscess, deep vein thrombosis (DVT), or foreign body	Radiation exposure Cost IV contrast in some cases
Ultrasound	Low cost Minimal patient discomfort No radiation Bedside availability, rapid May visualize abscess, foreign body	Availability of ultrasound Body habitus limitations Unable to exclude other serious underlying pathology

88

Foreign Body

Shefali Trivedi

Background

Soft tissue foreign bodies are a common and varied source of referrals to the emergency department. The causes range from deliberate to accidental, and the risks range from benign to deadly. The diagnosis of foreign bodies may be difficult if not visible to the eye and further imaging, including plain radiography, CT, or ultrasound, may be necessary. Retained soft tissue foreign bodies are a common cause of malpractice claims as well as morbidity from infectious complications. The majority of retained soft tissue foreign bodies are in pediatric patients and when the hands or feet are involved.

TABLE 88.1: Classic history and physical

Puncture or projectile injury
Puncture(s) through skin
Visible, palpable, or nonpalpable foreign body
Work-related mishap (pressure injector, nail gun, blast injury, etc.)
Region of redness or associated inflammatory changes
Skin tenting or edema

Ultrasound

- A high-frequency (7–10 MHz) linear probe provides high-resolution imaging of superficial soft tissue structures and foreign bodies
- The unaffected contralateral side should be imaged for comparison anatomy
- Image the area of interest in two planes/views
- Foreign bodies generally give a localized, hyperechoic signal with posterior shadowing
- Wooden and metallic foreign bodies can cause a reverberation artifact
- The foreign bodies may have a hypoechoic halo caused by edema, abscess, or granulation tissue
- A water bath or standoff pad may be used to image very superficial structures, as this increases the focal length between the probe and the object of interest and optimizing the image on the screen
- A water bath may be more comfortable for the patient, as there is less direct contact with the inflamed area

Classic Images

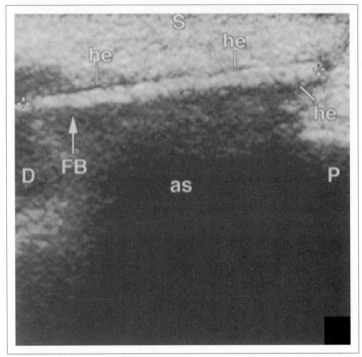

FIGURE 88.1: Hyperechoic foreign body (FB) in superficial soft tissue. Note the acoustic shadowing beyond the FB. (From Cosby KS and Kendall JL. The Practical Guide to Emergency Ultrasound. Philadelphia: Lippincott Williams & Wilkins, 2005.)

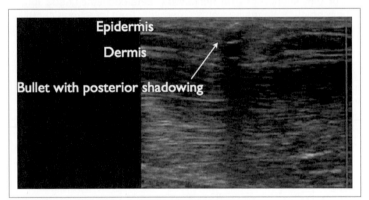

FIGURE 88.2: Superficial soft tissue foreign body with shadowing. (*Courtesy of Resa E. Lewiss, MD, Department of Emergency Medicine, St. Luke's Roosevelt Hospital, New York, NY.*)

X-Ray

- Materials that are visible on plain films include glass of all types, metallic objects (except aluminum), most animal bones and some large fish bones, some foods, mineral fragments, and some drugs (including chloral hydrate, heavy metals, iodides, phenothiazines, enteric coated pills, solvents)

- Materials that are not well visualized on plain films include most foods and drugs, most small fish bones, most wood, splinters, thorns, most plastics, and most aluminum objects
- Multiple views (anteroposterior and lateral or oblique) can increase the likelihood of foreign body visualization as well as localization

 TABLE 88.2: X-ray: foreign body

IV contrast	No
PO contrast	No
Amount of radiation	0.01 mSv (extremity)

Classic Images

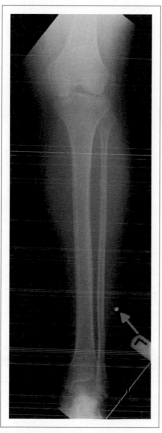

FIGURE 88.3: AP x-ray demonstrating BB in soft tissue lateral to left fibula (*arrow*). (*Courtesy of Bret Nelson, MD, Department of Emergency Medicine, Mt. Sinai Hospital, New York, NY.*)

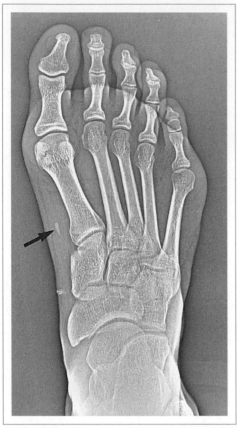

FIGURE 88.4: Glass foreign body, foot (*arrow*). (From Yochum TR and Rowe LJ. Essentials of Skeletal Radiology, 3rd ed. Philadelphia: Lippincott Williams & Wilkins, 2004.)

CT Scan

- CT can often identify objects that are radiolucent on plain radiography
- CT can also provide further information by indicating local anatomy, tissue reactions, abscess formation, and orientation of the foreign body

 TABLE 88.3: CT scan: foreign body

IV contrast	No, not necessary but will give information about surrounding tissue inflammation
PO contrast	No, bowel not organ of interest
Amount of radiation	Variable depending on site

Classic Images

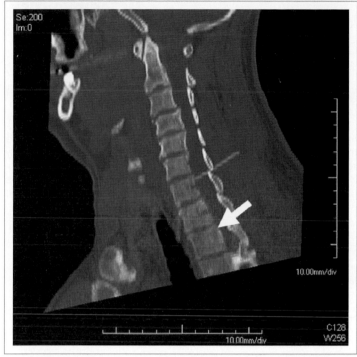

FIGURE 88.5: Sagittal reconstruction of acupuncture needle piercing soft tissues of the neck toward the cervical spine (*arrow*). (*Courtesy of Bret Nelson, MD, Department of Emergency Medicine, Mt. Sinai Hospital, New York, NY.*)

Basic Management

- Evaluate and document the neurovascular status of tissue involved, i.e., strength, sensation, capillary refill, pulses, etc.
- Consider imaging in cases where the entire foreign body is not well visualized or there is concern for additional trauma, infection, or multiple foreign bodies
- Consider repeat imaging after foreign body removal for documentation.
- Adequately irrigate and explore all wounds with good lighting
- Ensure that tetanus immunization status is up-to-date
- Consider prompt removal of foreign bodies that are painful, causing infection, or are made of noninert material (organic matter)
- Further imaging and surgical consultation are options for complex foreign bodies or in patients at higher risk of complications (diabetes, immunocompromised state, extremes of age, etc.)
- Consider prophylactic antibiotics for complex cases
- Empiric antibiotic treatment for infected foreign body cases

Summary

TABLE 88.4: Advantages and disadvantages of imaging modalities for subcutaneous foreign bodies

Imaging modality	Advantages	Disadvantages
Ultrasound	Low cost Minimal patient discomfort No radiation Bedside availability Less time consuming	Availability of ultrasound in the department of radiology Body habitus limitations Operator dependent
X-ray	Availability Low cost	Radiolucent foreign bodies Radiation exposure
CT scan	Availability Generally the most sensitive and specific test Evaluation of abscess, other complications	Increased cost Radiation exposure

89

Osteomyelitis

Mieka Close

Background

Osteomyelitis is an infection localized to bone that occurs as a result of hematogenous seeding, contiguous spread from adjacent soft tissues or joints, or direct inoculation from trauma or surgery. In children, the long bones are most often affected and osteomyelitis is most likely caused by hematogenous spread. The vertebrae are more commonly affected in adults. Contiguous spread occurs in younger patients as a result of trauma or surgery, and in older patients as a complication of decubitus ulcers or infected total joint arthroplasties. Osteomyelitis may be acute or chronic.

TABLE 89.1: Classic history and physical

Gradual onset of dull pain at affected site
Nonhealing ulcer, e.g., heel and sacrum
Sickle cell disease
Fever, rigors
Local tenderness, warmth, erythema, edema

TABLE 89.2: Potentially helpful laboratory test results

CBC: Leukocytosis
Erythrocyte sedimentation rate: Elevated, may be used to follow disease course
C-reactive protein: Elevated, may be used to follow disease course
Blood cultures (evaluate for hematogenous spread)

CBC, complete blood count.

X-Ray

- In early infection, findings may be subtle or absent. The earliest osseous change may be osteopenia and may take 1–2 weeks to become evident
- In chronic osteomyelitis, findings include cortical erosion, periosteal reaction, mixed lucency, and sclerosis
- Soft tissue swelling may be evident, particularly if cellulitis or abscess is present
- In patients with orthopedic hardware, fracture nonunion or periprosthetic lucency, suggesting loosening of hardware, may be apparent

 TABLE 89.3: X-ray: osteomyelitis

IV contrast	No
PO contrast	No
Amount of radiation	Variable depending on site

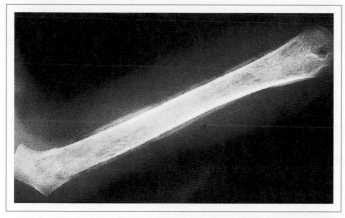

FIGURE 89.1: Radiograph of pediatric patient with osteomyelitis, demonstrating periosteal elevation and bony erosions. (From Fleisher GR, Ludwig S, and Baskin MN. Atlas of Pediatric Emergency Medicine. Philadelphia: Lippincott Williams & Wilkins, 2004.)

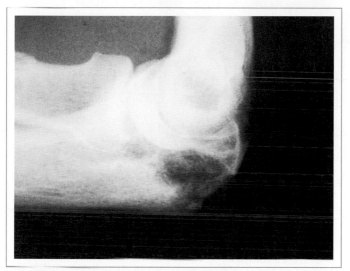

FIGURE 89.2: Radial osteomyelitis due to *Mycobacterium gordonae* group mycobacteria in a 47-year-old Caucasian man with chronic bursitis and intra-articular corticosteroid injections. (From Koopman WJ and Moreland LW. Arthritis and Allied Conditions: A Textbook of Rheumatology, 15th ed. Philadelphia: Lippincott Williams & Wilkins, 2005.)

Ultrasonography

- Although the physical properties of bone block ultrasound waves, ultrasound may be useful in demonstrating inflammatory changes superficial to cortical bone, such as periosteal thickening or pus exuding from bone as a subperiosteal collection
- Bone is typically bright white/hyperechoic; look for heterogeneity in bony cortex
- Look for cobble-stone changes in soft tissue superficial to the bony cortex suggesting soft tissue infection
- Look for a hypoechoic fluid collection superficial to the bony cortex consistent with periosteal reaction/fluid accumulation
- Ultrasound is more useful in pediatric patients in whom the periosteum is less adherent to the cortex
- This modality is helpful in the diagnosis of osteomyelitis in the setting of sickle cell disease

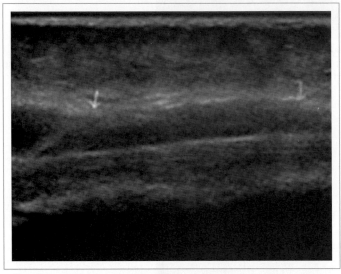

FIGURE 89.3: Sagittal view of focal subperiosteal collection over proximal tibial metaphysic (*arrows*). (From Mason LW, Carpenter EC, Morris E, and Davies J. Varicella zoster associated osteomyelitis. *Internet J Orthopedic Surg.* 11: 2009; 1.)

MRI

- MRI has high sensitivity and negative predictive value in the diagnosis of osteomyelitis
- Bone marrow edema may be evident on MRI 3–5 days following the onset of infection; however, this is a nonspecific finding and diagnosis must be based on the clinical picture
- MRI is the preferred imaging modality for suspected osteomyelitis of the vertebrae and of the foot in the case of diabetic ulcers
- Gadolinium contrast-enhanced MRI is helpful in the diagnosis of osteomyelitis complications, including sinus tracts, fistulas, abscesses, and vertebral discitis
- In vertebral osteomyelitis, T1-weighted images may demonstrate decreased signal intensity in the disk and adjacent vertebral bodies, as well as loss of endplate definition; similarly, T2-weighted images may demonstrate increased signal intensity in the disk and adjacent vertebral bodies

 TABLE 89.4: MRI: osteomyelitis

IV contrast	Yes, useful in diagnosis of complications of osteomyelitis
PO contrast	No, bowel not organ of interest
Amount of radiation	None

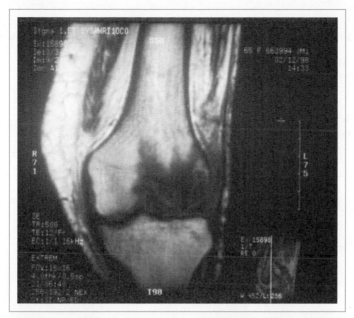

FIGURE 89.4: MRI of osteomyelitis of the femur. T1-weighted image demonstrating low-signal intensity. (From Koopman WJ and Moreland LW. Arthritis and Allied Conditions: A Textbook of Rheumatology, 15th ed. Philadelphia: Lippincott Williams & Wilkins, 2005.)

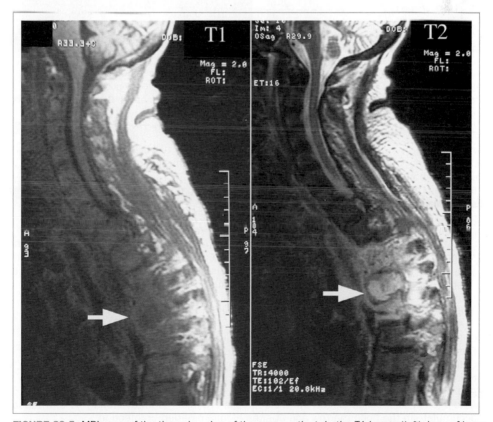

FIGURE 89.5: MRI scan of the thoracic spine of the same patient. In the T1 image (*left*), loss of bony structure in a vertebra is seen (*arrow*). In the T2 image (*right*), the high-signal intensity owing to water molecules shows edema and infiltrate in the same vertebra. (From Engleberg NC, Dermody T, and DiRita V. Schaecter's Mechanisms of Microbial Disease, 4th ed. Baltimore: Lippincott Williams & Wilkins, 2007.)

CT Scan

- CT findings in osteomyelitis include periosteal reaction, intraosseous gas, and the presence of sinus tracts
- CT is helpful in patients in whom MRI is contraindicated
- Metallic hardware may cause artifact, limiting the value of CT in these patients
- IV contrast-enhanced imaging is useful in the demonstration of adjacent soft tissue infection

 TABLE 89.5: CT scan: osteomyelitis

IV contrast	Yes, to evaluate for adjacent soft tissue inflammation
PO contrast	No, bowel not organ of interest
Amount of radiation	Variable

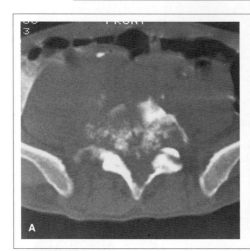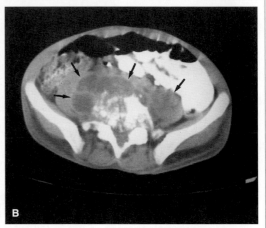

FIGURE 89.6: CT image of vertebral osteomyelitis and paraspinous abscess. **A:** Image demonstrating destructive process of L5 and paraspinal soft tissue mass anterior to vertebral body. **B:** IV contrast-enhanced image demonstrating multilocular abscess (*arrows*). (From Daffner RH. Clinical Radiology: The Essentials, 3rd ed. Philadelphia: Lippincott Williams & Wilkins, 2007.)

Nuclear Imaging

- Nuclear imaging studies are typically not performed in the emergency setting.
- Three-phase bone scan:
  - In this modality, a radionuclide tracer (technetium) accumulates in areas of bone turnover and increased osteoblast activity. A gamma camera is used to image the bone at three points after injection of tracer. In osteomyelitis, there is an intense uptake in all three phases (including the osseous phase) 4 hours after injection.
  - Sensitivity and specificity vary depending on radiographic findings. In the setting of normal radiographs, a positive bone scan approaches 95% sensitivity and specificity. False-positive results are more likely in the setting of radiographs showing noninfectious findings (fracture, Charcot arthropathy). Early osteomyelitis may result in a false-negative scan.
- Gallium scans:
  - In this modality, areas of inflammation are demonstrated by the affinity of gallium-67 to certain acute-phase reactants.
  - Gallium scans have a very high negative predictive value.
  - False positives may occur in the setting of fracture or neoplasm.
  - Gallium scans may be used in combination with a technetium-labeled three-phase bone scan to improve specificity.
- Tagged white blood cell scan:
  - Autologous radionuclide-tagged white blood cells are injected intravenously so that these accumulate in the bone marrow and at sites of inflammation or infection.
  - As with other nuclear modalities, specificity decreases in the setting of abnormal radiographic studies.
  - False-negative results can occur in chronic osteomyelitis.

TABLE 89.6: Bone scan: osteomyelitis

IV contrast	Yes, tracer used in nuclear imaging
PO contrast	No, bowel not organ of interest
Amount of radiation	6.3 mSv

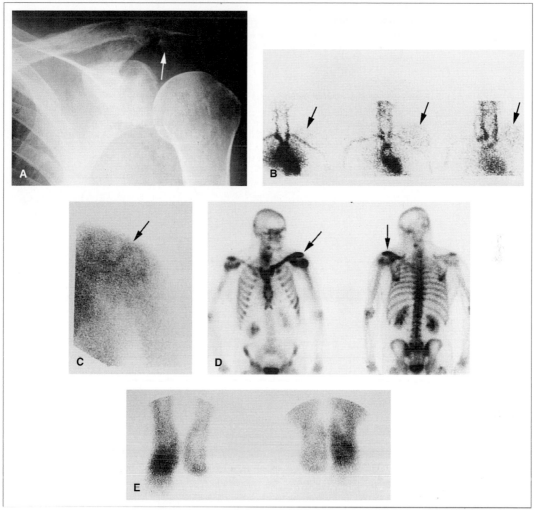

FIGURE 89.7: Radiographic and three-phase bone scan images of osteomyelitis of the shoulder. **A:** Radiograph demonstrating destruction and debris involving the acromioclavicular joint. **B:** Angiogram phase of bone scan showing increased vascular perfusion of left shoulder. **C:** Blood pool phase of bone scan showing increased tracer activity in left shoulder, indicating hyperemia. **D:** Delayed phase of bone scan demonstrating increased tracer activity in clavicle and acromioclavicular and glenohumeral joints, suggesting osteomyelitis. **E:** Bone Scan, Dorsal (Left) and Plantar (Right) Bilateral Foot. Observe the diffuse increased tracer activity in the right midfoot and forefoot, consistent with osteomyelitis. (*Courtesy of Michael A. Fox, MD, Memphis, TN.*) From Yochum TR and Rowe LJ. Yochum and Rowe's Essentials of Skeletal Radiology, 3rd ed. Philadelphia: Lippincott Williams & Wilkins, 2004.

Basic Management

- Surgical consultation for debridement of necrotic tissue, hardware placement or removal, and/ or revascularization
- Parenteral broad spectrum antimicrobial therapy
- Inpatient admission
- Hyperbaric oxygen and/or vacuum-assisted closure may be helpful in refractory osteomyelitis

Summary

TABLE 89.7: Advantages and disadvantages of imaging modalities in osteomyelitis

Imaging modality	Advantages	Disadvantages
X-ray	Useful in chronic osteomyelitis Inexpensive Low radiation exposure	Limited sensitivity and specificity
Ultrasonography	Excellent in the setting of sickle cell disease Helpful in pediatric patients No radiation exposure	Limited use in the imaging of adults
MRI	Preferred in evaluation of the vertebrae and osteomyelitis from diabetic foot infection No radiation exposure	Limited specificity Expensive Limited availability Contraindicated in patients with metallic implants
CT	Assesses complications of osteomyelitis	Radiation exposure Metallic hardware may cause artifact
Nuclear imaging	High negative predictive value	Limited specificity in setting of positive radiographic findings Time-consuming Not routinely available in ED

Section Editor: David Cherkas

90

Spine Trauma

Leah Honigman, Jeffrey P. Spear, and Carlo L. Rosen

Background

Spine trauma encompasses a wide range of injuries, from stable fractures to devastating spinal cord injury (SCI). Blunt trauma is the most common cause of SCI, typically resulting from motor vehicle collisions, falls, intentional violence, and sports-related activities. Approximately 3% of patients with blunt trauma have an injury to their spinal column. The cervical spine is the most frequently injured, affecting 11,000 Americans per year. The next most commonly injured area is the thoracolumbar junction, and 90% of the injuries to the thoracolumbar region occur between T11 and L4. Thoracic spine injuries are the least common. High-risk populations, including the elderly, patients on corticosteroids, and those with a history of metastatic cancer or other intrinsic spine diseases are predisposed to injury due to weakened bone or anatomic bony changes that make the cord more vulnerable. These patients should be carefully evaluated for spinal column injury, even with relatively minor trauma. It is also important to recognize that the cord can be injured in the absence of radiographic abnormality, a situation known as SCIWORA (spinal cord injury without radiographic abnormality).

TABLE 90.1: Classic history and physical

History of trauma mechanism
Neck or back pain and focal tenderness on examination
New onset of neurological deficits
Respiratory distress from C-spine injury
Risk factors for osteoporosis or neoplasm

TABLE 90.2: Potentially helpful laboratory tests

Urine or serum HCG: determine pregnancy status prior to imaging
BUN and creatinine: Evaluate renal function in event that IV contrast is needed

Cervical Spine

- Risk stratification: low risk patients can be identified by the NEXUS and Canadian C-spine Rules to determine those patients who do not need radiographic injuries (both rules have a high negative predictive value and can safely limit radiographic studies in certain populations)
- All patients who cannot be clinically cleared require radiographic evaluation
- The clinician should determine stability but assume unstable injury until radiographic proof is otherwise

TABLE 90.3: The NEXUS rule*

- No midline cervical tenderness
- No focal neurologic deficits
- Normal alertness
- No intoxication
- No painful distracting injury

*If all five criteria are met, patients are considered low risk and do not require imaging. From Hoffman et al. Validity of a Set of clinical criteria to rule out injury to the cervical spine in patients with blunt trauma. *N Engl J Med* 343: 2000; 94–99.

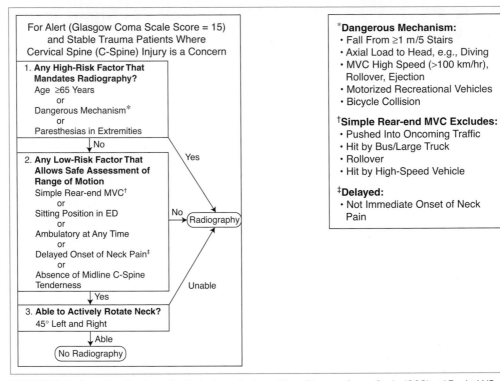

FIGURE 90.1: Canadian C-spine rule. Exclusion criteria: <16 yr, Glasgow Coma Scale (GCS) <15, abnl VS, injury >48-hr old, penetrating trauma, acute paralysis, known vertebral disease (ankylosing spondylitis, RA, spinal stenosis, or prev cervical surgery), return for same injury, or pregnant. (Redrawn from Stiell et al. The Canadian C-Spine rule for radiography in alert and stable trauma patients. *JAMA* 286(15): 2001; 1841–1848.)

Plain Films
- Readily available, quick, and portable
- Cervical spine:
  - three-view series—lateral, anteroposterior, and odontoid
  - requires correct exposure and positioning for adequate C-spine films—from base of skull to top of first thoracic vertebra; if incomplete or inadequate films, not possible to exclude injury
  - sensitivity of cervical x-ray is 90%
- Thoracolumbar:
  - Presence of one vertebral fracture mandates radiographic evaluation of the entire spine due to the high likelihood of other injuries
  - Sensitivity is 73% and specificity is 100%
- Sensitive in detecting the presence of injury, but often does not identify the specific injury
- Look for:
  - misalignment of the spinal column
  - soft tissue contour changes
- If plain films are abnormal, CT scan is necessary

TABLE 90.4: Plain films: spine trauma

IV contrast	No
PO contrast	No
Amount of radiation	0.2 mSv per view

Classic Images

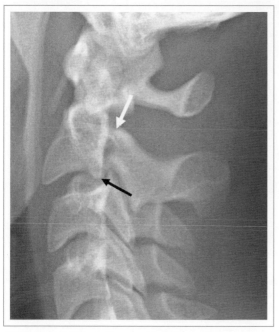

FIGURE 90.2: Traumatic spondylolisthesis (type 1) "Hangman fracture," bilateral fractures of par interarticularis, classified based on displacement of posterior ring and extreme hyperextension from abrupt deceleration. (From Schwartz ED and Flanders AE, eds. Spinal Trauma: Imaging, Diagnosis, and Management. Philadelphia: Lippincott Williams & Wilkins, 2007.)

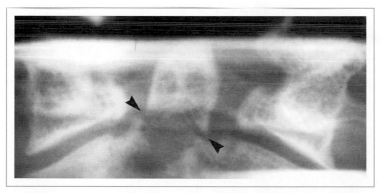

FIGURE 90.3: Type II dens fracture. From forceful flexion or extension of the head. (From Harris J and Harris W. The Radiology of Emergency Medicine, 4th ed. Philadelphia: Lippincott Williams & Wilkins, 2000.)

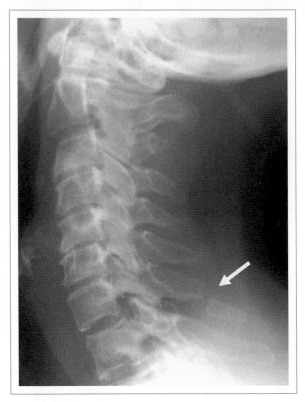

FIGURE 90.4: Spinous process fracture, C6. "Clay shoveler's fracture" results in avulsion fracture of spinous process from direct trauma or forced flexion. (From Schwartz ED, Flanders AE, eds. Spinal Trauma: Imaging, Diagnosis, and Management. Philadelphia: Lippincott Williams & Wilkins, 2007.)

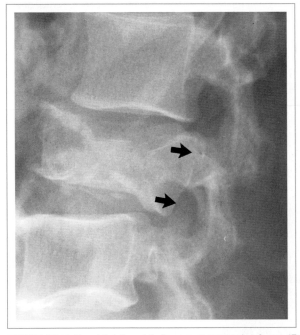

FIGURE 90.5: Burst fracture L1. From a compressive force. (From Harris J and Harris W. The Radiology of Emergency Medicine, 4th ed. Philadelphia: Lippincott Williams & Wilkins, 2000.)

Non-contrast CT Scan

- Has become the primary initial modality for screening spinal column injury after trauma in moderate to high risk patients
- Very sensitive (98%) and specific (97%) for bony injury, with a negative predictive value approaching 100%
- Should include coronal and sagittal reconstructions to increase sensitivity
- Injuries missed by CT include fractures of the dens, dislocations, or subluxations in the plane of the scanner, especially in older scanners
- Misses SCIWORA
- Similar in overall cost to plain films

 TABLE 90.5: CT scan: spine

IV contrast	No
PO contrast	No
Amount of radiation	6 mSv

Classic Images

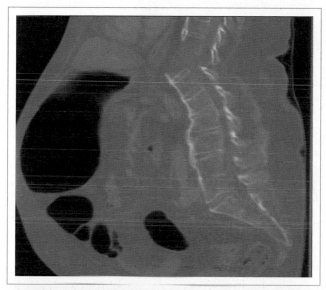

FIGURE 90.6: Complete fragmentation of the T11 vertebral body, with 60 degree anterior angulation and anterior distraction of the inferior elements. (*Courtesy of BIDMC PACS.*)

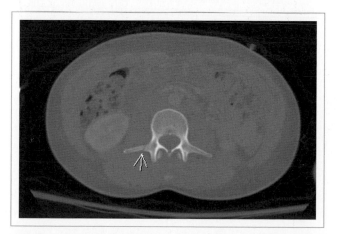

FIGURE 90.7: Minimally displaced right L3 transverse process fracture. (*Courtesy of BIDMC PACS.*)

MRI

- Best for soft tissue injuries as well as injury to the spinal cord, intervertebral disks, and paracervical tissues including ligaments
- Bony injuries often missed
- Helpful if pain or neurologic findings persist with negative plain films and CT
- Important in evaluation of occipitoatlantal subluxations and anterior subluxations
- Useful in patients with SCIWORA

TABLE 90.6: MRI: spine

IV contrast	No
PO contrast	No
Amount of radiation	None

Classic Images

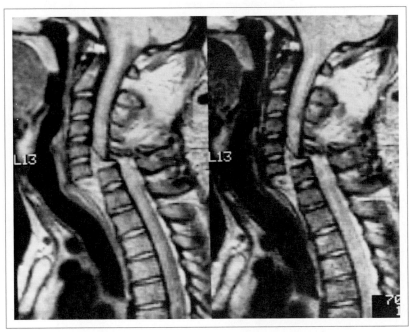

FIGURE 90.8: Fracture dislocation of C6–7 (MRI). (From Harris J and Harris W. The Radiology of Emergency Medicine, 4th ed. Philadelphia: Lippincott Williams & Wilkins, 2000.)

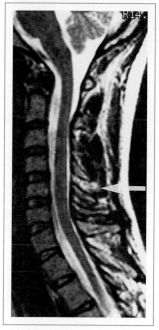

FIGURE 90.9: Anterior subluxation with ligamentous injury at C4–5. T2-weighted imaged with high-intensity signal showing damage to posterior ligament complex (*arrow*). (From Harris J and Harris W. The Radiology of Emergency Medicine, 4th ed. Philadelphia: Lippincott Williams & Wilkins, 2000.)

Basic Management

- Address ABCs
- Keep the patient in collar and on log roll precautions until spine is clinically or radiographically cleared
- Secure airway and maintain cervical spine precautions if the patient requires intubation and mechanical ventilation
- Maintain a high index of suspicion in all trauma patients for an injury to the spinal column or spinal cord
- Baseline neurologic evaluation
- Evaluate for other life-threatening conditions
- Assume unstable spine injury until proven otherwise
- Supportive care
- Evaluate for neurogenic shock; however, it is a diagnosis of exclusion and other etiologies of shock must be considered first
- Insertion of Foley catheter since patients with thoracic/lumbar/sacral injury often have urinary retention
- Consultation with a spine specialist or neurosurgeon if injury is present or suspected

Summary

TABLE 90.7: Advantages and disadvantages of imaging modalities in spine trauma

Imaging modality	Advantages	Disadvantages
Plain film	Rapid Portable	Low sensitivity compared to CT Can miss fractures Misses SCIWORA
CT scan	Widespread availability Rapid Highly sensitive Relatively low cost	Radiation Misses SCIWORA
MRI	Soft tissue injuries Images the cord well No radiation	Misses bony injuries Lengthy study time

SCIWORA, spinal cord injury without radiographic abnormality.

91

C1 (Atlas) Fractures

M. Tyson Pillow

Background

C1, or atlas fractures, make up approximately 2–13% of cervical fractures. There are two types of C1 fractures that can occur: burst fractures and posterior arch fractures.

Burst fractures, also known as Jefferson fractures, occur with vertical compression, or less commonly, hyperextension injuries that drive the lateral masses outward. Classically, this will lead to a four-part break in the anterior and posterior arches, but can also result in a two- or three-part fracture. These fractures can involve the transverse ligament and are considered unstable based on the extent of injury to the ligament. These fractures are very rare in children.

TABLE 91.1: Classic history and physical of burst fractures

Neck pain (usually without neurologic symptoms)
Diving into shallow water
Severe motor vehicle accidents, especially rollovers
Fall from playground equipment (pediatric)

Posterior arch fractures result from compression injury of the posterior neural arch between the occiput and spinous process of C2, usually from forced hyperextension. They are more common than burst fractures. These injuries are generally considered stable because the anterior arch and transverse ligaments are intact, but spinal cord injury is possible if there is significant anterior displacement (>1 cm).

TABLE 91.2: Associated injuries

Approximately, 50% of atlas fractures are associated with some other cervical spine fracture
Approximately, 33% of atlas fractures are associated with C2 (axis) fractures
Paralysis or lateral medullary syndrome from vertebral artery damage (extremely rare)

C-spine X-ray

- Standard views are AP, lateral, and open-mouth odontoid views
- Fracture may be difficult to identify on plain films if there is only minimal displacement
- C1 and C2 fractures are the most commonly missed fractures on plain radiographs

Burst Fractures

- Odontoid view:
  - The odontoid view may demonstrate the masses of C1 lateral to the outer margins of the articular pillars of C2
  - The transverse ligament is likely to be ruptured if the lateral displacement is >7 mm in adults
  - Overlapping lateral masses can be a normal variant in children and so this view cannot completely assess for stability
- Lateral view:
  - May show a widened predental space (between C1 and the dens)
  - Greater than 3 mm predental space in adults or 5 mm predental space in pediatric patients is considered abnormal
  - Greater than 6 mm pre-dental space in adults is considered to be transverse ligament rupture and considered unstable
- Flexion/extension view:
  - Atlantodental space of >3 mm indicates instability
  - Use is controversial and may only be of limited value

Posterior Arch Fractures
- Very difficult to visualize on odontoid views
- Lateral views may demonstrate the fracture line through the posterior arch

 TABLE 91.3: Plain film: cervical spine

IV contrast	No
PO contrast	No
Amount of radiation	0.2 mSv per view

Classic Images

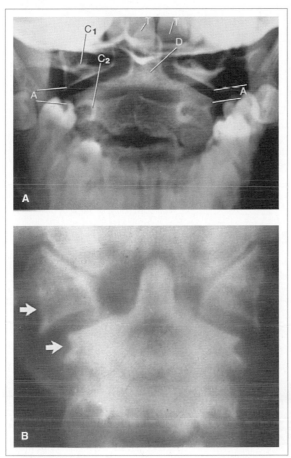

FIGURE 91.1: A: Normal anteroposterior (AP) (open-mouth, odontoid) view of C1 and C2. C1, first cervical vertebra (lateral mass); C2, second cervical vertebra; T, central incisors overlying dens D; A, normal relationship between lateral mass of C1 and vertebral body of C2. **B:** Jefferson fracture in AP view. Note the lateral offset of C1. (From Fleisher GR, Ludwig S, and Baskin MN. Atlas of Pediatric Emergency Medicine. Philadelphia: Lippincott Williams & Wilkins, 2004.)

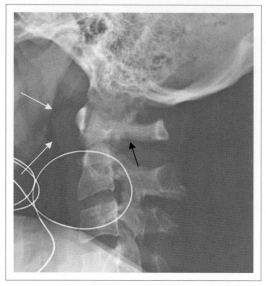

FIGURE 91.2: Jefferson fracture. Lateral radiograph shows soft tissue swelling anterior to C1 and the upper margin of C2 (*white arrows*). A fracture of the posterior C1 arch (*black arrow*), representing a part of a Jefferson fracture, is identified. Normal anterior atlantoaxial distance is noted. (From Schwartz ED and Flander AE. Spinal Trauma: Imaging, Diagnosis, and Management. Philadelphia: Lippincott Williams & Wilkins, 2007.)

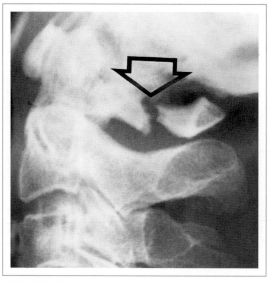

FIGURE 91.3: Isolated fracture of the posterior arch of C1. (From Harris J and Harris W. The Radiology of Emergency Medicine, 4th ed. Philadelphia: Lippincott Williams & Wilkins, 2000.)

Cervical Spine CT Scan

- CT scan of the C-spine will provide much more information about bony structures than plain radiographs
- CT can detect small ligament avulsion fractures better than x-ray
- If injury to C1 is suspected, a dedicated CT scan of C1 may be indicated

 TABLE 91.4: CT scan: cervical spine

IV contrast	No
PO contrast	No
Amount of radiation	3 mSv

Classic Images

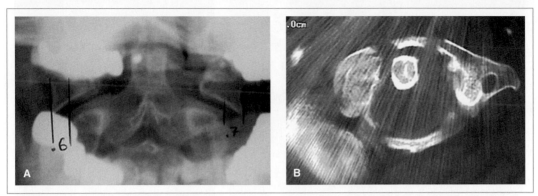

FIGURE 91.4: The open-mouth odontoid view shows a bilateral C1 lateral mass overhang relative to the C2 facets. As measured on the radiograph, the combined overhang amounts to 13 mm (**A**). The axial CT scan shows a true Jefferson fracture in the form of a four-part burst fracture of the atlas (**B**). This fracture is unstable due to traumatic transverse atlantal ligament disruption. (From Bucholz RW and Heckman JD. Rockwood & Green's Fractures in Adults, 5th ed. Lippincott, Williams & Wilkins, 2001.)

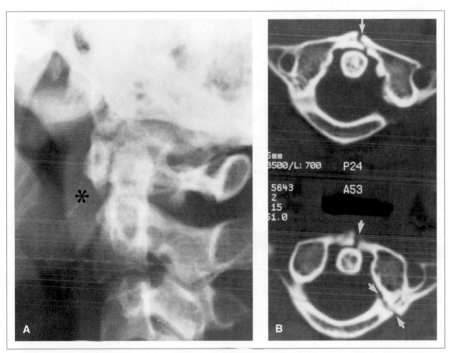

FIGURE 91.5: Eccentric Jefferson bursting fracture (JBF). The cervicocranial skeleton is normal on the contact lateral radiograph (**A**). The only abnormality on this examination is the convex prevertebral soft tissue contour (*asterisk*), which is consistent with a retropharyngeal hematoma in a posttrauma patient complaining of severe high neck pain and painful limitation of motion. The abnormal prevertebral soft tissue contour required further evaluation by CT, which demonstrated an eccentric JBF (*arrows,* **B**) caused by lateral tilt or vertical compression modified by left lateral tilt. (From Harris J and Harris W. The Radiology of Emergency Medicine, 4th ed. Philadelphia: Lippincott Williams & Wilkins, 2000.)

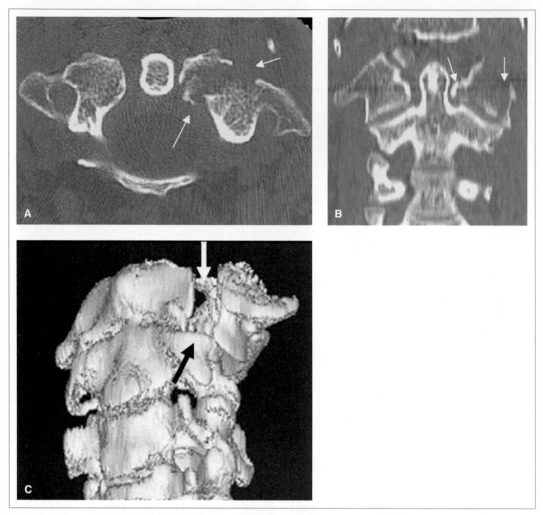

FIGURE 91.6: Lateral mass C1 fracture. **A:** Axial CT image shows a comminuted left lateral mass fracture of C1 (*arrows*) caused by lateral tilt. **B:** Coronal CT multiplanar reformation clearly demonstrates a comminuted fracture of the left lateral mass of C1 (*arrows*). **C:** Three-dimensional surface rendered frontal oblique view also demonstrates the left lateral mass of C1 fracture with fragment displacement (*arrows*). (From Schwartz ED and Flander AE. Spinal Trauma: Imaging, Diagnosis, and Management. Philadelphia: Lippincott Williams & Wilkins, 2007.)

MRI
- MRI is the study of choice to detect ligament instability or assess the spinal cord when there are associated neurologic deficits
- Must wait for radiologist to interpret study and determine results

Classic Images

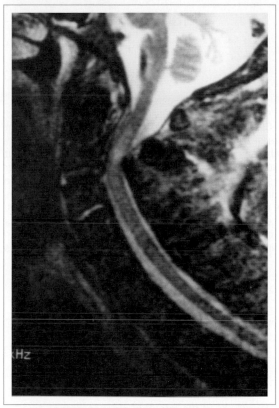

FIGURE 91.7: Sagittal T2-weighted MR image demonstrates mechanical impingement on the posterior aspect of the cervical spinal cord at the C2-C3 level. High signal in the cord itself indicates contusion. (From Chew FS. Musculoskeletal Imaging: A Teaching File. Philadelphia: Lippincott Williams & Wilkins, 2006.)

Basic Management

- Keep the cervical spine immobilized and in neutral position until fractures and injuries can be assessed
- Always evaluate the patient for concomitant spinal fractures and injuries
- Pain management with narcotic analgesics as needed
- Neurosurgical and/or orthopedic consultation as necessary
- Patients with a negative CT scan but persistent pain should have further imaging (i.e., MRI) or be discharged with a cervical collar and neurosurgical follow-up

Summary

TABLE 91.5: Advantages and disadvantages of imaging modalities in C1 fractures

Imaging modality	Advantages	Disadvantages
Plain films	Minimal radiation exposure Fast Inexpensive	Difficult to visualize C1 May miss minimally displaced fractures Moderate sensitivity
CT scan	Identifies bony structures much better than plain films Increased sensitivity	Radiation exposure Cannot visualize ligaments
MRI	No radiation Identifies soft tissue structures as well as spinal cord injuries	Expensive Time-consuming Not always readily accessible

92

Hangman's Fracture

Suzanne Bentley

Background

Hangman's fracture is defined as a bilateral C2 pars interarticularis fracture (the bone segment between the superior and inferior facet joints of the vertebrae). This fracture type is most commonly caused by hyperextension injury, such as during motor vehicle or diving accidents, but is named for its historic occurrence after judicial hangings caused by noose placement under the angle of the jaw. Hangman's fracture results when the occiput is forced down against the posterior arch of the atlas that is forced against the pedicles of C2. It results in traumatic spondylolisthesis of C2 anteriorly on C3 resulting in the loss of bony connection between C1 and C3. The anatomy of C2 results in passage of the superior facets anteriorly and the inferior facets posteriorly causing stress through the pars interarticularis. Because of the relatively large size of the spinal canal versus the size of the spinal cord at the cervical level, neurologic damage is rarely associated.

TABLE 92.1: Classic history and physical

Neck pain
Common mechanisms: motor vehicle accidents, falls, diving accidents, suspected hanging, and gunshot wounds

C-Spine X-Rays

- Initial radiography of the cervical spine should include a lateral view of the cervical spine down to T1, often performed portably
- The most frequently missed cervical spine fractures are of the odontoid process or the cervicothoracic junction
- If the cervicothoracic junction cannot be seen adequately on lateral views, additional views or a CT scan should be obtained
- More formal radiography should include cervical spine x-rays including anteroposterior, lateral, open-mouth, and right and left oblique views with the patient immobilized with spinal precautions during the studies
- Additionally, lateral flexion and extension views can be obtained to determine the stability of the cervical spine but are not routinely recommended in the initial examination
- When interpreting plain films, pay attention to the degree of displacement and angulation, as it determines the type of fracture in the Effendi classification

 TABLE 92.2: Plain film: cervical spine

IV contrast	No
PO contrast	No
Amount of radiation	0.2 mSv per view

Classic Images

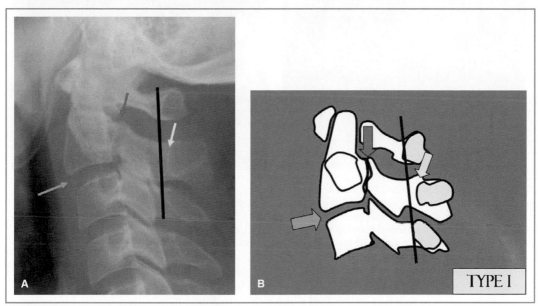

FIGURE 92.1: Type I Hangman's fracture. (**A**) Lateral radiograph and (**B**) type I Hangman's fracture illustration demonstrate a nondisplaced subtle fracture line through the pars interarticularis of the axis (*red arrow*) and posterior offset of the C2 spinolaminar line (*black line/yellow arrow*). The second intervertebral disk is intact (*green arrow*). (From Schwartz ED and Flanders AE. Spinal Trauma: Imaging, Diagnosis, and Management. Philadelphia: Lippincott Williams & Wilkins, 2007.)

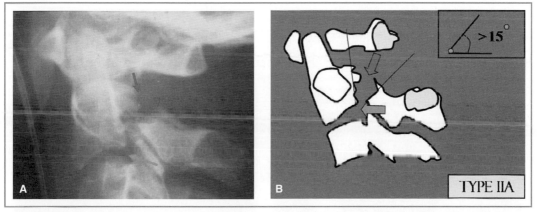

FIGURE 92.2: Type IIA Hangman's fracture. (**A**) Lateral radiograph and (**B**) type IIA Hangman's fracture illustration demonstrate a significant angulation (>15 degree) and displacement (>3 mm) at the fracture site (*red arrows*). Note the abnormal posterior widening of the C2–3 disk space (*green arrow*). (From Schwartz ED and Flanders AE. Spinal Trauma: Imaging, Diagnosis, and Management. Philadelphia: Lippincott Williams & Wilkins, 2007.)

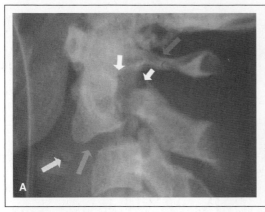
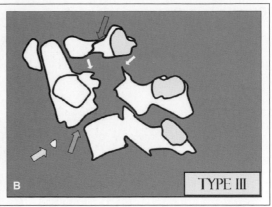

FIGURE 92.3: Type III Hangman's fracture. (**A**) Lateral radiograph and (**B**) type III Hangman's fracture illustration demonstrate a significant angulation (>15 degree) and displacement (>3 mm) at the fracture site (*white arrows*), bilateral interfacetal dislocation, disrupted C2–3 disk, posterior atlas ring fracture (*arrowhead*), massive prevertebral soft tissue swelling, and extension teardrop fracture of the axis (*black arrow*). (From Schwartz ED and Flanders AE. Spinal Trauma: Imaging, Diagnosis, and Management. Philadelphia: Lippincott Williams & Wilkins, 2007.)

Cervical Spine CT Scan

- CT scans without contrast can be used to clarify equivocal findings on plain radiographs, to reveal occult injury, and to further evaluate a known fracture
- CT scans are often utilized as first-line imaging in patients at high risk for cervical spine injuries (e.g., high-risk mechanism or abnormal examination findings)
- CT provides increased bony detail of fracture sites
- CT is helpful in evaluating the degree, if any, of spinal canal compromise

 TABLE 92.3: CT scan: cervical spine

IV contrast	No
PO contrast	No
Amount of radiation	3 mSv

Classic Images

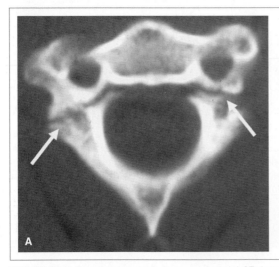
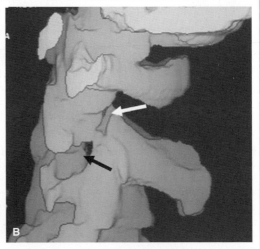

FIGURE 92.4: Type I Hangman's fracture. **A:** Axial CT demonstrates the bilateral pars fracture of C2 (*white arrows*) without significant fragment displacement. **B:** CT reformatted three-dimensional surface rendered lateral view shows the nondisplaced subtle fracture line through the pars interarticularis of the axis (*white arrows*) and normal C2–3 disk space (*black arrow*). (From Schwartz ED and Flanders AE. Spinal Trauma: Imaging, Diagnosis, and Management. Philadelphia: Lippincott Williams & Wilkins, 2007.)

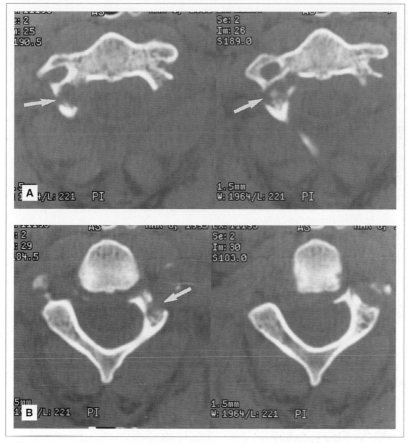

FIGURE 92.5: Traumatic spondylolisthesis. Axial CT images at two different levels (**A,B**) demonstrate bilateral pars fractures (*arrows*). (From Harris J and Harris W. The Radiology of Emergency Medicine, 4th ed. Philadelphia: Lippincott Williams & Wilkins, 2000.)

MRI

- MRI provides enhanced evaluation of the soft tissues, intervertebral disks, ligaments, and neural elements including the spinal cord itself
- Use of MRI is often limited by availability and time constraints and patients must be stable enough to undergo relatively lengthy MRI studies
- MRI use is contraindicated in patients with pacemakers or certain other types of metallic hardware including external fixation devices or cranial bolts in patients with concomitant head injury

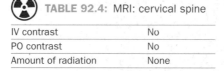 **TABLE 92.4:** MRI: cervical spine

IV contrast	No
PO contrast	No
Amount of radiation	None

Basic Management

- Hangman's fractures generally heal well with external immobilization
- Surgery is indicated if there is spinal cord compression or after failure of external immobilization
- Neurosurgical consultation is mandated when Hangman's fractures (like all cervical spine fractures) are identified
- Hangman's fracture classification types and treatment—which is based on the type of fracture—are listed in Table 92.5

- Whenever a C-spine injury is identified, remember to always consider and address associated injuries
- Additionally, consider angiography of neck vessels in the setting of Hangman's fracture

TABLE 92.5: Classification and treatment of Hangman's fractures

Classification	Description	Treatment
Type I	Hyperextension with or without additional axial load No angulation of the deformity and the fracture fragments are separated by less than 3 mm	Immobilization in a cervical collar or halo vest until union occurs
Type II	Hyperextension and axial load with secondary flexion causing displacement of the fracture	Reduction of anterior angulation of fracture, typically via traction therapy followed by use of a halo vest until union occurs
Type IIA	Same as type II with an additional component of distraction during injury that causes disruption of the C2–3 disc space making the fracture unstable	Immediate halo vest placement and traction should be avoided
Type III	Fracture through the neural arch, facet dislocation, and disruption of the C2–3 disc space making this fracture type unstable	Early closed reduction of the facet dislocation followed by halo vest to maintain reduction If closed reduction cannot be obtained or maintained, open reduction is indicated

From Shah K, Egan D, and Quaas J. Essential Emergency Trauma. Philadelphia: Lippincott Williams & Wilkins, 2010.

Summary

TABLE 92.6: Advantages and disadvantages of imaging modalities in Hangman's fracture

Imaging modality	Advantages	Disadvantages
X-ray	Low cost Readily available	Limited views in obtunded patient Body habitus limitations
CT scan	Readily available Excellent sensitivity for fractures	Limited assessment of spinal cord or soft tissues compared to MRI
MRI	Best evaluation of soft tissues, intervertebral disks, ligaments, and spinal cord	Time-consuming Limited availability Expensive

93

Odontoid Fractures

Emily Fontane

Background

The second cervical vertebra, one of two most common areas of injury in the cervical spine, is called the axis. It is the relationship of the odontoid process with the atlas (the first cervical vertebra) that allows for the majority of rotational movement of the head.

There are three types of odontoid fractures classified simply as types I, II, and III. Anderson and D'Alonzo are credited with developing this classification system.

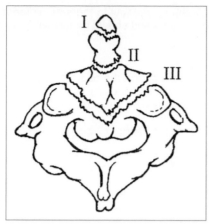

FIGURE 93.1: Three types of odontoid fractures. Type I: Fracture of the apical portion of the dens. Type II: Fracture of the dens at its base. Type III: Fracture of the dens extending into the body of C2. (From Blackbourne LH. Advanced Surgical Recall, 2nd ed. Baltimore: Lippincott Williams & Wilkins, 2004.)

Type I, the uncommon one, is an avulsion fracture of the tip of the odontoid process at the site of attachment of the alar ligament and is considered a stable fracture. Type II, the most common odontoid fracture (two-third of all odontoid fractures), is a fracture at the base of the odontoid and is considered unstable. Type III fractures extend from beneath the base of the odontoid up into the body of the axis and are generally considered stable fractures but can be unstable depending on the amount of displacement and angulation associated with the fracture.

Although spinal cord injury (SCI) most commonly occurs in association with fractures of the cervical vertebrae, odontoid fractures are an infrequent cause of SCI. One series found that only 7.5% of patients with odontoid fractures had SCI.

TABLE 93.1: Classic history and physical

Motor vehicle collisions, falls, and sports-related trauma
Neck pain
Midline cervical spine tenderness
Spinal cord injury: neurologic manifestations including extremity paresis or plegia, parthesias of the occipital region, and Brown Sequard syndrome

C-Spine X-Rays
- Standard views of the cervical spine including cross-table lateral cervical (CTLC), open mouth (OM), and anteroposterior (AP) views
- CTLC view alone can identify up to 80% of cervical spine injuries and adequate three views together can identify up to 95% of cervical spine injuries
- Certain abnormalities which may be noted on plain film:
  - 'Fat axis body'—axis ring disruption causes the axis body to look wider than normal
  - Abnormal prevertebral soft tissue contour or swelling suggests edema or hematoma of the prevertebral soft tissue; it is a nonspecific sign suggesting injury to any structure of the cervicocranium including the odontoid
- A number of shadows may interfere with the interpretation of plain radiographs:
  - Mach bands/lines are shadows caused by the overlap of the occiput and the inferior cortex of the posterior arch of the atlas, which may be mistaken for odontoid fractures (see example in Classic Images below)
  - Mach band/lines extend beyond the odontoid and axis body, which distinguish them from actual fractures
  - Nasogastric and endotracheal tubes may obscure the prevertebral soft tissue contour on a CTLC view

- The retropharyngeal space (distance from the posterior pharyngeal wall to the anteroinferior aspect of vertebrae) widening is concerning for a C-spine injury and should be further investigated by CT scan
  - At C2, it should measure 7 mm or less in adults
  - At C7, it should measure no more than 22 mm in adults
- OM view (also known as odontoid view) shows the odontoid process, the body of C-2, and the atlantoaxial joints; mouth opening is usually restricted by the cervical collar in the emergency setting; this view can only be obtained in conscious and cooperative patients

TABLE 93.2: Limitations

The AP view does not visualize the axis in adults
The OM view requires the patient to be conscious and cooperative
Plain radiographic investigation is often limited to the CTLC view
A CTLC view must show both the cervicocranial and cervicothoracic junctions to be useful
An adequate CTLC view is often not obtained in the emergency department on the first attempt

CTLC, cross-table lateral cervical; OM, open mouth.

TABLE 93.3: Plain film: cervical spine

IV contrast	No
PO contrast	No
Amount of radiation	0.2 mSv per view

Classic Images

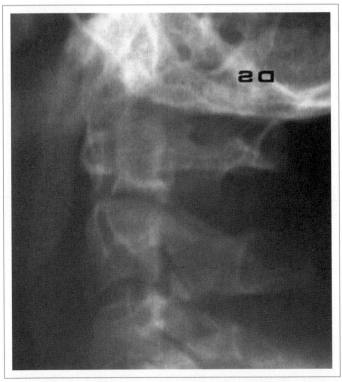

FIGURE 93.2: Cervical spine radiographs show a vertically distracted type II odontoid fracture. (From Bucholz RW and Heckman JD. Rockwood & Green's Fractures in Adults, 5th ed. Philadelphia: Lippincott Williams & Wilkins, 2001.)

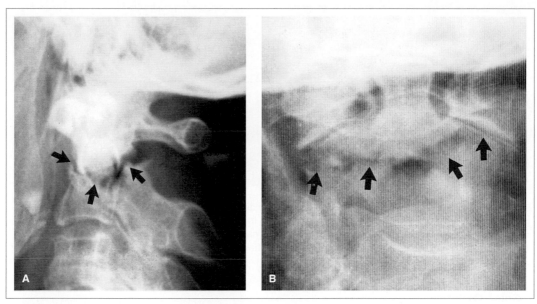

FIGURE 93.3: Obvious low dens fracture (*arrows*) in lateral (**A**) and frontal (**B**) projections. (From Harris J and Harris W. The Radiology of Emergency Medicine, 4th ed. Philadelphia: Lippincott Williams & Wilkins, 2000.)

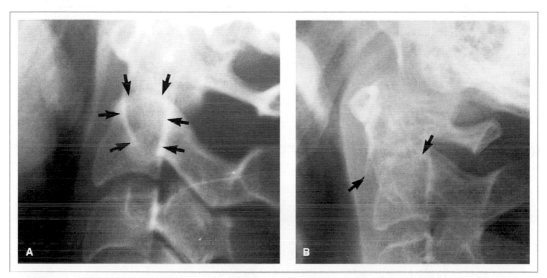

FIGURE 93.4: A: The normal axis "ring" (*arrows*). **B:** "Fat axis body" as a result of anterior and posterior disruption of the axis ring (*arrows*) suggests a low dens fracture. (From Harris J and Harris W. The Radiology of Emergency Medicine, 4th ed. Philadelphia: Lippincott Williams & Wilkins, 2000.)

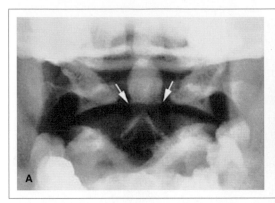
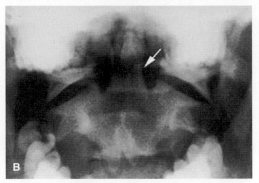

FIGURE 93.5: Mach effect. **A:** AP open mouth. The overlap density created from the posterior arch of the atlas crossing the base of the dens simulates a type II odontoid fracture or os odontoideum (*arrows*). **B:** AP open mouth. Overlap of the frontal incisor teeth has produced a pseudofracture line at the odontoid base (*arrow*). (From Yochum TR and Rowe LJ. Yochum and Rowe's Essentials of Skeletal Radiology, 3rd ed. Philadelphia: Lippincott Williams & Wilkins, 2004.)

C-Spine CT Scan
- It has supplanted plain radiography as the primary screening modality for suspected cervical spine injury after trauma
  - Delineates fractures more precisely than plain radiographs
  - Adds only a few additional minutes of time when the patient is obtaining a head CT
- Axial CT may occasionally fail to demonstrate a type II fracture in the axial plane but sagittal and coronal reconstructions should demonstrate the fracture

TABLE 93.4: CT scan: cervical spine

IV contrast	No
PO contrast	No
Amount of radiation	3 mSv

Classic Images

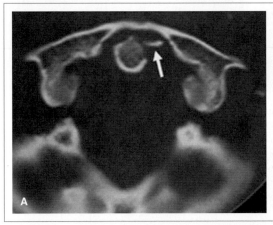
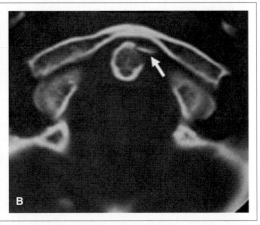

FIGURE 93.6: Type I odontoid fracture. **A** and **B:** Axial CT image. A small fracture fragment (*white arrows*) is avulsed from the left superolateral aspect of the dens. (From Schwartz ED and Flanders AE. Spinal Trauma: Imaging, Diagnosis, and Management. Philadelphia: Lippincott Williams & Wilkins, 2007.)

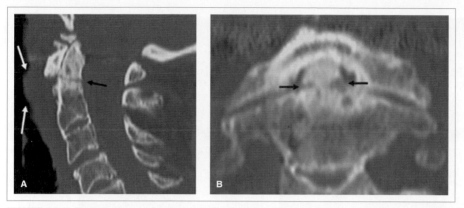

FIGURE 93.7: Type II odontoid fracture. (**A**) Sagittal and (**B**) coronal CT multiplanar reformations demonstrate a nondisplaced type II odontoid fracture (*black arrow*). Note the abnormal cervicocranial prevertebral soft tissue contour in (A) (*white arrows*). (From Schwartz ED and Flanders AE. Spinal Trauma: Imaging, Diagnosis, and Management. Philadelphia: Lippincott Williams & Wilkins, 2007.)

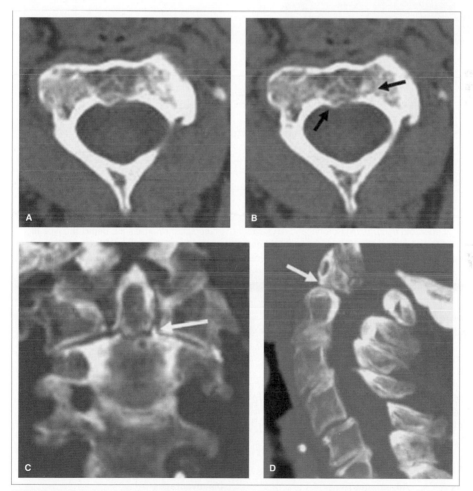

FIGURE 93.8: Subtle type II odontoid fracture. **A** and **B**: Axial CT images through the odontoid were nondiagnostic, demonstrating a questionable fracture line (*black arrows*). (**C**) Coronal and (**D**) lateral three-dimensional MIP reformations reveal the minimally displaced type II odontoid fracture (*white arrows*). (From Schwartz ED and Flanders AE. Spinal Trauma: Imaging, Diagnosis, and Management. Philadelphia: Lippincott Williams & Wilkins, 2007.)

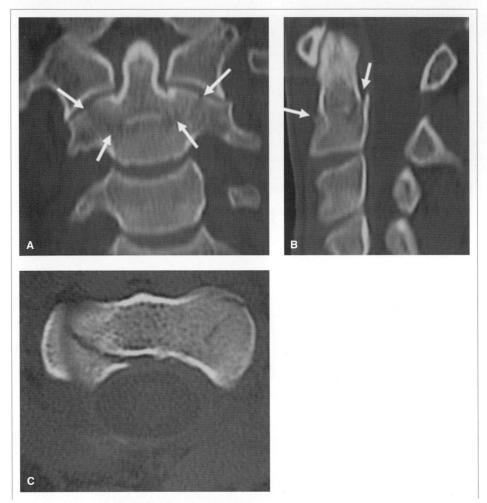

FIGURE 93.9: Type III odontoid fracture. (**A**) Coronal and (**B**) sagittal CT multiplanar reformations depict the type III odontoid fracture (*white lines*) through the base of odontoid extending into the body of axis. (**C**) Axial CT image confirms the disruption of the axis body. Anterior displacement of the rostral fragment (**B**) and the orientation of the axis fracture line are consistent with a flexion mechanism of injury. (From Schwartz ED and Flanders AE. Spinal Trauma: Imaging, Diagnosis, and Management. Philadelphia: Lippincott Williams & Wilkins, 2007.)

Basic Management

- Perform and document a detailed neurovascular examination
- In-line cervical spine stabilization immediately and at all times
- Spine/neurosurgical consultation
- Pain control
- Although there are, as of yet, no conclusive treatment standards or guidelines for odontoid fractures, recognition of fracture types is important for choosing management technique
- In general, external immobilization is commonly employed for type I and III fractures, whereas surgical options are more commonly employed for type II fractures

Summary

TABLE 93.5: Advantages and disadvantages of imaging modalities in odontoid fractures

Imaging modality	Advantages	Disadvantages
X-ray	Availability Low cost Less radiation	Mach bands/line interfere with interpretation Less sensitive than CT
CT scan	Availability Complex osseous injuries visible	Radiation exposure

94

Flexion Teardrop Fracture

Ram Parekh

Background

Flexion teardrop fractures represent the most severe fractures of the cervical spine. These fractures result from a combination of extreme flexion and compressive forces. They are often associated with acute anterior cervical cord syndrome, including quadriplegia and the loss of sensation. In adults, flexion teardrop fracture occurs most commonly at C5-C6. This fracture is unstable as result of complete disruption of both ligamentous and bony structures.

The vertebral body fracture is a triangular fragment off the anteroinferior body. There is posterior displacement of the involved vertebral bony fragments with varying degrees of compromise of canal diameter.

TABLE 94.1: Classic history and physical

Dive into shallow water
Fall from height
Motor vehicle collisions with severe neck flexion/compression
Quadriplegia or incomplete quadriplegia, though may be neurologically intact

X-Ray

- Obtain standard views of the cervical spine including cross-table lateral cervical (CTLC), open mouth (OM), and anteroposterior (AP) views
- The anterior aspect of the teardrop fragment is generally aligned with that of the vertebral body below, although in some cases it can be displaced and rotated anteriorly beyond the anterior vertebral line
- The posteroinferior aspect of the posterior fragment is displaced posteriorly in relation to the superior aspect of the vertebral body below; this displacement can vary from as little as 1 mm to the entire body width
- The superior aspect of the posterior fragment is typically, but not always, in normal alignment with the inferior aspect of the vertebral body above
- Findings suggestive of teardrop fracture (lateral view):
  - There is typically an anterior wedge deformity
  - Disk space between the posterior fragment and the vertebral body below in narrowed
  - The facet joint between the level of injury and the one below is widened
  - Interlaminar and interspinous spaces are typically widened
  - There is a varying degree of kyphotic deformity at the level of injury
  - Posterior displacement of upper column on lower column
  - Associated prevertebral soft tissue swelling is often seen
  - Varying degrees of canal diameter compromise
- Occurs most often at C5

 TABLE 94.2: Plain film: cervical spine

IV contrast	No
PO contrast	No
Amount of radiation	0.2 mSv per view

Classic Images

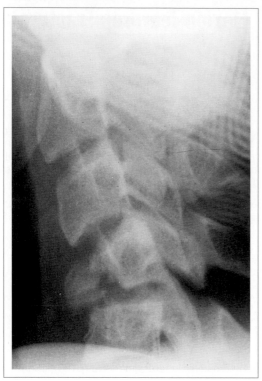

FIGURE 94.1: Flexion teardrop fracture of C4. (From Harris J and Harris W. The Radiology of Emergency Medicine, 4th ed. Philadelphia: Lippincott Williams & Wilkins, 2000.)

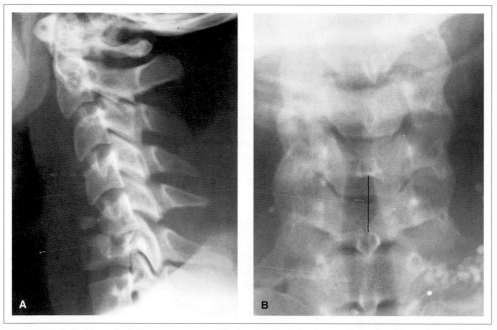

FIGURE 94.2: A: Characteristic appearance of flexion teardrop fracture on lateral radiograph. **B:** The C5-6 interspinous space is abnormally wide (*solid line*) on the AP radiograph. (From Harris J and Harris W. The Radiology of Emergency Medicine, 4th ed. Philadelphia: Lippincott Williams & Wilkins, 2000.)

CT Scan

- More sensitive in the detection of fractures than plan radiography
- Classic finding: sagittal fracture through the vertebral body

TABLE 94.3: CT scan: cervical spine

IV contrast	No
PO contrast	No
Amount of radiation	3 mSv

Classic Images

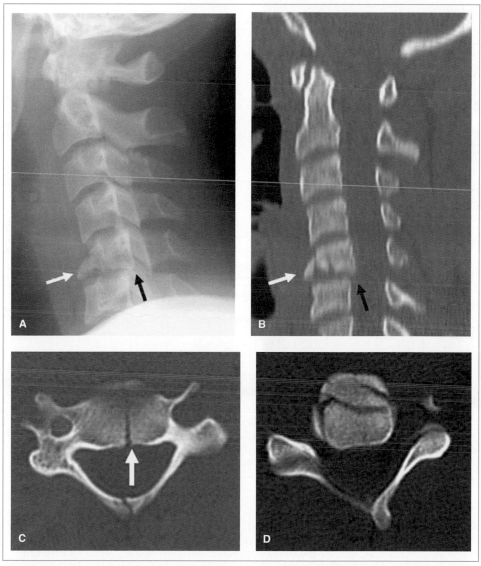

FIGURE 94.3: Flexion teardrop fracture of C5. Lateral radiographs of cervical spine (**A**) and sagittal multiplanar CT reformation (**B**) show compression of the body of C5 associated with a mild posterior subluxation of C5 upon C6 (*black arrows*). The fragment from the anteroinferior surface of C5 (*white arrow*) is the "teardrop." **C:** Axial CT image through the top of C5 demonstrates a sagittal fracture of the vertebral body (white line) and sagittal fracture of the spinous process. **D:** Axial CT image through the lower half of C5 shows a comminuted fracture of the anteroinferior end plate. (From Schwartz ED and Flanders AE. Spinal Trauma: Imaging, Diagnosis, and Management. Philadelphia: Lippincott Williams & Wilkins, 2007.)

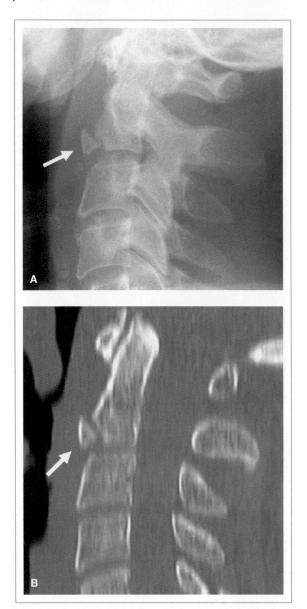

FIGURE 94.4: Hyperextension teardrop fracture of C2. Plain X-ray (**A**) and Sagittal multiplanar CT reformation (**B**) shows a triangular fragment arising from the anteroinferior margin of C2 (*white arrows*). (From Schwartz ED and Flanders AE. Spinal Trauma: Imaging, Diagnosis, and Management. Philadelphia: Lippincott Williams & Wilkins, 2007.)

MRI

- Technique of choice for evaluating the spinal cord, differentiating edema from hemorrhage, and defining cord impingement from extradural lesions such as bone or disk
- Superior in diagnosing disk, ligamentous, and associated vascular injuries, such as vertebral artery occlusion after cervical spine trauma
- Not considered reliable enough to detect and delineate fractures in comparison with CT and plain radiography, as MRI is relatively insensitive to cortical disruption
- Fracture may not be visualized but secondary effects are apparent in the form of marrow signal changes, soft tissue hematoma, and edema adjacent to fractures

Classic Images

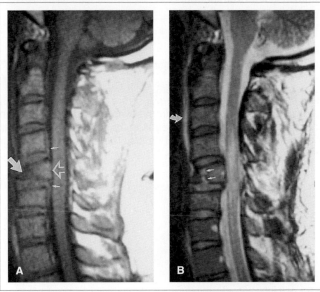

FIGURE 94.5: Flexion teardrop fracture of C5. **A:** Sagittal T1-weighted image shows loss of height of the C5 vertebral body anteriorly (*large arrow*). The marrow signal of the compressed segment is hypointense. The posterior aspect of the vertebral body is retropulsed into the spinal canal (*open arrow*). There is associated elevation of the posterior longitudinal ligament (*small arrows*) and there is mild swelling of the spinal cord. **B:** Sagittal FSE T2-weighted image depicts the hyperintense vertically oriented fracture line that interrupts the inferior endplate (*small arrows*). A small amount of prevertebral edema is also present (*curved arrow*). There is edema in the spinal cord without a discrete focus of hemorrhage. (Hypointense focus in brainstem is artifactual.) (From Flanders AE and Croul SE. Spinal trauma. In: Atlas SW, ed. Magnetic Resonance Imaging of the Brain and Spine. 3rd ed. Philadelphia: Lippincott Williams & Wilkins; 2002:1776.)

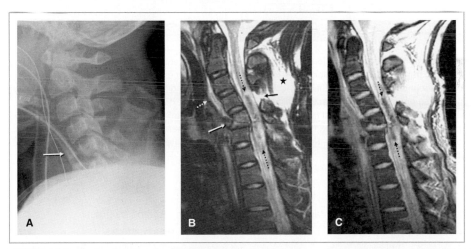

FIGURE 94.6: Flexion teardrop fracture of C5 with severe spinal cord injury. **A:** Lateral radiograph shows the typical teardrop configuration of the C5 vertebral body (*arrow*) in which a large anterior bone fragment is disassociated from the vertebral body from combined axial loading and flexion. **B:** Sagittal FSE T2-weighted image shows a flexion teardrop fracture of the C5 vertebral body with avulsion of a fragment ventrally (*white arrow*). There is prevertebral soft tissue swelling (*dotted white arrow*). The ligamentum flavum and posterior ligamentous complex is ruptured (*small black arrow*) and the posterior musculature is edematous (*asterisk*). An extensive intramedullary hemorrhage is present (*dotted black arrows*). **C:** Sagittal gradient echo image shows the extensive hypointense intramedullary hemorrhage (*dotted black arrows*). (From Schwartz ED and Flanders AE. Spinal Trauma: Imaging, Diagnosis, and Management. Philadelphia: Lippincott Williams & Wilkins, 2007.)

Basic Management

- Perform and document a detailed neurovascular examination
- In-line cervical spine stabilization immediately and at all times
- Spine/neurosurgical consultation
- Pain control
- Consider MRI to assess for cord and ligamentous injury
- Admission for possible surgical fusion depending on extent of injury

Extension Teardrop Fracture

Extension teardrop fracture is a fracture of the anteroinferior corner of the body (typically of C2) avulsed by the intact anterior longitudinal ligament that results from severe hyperextension. The vertical height of the extension teardrop fragment equals or exceeds its horizontal width. This is generally a stable injury and is not associated with neurological deficit. This fracture may occur in isolation or be associated with a Hangman's fracture.

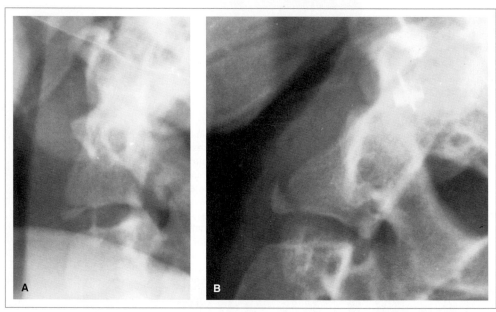

FIGURE 94.7: Comparison of the typical avulsion fracture fragment of hyperextension dislocation (**A**) with that of the hyperextension teardrop fragment (**B**). The avulsion fracture, the fragment of hyperextension dislocation (**A**), involves the anterior aspect of the inferior endplate of the axis vertebra. The transverse dimension of the fragment exceeds its vertical height. Diffuse prevertebral soft tissue swelling is present. In hyperextension teardrop fracture (**B**), the fragment avulsed by the intact anterior longitudinal ligament comprises the entire anteroinferior corner of the axis vertebra, and its vertical height equals or exceeds its transverse diameter. Prevertebral soft tissue swelling is focal and minimal. (From Harris J and Harris W. The Radiology of Emergency Medicine, 4th ed. Philadelphia: Lippincott Williams & Wilkins, 2000.)

Summary

TABLE 94.4: Advantages and disadvantages of imaging modalities in teardrop fractures

Imaging modality	Advantages	Disadvantages
X-ray	Availability Low cost Less radiation	Less sensitive than CT
CT scan	Availability Complex osseous injuries visible	Radiation exposure
MRI	Gold standard for cord, ligamentous, and disk injuries	Availability Time-consuming Insensitive for fracture detection Cost

95

Clay-Shoveler's Fracture

Greg Buehler

Background

The clay-shoveler's fracture is an avulsion fracture of one or more of the spinous processes of the lower cervical or upper thoracic spine (most commonly C6, C7, or T1). First described in the 1930s in Australian relief workers, the fracture occurs as the result of abrupt flexion of the head and neck against tensed ligaments of the posterior neck or forceful contraction of the posterior neck muscles that insert on the spinous processes. Most commonly, the miners would sustain the injury when clay would stick to the shovel while attempting to throw it, causing sudden flexion of the head and neck. It has since also been described in metal dippers, whiplash injuries, and sports injuries. Atypically, extension of the fracture into the lamina has been described in cases of whiplash or direct trauma to the posterior neck.

TABLE 95.1: Classic history and physical

Sudden onset of pain between shoulders after hyperflexion of the neck
May feel or hear "pop" between shoulders
Tenderness of spinous process at site of fracture (avulsed fragment may be mobile)
Head held in slight flexion with elevation of shoulders in attempt to immobilize the interscapular area

Cervical Spine X-Rays

- Cervical spine x-rays are the diagnostic study recommended in the evaluation of patients with suspected clay-shoveler's fracture
- Classic appearance on lateral view is a fracture line with horizontally oblique orientation through the spinous process and caudal displacement of the avulsed fragment
- On AP view, this caudally displaced fragment creates the double shadow sign

 TABLE 95.2: Plain film: cervical spine

IV contrast	No
PO contrast	No
Amount of radiation	0.2 mSv per view

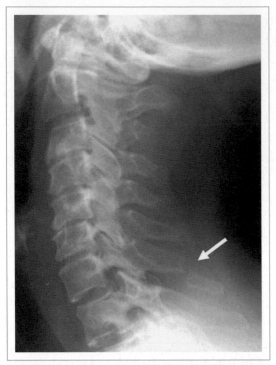

FIGURE 95.1: Typical clay-shoveler's fracture of the spinous process of C7 (*white arrow*). (From Schwartz ED and Flanders AE. Spinal Trauma: Imaging, Diagnosis, and Management. Philadelphia: Lippincott Williams & Wilkins, 2007.)

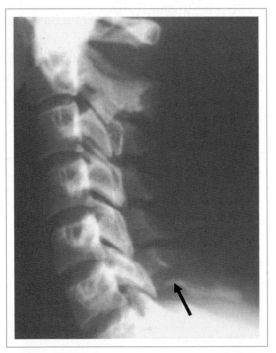

FIGURE 95.2: Atypical clay-shoveler's fracture of C6. The fracture line extends beyond the spinous process into the lamina (*black arrow*). Spinal cord injury is possible with this fracture. (From Schwartz ED and Flanders AE. Spinal Trauma: Imaging, Diagnosis, and Management. Philadelphia: Lippincott Williams & Wilkins, 2007.)

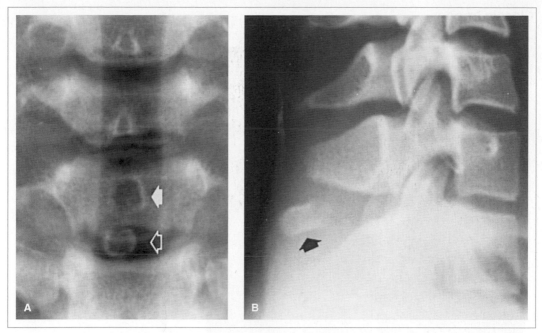

FIGURE 95.3: Clay-shoveler's fracture. **A:** Frontal view of the cervical spine shows the characteristic double–spinous-process sign resulting from the caudad displacement of the avulsed fragment (*open arrow*) with respect to the normal position of the major portion of the spinous process (*closed arrow*). **B:** A lateral view clearly shows the avulsed fragment (*arrow*). (From Eisenberg RL. An Atlas of Differential Diagnosis, 4th ed. Philadelphia: Lippincott Williams & Wilkins, 2003.)

CT Scan

- Although cervical spine x-rays are usually adequate to identify a clay-shoveler's fracture, CT scan of the cervical spine is a commonly used diagnostic study for undifferentiated evaluation after neck injury
- As on x-ray, a fracture line would be seen in the spinous process of the lower cervical or upper thoracic vertebrae

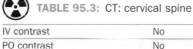 TABLE 95.3: CT: cervical spine

IV contrast	No
PO contrast	No
Amount of radiation	3 mSv

Classic Images

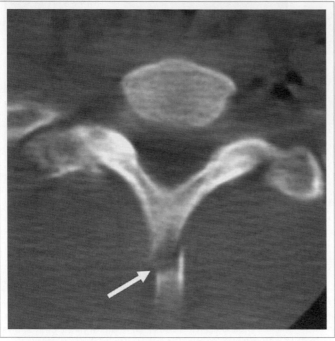

FIGURE 95.4: Axial CT image shows a typical clay-shoveler's fracture of the spinous process of T1 (*white arrow*). (From Schwartz ED and Flanders AE. Spinal Trauma: Imaging, Diagnosis, and Management. Philadelphia: Lippincott Williams & Wilkins, 2007.)

Basic Management
- Typically, treatment is conservative, as this fracture is both mechanically and neurologically stable
  - Cervical brace for comfort
  - Pain management
- Rarely, when extension of the fracture into the lamina involves the spinal canal, the potential for instability and spinal cord injury exists

Summary

TABLE 95.4: Advantages and disadvantages of imaging modalities

Imaging modality	Advantages	Disadvantages
X-ray	Low cost Readily available	Limited views in obtunded patient Body habitus limitations
CT scan	Readily available Excellent sensitivity for fractures	Limited assessment of spinal cord or soft tissues compared to MRI

96

Thoracolumbar Fractures

Crystal Cassidy

Background

It is estimated that approximately 4,000 traumatic thoracolumbar (TL) fractures are diagnosed each year in the United States. Most nontraumatic lumbar fractures are osteoporotic in origin. The classification of these fractures is based on the three-column theory, which includes the anterior, middle, and posterior spinal columns, and the associated ligamentous and soft-tissue elements. Instability occurs when there is disruption in two of the three columns.

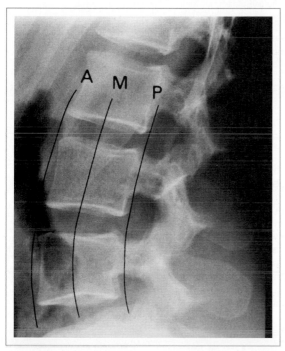

FIGURE 96.1: Lateral radiographs demonstrating the three columns proposed by Denis. Anterior-anterior longitudinal ligament, anterior disc, and vertebral body. Middle-posterior disc, body, and posterior longitudinal ligament. Posterior-facet joints, ligamentum flavum, interspinous, and supraspinous ligaments. (From Berquist TH. Musculoskeletal Imaging Companion, 2nd ed. Philadelphia: Lippincott Williams & Wilkins, 2007.)

Wedge Fractures

Wedge fracture is the most common type of lumbar fracture and accounts for 50–70% of all TL fractures. Wedge fractures are a type of anterior compression fractures that are seen in traumatic injuries, malignancy, and osteoporosis.

Flexion and Distraction Injuries

Flexion and distraction injuries are most commonly associated with the use of a lap belt (without the associated use of the shoulder strap) in motor vehicle collision, where there is disruption in the posterior column and the associated posterior ligaments. In the setting of trauma, this injury is may also be associated with intestinal perforation.

A chance fracture refers to a spinal fracture that occurs with hyperflexion. The fracture line extends through the body of the vertebra in a horizontal fashion. These fractures occur most commonly at the T12, L1, or L2 level and tend to be stable fractures.

Burst Fractures

Burst fractures occur by compressive forces and can be stable or unstable. They account for approximately 14% of TL injuries. Because of the possible retropulsion of bony fragments into the spinal canal, neurologic deficits are common with this injury.

Translational Spinal Column Injury

Translational spinal column injury occurs from massive direct trauma to the back. This injury can cause disruption of all the spinal columns and frequently results in neurologic deficits.

TABLE 96.1: Classic history and physical

High-risk injury mechanism
▪ Fall greater than 3 m
▪ Moderate to high velocity motor vehicle crash
▪ Ejection from a vehicle
▪ Auto versus pedestrian
Fall with history of osteoporosis
Prostate or breast cancer, multiple myeloma, or other history of cancer known to metastasize to the spine
Midline tenderness
Visible injury; step-off, bruising, hematoma
Neurologic deficit
Presence of another spine injury

Plain X-ray

- AP and lateral plain films is an acceptable screening tool for low impact or nontraumatic mechanism in the neurologically intact patient
- Plain films are cost-effective with lower mean overall spinal imaging charge than CT
- Evaluation of the entire spine should be considered when a fracture is identified because of the high incidence of multiple fractures
- Spinal instability should be considered when:
  - compression fracture has greater than 50% loss of height
  - compression fracture has greater than 30% angulation
  - burst fracture has greater than 25% angulation
  - neurologic deficit present
- Any concern for spinal instability warrants CT evaluation

TABLE 96.2: Plain x-ray: thoracolumbar

PO contrast	No
IV contrast	No
Amount of radiation T-spine	1 mSv per view
Amount of radiation L-spine	1.5 mSv per view

Classic Images

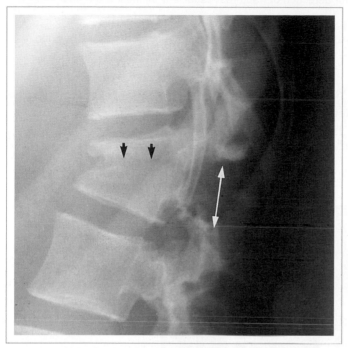

FIGURE 96.2: Chance fracture of L1. Lateral radiograph demonstrates the horizontal fracture line (*short arrows*) as well as the posterior distraction (*double arrow*) that occurs with this injury. (From Daffner RH. Clinical Radiology: The Essentials, 3rd ed. Philadelphia: Lippincott Williams & Wilkins, 2007.)

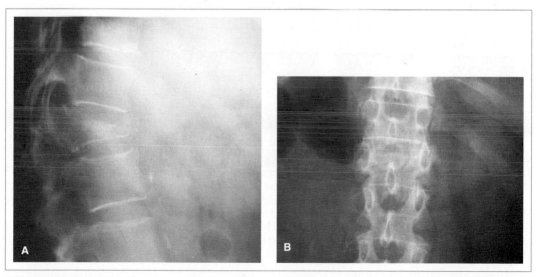

FIGURE 96.3: This woman in her early fifties experienced a high-energy L-1 burst fracture with severe fracture deformity and comminution without neurologic deficit in a boating accident. (From Frymoyer JW, Wiesel SW, et al. The Adult and Pediatric Spine. Philadelphia: Lippincott Williams & Wilkins, 2004.)

CT Scan

- More sensitive than plain film for detection of fractures, especially injuries to the posterior elements
- Visualizes the spinal canal for bony fragments and integrity
- Avoid additional radiation exposure by using reformatted chest, abdomen/pelvis CTs when available, e.g., trauma setting

 TABLE 96.3: CT scan: thoracolumbar

IV contrast	No
PO contrast	No
Amount of radiation	3 mSv

Classic Images

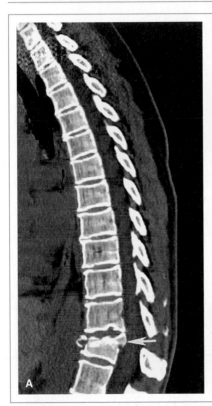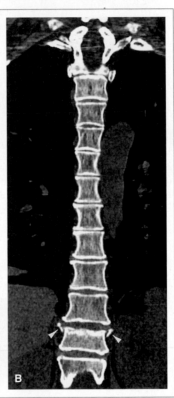

FIGURE 96.4: Lower thoracic burst fracture. Reformatted sagittal (**A**) and coronal (**B**) CT images demonstrate vertebral compression with outward displacement of fragments on the coronal image (*arrowheads*) and posterior displaced fragments on the sagittal image (*arrow*). Axial image demonstrates displaced anterior fragments and posterior extension into the spinal canal (*open arrow*). (From Berquist TH. Musculoskeletal Imaging Companion, 2nd ed. Philadelphia: Lippincott Williams & Wilkins, 2007.)

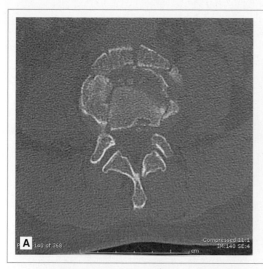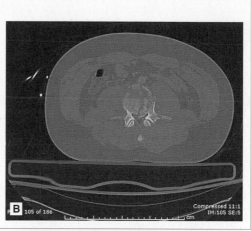

FIGURE 96.5: CT of lumbar spine in axial view demonstrating compression fracture (**A**) without retropulsion and (**B**) with retropulsion. (*Courtesy of Crystal Cassidy, MD, and Ben Taub Hospital, Houston, TX.*)

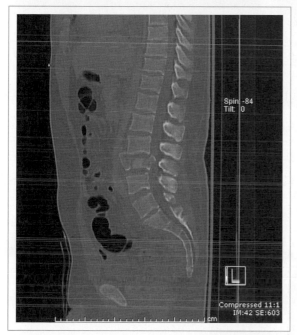

FIGURE 96.6: CT of lumbar spine in sagittal view demonstrating a compression fracture with retropulsion. (*Courtesy of Crystal Cassidy, MD, and Ben Taub Hospital, Houston, TX.*)

MRI
- Indicated in the nontraumatic presentation of lower extremity motor or sensory loss
- Indicated in the evaluation of radicular pain
- Most sensitive in evaluation of hemorrhage, tumor, and infection

 TABLE 96.4: MRI: thoracolumbar

IV contrast	No
PO contrast	No
Amount of radiation	None

Classic Images

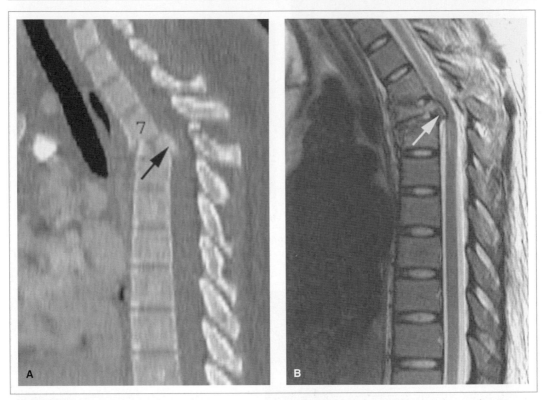

FIGURE 96.7: Utility of MR imaging in vertebral trauma. **A:** Sagittal reconstructed CT image shows a burst fracture of T1 with retropulsion of a bone fragment into the vertebral canal (*arrow*). **B:** T2-weighted sagittal MR image shows the cord compression (*arrow*). (From Daffner RH. Clinical Radiology: The Essentials, 3rd ed. Philadelphia: Lippincott Williams & Wilkins, 2007.)

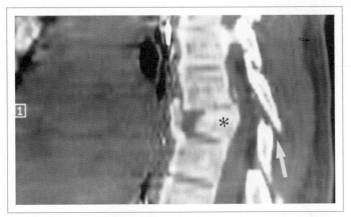

FIGURE 96.8: Wedge compression fracture with retropulsion of fragments. MRI demonstrates spinal cord compression with extensive high-intensity signals of cord edema (*arrows*). (From Harris J and Harris W. The Radiology of Emergency Medicine, 4th ed. Philadelphia: Lippincott Williams & Wilkins, 2000.)

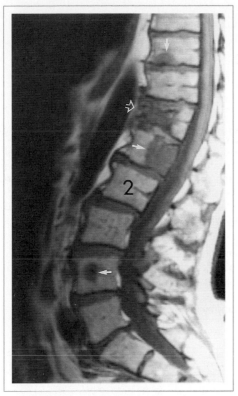

FIGURE 96.9: Metastases (*solid arrows*) and pathologic collapse (*open arrow*) of T12 as demonstrated on a T1-weighted MR image. The abnormal signal in the collapsed vertebra extends throughout the vertebra, typical of metastases. (From Daffner RH. Clinical Radiology: The Essentials, 3rd ed. Philadelphia: Lippincott Williams & Wilkins, 2007.)

Basic Management
- Perform and document a detailed neurovascular examination
- In-line cervical spine stabilization immediately and at all times
- Spine/neurosurgical consultation
- Pain control
- Log-roll when necessary

Summary

TABLE 96.5: Advantages and disadvantages of imaging modalities in thoracolumbar fractures

Imaging modality	Advantages	Disadvantages
Plain x-ray	Availability Lowest mean cost	Higher radiation than most plain films
CT scan	Overall, most cost-effective in polytrauma Can be examined from reformatted chest/abdomen/pelvis scan Visualizes spinal canal	High cost if used as a screening study in isolated low-mechanism injuries
MRI	Most sensitive for hemorrhage, tumor, and infection Better visualization of the spinal cord and ligamentous structures	Availability Time-consuming Cost

97

Coccyx Fracture

David Nguyen

Background

The coccyx is the most inferior bone in the spine and is usually made up of four coccygeal vertebrae. Fractures of the coccyx most commonly occur after a fall with the patient landing in the sitting position. Simple coccyx fractures are often diagnosed clinically and radiologic studies are unnecessary in many of these cases. There is limited data on the true incidence of these fractures. Coccydynia or coccygodynia, which are nonspecific terms defined as pain in the localized region of the coccyx, can often be chronic after a coccyx fracture. Healing can be prolonged, as movement prevents rapid healing of this fracture.

Postacchini and Massobrio (1983) studied 120 asymptomatic people and analyzed their coccyx anatomy radiographically. They were able to classify each coccyx shape into four different categories (see Table 97.1).

TABLE 97.1: Classification of normal coccyx anatomy by Postacchini and Massobrio

Coccyx type	Description of coccyx anatomy	Frequency
I	Coccyx has a slight forward curvature	68
II	Coccyx is curved forward and the apex of the coccyx is pointing forward	17
III	Coccyx has a sharp anterior angulation	6
IV	Coccyx shows a subluxation at either the intercoccygeal joints or the sacrococcygeal joints	9

TABLE 97.2: Classic history and physical

Pain occurring usually after a fall, with patient landing in the sitting position
Significant pain in coccygeal region
Pain is exacerbated by sitting or leaning backward
Direct palpation or rectal exam can reproduce pain

Plain X-Ray

- Plain films of the coccyx are the first recommended radiographic images in a suspected fracture
- The anteroposterior (AP) and lateral images of the sacrococcygeal spine with a coned-down lateral view of the coccyx often help determine if a fracture is present
- The hips should be flexed in the lateral view to allow increased visibility of the coccyx

 TABLE 97.3: Plain x-ray: coccyx

IV contrast	No
PO contrast	No
Amount of radiation	1.2 mSv per view

Classic Images

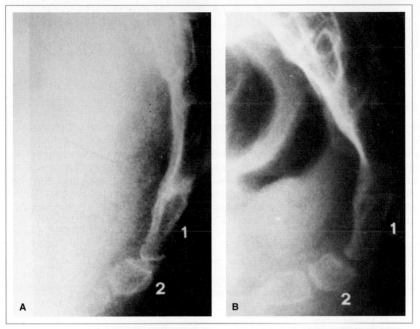

FIGURE 97.1: A: Type I configuration consists of three bony segments with a gentle forward-flexed attitude. **B:** Type II configuration of the coccyx with a more acute forward-flexed attitude. 1, last fused coccygeal segments; 2, mobile coccygeal segment. (Adapted with permission from Postacchini F and Massobrio M. Idiopathic coccygodynia. Analysis of fifty-one operative cases and a radiographic study of the normal coccyx. *J. Bone Joint Surg.* 65A(8): 1983; 1116–1124.)

CT Scan
- CT scanning of the coccyx can help further visualize the area and determine if a fracture is present
- CT scans also allow the clinician to visualize the surrounding coccygeal structures and determine any adjacent injuries
- CT scans expose the patient to increased amounts of radiation compared to plain radiographs

 TABLE 97.4: Noncontrast CT scan: pelvis

IV contrast	No
PO contrast	No
Amount of radiation	6 mSv

Basic Management
- Pain control with NSAIDs and/or narcotics may be necessary
- Donut- or wedge-shaped pillows are often used to prevent direct pressure on coccyx
- Most cases resolve with conservative treatment
- Orthopedic (and/or pain management) referral is indicated for intractable pain despite conservative management

Summary

TABLE 97.5: Advantages and disadvantages of imaging modalities in coccyx fracture

Imaging modality	Advantages	Disadvantages
Plain radiography	Inexpensive Rapid Widely available	Radiation exposure
Noncontrast CT scan	Rapid Widely available Helps detect surrounding injuries	Radiation exposure Costly

98 Ligamentous Injury and Subluxation

Gregory Rumph

Background

Subluxation is the abnormal movement of one body part with respect to another. Classically, in the cervical spine it is the anteroposterior movement of vertebral bodies with respect to one another or at the craniocervical junction. Hyperflexion and rotation-flexion mechanisms are the most likely causes of injury in the cervical spine. Injury to the anterior or posterior ligaments, the atlanto-occiptal/atlantoaxial ligament complex, or the ligaments connecting to the dens can be catastrophic, allowing the spinal cord to be compressed or even transected. The risk of spinal cord injury and ligamentous injury in patients with head injuries range from 1.4% for mild (GCS ≥13), 6.8% for moderate (GCS ranging 9–12), and 10.2% for severe (GCS ≤8).

TABLE 98.1: Classic history and physical

Rear-end motor vehicle collision causing hyperflexion
Hanging injury, causing sudden hyperextension
Blunt trauma to head and neck
Midline neck pain
Pain with flexion or extension of the neck
Central cord syndrome: weakness of the upper extremities compared to the lower and tingling and numbness of arms and hands

TABLE 98.2: Pediatric and anatomic variances

Pseudosubluxation: Common in up to 40% of children; typical at C2-C3 and C3-C4
Swischuk line: Line on anterior cortical margin of the spinous process at C1 to the same at C3
C2 anterior cortical margin should be on that line or less than 2 mm displaced (pseudosubluxation)
Os odontoideum: Dens is discontinuous from C2, attached by fibrous tissue only

Plain Film X-Rays

- Indicated for low-risk injuries: low-speed MVC, fall from standing position, and the awake, alert, or oriented patient without neurologic deficits
- Three view series: AP, lateral, and odontoid views
- Lateral films are no longer needed for major trauma undergoing CT cervical spine due to the ability to reconstruct images in three-dimensions
- Sensitivity for fracture is 60–80% and is lower for craniocervical junction injuries

TABLE 98.3: Findings suggestive of ligamentous injury

X-ray view	Findings suggestive of ligamentous injury
Lateral cervical spine	Prevertebral soft tissue 6 mm or more at C2 and 2 cm or more at C6 Anterior, posterior, and spinolaminar lines not intact Widening or fanning of spinous processes may indicate ligamentous injury Anterior interdental space C1-dens >3 mm
AP cervical spine	Distraction of vertebral bodies in inferosuperior direction Rotated pedicles Spinous process rotated out of midline
Odontoid	Lateral masses of C1 not symmetric around the dens Edges of C1 not aligning symmetrically over C2 Dens fracture or asymmetry of interdental spaces to C1
Flexion-extension (not typically done acutely)	Anterior interdental space C1-dens >3 mm in adults and >3.5 mm in children Anterior subluxation of vertebral bodies Pain with attempted movement

 TABLE 98.4: Plain film: cervical spine

IV contrast	No
PO contrast	No
Amount of radiation	0.2 mSv per view

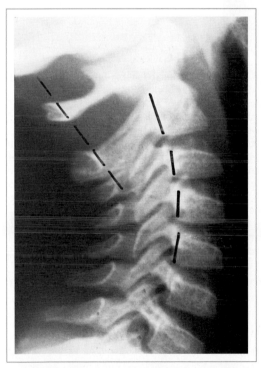

FIGURE 98.1: Normal relationship of the posterior laminar line of the axis to the posterior spinal line in neutral neck position. (From Harris J and Harris W. The Radiology of Emergency Medicine, 4th ed. Philadelphia: Lippincott Williams & Wilkins, 2000.)

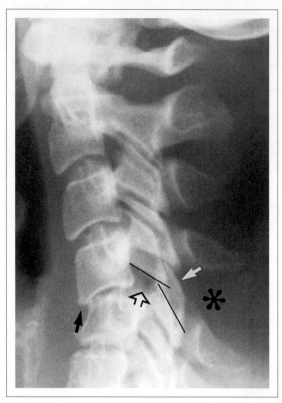

FIGURE 98.2: Anterior subluxation (AS) of C4 on C5 shown on the cross-table lateral radiograph of a patient in a rigid cervical collar. The signs of AS are unusually obvious in this patient in spite of recumbency and cervical immobilization. The most obvious sign of AS on the lateral radiograph is a hyperkyphotic angulation at the site of the posterior ligament complex tear. The "infrastructure" signs of AS inherent in the hyperkyphotic angulation include, from posterior to anterior, "fanning" (widening of the intraspinous, but more reliably the intralaminar, space) (*asterisk*); subluxation of the interfacetal joints at the level of injury characterized by partial uncovering of the superior facets of the subjacent vertebra (*white arrow*) and incongruity of the contiguous facets (*black arrows*); widening of the space between the posterior cortex of the subluxated vertebral body and the articular process of the subjacent vertebra (*open arrow*); widening of the involved disk space posteriorly and reciprocal narrowing anteriorly; and varying degrees of anterior translation (displacement) of the subluxated vertebra (*black arrow*) which is characteristically less than the translation associated with unilateral interfacetal dislocation. Indeed, anterior translation is not a prerequisite sign of AS. (From Harris J and Harris W. The Radiology of Emergency Medicine, 4th ed. Philadelphia: Lippincott Williams & Wilkins, 2000.)

Classic Images

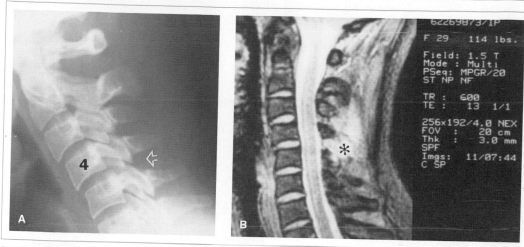

FIGURE 98.6: Subtle acute anterior subluxation (AS) established by MRI. AS of C4 on C5 (*open arrow*) could only be suspected on the flexion lateral radiograph (**A**) of this patient who sustained a "whiplash" injury. The T2-weighted magnetic resonance image (**B**) obtained the same day shows the high-intensity signal (*asterisk*) of edema indicating acute disruption of the posterior ligament complex. (From Harris J and Harris W. The Radiology of Emergency Medicine, 4th ed. Philadelphia: Lippincott Williams & Wilkins, 2000.)

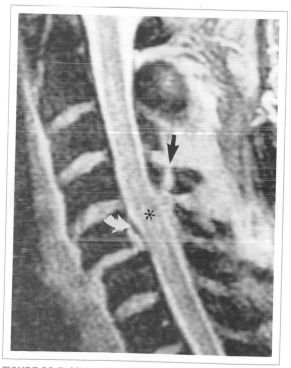

FIGURE 98.7: Midsagittal MRI of a stage IV pedicolaminar fracture separation shows the C4 spinous process fracture (*arrow*), compression and swelling of the cord at the C5 level (*asterisk*), and anterior translation of C5 with avulsion of the posterior longitudinal ligament (*curved arrow*). (From Harris J and Harris W. The Radiology of Emergency Medicine, 4th ed. Philadelphia: Lippincott Williams & Wilkins, 2000.)

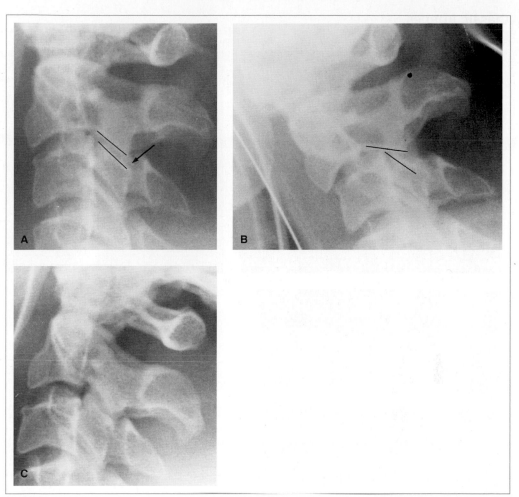

FIGURE 98.3: Anterior subluxation (AS) of C2. The neutral lateral radiograph (**A**) of this intubated major trauma patient suggested AS by minor widening of the C2-3 interlaminar space, minimal uncovering of the superior facets of C3 (*arrow*), and subtle incongruity of the contiguous C2-3 facets (*lines*). Radiologist-controlled flexion (**B**) and extension (**C**) lateral radiographs obtained in the trauma room confirmed AS by anterior translation of C2 (*arrow*) and the gross incongruity of the C2-3 facets (*lines*, B). The extension lateral (**C**) shows normal C2-3 relations, which is also characteristic of AS. (From Harris J and Harris W. The Radiology of Emergency Medicine, 4th ed. Philadelphia: Lippincott Williams & Wilkins, 2000.)

CT Scan

- Used routinely in multitrauma with moderate or major injury or mechanism
- Modern helical CT scanners quickly provide reconstruction images allowing three-dimensional representation of the spine, with estimated 97–99% sensitivity for fractures
- Best used for detecting fracture, dislocation, and obvious ligamentous injuries
- CT scan for ligamentous injury is 32% sensitive
- Contrast CT cervical spine angiography may be done to assess injury to carotids and vertebral arteries
- In the setting of fracture with subluxation, there is a higher rate of vascular injury

 TABLE 98.5: CT: cervical spine

IV contrast	No, unless suspicion of vascular injury
PO contrast	No
Amount of radiation	3 mSv

Classic Images

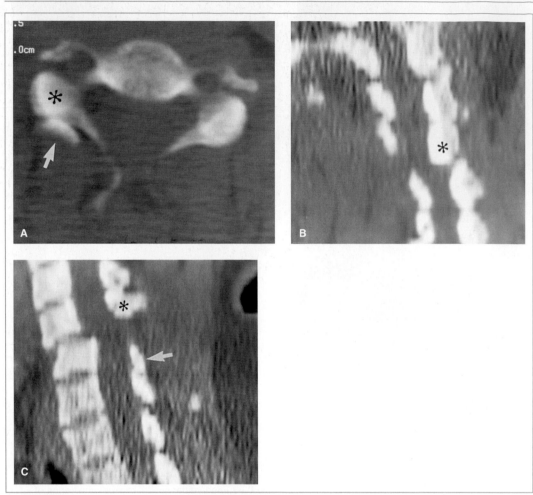

FIGURE 98.4: Unilateral interfacetal dislocation as seen by multiplanar CT. On the axial CT image (**A**), the dislocated articular mass (*asterisk*) lies anterior to the superior articular process of the subjacent articular mass, leaving its superior facet uncovered ("naked facet") (*arrow*). The sagittal reformation of the side of dislocation (**B**) clearly shows the dislocated articular mass (*asterisk*) anterior to its subjacent counterpart. On the sagittal reformation of the opposite side (**C**), the articular mass (*asterisk*) is subluxated with respect to the subjacent lamina (*arrow*). (From Harris J and Harris W. The Radiology of Emergency Medicine, 4th ed. Philadelphia: Lippincott Williams & Wilkins, 2000.)

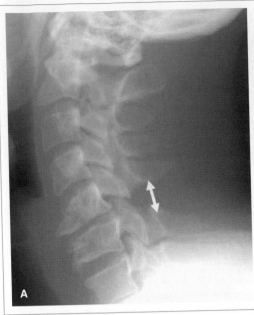
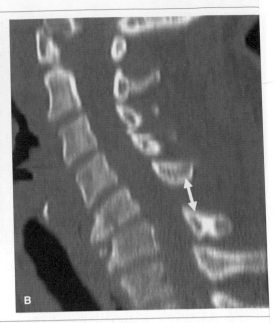

FIGURE 98.5: Anterior subluxation of C5. Lateral radiographs of the cervical spine (**A**) and sagittal multiplanar reformation (**B**) show widening of the interspinous distance at C5-6 ("fanning") (*white arrows*) and subtle localized hyperkyphotic angulation at C5-6. (From Schwartz Ed and Flanders AE. Spinal Trauma: Imaging, Diagnosis, and Management. Philadelphia: Lippincott Williams & Wilkins, 2007.)

MRI
- Gold standard test for ligamentous injury
- Most commonly performed 3 days or more after initial injury
- Typically performed without contrast

TABLE 98.6: Indications for MRI

Neurologic deficit
Obvious subluxation on x-ray or CT scan
Subluxation or abnormality on flexion-extension x-rays
Persistent pain in cervical spine with limited neck movement posttrauma

 TABLE 98.7: MRI: cervical spine

IV contrast	No
PO contrast	No
Amount of radiation	None

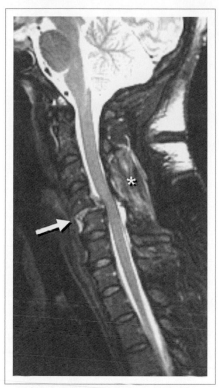

FIGURE 98.8: Unilateral interfacetal dislocation at C4-5. Sagittal T2-weighted image with fat suppression shows anterior subluxation of C4 on C5 with disk disruption and anterior herniation of disk material (*arrow*). Note that the edema in the posterior paraspinal musculature (*asterisk*) is related to the rotational component of the injury. (From Schwartz ED and Flanders AE. Spinal Trauma: Imaging, Diagnosis, and Management. Philadelphia: Lippincott Williams & Wilkins, 2007.)

Basic Management

- Maintain cervical spine precautions with cervical collar
- Patients requiring airway protection should be intubated without spinal manipulation
- Perform a thorough neurologic examination
- When subluxation or ligamentous injury is identified, obtain spine consultation from either neurosurgeon or spine orthopedic surgeon to determine further management

Summary

TABLE 98.8: Advantages and disadvantages of imaging modalities in ligamentous cervical injury

Imaging modality	Advantages	Disadvantages
Plain x-ray	Low cost Minimal patient discomfort	Poor sensitivity Difficult to obtain in obtunded patients
CT scan	Readily available Fracture/dislocation evaluation Other diagnoses also possible	Radiation exposure Poor sensitivity for ligamentous injury
MRI	Gold standard	Time-consuming Often difficult to obtain rapidly

99

Boxer's Fracture

Michael Barra and Sanford Sineff

Background

Boxer's fractures are fractures of the neck of the metacarpal bones typically the fourth or fifth metacarpal. Volar angulation the fracture fragment occurs with resultant rotational deformity.

TABLE 99.1: Classic history and physical

Sudden pain near the base of the fifth or fourth finger after an impaction force, i.e., punch into an unyielding surface such as a wall, window, or skull

Swelling, tenderness, erythema, or ecchymosis over the ulnar aspect of the hand

Deformity with volar angulation on the ulnar aspect of the hand

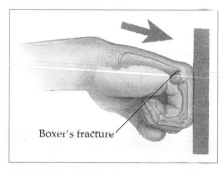

FIGURE 99.1: Mechanism for a boxer's fracture. (Anatomical Chart Company, Upper extremity disorders.)

Hand X-ray

- Order three views (PA, lateral, and oblique) of the hand to assess fracture deformity and angulation
- Look for an interruption of the metacarpal's radiopaque cortex near the neck/head junction of the fourth or fifth digit
- Assess angulation of the distal fracture fragment

 TABLE 99.2: Hand x-ray: boxer's fracture

IV contrast	No
PO contrast	No
Amount of radiation	0.005 mSv per view

Classic Images

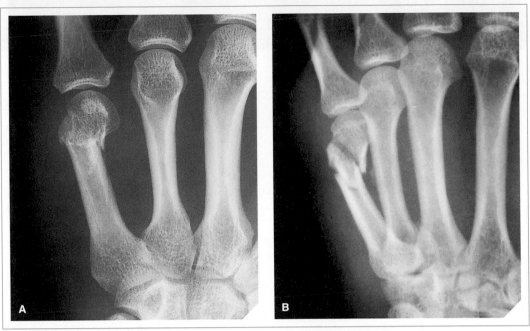

FIGURE 99.2: Boxer's fracture. **A:** Dorsovolar radiograph of the right hand demonstrates a fracture of the fifth metacarpal with volar angulation of the distal fragment—a simple boxer's fracture. When comminution is present, it is essential for its prognostic value to demonstrate the extent of fracture lines because such fractures are frequently unstable. **B:** The oblique projection usually suffices to determine the extent of comminution. (From Greenspan A. Orthopedic Imaging: A Practical Approach, 4th ed. Philadelphia: Lippincott Williams & Wilkins, 2004.)

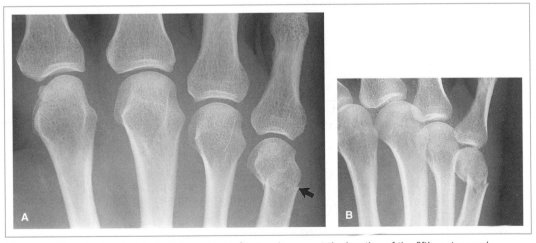

FIGURE 99.3: A: PA hand. Note that a transverse fracture is seen at the junction of the fifth metacarpal head and shaft (*arrow*). Some slight radial displacement of the head is also present. **B:** PA oblique hand. Note that this view reveals the significant anterior displacement of the metacarpal head, which is common in these injuries. (From Yochum TR and Rowe LJ. Yochum and Rowe's Essentials of Skeletal Radiology, 3rd ed. Philadelphia: Lippincott Williams & Wilkins, 2004.)

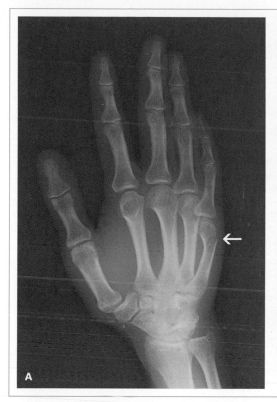 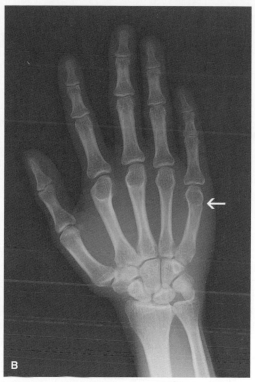

FIGURE 99.4: A: Oblique view with fracture of the fifth metatarsal (*arrow*). **B:** Frontal view with fracture of the fifth metatarsal (*arrow*) (*Courtesy of Washington University Hospital, St. Louis, MO.*)

Basic Management
- Evaluate and document a neurovascular examination both before and after reduction is performed and splint applied
- Pain control
- Open fracture
  - Higher risk of infection if impact was with the mouth or teeth
  - Consult orthopaedics
- Fracture reduction if angulation is >20 degrees for the fourth metacarpal and >40 degrees for the fifth metacarpal
- Splint with the wrist in 20 degrees of extension and the metacarpophalangeal joint flexed to 90 degrees

Summary

TABLE 99.3: Advantages and disadvantages of x-ray in boxer's fracture

Advantage	Disadvantage
Fast	May not delineate fracture or extent of fracture
Low cost	Cannot assess rotational deformity
Minimal radiation	

100

Scaphoid (Navicular) Fracture

Nick Rathert and David Seltzer

Background

Scaphoid fractures are the most common carpal fractures accounting for approximately 70% and occurring most commonly in young adults. Radiographic diagnosis can be difficult as film radiography misses up to 15% of acute fractures. The major blood supply is from the scaphoid branch of the radial artery, which supplies 70–80% of this bone including the proximal pole. Most fractures occur at the waist or middle pole of the bone. Because of the vascular supply, fractures through the proximal two-thirds are at risk for avascular necrosis (15–50%). Other complications of these fractures include delayed union or malunion and degenerative arthritis.

TABLE 100.1: Classic history and physical

Fall on outstretched hand
Pain and tenderness over distal radius
Subacute or chronic wrist pain (e.g., in athletes)
Anatomic snuff box tenderness (especially in ulnar deviation)
Pain with axial loading of first metacarpal
Pain elicited with resisting supination and pronation of hand
Reduced grip strength
Mild limited range of motion of first metacarpal
Swelling and ecchymosis rarely

Plain Radiographs

- Because scaphoid fractures can be subtle, precise positioning for x-ray is important
- Anteroposterior (AP) and lateral views of the wrist have a sensitivity of only 65–70%; order a dedicated scaphoid view to increase sensitivity
- Standard views: posteroanterior, true lateral, and semipronated oblique
- Look for a lucent line with a disrupted cortex
- Look for disruption of the scaphoid fat pad
- Look for soft tissue swelling
- On AP view, look for humpback deformity:
  - Angulation of the scaphoid at the fracture—proximal fragment dorsiflexes and distal fragment volarflexes causing dorsal apical angulation
  - Associated with mal- or non-union and arthritis
- On lateral view, look for excessive dorsiflexion (dorsal tilting) of the lunate:
  - Displacement of a scaphoid waist fracture is one etiology
  - Dorsal intercalated segment instability is another etiology
- Measure the scapholunate angle: a normal scapholunate angle is 47 degrees and >60 degrees represents injury
- Measure the intrascaphoid angles (see Figure 100.1) to determine severity of injury
- Draw lines through the extremes of the articular surfaces of both the proximal scaphoid and the distal scaphoid
- Draw an additional line perpendicular to these initial lines
- The angle between these lines should be <35 degrees, with angulation >45 degrees prognostic for poor outcomes

 TABLE 100.2: Wrist x-ray: scaphoid fracture

IV contrast	No
PO contrast	No
Amount of radiation	0.005 mSv per view

Classic Images

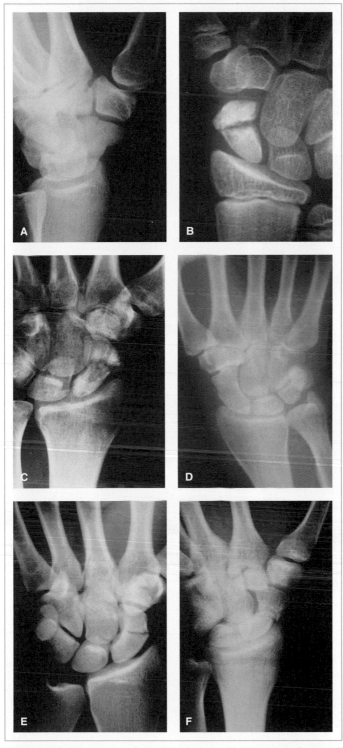

FIGURE 100.1: Locations of scaphoid fracture. Distal tubercle fracture (**A**). Distal body fracture in a child (**B**) and in an adult (**C**). Scaphoid waist fracture, nondisplaced (**D**), minimally displaced and angulated (**E**), or widely displaced (**F**). (From Bucholz RW and Heckman JD. Rockwood and Green's Fractures in Adults, 5th ed. Philadelphia: Lippincott Williams & Wilkins, 2001.)

Carpal Bones CT Scan

- Thin section multidetector CT preferred
- Details complications associated with fractures and useful for monitoring healing
- Affected areas of fracture show increased areas of density

 TABLE 100.3: CT carpal bones: scaphoid fracture

IV contrast	No
PO contrast	No
Amount of Radiation	0.1 mSv

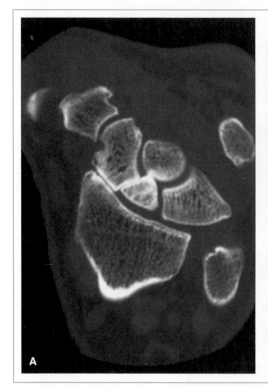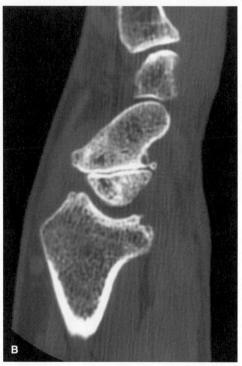

FIGURE 100.2: CT of ununited scaphoid fracture. Coronal (**A**) and sagittal (**B**) CT images showing nonunion of a scaphoid fracture. Note the sclerotic edges and gap between the fractured fragments. (From Greenspan A. Orthopedic Imaging: A Practical Approach, 4th ed. Philadelphia: Lippincott Williams & Wilkins, 2004.)

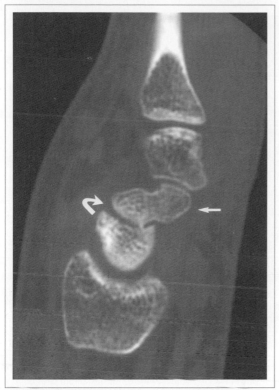

FIGURE 100.3: Humpback deformity. A sagittal reformatted CT image showing a humpback deformity of a fractured scaphoid. Note the palmar flexion of the distal fragment (*arrow*) and dorsal apex angulation (*curved arrow*). (From Greenspan A. Orthopedic Imaging: A Practical Approach, 4th ed. Philadelphia: Lippincott Williams & Wilkins, 2004.)

Bone Scan

- Rarely performed modality in the emergency department
- Not for acute injuries
- 100% sensitivity and 98% specificity

 TABLE 100.4: Bone scan: scaphoid fracture

IV radiotracer	As required by modality
PO contrast	No
Amount of radiation	3 mSv

MRI

- Considered the gold standard study
- Demonstrates fracture line not apparent with other modalities
- Diagnoses many other injuries, both bony and ligamentous
- Most sensitive and specific of all imaging modalities for scaphoid fracture diagnosis

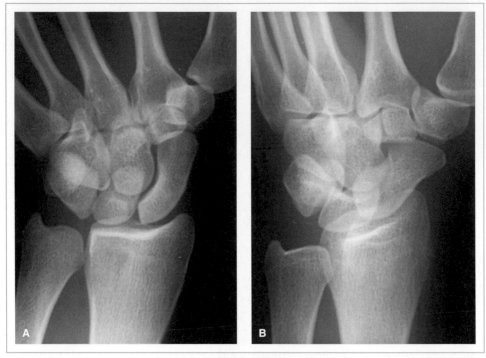

FIGURE 100.4: MRI of scaphoid fracture. Dorsovolar (**A**) in ulnar deviation and oblique (**B**) radiographs (as well as conventional dorsovolar and lateral views, not shown here) were normal. (From Greenspan A. Orthopedic Imaging: A Practical Approach, 4th ed. Philadelphia: Lippincott Williams & Wilkins, 2004.)

Table 100.5: Comparison of examination modalities

Test	Sensitivity (%)	Specificity (%)	Radiation dose (mSv)
Physical examination		74–80	
Plain film	65–70	90	0.03
Bone scan	100	98	3
CT (multidetector)	85–95	100	0.02
MRI	95–100	100	0

Basic Management

- Evaluate and document the neurovascular status
- Pain control
- Any fracture or suspected fracture (i.e., "snuff box tenderness") should be treated with immobilization using a thumb spica splint
- Long-arm thumb spica (vs. short-arm) immobilization may reduce nonunion and decrease healing time
- Close outpatient follow-up with an orthopedic surgeon
- If greater than 1 mm step off or >60 degree angle, consult orthopedic surgeon in emergency department

Summary

TABLE 100.6: Advantages and disadvantages of imaging modalities in scaphoid fracture

Imaging modalities	Advantages	Disadvantages
X-ray	Accessible	Often nondiagnostic
CT	Often accessible	Unable to evaluate ligaments
Bone scan	Highly diagnostic	Limited access Not for acute injury
MRI	Superior diagnostic ability	Costly Limited access

101 Lunate and Perilunate Dislocation

Patrick Kennedy and Brian Cohn

Background

Lunate and perilunate dislocations are the most common carpal bone dislocations. These can be purely ligamentous injuries or can involve fractures of the surrounding carpal bones. When the fracture is associated with a carpal dislocation, the term "trans" refers to the fractured bone. A transscaphoid perilunate dislocation is most common. The injuries represent a spectrum of ligamentous and bony disruption. Potential complications include degenerative arthritis, delayed union or malunion, avascular necrosis, or carpal tunnel median nerve compression.

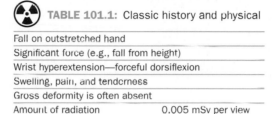

TABLE 101.1: Classic history and physical

Fall on outstretched hand	
Significant force (e.g., fall from height)	
Wrist hyperextension—forceful dorsiflexion	
Swelling, pain, and tenderness	
Gross deformity is often absent	
Amount of radiation	0.005 mSv per view

Wrist X-ray

- Obtain anteroposterior (AP), lateral, and oblique views—neutral position is usually sufficient
- "3 C's" sign: normal alignment on lateral view of the distal radius, lunate, and capitate; a break in this lateral alignment is pathognomonic of a subluxation or dislocation
- "Terry-Thomas" sign: widened space between the scaphoid and the lunate (normally <2 mm); especially apparent on ulnar deviation view
- "Signet ring" sign: abnormal finding of cortical ring shadow of the scaphoid on dorsovolar AP view; look for the scaphoid's tuberosity viewed on end, apparent in neutral or ulnar deviation view
- Lunate dislocation:
  - Capitate is in normal alignment, lunate is angled away from distal radial surface (lateral view)
  - "Spilled teacup" sign: the lunate normally is shaped like an upward facing cup; when dislocated, the "cup" tips toward the palmar surface of the wrist (lateral view)
  - "Piece of pie" sign: the lunate will appear as a quadrangle normally; when dislocated it will look triangular (AP view)
- Perilunate dislocation:
  - Dorsal or volar angulation of the capitate with the lunate and distal radius aligned (lateral view)
  - The "teacup" lunate is upright on lateral view, but the capitate will not articulate with the "cup" surface of the lunate; the capitate is most often displaced dorsally and will sit on top of the radius

Classic Images

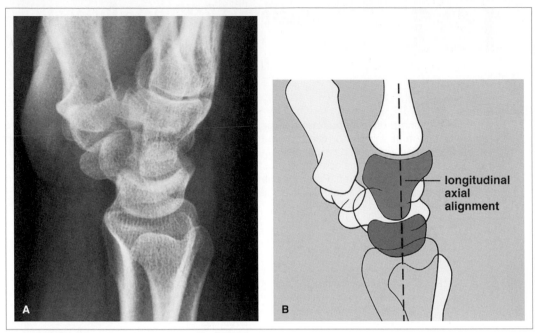

FIGURE 101.1: Longitudinal axial alignment. On the lateral view of the wrist, the central axes of the radius, the lunate, the capitate, and the third metacarpal normally form a straight line. (From Greenspan A. Orthopedic Imaging: A Practical Approach, 4th ed. Philadelphia: Lippincott Williams & Wilkins, 2004.)

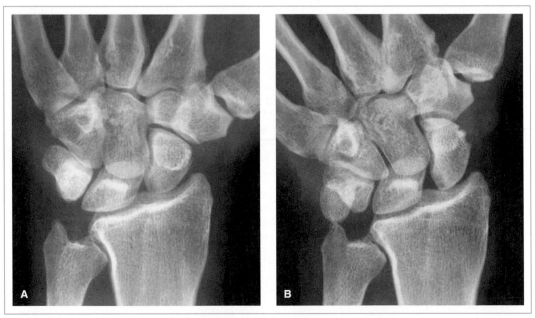

FIGURE 101.2: Scapholunate dissociation. (**A**) On the dorsovolar projection of the wrist in the neutral position, a gap between the scaphoid and the lunate is not well demonstrated. (**B**) On ulnar deviation, however, the gap becomes apparent, indicating scapholunate dissociation. (From Greenspan A. Orthopedic Imaging: A Practical Approach, 4th ed. Philadelphia: Lippincott Williams & Wilkins, 2004.)

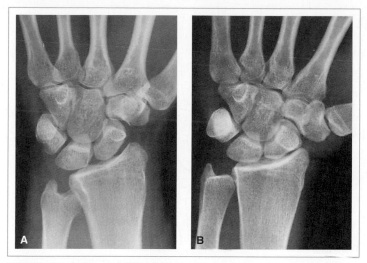

FIGURE 101.3: Signet-ring sign. (**A**) On the dorsovolar view of the wrist in the neutral position, rotary subluxation of the scaphoid can be recognized by the cortical ring shadow that appears projecting over the scaphoid. This phenomenon is caused by the bone's volar tilt and rotation, which cause it to appear foreshortened and its tuberosity to be seen on end. (**B**) A similar picture can be seen on the dorsovolar view of the wrist in radial deviation, but this apparent ring shadow is caused by the normal volar tilt of the scaphoid exaggerated by radial deviation. (From Greenspan A. Orthopedic Imaging: A Practical Approach, 4th ed. Philadelphia: Lippincott Williams & Wilkins, 2004.)

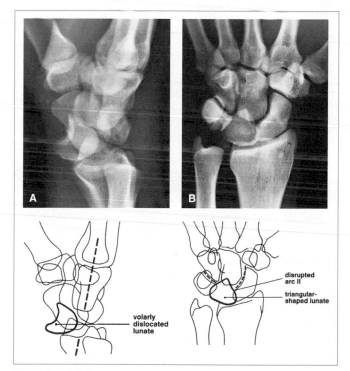

FIGURE 101.4: Lunate dislocation. (**A**) On the lateral view of the wrist, lunate dislocation is evident from the break in the longitudinal alignment of the third metacarpal and the capitate over the distal radial surface at the site of the lunate, which is volarly rotated and displaced. (**B**) Dorsovolar projection shows a disrupted arc II at the site of the lunate, indicating malalignment. Note also the triangular appearance of the lunate, a finding virtually pathognomonic of dislocation of this bone. (From Greenspan A. Orthopedic Imaging: A Practical Approach, 4th ed. Philadelphia: Lippincott Williams & Wilkins, 2004.)

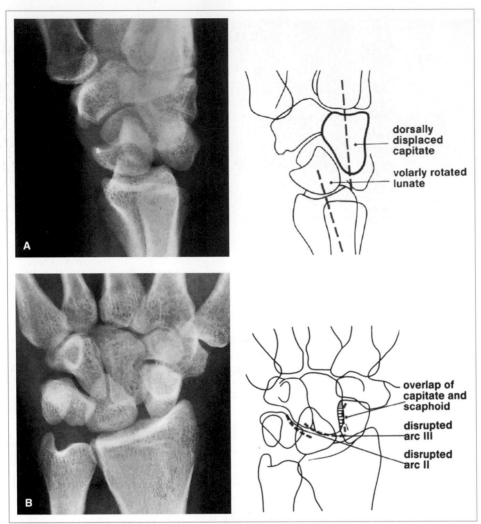

FIGURE 101.5: Perilunate dislocation. (**A**) Lateral radiograph of the wrist demonstrates perilunate dislocation characterized by displacement of the capitate dorsal to the lunate, which, although slightly volarly rotated, remains in articulation with the distal radius. Note the break in the longitudinal alignment of the third metacarpal and the capitate with the lunate and the distal radial surface. On the dorsovolar projection (**B**), perilunate dislocation is evident from the overlapping proximal and distal carpal rows and the resulting disruption of arcs II and III. (From Greenspan A. Orthopedic Imaging: A Practical Approach, 4th ed. Philadelphia: Lippincott Williams & Wilkins, 2004.)

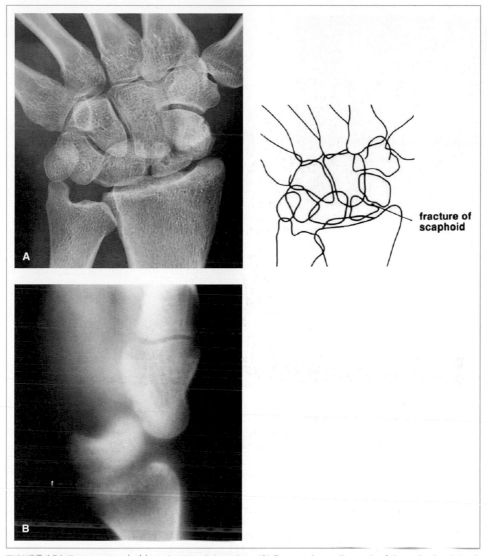

fracture of scaphoid

FIGURE 101.6: Transscaphoid perilunate dislocation. (**A**) Dorsovolar radiograph of the wrist in ulnar deviation clearly shows scaphoid fracture, but the disruptions in the distal carpal arcs are unclear as to the type of dislocation. The lateral view was also inconclusive. (**B**) Lateral tomogram demonstrates that the capitate is displaced dorsal to the lunate, which remains in articulation with the distal radius—the classic appearance of perilunate dislocation. (From Greenspan A. Orthopedic Imaging: A Practical Approach, 4th ed. Philadelphia: Lippincott Williams & Wilkins, 2004.)

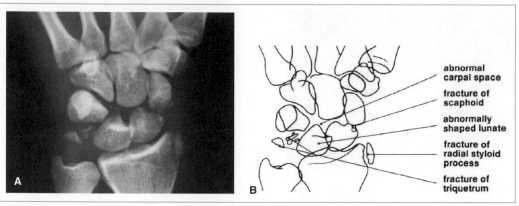

FIGURE 101.7: Transradial, transscaphoid, transtriquetral lunate dislocation. Dorsovolar view of the wrist clearly reveals fractures of the radial styloid process, the scaphoid, and the triquetrum. The wide space separating the proximal and distal carpal rows and the triangular shape of the lunate indicate the possibility of lunate dislocation. Note the disruption in arcs I and II. The lateral view confirmed volar displacement of the lunate and the normal position of the capitate. This abnormality can be described as a transradial, transscaphoid, and transtriquetral lunate dislocation. (From Greenspan A. Orthopedic Imaging: A Practical Approach, 4th ed. Philadelphia: Lippincott Williams & Wilkins, 2004.)

Basic Management

- Analgesia
- Hand/orthopedic surgery consultation
- Closed reduction may be attempted followed by splinting
- Primary or delayed surgical intervention is the definitive treatment, and may consist of open or percutaneous pin fixation

Summary

TABLE 101.2: Advantages and disadvantages of x-ray in lunate-perilunate dislocation

Advantages	Disadvantages
Fast	Pain with manipulation to obtain all views
Low cost	
Minimal radiation	

102

Colles' Fracture

Caleb Trent and Julie McManemy

Background

Distal radius fractures are the most common pediatric and adult fractures of the upper extremity, with fractures of the radius and/or ulna accounting for up to 44% of fractures in the emergency department. Abraham Colles originally described an impacted metaphyseal fracture with dorsal displacement of the distal fragment ("silver fork deformity"). Commonly, an ulnar styloid fracture is present. A distal radius fracture with a volarly displaced distal fragment is referred to as a Smith's fracture (see Chapter 103) or a reverse Colles' fracture. Acute complications associated with a Colles' fracture may include injury to the median nerve or to the triangular fibrocartilage complex when there is concomitant ulnar styloid fracture Long-term complications may include malunion, joint instability, or post-traumatic arthritis.

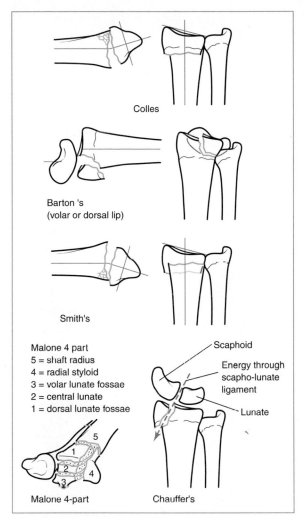

FIGURE 102.1: Eponymic classification of five basic types of distal radius fractures: four classic (Colles, Barton, Smith, and chauffeur's) fracture descriptions, and the Malone four-part fracture, which was described more recently and represents an increasing understanding of the importance of the distal radioulnar joint and the ulnar column of the radius. (From Egol K, Koval KJ, and Zuckerman JD. Handbook of Fractures, 4th ed. Philadelphia: Lippincott Williams & Wilkins, 2010.)

TABLE 102.1: Classic history and physical

Fall on an outstretched hand with the wrist in extension and forearm pronated
Wrist tenderness, swelling, decreased range of motion, and associated deformity
Palmar numbness or paresthesias (median nerve injury)

Wrist X-ray

- Obtain anteroposterior (AP) lateral and oblique views of the wrist
- Measure the radial inclination, height, and volar tilt
- Standard measurements include:
    - Radial inclination of 20–25 degrees
    - Radial height of 10–13 mm
    - Volar tilt of 2–20 degrees with an average of 11 degrees on the lateral x-ray
- Look for ulnar styloid process or ulnar head fractures
- Look for a distal metaphyseal fracture of the radius appearing shortened from angulation or comminution (AP view)
- Look for dorsal angulation and comminution (lateral view)

- Complicated fracture characteristics:
  - \>20 degrees angulation
  - Comminution
  - \>1-cm shortening
  - Intra-articular involvement

 TABLE 102.2: Wrist x-rays: distal radial fracture

IV contrast	No
PO contrast	No
Amount of radiation	0.005 mSv per view

Classic Images

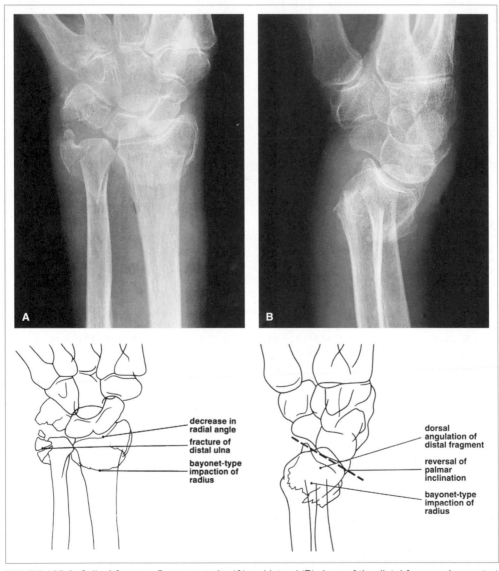

FIGURE 102.2: Colles' fracture. Posteroanterior (**A**) and lateral (**B**) views of the distal forearm demonstrate the features of Colles' fracture. On the posteroanterior projection, a decrease in the radial angle and an associated fracture of the distal ulna are evident. The lateral view reveals the dorsal angulation of the distal radius, as well as a reversal of the palmar inclination. On both views, the radius is foreshortened secondary to bayonet-type displacement. The fracture line does not extend to the joint (Frykman type II). (From Greenspan A. Orthopedic Imaging: A Practical Approach, 4th ed. Philadelphia: Lippincott Williams & Wilkins, 2004.)

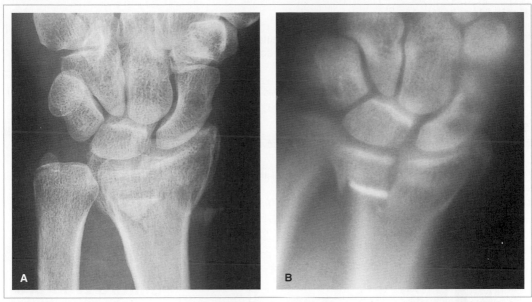

FIGURE 102.3: Intra-articular fracture of the distal radius. Posteroanterior radiograph of the distal forearm (**A**) and trispiral tomogram (**B**) show Frykman type IV fracture. The fracture extends into the radiocarpal joint, the distal radioulnar joint is spared, and there is an associated fracture of the ulnar styloid. (From Greenspan A. Orthopedic Imaging: A Practical Approach, 4th ed. Philadelphia: Lippincott Williams & Wilkins, 2004.)

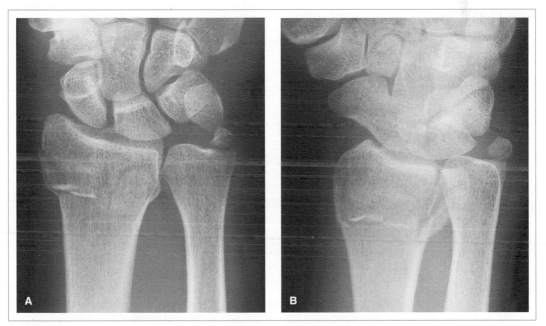

FIGURE 102.4: Intra-articular fracture of the distal radius. Posteroanterior (**A**) and oblique (**B**) radiographs of the distal forearm show Frykman type VI fracture. The fracture line extends into the distal radioulnar joint and in addition, there is a fracture of the ulnar styloid. (From Greenspan A. Orthopedic Imaging: A Practical Approach, 4th ed. Philadelphia: Lippincott Williams & Wilkins, 2004.)

Basic Management
- Analgesia
- Perform and document a detailed neurovascular examination pre- and postreduction
- Accurate anatomic reduction for displaced fractures
- Perform a postreduction x-ray
- Initial immobilization with splinting
- Orthopedic consultation should be considered for complicated or open fractures, neurovascular compromise, or difficulty in fracture reduction

Summary

TABLE 102.3: Advantages and disadvantages of x-ray in Colles' fracture

Advantages	Disadvantages
Minimal radiation	Pain with manipulation to obtain all views
Minimal cost	
Fast	
Easy to obtain	

103

Smith's Fracture

Michael Lohmeier and Chris Sampson

Background

Named after the orthopedic surgeon Robert William Smith, a Smith's fracture (also called a garden spade deformity or a reverse Colle's fracture) describes a transverse distal radius fracture with volar angulation of the distal fragment.

The radioulnar joint is typically not involved. Complications are seen infrequently, but can include Volkmann's ischemic contracture, acute carpal tunnel syndrome, compressive neuropathy, and post-traumatic osteoarthritis.

TABLE 103.1: Classic history and physical

Fall or direct blow on the dorsum of the hand or wrist
Punch with clenched fist and wrist slightly flexed
Backward fall onto outstretched palm with forced pronation
Pain over the distal aspect of the forearm, with volar displacement of the hand and wrist
Hand appears as a garden spade

TABLE 103.2: Classification of Smith's fracture

Type I: Transverse fracture remaining extra-articular
Type II: Involves the dorsal articular surface
Type III: Enters the radiocarpal joint

Wrist X-ray
- Order anteroposterior (AP), lateral, and oblique views of the wrist
- AP view appears similar to a Colle's fracture with a shortened and perhaps comminuted distal metaphyseal radius
- The lateral view demonstrates volar angulation (in contrast to a Colle's fracture) of the displaced distal fracture fragment sometimes involving the radiocarpal joint
- Lateral view best assesses the fracture line obliquity

 TABLE 103.3: Wrist x-rays: Smith's Fracture

IV contrast	No
PO contrast	No
Amount of radiation	0.005 mSv per view

Classic Images

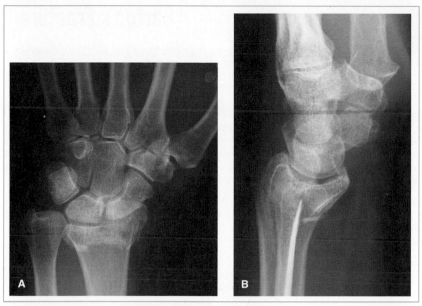

FIGURE 103.1: Smith's fracture of distal radius. On AP view (**A**), a shortened distal metaphyseal distal radius is seen. On lateral view (**B**), volar angulation is seen. (*Courtesy of Washington University School of Medicine, St. Louis, MO.*)

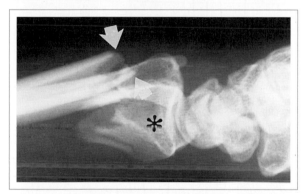

FIGURE 103.2: Smith's fracture characterized by a transverse fracture (*arrows*) of the distal radius, with volar and proximal displacement of the distal radial fragment (*asterisk*). (From Harris JH Jr and Harris WH. The Radiology of Emergency Medicine, 3rd ed. Philadelphia: Lippincott-Raven, 2000:386, with permission.)

Basic Management
- Perform and document a detailed neurovascular examination pre- and postreduction
- In type I fractures, closed reduction may be attempted
- Place a long-arm splint with the forearm in supination and the wrist in neutral or slight extension
- Type II and III fractures require open reduction and internal fixation
- CT and MRI can better evaluate complex distal radius fractures to assess for associated injuries and may be requested by the consultative service but are not routinely ordered from the emergency department

Summary

TABLE 103.4: Advantages and disadvantages of x-ray in Smith's fracture

Advantages	Disadvantages
Fast and available	Pain with manipulation to obtain all views
Inexpensive	May not delineate subtle fractures or extent of fracture
Minimal radiation	

Background

Barton's fracture (BF) is an unstable distal radiocarpal fracture dislocation named after John Rhea Barton (1794–1871), an American surgeon who first described this injury in 1814. BF is caused by a fall on a dorsiflexed and pronated wrist increasing carpal compression force on the dorsal rim. It is the most common fracture-dislocation of the wrist joint and results from shearing of the carpal bones against the anterior or dorsal lip of the radial articular surface.

BF does not violate the volar surface of the radius. A reverse BF involves the volar rim of the distal end of the radius. Complications of BF include radial shortening and angulation leading to deformity, inferior radioulnar joint subluxation or dislocation, reflex sympathetic dystrophy, osteoarthritis, and tendon rupture.

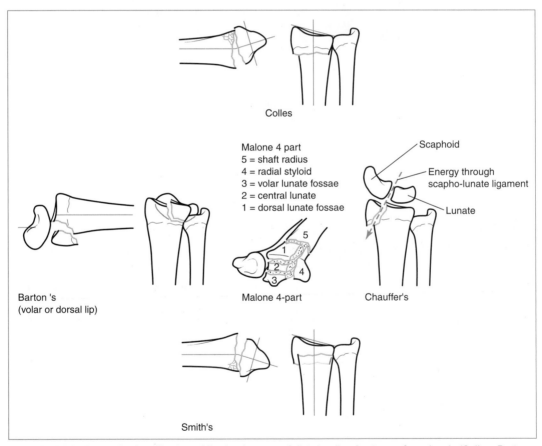

FIGURE 104.1: Eponymic classification of five basic types of distal radius fractures: four classic (Colles, Barton, Smith, and chauffeur's) fracture descriptions and the Melone four-part fracture, which was described more recently and represents an increasing understanding of the importance of the distal radioulnar joint (DRUJ) and the ulnar column of the radius. (From Bucholz RW and Heckman JD. Rockwood and Green's Fractures in Adults, 5th ed. Philadelphia: Lippincott Williams & Wilkins, 2001.)

TABLE 104.1: Classic history and physical

Fall on an outstretched hand
Limited range of motion at the wrist
Soft tissue swelling, deformity, and tenderness at the wrist

Wrist X-ray

- Order anteroposterior (AP) lateral and oblique views of the wrist
- AP view typically shows a comminuted distal radius
- Lateral view typically shows an intra-articular fracture of the dorsal (or volar [reverse BF]) rim
- Carpal bones often sublux in the same direction as the fracture
- Check the normal anatomic alignments
  - Lateral: radio-carpal joint normally has 11 degrees of palmar angulation with range of 1–23 degrees
  - AP: Ulnar angulation is normally 15–30 degrees
  - Radial length (distance between the ulnar aspect of the distal radius and the tip of the radial styloid) normally measures 11–12 mm
- Look for an associated ulnar styloid fracture
- Look for involvement of the radiocarpal joint
- If the radius appears to be angulated and/or displaced significantly, maintain a high degree of suspicion for a concomitant fracture of the ulna

 TABLE 104.2: Wrist x-ray: Barton's fracture

IV contrast	No
PO contrast	No
Amount of radiation	0.005 mSv per view

Classic Images

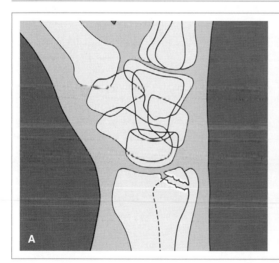 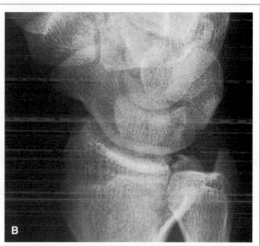

FIGURE 104.2: Barton's fracture (BF). Schematic (**A**) and oblique radiograph (**B**) showing the typical appearance of BF. The fracture line in the coronal plane extends from the dorsal margin of the distal radius into the radiocarpal articulation. (From Greenspan A. Orthopedic Imaging: A Practical Approach, 4th ed. Philadelphia: Lippincott Williams & Wilkins, 2004.)

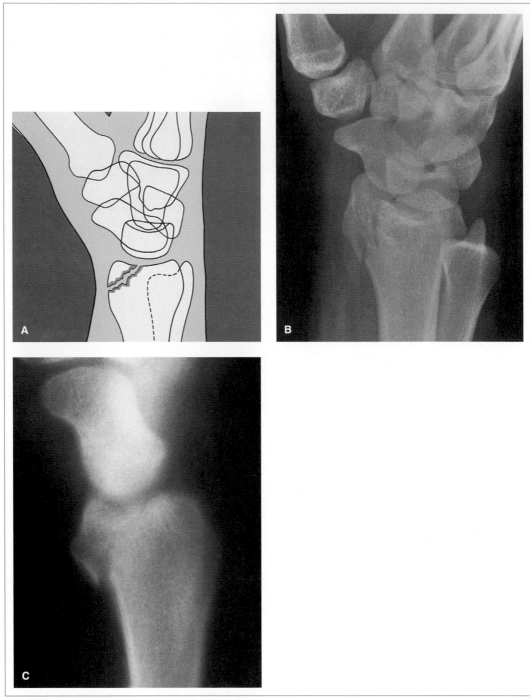

FIGURE 104.3: Reverse Barton's fracture (BF). Schematic (**A**), oblique radiograph (**B**), and lateral trispiral tomogram (**C**) showing reverse (or volar) BF; the fracture line is also oriented in the coronal plane, but extends from the volar margin of the radial styloid process into the radiocarpal joint. (From Greenspan A. Orthopedic Imaging: A Practical Approach, 4th ed. Philadelphia: Lippincott Williams & Wilkins, 2004.)

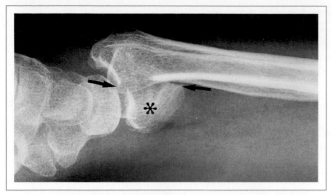

FIGURE 104.4: Classic volar Barton's fracture. The oblique intra-articular fracture (*arrows*) involves the volar aspect of the distal radius. The separate fragment (*asterisk*) and the bones of the wrist and hand are volarly and proximally displaced. (From Harris JH Jr and Harris WH. The Radiology of Emergency Medicine, 3rd ed. Philadelphia: Lippincott-Raven, 2000.)

Basic Management
- Analgesia
- Perform and document a detailed neurovascular examination pre- and postreduction
- Early anatomic closed reduction, splint, and stabilization
- Orthopaedic surgery consultation
  - Carpal subluxation
  - >50% involvement of the articular surface
  - Open reduction internal fixation is common

Summary

TABLE 104.3: Advantages and disadvantages of x-ray in Barton's fracture

Advantages	Disadvantages
Easy	Pain with manipulation to obtain all views
Inexpensive	Difficult to visualize lack detail of articular disruption
Low radiation	

105

Chauffeur's Fracture

Sreeja Natesan and Mark Levine

Background

Chauffeur's fracture or Hutchinson fracture is a fracture of the radial styloid caused by tension forces applied during ulnar deviation with supination of the wrist.

The name originates from a fracture a chauffeur would sustain when hand-cranking to start an automobile. A backfire of the crank would cause a direct injury to the thenar side of the wrist resulting in an intra-articular fracture at the base of the radial styloid.

TABLE 105.1: Classic history and physical

Sudden deceleration with hands on steering wheel
Direct blow to radial aspect of the wrist
Fall back onto outstretched hand
Forced ulnar deviation and wrist supination
Soft tissue swelling, deformity, and radial side of wrist tenderness

Wrist X-ray

- Obtain three views (anteroposterior, lateral, oblique) of the wrist to clearly visualize the radial styloid and associated carpal bones
- Look for an interruption in the radio-opaque cortex of the radial styloid
- Look for a concomitant fracture of the scaphoid, the lunate, or a scapholunate dislocation

 TABLE 105.2: Wrist x-ray: chauffeur's fracture

IV contrast	No
PO contrast	No
Amount of radiation	0.005 mSv per view

Classic Images

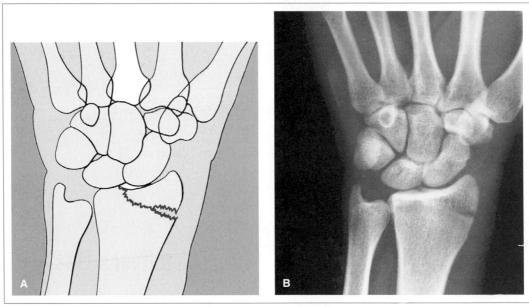

FIGURE 105.1: Hutchinson fracture. Schematic (**A**) and dorsovolar radiograph (**B**) showing classic appearance of Hutchinson fracture. The fracture line in the sagittal plane extends through the radial margin of the radial styloid process into the radiocarpal articulation. (From Greenspan A. Orthopedic Imaging: A Practical Approach, 4th ed. Philadelphia: Lippincott Williams & Wilkins, 2004.)

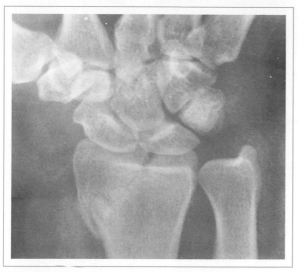

FIGURE 105.2: Chauffeur's fracture. Complete fracture extending diagonally across the base of the radial styloid. (From Eisenberg RL. An Atlas of Differential Diagnosis, 4th ed. Philadelphia: Lippincott Williams & Wilkins, 2003.)

Basic Management
- Analgesia
- Evaluate and document a neurovascular examination both before and after splinting is performed
- Immobilize the patient in a thumb spica splint and refer to an orthopedic hand specialist for expectant operative fixation
- With neurovascular compromise, reduction and immediate orthopedic consultation are indicated
- CT or MRI is not indicated but may be requested by the consultative service

Summary

TABLE 105.3: Advantages and disadvantages of x-ray in chauffeur's fracture

Advantages	Disadvantages
Fast	Pain with manipulation to obtain all views
Minimal radiation	May not delineate fracture or extent of fracture

106
Galeazzi Fracture-Dislocation
Jeff Spencer and Randall Howell

Background

The Galeazzi fracture-dislocation (GFD), also known as a reverse Monteggia fracture, is an injury pattern involving a fracture of the junction of the middle and distal thirds of the radius with an associated subluxation or dislocation of the distal radioulnar joint (DRUJ). First described by Cooper in 1842, this fracture became synonymous with the name of Italian surgeon Ricardo Galeazzi (1866–1952) who presented this pattern as a compliment to the Monteggia fracture. GFDs account for 3–7% of all forearm fractures, are more common in men, and can present a difficult diagnosis for acute care providers. This injury occurs during extremes of wrist extension and pronation. Nondiagnosis can lead to long-term functional impairment of the affected wrist, most notably chronic pain and limited pronation and supination.

TABLE 106.1: Classic history and physical

Fall on an outstretched hand with the elbow flexed and forearm pronated
Direct blow to the dorsolateral aspect of the wrist
Swelling and tenderness over the DRUJ
Tenderness and dorsal swelling or deformity of the mid to distal ulna
AIN palsy with loss of the pinch mechanism between the thumb and index finger but with preserved sensation
Concave deformity on the radial aspect of the wrist and/or tenting of the skin

AIN, anterior interosseous nerve; DRUJ, distal radioulnar joint.

Forearm X-ray

- Obtain anteroposterior and true lateral views of the forearm, wrist, and elbow
- Radiographs of the contralateral extremity may be helpful for comparison
- Indications of a GFD:
  - Type 1: extra-articular distal radial fracture
  - Type 2: comminuted distal radius fracture involving the radiocarpal joint
  - Look for a dorsally displaced proximal end of the radial fracture fragment and a medially and dorsally displaced ulna
  - Fracture at the base of the ulnar styloid is the functional equivalent of triangular fibrocartilage rupture
  - Anteroposterior widening of the DRUJ (no absolute width defines a dislocation)
  - Complete radioulnar dislocation with widening of the DRUJ and dorsal prominence of the distal ulna
  - Lateral view:
    - Look for disassociation of the radius and ulna
    - Distal radius and ulna no longer lie in the same vertical plane
    - Ulna is displaced dorsally
  - There is 5 mm of radial shortening (comparison films are helpful)

 TABLE 106.2: Upper extremity x-ray: Galeazzi fracture-dislocation

IV contrast	No
PO contrast	No
Amount of radiation	0.005 mSv per view

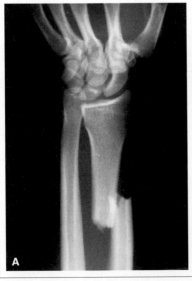 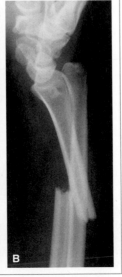

FIGURE 106.1: Galeazzi fracture-dislocation (GFD). Posteroanterior (**A**) and lateral (**B**) radiographs of the distal forearm show type I GFD. The simple fracture of the radius affects the distal third of the bone, and the proximal end of the distal fragment is dorsally displaced and angulated. In addition, there is dislocation in the distal radioulnar joint. (From Greenspan A. Orthopedic Imaging: A Practical Approach, 4th ed. Philadelphia: Lippincott Williams & Wilkins, 2004.)

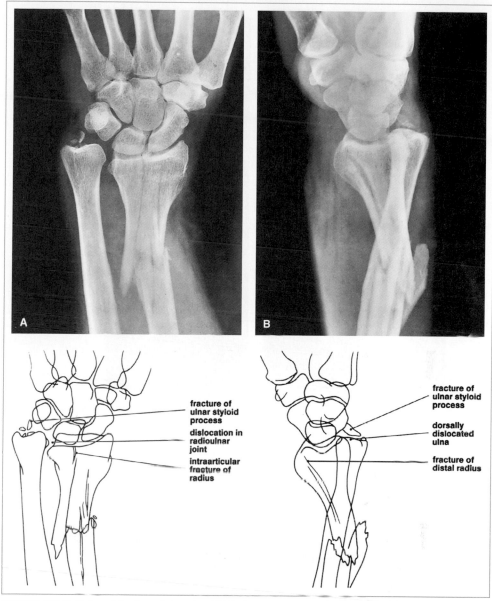

FIGURE 106.2: Galeazzi fracture-dislocation (GFD). Posteroanterior (**A**) and lateral (**B**) projections of the distal forearm demonstrate the two components of type II GFD. The posteroanterior view clearly reveals the fracture of the distal radius, which in this case is a comminuted fracture extending into the radiocarpal joint. The distal fragment has a slight lateral angulation. Note also the associated comminuted fracture of the ulnar styloid process and the dislocation in the radioulnar joint. These features are also seen on the lateral projection, but this view provides in addition a better demonstration of the dorsal dislocation of the distal ulna. (From Greenspan A. Orthopedic Imaging: A Practical Approach, 4th ed. Philadelphia: Lippincott Williams & Wilkins, 2004.)

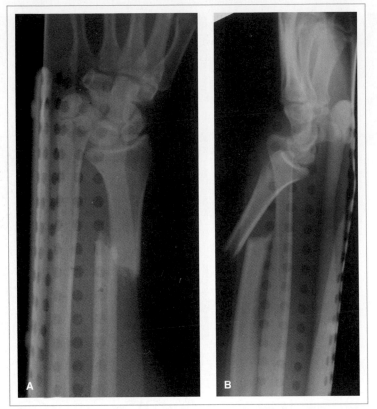

FIGURE 106.3: GFD. Anteroposterior (**A**) and lateral (**B**) views show a short oblique or transverse fracture of the radius with associated dislocation of the distal ulna. The dislocation results from the disruption of the distal radioulnar joint. (*Courtesy of Washington University School of Medicine. St. Louis, MO.*)

Basic Management

- Evaluate and document a detailed neurovascular examination both before and after reduction is performed and splint is applied
- Analgesia, immobilization, and orthopedic consultation
- Closed reduction and long-arm splint with the forearm in supination
- If unable to reduce, urgent orthopedic consultation
- Open fractures require tetanus immunization and prophylactic antibiotics
- Open reduction internal fixation is common

Summary

TABLE 106.3: Advantages and disadvantages of x-ray in Galeazzi fracture-dislocation

Advantages	Disadvantages
Fast	Pain with manipulation to obtain all views
Low cost	May not delineate fracture or extent of fracture
Minimal radiation	

107

Monteggia Fracture-Dislocation

Jake Keeperman and Richard T. Griffey

Background

Giovanni Battista Monteggia (1762–1815) first described a fracture of the proximal third of the ulna with dislocation of the radial head, giving this fracture-dislocation its name. While these injuries are relatively uncommon, accounting for less than 5% of all forearm fractures, there can be significant morbidity with missed injuries. It is thus imperative to properly evaluate and treat these fractures in a timely fashion. Several classification schemes have been proposed for Monteggia fractures, but the Bado classification system (proposed by Jose Luiz Bado) is the most widely used. Adults with Monteggia fractures-dislocations may have long-term complications including loss of range of motion.

TABLE 107.1: Classic history and physical

Fall on an outstretched hand with forearm in pronation
Direct blow to the dorsal forearm
Soft tissue swelling, pain and limited range of motion at the elbow
Obvious forearm deformity; tenting of the skin or ecchymosis
Impaired extension of the digits at the metacarpophalangeal joint or at the interphalangeal joint of the thumb with injury to the posterior interosseous nerve

TABLE 107.2: Bado Classification

Type	%	Dislocation direction of the radial head	Fracture location
I	60	Anterior	Proximal or middle third of the ulna
II	15	Posterior	Proximal or middle third of the ulna
III	20	Lateral	Ulnar metaphysis
IV	5	Anterior	Proximal or middle third of the ulna and radius

Upper Extremity X-ray

- Obtain two views of the forearm in orthogonal planes, including the elbow and wrist joints
- Obtain three-view views of the elbow (anteroposterior, lateral, and oblique) especially with isolated proximal or midshaft ulnar fractures and look for a radial head fracture
- In order to assess the radiocapitellar joint, a line down the long axis of the radius should bisect the capitellum on any projection of the elbow; discordance with this line and the capitellum suggests a possible radial head dislocation

 TABLE 107.3: Forearm and elbow x-rays: Monteggia fracture-dislocation

IV contrast	No
PO contrast	No
Amount of radiation	0.005 mSv per view

Classic Images

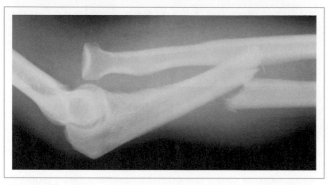

FIGURE 107.1: Monteggia fracture-dislocation. Lateral radiograph of the elbow joint and proximal third of the forearm shows type I Monteggia fracture-dislocation; anteriorly angulated fracture is at the proximal third of the ulna, associated with anterior dislocation of the radial head. (From Greenspan A. Orthopedic Imaging: A Practical Approach, 4th ed. Philadelphia: Lippincott Williams & Wilkins, 2004.)

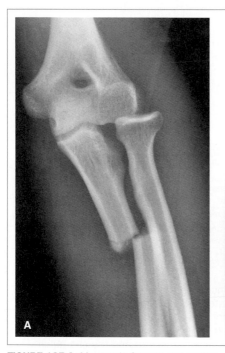
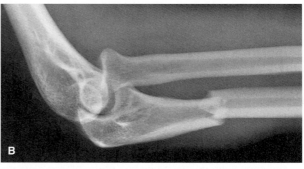

FIGURE 107.2: Monteggia fracture-dislocation. Anteroposterior (**A**) and lateral (**B**) views of the elbow that include the proximal third of the forearm demonstrate the typical appearance of type III Monteggia fracture-dislocation; fracture is at the proximal third of the ulna, associated with anterolateral dislocation of the radial head. (From Greenspan A. Orthopedic Imaging: A Practical Approach, 4th ed. Philadelphia: Lippincott Williams & Wilkins, 2004.)

Basic Management
- Evaluate and document a detailed neurovascular examination both before and after reduction is performed and splint applied
- Analgesia, immobilization, and orthopedic consultation
- Successful closed reduction and splinting can be followed by evaluation for elective surgical management
- If unable to reduce, urgent orthopedic consultation for likely operative management
- Open fractures also require tetanus immunization and prophylactic antibiotics

Summary

TABLE 107.4: Advantages and disadvantages of x-rays in Monteggia fracture-dislocation

Advantages	Disadvantages
Fast	Manipulation for views may be painful
Low cost	
Minimal radiation	

108

Radial Head Fracture

Betty Chen and Richard T. Griffey

Background

Radial head fractures occur in approximately 20% of all elbow fractures. Injury usually results when an axial load injury, for example, fall on an outstretched hand, causes the radial head to collide with the capitellum. Radial head fractures can occur in conjunction with other structural injuries such as the radioulnar or interosseous membranes. A nondisplaced radial head fracture accounts for 50% of all elbow fractures.

TABLE 108.1: Classic history and physical

Fall on an outstretched hand
Limited range of motion at the elbow
Soft tissue swelling and ecchymosis at the elbow
Crepitance and pain elicited at the radial head especially with forearm rotation

TABLE 108.2: Mason classification of radial head fractures

Type I	Nondisplaced fracture
Type II	Single displaced fragment
Type III	Comminuted fracture
Type IV	Radial head fracture associated with elbow dislocation

Elbow X-ray

- Order anteroposterior (AP) and lateral views of the elbow and consider wrist views with concern for associated injury or any tender bony part of the extremity
- A positive fat pad sign (anterior, posterior, or both) is seen on lateral radiograph as a triangular or sail shaped radiolucent triangle proximal to the joint on anterior and/or posterior surfaces of the distal humerus
- A fat pad sign indicates hemarthrosis from an intra-articular fracture and may be the only indication of a fracture
- The double cortical sign is the result of an impaction fracture from the capitellum into the radial head, which displaces the radial head cortex distally
- Fractures may be difficult to identify if they are small and nondisplaced. Consider imaging in patients with persistent pain even with subacute injury
- Normal radiographic examination findings demonstrate that the radial head is aligned with the capitellum on all views
- For the normal elbow, a line drawn through the radial head and shaft should always line up with the capitellum, and with a supinated lateral view, lines drawn tangential to the head anteriorly and posteriorly should enclose the capitellum; with a radial head dislocation, these radiographic findings are disrupted

TABLE 108.3: Elbow x-ray: radial head fracture

IV contrast	No
PO contrast	No
Amount of radiation	0.005 mSv per view

Classic Images

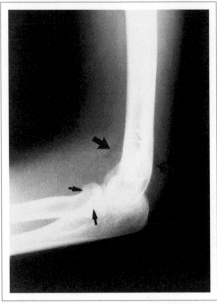

FIGURE 108.1: Anterior and posterior fat pad signs are indicated by the large arrows. *Small arrows* indicate the radial head fracture that produced the effusion displacing the fat pads. (From Harwood-Nuss. Clinical Practice of Emergency Medicine. Wolfson AB (ed). 3rd ed. Philadelphia: Lippincott Williams & Wilkins 2001.)

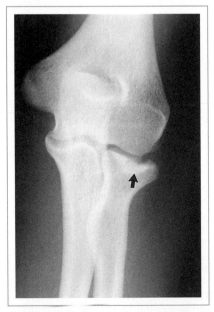

FIGURE 108.2: Radial head fracture. Double cortical sign. Observe the increased density of the articular cortex of the radial head, with projection of the opacity below the articular surface (*arrow*). Posteriorly, a fracture line is identified as a linear radiolucency. This double cortical sign may be the only sign of a radial head fracture. (From Yochum TR and Rowe LJ. Yochum and Rowe's Essentials of Skeletal Radiology, 3rd ed. Philadelphia: Lippincott Williams & Wilkins, 2004.)

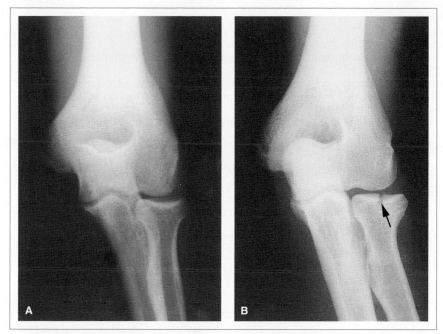

FIGURE 108.3: Occult radial head fracture. **A:** AP elbow. Note there is no evidence of fracture in the radial head. **B:** Two-month follow-up, AP elbow. Note that a vertical fracture line is now apparent (chisel fracture) (*arrow*). (From Yochum TR and Rowe LJ. Yochum and Rowe's Essentials of Skeletal Radiology, 3rd ed. Philadelphia: Lippincott Williams & Wilkins, 2004.)

Elbow CT Scan
- In rare instances, CT may be useful in defining fracture patterns and aiding in preoperative planning
- CT can be especially useful in fractures involving the articular surface

 TABLE 108.4: CT scan: radial head fracture

IV contrast	No
PO contrast	No
Amount of radiation	0.2 mSv

Classic Images

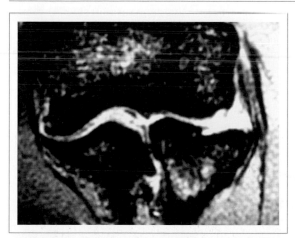

FIGURE 108.4: CT image demonstrating articular step off. (From Bucholz RW and Heckman JD. Rockwood and Green's Fractures in Adults, 5th ed. Philadelphia: Lippincott Williams & Wilkins, 2001.)

Basic Management

- Analgesia, ice and elevation
- Evaluate and document a thorough neurovascular examination
- Type I fractures are treated nonoperatively with a sling or a splint and early range of motion exercises
- Type II fractures with near-normal range of motion, minimal step off, and without associated injury are treated nonsurgically; if there is a large limitation in range of motion or elbow instability, consult orthopedic surgery
- Type III and IV fractures require orthopedic surgery consultation and surgical management

Summary

TABLE 108.5: Advantages and disadvantages of imaging modalities in radial head fracture

Imaging modalities	Advantages	Disadvantages
X-ray	Fast Low cost Minimal radiation	Manipulation to obtain all views may be painful May not delineate fracture or extent of fracture
CT scan	May delineate extent of fracture; aids surgical planning	Radiation exposure Expensive

109

Olecranon Fractures

Joy English and Brian Cohn

Background

Olecranon fractures account for approximately 4–6% of elbow fractures and occur often either in the elderly or in younger active athletes. There is no one universally accepted classification system for olecranon fractures. The Mayo classification is based on displacement, comminution, and subluxation.

The main complications associated with olecranon fractures include loss of range of motion, non-union, delayed union, compartment syndrome, nerve compression, and post-traumatic arthritis.

TABLE 109.1: Classic history and physical

Fall onto a semiflexed elbow with forearm supinated (triceps snaps the olecranon)
Direct trauma to the point of the elbow
Athletes (e.g., gymnast, pitcher) with repetitive extension at that elbow
Pain with range of motion, inability to fully extend at the elbow
Swelling and tenderness over the elbow
Weakness or numbness in ulnar nerve distribution

Elbow X-ray

- Obtain true anteroposterior and lateral views of the elbow
- Look for the fracture line, comminution, and articular surface involvement
- Thirty-two percent have an associated fracture typically of the radial head or neck
- A radiocapitellar view may further delineate associated radial head and capitellar fractures

 TABLE 109.2: Elbow x-ray: olecranon fracture

IV contrast	No
PO contrast	No
Amount of radiation	0.005 mSv per view

Classic Images

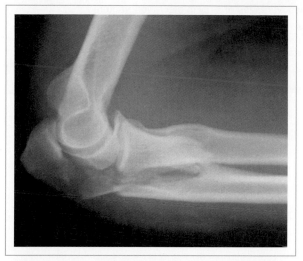

FIGURE 109.1: A 41-year-old man fell on his flexed elbow and sustained a type IIB (Horne and Tanzer classification) comminuted olecranon fracture, well demonstrated on this lateral radiograph. (From Greenspan A. Orthopedic Imaging: A Practical Approach, 4th ed. Philadelphia: Lippincott Williams & Wilkins, 2004.)

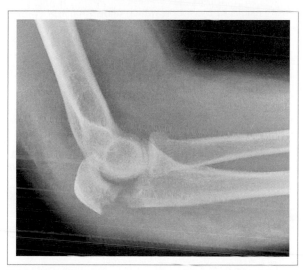

FIGURE 109.2: A 52-year-old woman fell on her outstretched arm and sustained a type III (Horne and Tanzer classification) olecranon fracture, effectively demonstrated on the lateral view of the elbow. Note the positive anterior and posterior fat pad sign. (From Greenspan A. Orthopedic Imaging: A Practical Approach, 4th ed. Philadelphia: Lippincott Williams & Wilkins, 2004.)

Basic Management
- Analgesia
- Evaluate and document a thorough neurovascular examination with particular attention to the ulnar nerve
- According to the Mayo classification system:
  - Type 1 fractures should be immobilized in a long-arm cast for 7–10 days with return to active motion as tolerated thereafter
  - Type II and III fractures involve surgical intervention with placement of hardware
  - For nondisplaced fractures <2 mm in both flexion and extension, splint with the elbow in 45 degrees of flexion
  - For displaced fractures >2 mm, obtain orthopedic surgery consultation

Summary

TABLE 109.3: Advantages and disadvantages of x-ray in olecranon fracture

Advantages	Disadvantages
Fast	Manipulation to obtain all views may be painful
Low cost	May not delineate fracture or extent of fracture
Minimal radiation	

110

Supracondylar Fractures

Joy English and Julie McManemy

Background

A supracondylar fracture is the most common fracture of the elbow in children. The incidence is higher in boys, the nondominant side is more often affected, a fall from a height is the most common mechanism and 5–7 years is the peak age.

Early in childhood increased ligamentous laxity exists at the elbow, which allows for hyperextension when a child falls on an outstretched arm. This pattern places the olecranon in a more protected space and increases stress in the supracondylar region accounting for the large number of supracondylar fractures.

An extension mechanism accounting for 92–98% of fractures causes posterior displacement of the fracture fragment and flexion causes anterior displacement of the fracture fragment.

Nerve injury occurs in approximately 7% of fractures. Posteromedial displacement is a risk factor for median nerve injury and vascular compromise with shearing of the brachial artery. Posterolateral displacement is a risk factor for radial nerve injury.

Long-term morbidity mainly occurs from varus deformity of the elbow and from Volkmann's contracture, an ischemic injury causing muscle and nerve necrosis as arterial and venous blood flows are impeded.

TABLE 110.1: Classic history and physical

Elbow pain after falling on the nondominant arm in extension
Elbow pain after a direct anterior force against a flexed elbow
Elbow pain, swelling, and resistance to range of motion
Depression proximal to the elbow at the triceps muscle area
Faint distal pulses, dusky fingertips, delayed capillary refill, pain out of proportion to examination, paresthesias, tense swollen antecubital fossa

Elbow X-ray

- Image the elbow in both anteroposterior (AP) and lateral views; the lateral film should be taken with the humerus in its anatomic position and not externally rotated
- A posterior fat pad (radiopaque triangle shape on the posterior surface of the distal humerus) may be visualized; less commonly an anterior pad may be present as well
- AP view usually demonstrates a transverse fracture line
- With a high index of suspicion for a fracture and no fracture line visualized, obtain oblique elbow views
- If it is difficult to delineate whether a finding is an anatomic variant, obtain comparison views of the unaffected side
- The distal fracture fragment is displaced anterior to the humerus in flexion injuries and often results in an open fracture

TABLE 110.2: Elbow x-rays

IV contrast	No
PO contrast	No
Amount of radiation	0.005 mSv per view

Classic Images

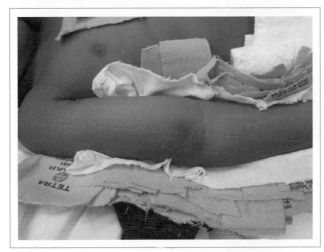

FIGURE 110.1: Pucker sign due to entrapment of the brachialis muscle. The anteriorly displaced fragment may have penetrated the brachialis muscle. (*Courtesy of J. McManemy, Washington University School of Medicine, St. Louis, MO.*)

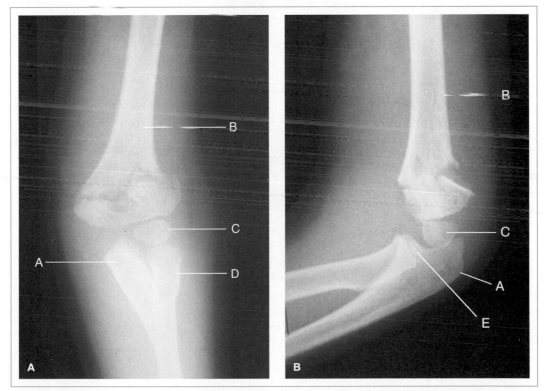

FIGURE 110.2: Supracondylar humerus fractures: operative management. Type II extension supracondylar humerus fracture (left elbow). **A:** Anterior-posterior. **B:** Lateral. A, ulna; B, humerus; C, capitellar epiphysis; D, radius; E, radial head. (From Koval KJ and Zuckerman JD. Atlas of Orthopaedic Surgery: A Multimedial Reference. Philadelphia: Lippincott Williams & Wilkins, 2004.)

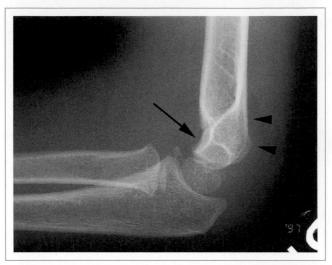

FIGURE 110.3: Type I supracondylar fracture on lateral view. The radiograph shows a posterior fat pad (*arrowheads*) and a subtle cortical defect is visible (*arrow*) on the anterior surface of the distal humeral metaphysis. (From Fleisher GR, Ludwig S, and Baskin MN. Atlas of Pediatric Emergency Medicine. Philadelphia: Lippincott Williams & Wilkins, 2004.)

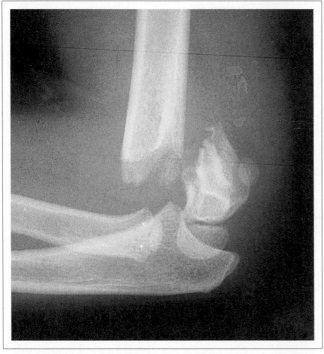

FIGURE 110.4: Supracondylar fracture of the humerus. Note the complete comminuted fracture through the supracondylar region of the humerus. Significant posterior displacement of the distal fragment has also occurred. (From Yochum TR and Rowe LJ. Yochum and Rowe's Essentials of Skeletal Radiology, 3rd ed. Philadelphia: Lippincott Williams & Wilkins, 2004.)

Management

- Analgesia
- Evaluate and document a thorough neurovascular examination
- Signs and symptoms of neurovascular injury and/or compartment syndrome require emergent orthopedic consultation
- Type I fractures (non-displaced or minimally displaced) can be splinted with a posterior splint in 60–90 degrees of flexion followed by outpatient follow-up with orthopedics
- Type II fractures (displacement but cortex intact) should be reduced into anatomic alignment and placed in a splint just as in type I fractures; consider orthopedic consultation
- Type III fractures (displacement with cortical disruption) require immediate orthopedic consultation for operative reduction and stabilization
- CT or MRI is not indicated but may be requested by the consultative service

Summary

TABLE 110.3: Advantages and disadvantages of plain films in supracondylar fracture

Advantages	Disadvantages
Fast and available	Manipulation to obtain all views may be painful
Inexpensive	May not delineate subtle fracture or extent of fracture
Minimal radiation	

111

Elbow Dislocation

Sanford Sineff and Sean Stickles

Background

The elbow is the most commonly dislocated major joint in children and the second most commonly dislocated major joint in adults. The annual incidence of elbow dislocations is around 6 per 100,000 individuals. While dislocation of the elbow joint is often an isolated injury, this may be associated with radial head and neck fractures in 5–10%, medial or lateral epicondyle avulsion fractures in 12%, and coronoid fractures in 10% of dislocations. Children have a high incidence of associated fractures of up to 50%. Ligamentous, vascular (brachial artery), and nerve injury (ulnar most common) may also be associated with dislocations. Dislocations depend on the resting position of the distal bones (radius and ulna). The vast majority of dislocations are posterior or posterolateral to the radius and ulna.

TABLE 111.1: Classic history and physical

Fall onto outstretched hand (FOOSH)
Forced pronation of the forearm during a fall or direct blow
Obvious deformity of elbow joint, often palpable bulge of olecranon posteriorly
Elbow held in 45 degrees of flexion
Tenderness over elbow joint

Elbow X-ray

- Obtain anteroposterior (AP) and lateral views
- Include the entire forearm in the image to look for an associated ulnar fracture
- The initial and often only imaging study necessary
- On lateral view, look for posteriorly displaced radius and ulna
- On AP view, look for lateral or medial displacement with the ulna and radius in normal relationship to each other
- Identify any other associated fractures that may be present
- After attempted reduction, postreduction films assess anatomic alignment

TABLE 111.2: X-rays: elbow dislocation

IV contrast	No
PO contrast	No
Amount of radiation	0.005 mSv per view

Classic Images

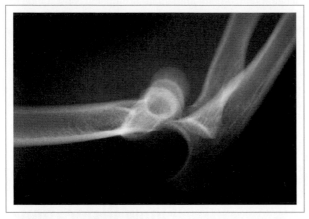

FIGURE 111.1: Posterior dislocation of elbow showing posteriorly displaced olecranon without associated fracture. (From Fleisher GR, Ludwig S, and Baskin MN. Atlas of Pediatric Emergency Medicine. Philadelphia: Lippincott Williams & Wilkins, 2004.)

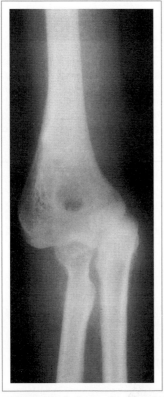

FIGURE 111.2: A late discovered (6 weeks) medial elbow dislocation. (From Bucholz RW and Heckman JD. Rockwood and Green's Fractures in Adults, 5th ed. Philadelphia: Lippincott Williams & Wilkins, 2001.)

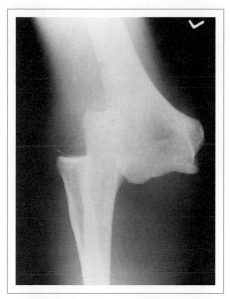

FIGURE 111.3: AP view of a lateral dislocation of elbow with the olecranon completely displaced from the trochlea. (From Bucholz RW and Heckman JD. Rockwood and Green's Fractures in Adults, 5th ed. Philadelphia: Lippincott Williams & Wilkins, 2001.)

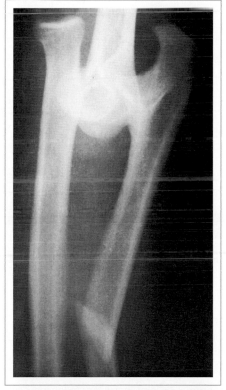

FIGURE 111.4: Divergent dislocation of elbow with the ulna displaced posteriorly and radius displaced anteriorly (as well as a mid-shaft ulna fracture). (From Bucholz RW and Heckman JD. Rockwood and Green's Fractures in Adults, 5th ed. Philadelphia: Lippincott Williams & Wilkins, 2001.)

CT
- Typically not necessary in the initial evaluation of elbow dislocation
- Useful for evaluating associated fracture extension and for operative planning
- CT angiography evaluates brachial artery injury if suspected (particularly in posterior dislocations)

 TABLE 111.3: CT scan: elbow dislocation

IV contrast	No for musculoskeletal protocol; Yes for angiography
PO contrast	No
Amount of Radiation	0.2 mSv per view

Classic Images

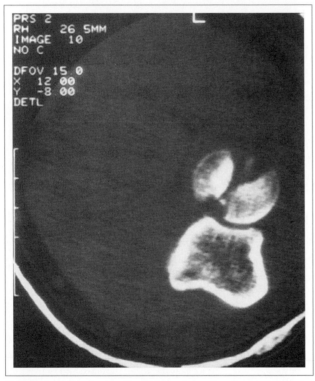

FIGURE 111.5: CT scan of radial head showing size of fragments in elbow dislocation with associated radial head fracture. (From Bucholz RW and Heckman JD. Rockwood and Green's Fractures in Adults, 5th ed. Lippincott Williams & Wilkins, 2001.)

Basic Management
- Analgesia
- Keep NPO as sedation will likely be required for reduction
- Evaluate and document initial and postreduction neurovascular status
- Once confirming type of dislocation, prompt reduction using traction-countertraction to realign the articular surfaces-palpable "clunk" is felt
- Orthopedic consultation for complicated dislocations, fractures, or joint instability following reduction; otherwise outpatient orthopedic surgery referral the following day to check neurovascular status
- Although traditionally extended immobilization in a sling and posterior mold (up to 4 weeks) was recommended, recent studies suggest that early mobilization (as soon as 3 days) has better functional outcome

Summary

TABLE 111.4: Advantages and disadvantages of imaging modalities in elbow dislocation

Imaging modalities	Advantages	Disadvantages
X-ray	Low amount of radiation Quick Widely available Often only test needed	May not fully evaluate fractures/soft tissues/vessels Pain with manipulation for obtaining all views
CT scan	Better visualization of fracture extension Can evaluate vessel injury	Radiation exposure IV contrast needed for angiography

112

Humeral Shaft Fractures

Joseph M. Fuentes and Brian Wessman

Background

Over 65,000 humeral fractures occur annually in the United States, accounting for approximately 3% of all fractures. Incidence has a bimodal age distribution, with peaks in the third and seventh decade of life. Most humeral fractures occur in the middle one third of the bone. Neurovascular injuries to the brachial artery and vein or the radial, ulnar, or median nerve can occur. Spiral fractures (Holstein-Lewis fracture) commonly produce radial nerve injury, which is the most common complication (10–20%) of humeral shaft fractures. Rates of nonunion range from 1% to 15%, more commonly with transverse and open fractures.

TABLE 112.1: Classic history and physical

Direct blow to the humerus in sports or with a blunt object
Fall on an outstretched hand
History of breast cancer or Paget's disease
Pain, swelling, deformity, ecchymosis, and/or crepitance at site
Foreshortened arm with loss of function
Wrist drop and altered sensation of the dorsal first web space

Humerus X-ray

- Obtain anteroposterior (AP) and lateral views of the humerus
- Consider imaging the shoulder and elbow
- Look for a transverse fracture with bending of the fracture fragment common with a direct blow as the mechanism of injury
- Look for a spiral fracture common with a fall on an outstretched hand as the mechanism of injury causing a torsion force
- A butterfly fragment may be seen with a comminuted oblique fracture
- Look for pathological fractures (e.g., metastatic disease)

 TABLE 112.2: X-ray: humeral shaft fracture

IV contrast	No
PO contrast	No
Amount of radiation	0.005 mSv per view

Classic Images

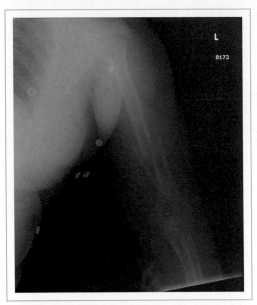

FIGURE 112.1: AP view. Comminuted fracture of left mid-shaft humerus. (*Courtesy of Washington University School of Medicine St. Louis, MO.*)

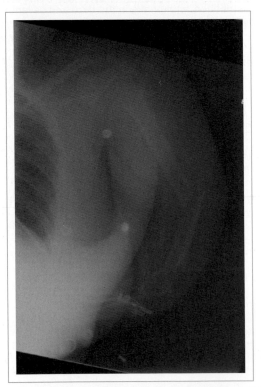

FIGURE 112.2: Lateral view. Comminuted fracture of left humerus. (*Courtesy of Washington University School of Medicine St. Louis, MO.*)

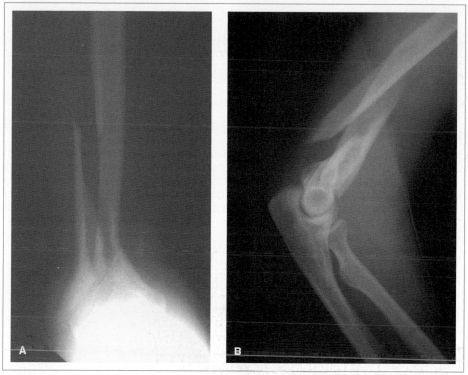

FIGURE 112.3: Posteroanterior (**A**) and lateral (**B**) radiographs of a Holstein-Lewis fracture of the distal third of the humerus. (From Strickland JW and Graham TJ. Master Techniques in Orthopaedic Surgery: The Hand, 2nd ed. Philadelphia: Lippincott Williams & Wilkins, 2005.)

Basic Management

- Evaluate and document a neurovascular examination
- Ice, analgesia
- Immobilization with sling and swathe for simple fractures
- Reduction with reevaluation of neurovascular status
- Coaptation or sugar tong splint for fracture fragments within 1–2 inches following reduction
- Orthopedic consultation for complicated fractures and unsuccessful reductions
- Consider CT, MRI, or technetium-labeled bone scan for further evaluation of pathological fractures

Summary

TABLE 112.3: Advantages and disadvantages of x-rays in humeral shaft fracture

Advantages	Disadvantages
Low cost	Radiation exposure
Rapid	Pain with manipulation to obtain views
	May not delineate extent of pathological fractures

113

Humeral Head Fractures

Delwin Merchant and Brian Wessman

Background

Fractures of the humeral head represent 5% of fractures seen in the emergency department. They are most commonly seen in the elderly and osteoporotic. These fractures may be complicated by shoulder dislocation (e.g., greater tuberosity fracture in setting of anterior shoulder dislocation or lesser tuberosity fracture in setting of posterior shoulder dislocation), by axillary nerve or brachial plexus damage (e.g., angulated surgical neck fractures), and in the long term by avascular necrosis.

TABLE 113.1: Classic history and physical

Trauma or fall on an outstretched hand
Seizure, electrical shock, or injury playing sports
Point tenderness at proximal humerus or shoulder
Swelling, crepitus, and ecchymosis at/around shoulder
Arm held close to the chest wall

Humerus X-rays

TABLE 113.2: Common humerus x-ray views

Anterior-posterior view	Identifies most fractures
Lateral view in the scapular plane (Y view)	Identifies fracture-dislocations Helps delineate degree of displacement/angulation of bony fragments
Velpeau modified axillary view	Identifies fracture-dislocations

TABLE 113.3: Fracture parts classification

One	No to minimal angulation (<45 degrees) No to minimal displacement (<1 cm) of the fracture fragments Any of the four portions of the proximal humerus may be fractured Accounts for 80% of fractures
Two	Three nondisplaced and one displaced fracture fragment Accounts for 10% of fractures
Three	Two displaced and two nondisplaced fracture parts Lesser or greater tuberosity must be involved
Four	Three displaced fracture fragments Avascular necrosis is common

 TABLE 113.4: Shoulder x-ray: humeral head fracture

IV contrast	No
PO contrast	No
Amount of radiation	0.01 mSv per view

Classic Images

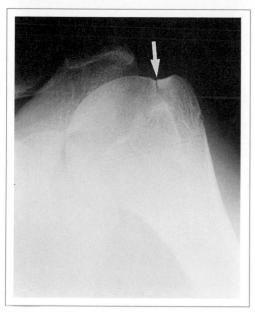

FIGURE 113.1: Flap fracture: greater tuberosity. Anteroposterior shoulder. Note the displaced fracture of the greater tuberosity of the humerus, which is recognized by the presence of a radiolucent line (*arrow*). (From Yochum TR and Rowe LJ. Yochum and Rowe's Essentials of Skeletal Radiology, 3rd ed. Philadelphia: Lippincott Williams & Wilkins, 2004.)

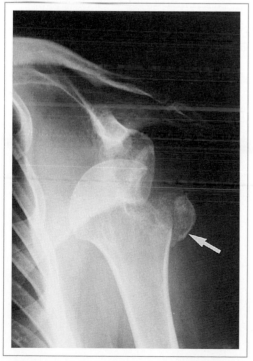

FIGURE 113.2: Flap fracture associated with anterior glenohumeral dislocation. Note that the humeral head is dislocated anteriorly and inferiorly to a subcoracoid position. This is associated with an avulsion fracture of the greater tuberosity of the humerus (flap fracture) (*arrow*). (From Yochum TR and Rowe LJ. Yochum and Rowe's Essentials of Skeletal Radiology, 3rd ed. Philadelphia: Lippincott Williams & Wilkins, 2004.)

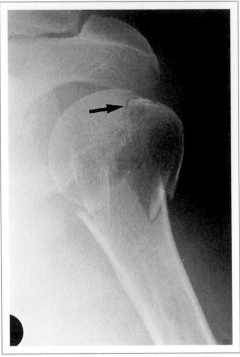

FIGURE 113.3: Surgical neck fracture: shoulder. Observe that a transverse comminuted fracture has occurred through the surgical neck of the humerus. There has been extension of the fracture line to involve the greater tuberosity (flap fracture) (*arrow*). (From Yochum TR and Rowe LJ. Yochum and Rowe's Essentials of Skeletal Radiology, 3rd ed. Philadelphia: Lippincott Williams & Wilkins, 2004.)

Basic Management

- Evaluate and document a neurovascular examination especially of the axillary nerve injury and deltoid muscle
- Pain control
- Initial immobilization may be achieved with a sling, shoulder immobilizer, or a sling with an accompanying swathe
- Orthopedic consultation urgently/emergently for 2 or more fracture parts, fracture-dislocations, or neurovascular compromise for closed reduction and further surgical management
- CT or MRI may be requested by the consultative service for better delineation of the injuries

Summary

TABLE 113.5: Advantages and disadvantages of plain films in humeral head fracture

Advantages	Disadvantages
Low cost	May not delineate extent of pathological fractures
Fast	
Minimal radiation	

114

Shoulder Dislocation

Sanford Sineff and Hawnwan Moy

Background

The shoulder, unlike the hip, is an inherently unstable joint. The joint must be flexible enough for the wide range of motion required in the arms and hands, yet strong enough to allow for actions such as pushing, pulling, and lifting. The compromise between these two functions results in a decrease in stability. Subluxation occurs when the humeral head partially slips out of the fossa, whereas a dislocation occurs when the head slips *completely* off the glenoid so that articular surfaces are not in contact. Anterior dislocations of the glenohumeral joint are the most common major joint dislocations (95–97% of cases). Posterior dislocations occur in 2–5% of cases. Inferior and superior dislocations are even more rare (less than 1%). Acute and chronic complications include injury to the axillary nerve or artery, recurrent dislocations, rotator cuff injuries, and post-traumatic arthritis.

TABLE 114.1: Classic history and physical

Anterior dislocation
Combination of abduction, extension, and external rotational force causing injury
Arm in slight abduction, external rotation, and elbow flexed
Shoulder is "squared off" (acromioclavicular step off), lacking normal rounded contour
The patient resists abduction and internal rotation
Decreased sensation over the lateral deltoid (axillary nerve injury)

Posterior dislocation
Forceful internal rotation and adduction from a fall, seizure, or electric shock
Fall on outstretched hand
Direct blow to shoulder
Arm is in adduction and internally rotated
The anterior shoulder is flat and the posterior aspect full
Coracoid process is prominent
The patient will not allow external rotation or abduction because of severe pain

Inferior dislocation
Hyperabduction levers the neck of the humerus against the acromion, forcing the inferior
    capsule to tear, forcing the head out inferiorly
Humerus is fully abducted, elbow is flexed, hand is on or behind the head
Humeral head may be palpated on the lateral chest wall

Shoulder X-ray

- Obtain three views: anteroposterior (AP), true lateral (Y view), and axillary
- Look for Hills-Sachs deformity
  - Seen in AP view
  - Hatchet-like defect of humeral head
  - Posterolateral aspect of humeral head at junction with neck
  - Suggests previous anterior dislocations
- Look for Bankart lesion
  - Seen in AP view
  - Suggests previous anterior dislocations
  - Avulsion fracture of the anterior portion of the inferior glenoid rim
- Look for trough sign
  - Seen in AP and axillary views
  - Compression fracture of anteromedial portion of humeral head
  - Vertical or arch-like line within the humeral head cortex projecting lateral and parallel to the articular end of the bone

- Look at the true lateral view for the humeral head laying on the "Y"
  - Infraspinous portion of the scapula, the acromion, and the coracoid processes form two arms of a "Y"; the humeral head should be superimposed on the glenohumeral fossa which is centered at the junction of these portions
- Suspected posterior dislocation:
  - AP view may appear normal with the humeral head beside/overlapping the glenoid
  - Humeral head will be clearly posteriorly located on the "Y view"

 TABLE 114.2: X-ray: shoulder dislocation

IV contrast	No
PO contrast	No
Amount of radiation	0.01 mSv per view

Classic Images

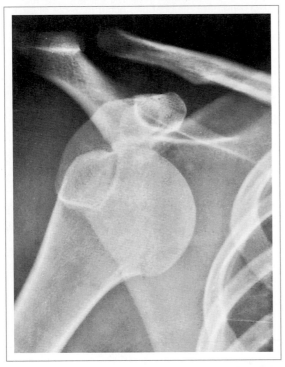

FIGURE 114.1: Anterior shoulder dislocation. AP film of the shoulder shows the typical appearance of anterior dislocation. The humeral head lies beneath the inferior rim of the glenoid. (From Greenspan A. Orthopedic Imaging: A Practical Approach, 4th ed. Philadelphia: Lippincott Williams & Wilkins, 2004.)

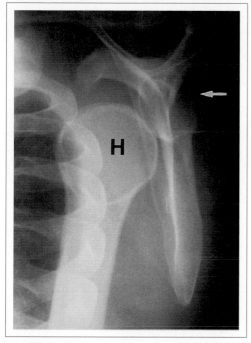

FIGURE 114.2: Anterior shoulder dislocation. A dislocation is well demonstrated on this trans-scapular (or Y) projection of the shoulder girdle. An *arrow* is pointing to the empty glenoid fossa. The humeral head (*H*) is medially and anteriorly displaced. (From Greenspan A. Orthopedic Imaging: A Practical Approach, 4th ed. Philadelphia: Lippincott Williams & Wilkins, 2004.)

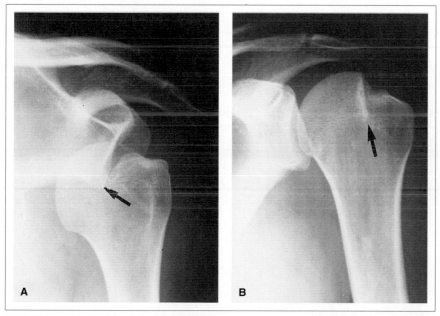

FIGURE 114.3: Hill-Sachs deformity associated with anterior humeral dislocation. (**A**) AP shoulder. Note that an anteroinferior dislocation of the humerus has resulted in an impaction between the inferior glenoid rim and the opposing humeral head (*arrow*). The impaction by the angular surface of the inferior glenoid rim produces the articular defect that has been referred to as the hatchet deformity (Hill-Sachs defect). (**B**) Postreduction, AP shoulder. Note that after repositioning of the humeral head within the glenoid fossa, the residual effect of compression of the articular surface is clearly identified (*arrow*). (From Yochum TR and Rowe LJ. Yochum and Rowe's Essentials of Skeletal Radiology, 3rd ed. Philadelphia: Lippincott Williams & Wilkins, 2004.)

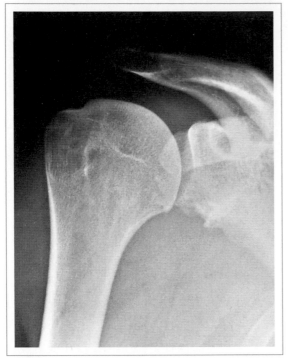

FIGURE 114.4: Bankart lesion. AP view of the shoulder shows compression fracture of the anterior aspect of the inferior portion of the glenoid, known as the Bankart lesion. (From Greenspan A. Orthopedic Imaging: A Practical Approach, 4th ed. Philadelphia: Lippincott Williams & Wilkins, 2004.)

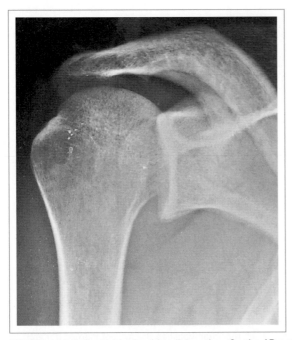

FIGURE 114.5: Posterior shoulder dislocation. On the AP projection of the shoulder obtained by rotating the patient 40 degrees toward the affected side (Grashey view), overlap of the medially displaced humeral head with the glenoid is virtually diagnostic of posterior dislocation. (From Greenspan A. Orthopedic Imaging: A Practical Approach, 4th ed. Philadelphia: Lippincott Williams & Wilkins, 2004.)

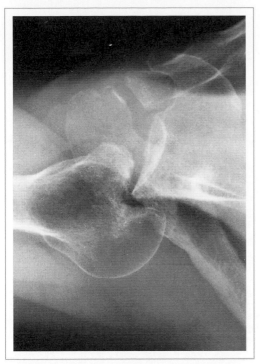

FIGURE 114.6: Posterior shoulder dislocation. Axillary projection of the shoulder demonstrates posterior dislocation. Note the associated compression fracture of the anteromedial aspect of the humeral head. (From Greenspan A. Orthopedic Imaging: A Practical Approach, 4th ed. Philadelphia: Lippincott Williams & Wilkins, 2004.)

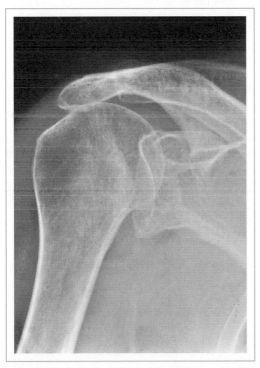

FIGURE 114.7: Posterior shoulder dislocation. AP view of the shoulder demonstrates posterior dislocation in the glenohumeral joint. Note the trough line impaction on the anteromedial aspect of the humeral head. (From Greenspan A. Orthopedic Imaging: A Practical Approach, 4th ed. Philadelphia: Lippincott Williams & Wilkins, 2004.)

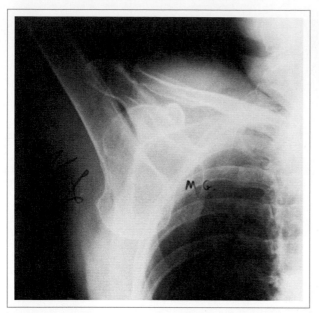

FIGURE 114.8: AP x-ray film of the inferior dislocation reveals that the entire humeral head and surgical neck of the humerus are inferior to the glenoid fossa. (From Bucholz RW and Heckman JD. Rockwood and Green's Fractures in Adults, 5th ed. Lippincott Williams & Wilkins, 2001.)

Shoulder CT Scan
- Effective at demonstrating dislocation
- Likely unnecessary for evaluation of dislocation
- Maybe helpful in cases of uncertainty or for preoperative planning
- If MRI is available, it would be the preferred imaging test over CT to better delineate the injuries

Shoulder MRI
- MRI may be useful to evaluate soft tissue injuries such as those to the labrum or glenohumeral ligament

 TABLE 114.3: MRI: shoulder dislocation

IV contrast	No
PO contrast	No
Amount of radiation	None

Basic Management
- Evaluate and document a neurovascular examination
- Adequate analgesia
- Reduce dislocation
- Re-evaluate and document a neurovascular examination
- Simple sling or shoulder immobilizer
- Return to normal activity after a few weeks
- After full range of motion is achieved, strength training exercises will help with recovery

Summary

TABLE 114.4: Advantages and disadvantages of imaging modalities in shoulder dislocation

Imaging modalities	Advantages	Disadvantages
X-ray	Quick Inexpensive	Minimal radiation Manipulation for views may cause pain
MRI	Useful in diagnosing occult injury or soft tissue injuries	Expensive Time-consuming

115

Scapular Fracture

Irena Vitkovitsky and Christopher Sampson

Background

A fracture of the scapula is an uncommon injury. When such an injury occurs, it most commonly involves the body of the scapula, and least commonly the coracoid process. Because of the high energy required to fracture the scapula, up to 96% of fractures have other associated injuries most commonly to the lung (e.g., pneumothorax), thoracic cage (e.g., rib or clavicle fractures), or shoulder girdle (e.g., humeral head fractures, anterior or posterior shoulder dislocations). Fractures are classified by their anatomic location and most commonly occur in the body and the glenoid neck.

TABLE 115.1: Classic history and physical

High mechanism motor vehicle accident, fall from a height or trauma
Direct blunt force to the shoulder
Soft tissue swelling and limited range of motion at the shoulder
Flattened appearance to shoulder
Deformity, splinting, shortness of breath

Shoulder X-ray

- Order anteroposterior (AP), lateral, and Y views of the shoulder
- AP view: look specifically for intra-articular fractures
- Y view: look for displaced fracture fragments
- Additional views:
  - Axillary: evaluate location of humeral head in the glenoid fossa
  - AP shoulder with 45-degree cephalic tilt: evaluate coracoid process
  - Apical oblique (Garth view): evaluate glenoid rim
  - Chest x-ray: evaluate clavicle, ribs, lung, shoulder symmetry

 TABLE 115.2: Shoulder x-ray: scapula fracture

IV contrast	No
PO contrast	No
Amount of radiation	0.01 mSv per view

Classic Images

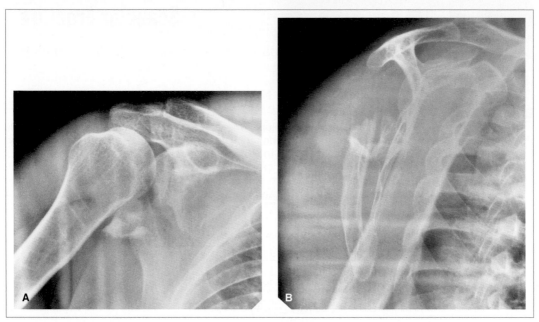

FIGURE 115.1: Fracture of the scapula. A 52-year-old man was injured in a motorcycle accident. (**A**) On the anteroposterior view of the right shoulder, a comminuted fracture of the scapula is evident. Displacement of the fragments, however, cannot be evaluated. (**B**) Transscapular (Y) view demonstrates lateral displacement of the body of the scapula. (From Greenspan A. Orthopedic Imaging: A Practical Approach, 4th ed. Philadelphia: Lippincott Williams & Wilkins, 2004.)

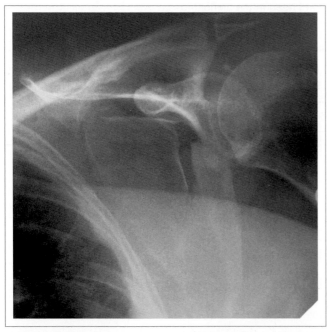

FIGURE 115.2: Fracture of the scapula. A 57-year-old woman sustained an injury to the left shoulder in a motorcycle accident. Anteroposterior view shows a comminuted fracture of the left scapula. The glenohumeral joint cannot be properly assessed in this study. (From Greenspan A. Orthopedic Imaging: A Practical Approach, 4th ed. Philadelphia: Lippincott Williams & Wilkins, 2004.)

Chest CT Scan
- Look for displaced fracture fragments
- Better evaluates intra-articular glenoid fractures
- Enables thoracic cage and lung parenchyma evaluation

 TABLE 115.3: Chest CT: scapula fracture

IV contrast	No
PO contrast	No
Amount of radiation	7 mSv

Classic Images

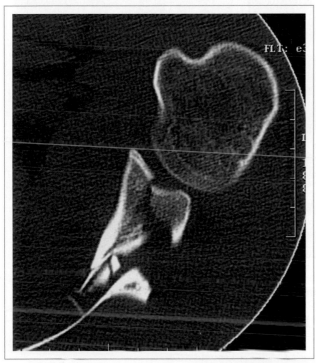

FIGURE 115.3: Comminuted fracture of the glenoid. Axial CT section through the shoulder joint shows a comminuted, displaced fracture of the glenoid fossa extending across the entire scapula. (From Greenspan A. Orthopedic Imaging: A Practical Approach, 4th ed. Philadelphia: Lippincott Williams & Wilkins, 2004.)

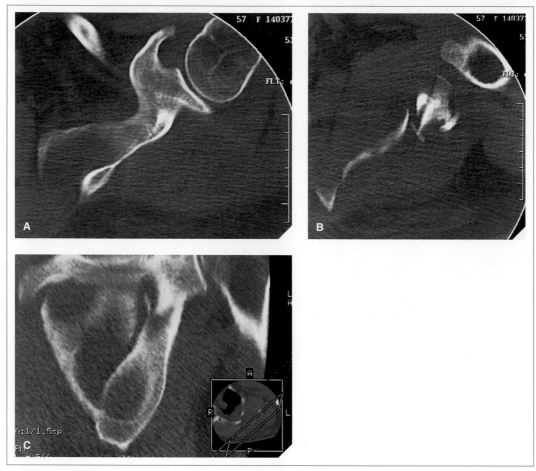

FIGURE 115.4: Fracture of the scapula. A 57-year-old woman sustained an injury to the left shoulder in a motorcycle accident. Two axial CT sections, one at the level of the glenohumeral joint (**A**) and the other at the level of the body of the scapula (**B**) and reformatted coronal image (**C**) show to better advantage the configuration of various displaced fragments as well as an intact glenohumeral joint. (From Greenspan A. Orthopedic Imaging: A Practical Approach, 4th ed. Philadelphia: Lippincott Williams & Wilkins, 2004.)

Basic Management
- Evaluate and document a thorough neurovascular examination with particular attention to the brachial plexus
- Evaluate and document the examination of the cervical and thoracic spines
- Ice and pain control
- Sling
- Consultation (e.g., trauma surgery, orthopedic surgery) for significant associated injuries or significant/displaced fractures of the glenoid, acromion, or coracoid

Summary

TABLE 115.4: Advantages and disadvantages of imaging modalities in scapular fracture

Imaging modalities	Advantages	Disadvantages
X-ray	Availability Low cost Minimal radiation	May not delineate fracture or extent of fracture Painful to obtain all views
CT scan	Delineates extent of fracture and injury to associated structures	Radiation exposure Expensive

116

Clavicle Fracture

Daniel A. Kopp and Doug Char

Background

Fractures of the clavicle account for 2.6–5% of all adult fractures and 35–44% of all shoulder girdle injuries. The incidence of clavicle fractures follows a bimodal distribution, with peaks being in males under age 40 and in males and females over age 70.

The middle third of the shaft of the clavicle is the thinnest, least supported and consequently most commonly fractured portion of the clavicle followed by the lateral and then proximal thirds. Fractures of the lateral third of the clavicle are relatively common in children.

TABLE 116.1: Classic history and physical

Trauma to the lateral shoulder
Fall from standing or from a bicycle
Direct blow to the clavicle
Fall onto an outstretched hand
Shoulder pain relieved by holding the arm supported in adduction
Ecchymosis, edema, or tenting of the skin
A sagging shoulder
Tenderness or crepitance over clavicle
Deformity and shortening

Clavicle X-ray

- Look for a cortical break/step off in the radio-opaque bony cortex
- Order shoulder and scapular x-rays when the mechanism is concerning or if severe diastasis of the clavicle is present
- Order a chest x-ray to exclude a pneumothorax and rib fractures and to provide a comparison view of the opposite shoulder

TABLE 116.2: Utility of various radiographic views of the clavicle

View	Utility
Anteroposterior	Sufficient for most clavicle fractures
45 degrees cephalad	Assesses degree of displacement and comminution
40 degrees cephalic (serendipity view)	Assesses the sternoclavicular joints and medial one third of the clavicles for fractures or dislocation
Stress	Assesses lateral third fractures and integrity of the coracoclavicular ligaments

 TABLE 116.3: Clavicle x-ray: clavicle fracture

IV contrast	No
PO contrast	No
Amount of radiation	0.01 mSv per view

Classic Images

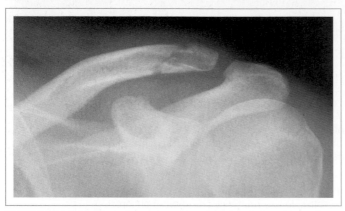

FIGURE 116.1: Fracture of the acromial end of the clavicle. Type I fracture of the distal third clavicle. There is no displacement of the fractured fragment. (From Greenspan A. Orthopedic Imaging: A Practical Approach, 4th ed. Philadelphia: Lippincott Williams & Wilkins, 2004.)

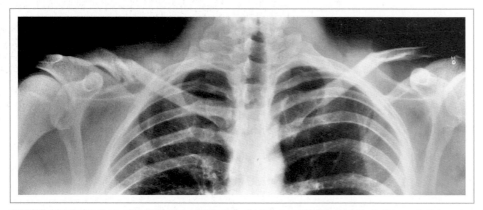

FIGURE 116.2: Fracture of both clavicles. Anteroposterior view of both shoulders demonstrates a comminuted fracture of the middle third of the right clavicle and a simple fracture of the middle third of the left. (From Greenspan A. Orthopedic Imaging: A Practical Approach, 4th ed. Philadelphia: Lippincott Williams & Wilkins, 2004.)

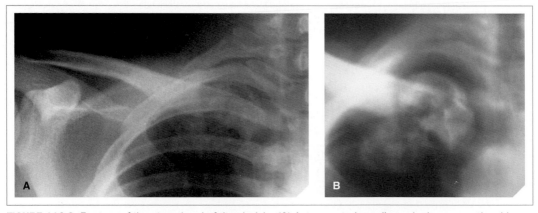

FIGURE 116.3: Fracture of the sternal end of the clavicle. (**A**) Anteroposterior radiograph shows questionable lesion of the medial end of the clavicle; however, the abnormality is not well demonstrated. (**B**) A trispiral tomogram clearly shows healing fracture of the medial clavicle. (From Greenspan A. Orthopedic Imaging: A Practical Approach, 4th ed. Philadelphia: Lippincott Williams & Wilkins, 2004.)

CT Scan

- Useful in medial third fractures with posterior displacement of fragments or dislocation of the sternoclavicular joint
- Evaluates compression of the mediastinal structures and angiography evaluates suspected vascular injury
- Useful in distal third fractures to assess the degree of comminution and position of fragments

 TABLE 116.4: CT scan: clavicle fracture

IV contrast	No
PO contrast	No
Amount of radiation	7.0 mSv

Classic Images

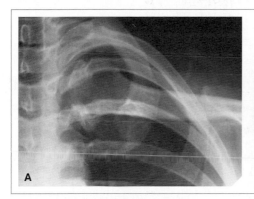
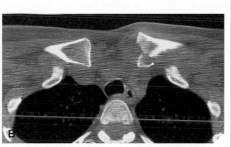

FIGURE 116.4: Fracture of the sternal end of the clavicle. (**A**) Anteroposterior radiograph is suggestive of a fracture of the medial end of the clavicle, but the fracture line is not well demonstrated. (**B**) A CT section shows a fracture of the left sternal end of the clavicle and associated soft tissue swelling. (From Greenspan A. Orthopedic Imaging: A Practical Approach, 4th ed. Philadelphia: Lippincott Williams & Wilkins, 2004.)

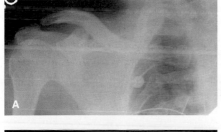
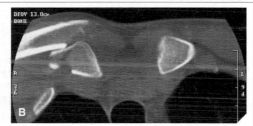
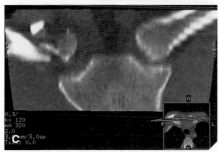

FIGURE 116.5: Fracture of the sternal end of the clavicle. (**A**) Anteroposterior radiograph of the right shoulder and upper chest shows multiple rib fractures. The medial portion of the clavicle is not adequately visualized. Axial CT scan (**B**) and coronal reformatted image (**C**) show a comminuted fracture of the sternal end of the right clavicle with anterior displacement and overriding of the fragments. (From Greenspan A. Orthopedic Imaging: A Practical Approach, 4th ed. Philadelphia: Lippincott Williams & Wilkins, 2004.)

Basic Management

- Perform and document a neurovascular examination
- Pain control
- Immobilization in a sling is favored over a figure-of-eight splint for comfort
- Progression to range of motion pendulum exercises as tolerated
- Inform patient that callous formation may cause a cosmetic defect (usually temporary during healing process)
- Consult orthopedics for:
  - Tenting of the skin that may cause skin necrosis
  - Posterior displacement of the medial segment with vascular compromise or neurologic deficit
  - Type II, IV, and V distal third fractures
  - Determining need for shoulder spica splint
  - Determining need for open reduction internal fixation

Summary

TABLE 116.5: Advantages and disadvantages of imaging modalities in clavicle fracture

Imaging modalities	Advantages	Disadvantages
X-ray	Fast Low cost Minimal radiation	May not delineate fracture or extent of fracture
CT scan	Delineates extent of fracture Evaluates for vascular injury Aids surgical planning	Contrast exposure Radiation exposure Expensive

Section Editor: Azita Hamedani

117 Pelvic Ring and Sacroiliac Joint Fracture

Kyle Minor, Lauren Wade, Janis P. Tupesis,
and James Svenson

Background

Pelvic ring fractures are a common cause of morbidity and mortality in the context of trauma. The overall mortality rate has been reported to be as high as 20%. Uncontrolled pelvic hemorrhage accounts for 40% of these deaths, as disruption of pelvic veins and/or arteries occurs in many patients. The classification system that is most commonly used is the Young-Burgess classification: anterior-posterior compression, lateral compression, vertical sheer, and combination fractures. This classification system not only provides descriptions of various mechanisms that cause pelvic injuries, but also provides context for the concomitant injuries (e.g., urethral and bowel) and has prognostic potential. This chapter will focus on pubic symphysis and sacroiliac dislocations associated with anterior-posterior and lateral compression fractures as well as isolated pubic rami fractures and acetabular fractures.

TABLE 117.1: Young-Burgess classification system for pelvic fractures

Mechanism and type	Characteristics	Hemipelvis displacement	Stability
APC–I	Pubic diastasis <2.5 cm	External rotation	Stable
APC–II	Pubic diastasis >2.5 cm, anterior sacroiliac joint disruption	External rotation	Rotationally unstable, vertically stable
APC–III	Type II plus posterior sacroiliac joint disruption	External rotation	Rotationally unstable, vertically unstable
LC-I	Ipsilateral sacral buckle fractures, ipsilateral horizontal pubic rami fractures (or disruption of symphysis with overlapping pubic bones)	Internal rotation	Stable
LC-II	Type I plus ipsilateral iliac wing fracture or posterior sacroiliac joint disruption	Internal rotation	Rotationally unstable, vertically stable
Vertical shear	Vertical pubic rami fractures, sacroiliac joint disruption ± adjacent fractures	Vertical (cranial)	Rotationally unstable, vertically unstable

APC, anterior-posterior compression; LC, lateral compression.

TABLE 117.2: Classic history and physical

High-speed motor vehicle collisions
Significant falls in the elderly
Instability on palpation of bony elements of pelvis
Rectal and genitourinary findings (e.g., vaginal bleeding, palpation of fracture edge on pelvic examination, blood at the urethral meatus, scrotal hematoma, palpation of bony spicules on rectal examination, gross blood on rectal examination)

TABLE 117.3: Potentially helpful laboratory tests

Complete blood count	Hemoglobin and hematocrit may be normal initially, even with active hemorrhage; serial levels indicated
Coagulation studies	May indicate need for FFP or vitamin K in a patient with coagulopathy
Type and screen	To expedite transfusion and as part of preoperative workup
Urinalysis	Presence of blood may indicate kidney or urethral injury
Lactate	Marker of hypoperfusion and reflective of adequacy of resuscitation

FFP, fresh frozen plasma.

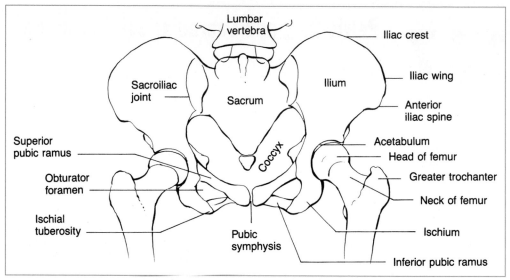

FIGURE 117.1: Bony anatomy of pelvis in an adult. (From Harwood-Nuss A, Wolfson AB, Hendey GW, Hendey PL. The Clinical Practice of Emergency Medicine, 3rd ed. Philadelphia, PA: Lippincott Williams & Wilkins, 2001.)

Pelvis X-ray

- Anteroposterior (AP) pelvic radiograph is the initial imaging modality of choice; it identifies up to 90% of fractures
- Posterior sacroiliac ligament disruption may be difficult to diagnose
- In the past, inlet and outlet pelvic views (taken with beam 45 degrees caudally or cephalad, respectively) were used to demonstrate posterior dislocation of pelvic ring and opening of pubic symphysis; these views are now replaced by CT imaging

 TABLE 117.4: Pelvis x-ray: pelvis fracture

IV contrast	No
PO contrast	No
Amount of radiation	0.6 mSv

CT Scan

- Provides optimal imaging for evaluation of bony pelvic anatomy, while also providing information on pelvic, retroperitoneal, and intraperitoneal bleeding
- In patients with a significant mechanism of injury, a CT of the abdomen/pelvis is often performed
- Intravenous contrast may highlight active hemorrhage and indicate source for hemodynamic instability
- CT scan can also confirm hip dislocation associated with an acetabular fracture

 TABLE 117.5: Pelvis CT scan: pelvic ring fracture

IV contrast	Yes, will demonstrate "blush" (contrast extravasation) that indicates active bleeding
PO contrast	No
Amount of radiation	6 mSv

MRI

- More sensitive for detecting ligamentous injury
- Time-consuming and often requires patient to leave the emergency department, and is therefore not recommended in the initial evaluation

 TABLE 117.6: MRI: pelvic ring fracture

IV contrast	No
PO contrast	No
Amount of radiation	None

Anterior-Posterior Compression-I

- The sacrotuberous and sacrospinous ligaments typically remain intact if the pubic symphysis is displaced by less than 2.5 cm
- Patients with anterior-posterior compression-I (APC-I) injuries can have severe hemorrhage (1%), bladder rupture (8%), and urethral injury (12%)
- Typically, these patients are managed nonoperatively

Anterior-Posterior Compression-II

- The pubic symphysis is often wider than 2.5 cm
- Patients with APC-II injuries can have severe hemorrhage (28%), bladder rupture (11%), and urethral injury (23%)
- Because the posterior ligaments are intact, surgical repair is typically limited to plating of the pubic symphysis

Anterior-Posterior Compression-III

- Patients with APC-III injuries can have severe hemorrhage (53%), bladder rupture (14%), and urethral injury (36%)
- As a result of posterior ligament disruption, simply reducing the pubic symphysis is inadequate
- These patients need to have surgical reduction of their widened sacroiliac joint

Lateral Compression-I

- Patients with lateral compression-I (LC-I) injuries can have severe hemorrhage (0.5%), bladder rupture (4%), and urethral injury (2%)
- Management depends on the extent of the sacral fracture and should be determined by an orthopedic surgeon

Lateral Compression-II

- Patients with LC-II injuries can have severe hemorrhage (36%) and bladder rupture (7%)
- These fractures typically require internal fixation with multiple screws

Lateral Compression-III

- An LC-III injury is essentially a combination of an LC-II and an APC-II or an APC-III
- Patients with LC-III injuries can have severe hemorrhage (60%), bladder rupture (20%), and urethral injury (20%)

Pubic Rami Fractures

- Isolated pubic ramus fractures are not included in the Young-Burgess classification system
- If treated conservatively most will heal well; this is due to the stabilization by the inguinal ligament that runs parallel to the superior pubic ramus
- Surgical repair is controversial but may give patients improved pain relief and early mobilization

Acetabular Fractures

- Acetabular fractures are also not included in the Young-Burgess classification system
- These fractures require orthopedic consultation for surgical repair; patients cannot bear weight on these injuries
- The initial AP radiograph should be taken without traction placed on the involved extremity to make fractures more evident; after the radiograph is taken, traction may be applied for patient comfort

Classic Images

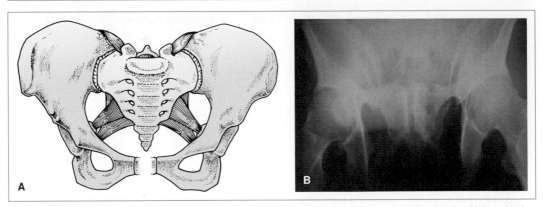

FIGURE 117.2: (**A**) Schematic and (**B**) outlet radiograph of a typical anterior-posterior compression-I injury. Notice that both the sacrotuberous and sacrospinous ligaments are intact bilaterally. (From Bucholz RW, Heckman JD, Court-Brown CM, et al. Rockwood and Green's Fractures in Adults, 7th ed. Philadelphia, PA: Lippincott Williams & Wilkins, 2010.)

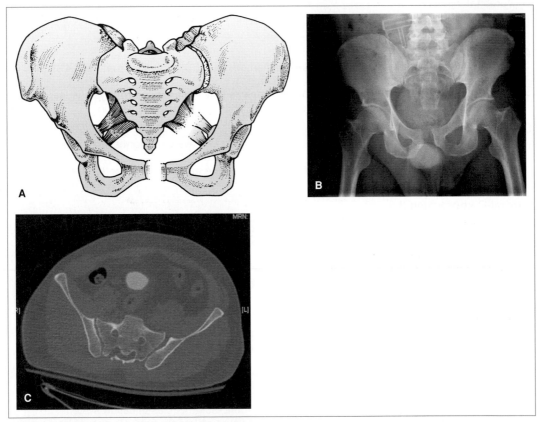

FIGURE 117.3: (**A**) Schematic and (**B**) Anteroposterior radiograph with (**C**) CT scan of a typical anterior-posterior compression-III injury. Notice that both the sacrotuberous and sacrospinous ligaments are disrupted but the posterior sacroiliac ligament remains intact. (From Bucholz RW, Heckman JD, Court-Brown CM, et al. Rockwood and Green's Fractures in Adults, 7th ed. Philadelphia, PA: Lippincott Williams & Wilkins, 2010.)

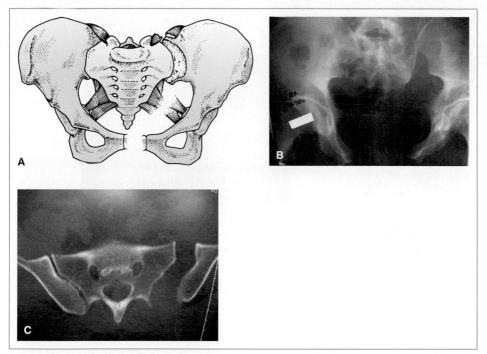

FIGURE 117.4: (**A**) Schematic and (**B**) Anteroposterior radiograph with (**C**) CT scan of a typical anterior-posterior compression-III injury. (From Bucholz RW, Heckman JD, Court-Brown CM, et al. Rockwood and Green's Fractures in Adults, 7th ed. Philadelphia, PA: Lippincott Williams & Wilkins, 2010.)

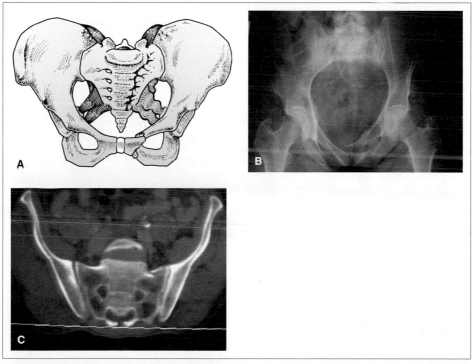

FIGURE 117.5: (**A**) Schematic and (**B**) inlet radiograph with (**C**) CT scan demonstrating a typical lateral compression (LC)-I injury with a sacral impaction fracture posteriorly and rami fractures anteriorly. All of the ligaments are intact. There is a left-sided sacral compression fracture, which is the distinguishing characteristic of an LC-I fracture, as well as left-sided superior and inferior pubic rami fractures, and no iliac fracture. (From Bucholz RW, Heckman JD, Court-Brown CM, et al. Rockwood and Green's Fractures in Adults, 7th ed. Philadelphia, PA: Lippincott Williams & Wilkins, 2010.)

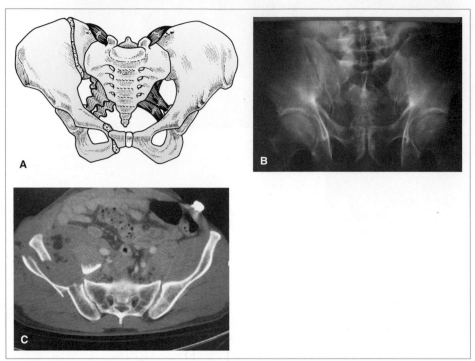

FIGURE 117.6: (**A**) Schematic and (**B**) Anteroposterior radiograph with (**C**) CT scan of a typical lateral compression (LC)-II injury associated with an iliac wing fracture. All of the ligaments are intact, but there is a right-sided iliac wing fracture (which is the distinguishing characteristic of an LC-II fracture), as well as pubic rami fractures. (From Bucholz RW, Heckman JD, Court-Brown CM, et al. Rockwood and Green's Fractures in Adults, 7th ed. Philadelphia, PA: Lippincott Williams & Wilkins, 2010.)

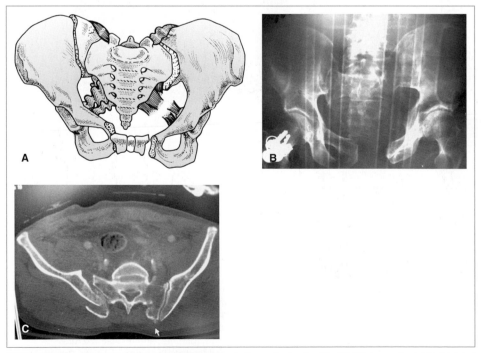

FIGURE 117.7: (**A**) Schematic and (**B**) Anteroposterior radiograph with (**C**) CT scan of a typical lateral compression-III injury. (From Bucholz RW, Heckman JD, Court-Brown CM, et al. Rockwood and Green's Fractures in Adults, 7th ed. Philadelphia, PA: Lippincott Williams & Wilkins, 2010.)

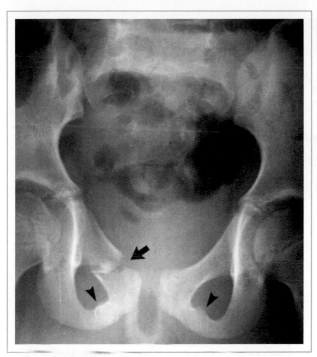

FIGURE 117.8: The comminuted, slightly displaced fracture of the superior pubic ramus (*arrow*) is the only site of pelvic ring fracture in this 6-year-old child. The bulging ischiopubic synchondroses (*arrowheads*) are normal for a child of this age, and neither should be misinterpreted as a fracture site. (From Harris J and Harris W. The Radiology of Emergency Medicine, 4th ed. Philadelphia, PA: Lippincott Williams & Wilkins, 2000.)

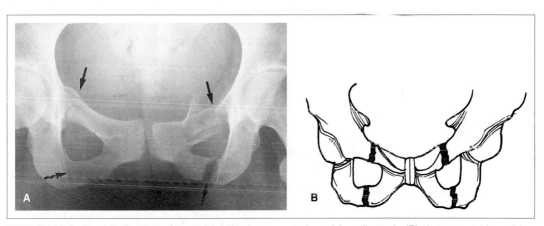

FIGURE 117.9: Straddle fracture of the pelvis. (**A**): Anteroposterior pelvis radiograph. (**B**): Anteroposterior pelvis (diagram). Note the double vertical fractures involving both the superior pubic rami and the ischiopubic junction bilaterally (*arrows*). (From Yochum TR and Rowe LJ. Yochum and Rowe's Essentials of Skeletal Radiology, 3rd ed. Philadelphia, PA: Lippincott Williams & Wilkins, 2004.)

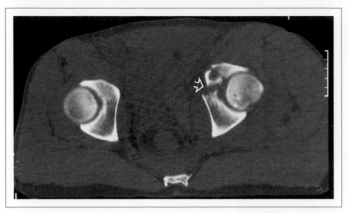

FIGURE 117.10: A posterior wall acetabular fracture is present (*arrow*). (From Bucholz RW and Heckman JD. Rockwood and Green's Fractures in Adults, 5th ed. Philadelphia, PA: Lippincott Williams & Wilkins, 2001.)

Basic Management

- Follow advanced trauma life support (ATLS) algorithm as appropriate
- Avoid excessive movement of the pelvis
- Consider stabilization of the pelvis with a sheet or pelvic binder prior to transport or upon arrival to the emergency department
- In obese patients where a compression binder may not be as effective, internal rotation of the knees and taping of knees together may be effective
- Consider FAST examination to identify other bleeding sources, especially in a hemodynamically unstable patient; of note, uroperitoneum may be confused with hemoperitoneum on FAST examination
- Early orthopedic surgery consultation for operative management or placement of an external fixator
- Angiography and arterial embolization should be considered in cases where hemodynamic instability is likely due to pelvic bleeding
- Avoid urinary catheter insertion in patients with possible urethral injury
- Achieve adequate pain control with opioid analgesics

Summary

TABLE 117.7: Advantages and disadvantages of imaging modalities in pelvic ring fractures

Imaging modalities	Advantages	Disadvantages
AP pelvis x-ray	Quick Demonstrates most injury patterns Standard component of initial trauma evaluation Low cost Bedside availability	Difficulty determining posterior sacroiliac ligament disruption Does not indicate active hemorrhage Not useful for identifying associated solid organ injury or bleeding May miss subtle fractures or dislocations
CT scan	May demonstrate posterior sacroiliac ligament disruption May demonstrate active hemorrhage Demonstrates other intra-abdominal injuries Allows for better operative planning	Time-consuming May require the patient to leave the emergency department Radiation exposure Cannot be obtained in unstable patients
MRI	Theoretically better at detecting ligament damage; however, edema often complicates diagnosis	Most time-consuming Decreased availability Does not have significant benefit over CT scan in the acute setting

118

Malgaigne Fracture

Ashley Peko and Jill Lehrman

Background

The Malgaigne fracture was first described by the French surgeon Joseph-Francois Malgaigne in 1859. This type of injury consists of vertically oriented fractures through the anterior *and* posterior aspects of the pelvis in addition to superior displacement of the lateral acetabulum containing portion of the pelvis. Furthermore, there is associated rupture of the entire pelvic floor including the posterior sacroiliac complexes and the sacrospinous and sacrotuberous ligaments. Together this causes a very unstable fracture pattern, with a high rate of morbidity and mortality. These fractures can be unilateral or bilateral and have several variant patterns.

TABLE 118.1: Classic history and physical

Fall from height onto lower limbs
Heavy load delivered across the head, shoulders, or back (e.g., hit by a falling tree)
Less often from crush injuries
Concomitant head and thoracic injuries are common
Significant hypotension due to arterial or venous plexus hemorrhage in the pelvis
Vertical displacement of the contralateral limb when applying pressure to the pelvic iliac crest and traction to the contralateral leg
Neurological deficit in the fifth lumbar and first sacral nerve root distribution

TABLE 118.2: Potentially helpful laboratory tests

Complete blood count—serial hemoglobin and hematocrit
Coagulation studies—may indicate need for FFP or vitamin K in a patient with coagulopathy
Blood type and cross

FFP, fresh frozen plasma.

Pelvis X-ray

- Anteroposterior (AP) pelvic radiograph is the initial imaging modality of choice; it identifies up to 90% of fractures
- Pelvic inlet and outlet radiographs can be obtained to further classify fractures seen on the AP view; degree of vertical displacement is best seen on outlet view while the degree of posterior displacement is best seen on inlet view; however, these views are rarely obtained in the setting of major trauma while in the emergency department
- Cryer's criteria: vascular injury and significant hemorrhage should be suspected with any displacement of >5 mm at any fracture site in the pelvic ring and acetabulum as seen on the AP image

TABLE 118.3: Anterior ring fractures

Disruption of the pubic symphysis
Disruption of the inferior and superior pubic rami
Disruption of all four rami
Disruption of two rami plus the pubic symphysis

TABLE 118.4: Posterior ring fractures

Fracture of the ileum
Dislocation or fracture dislocation of the sacroiliac complex
More that 5–15 mm of cephalic displacement of the posterior sacroiliac complex on an x-ray outlet view
Fracture of the fourth or fifth lumbar transverse process (attachment sites of the iliolumbar and lateral lumbosacral ligaments)
Detachment of the bony insertion of the sacrospinous ligaments from either the sacrum or the ischial spine
Fracture of the sacrum

 TABLE 118.5: Pelvis x-ray: Malgaigne fracture

IV contrast	No
PO contrast	No
Amount of radiation	0.6 mSv per view

Classic Images

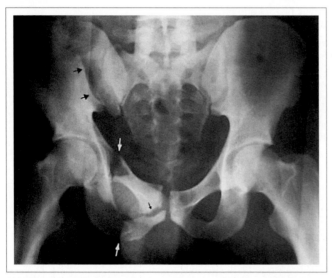

FIGURE 118.1: Malgaigne fracture. There are fractures of the right superior and inferior pubic rami (*white arrows*) and wide separation of the ipsilateral sacroiliac joint (*large black arrows*). There is also some sacroiliac joint separation, an avulsion of the L5 transverse process on the left, and a fracture of the right pubic symphysis (*small black arrow*). (From Eisenberg RL. An Atlas of Differential Diagnosis, 4th ed. Philadelphia, PA: Lippincott Williams & Wilkins, 2003.)

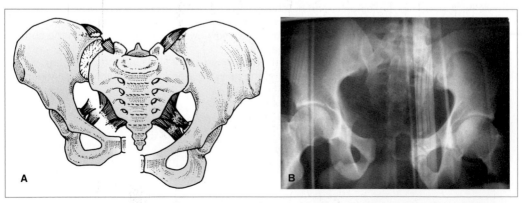

FIGURE 118.2: (**A**) Schematic and (**B**) AP radiograph of a typical vertical shear injury. (From Bucholz RW, Heckman JD, Court-Brown CM, et al. Rockwood and Green's Fractures in Adults, 7th ed. Philadelphia, PA: Lippincott Williams & Wilkins, 2010.)

CT Scan
- Provides detailed imaging of ligamentous injuries, sacroiliac complex, and sacrum
- Provides more precise measurements of displacements
- Pelvic inlet and outlet views on plain film have basically been replaced with CT imaging
- CT scans and reconstructions not only allow for detailed identification of fractures but also identify the presence of retroperitoneal hematomas

 TABLE 118.6: Pelvis CT scan: Malgaigne fracture

IV contrast	Yes, for evaluation of vascular injury
PO contrast	No
Amount of radiation	6 mSv

Classic Images

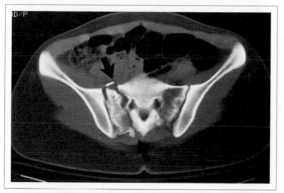

FIGURE 118.3: Fracture through the sacrum (*arrow*) on CT scan. (From Harris J and Harris W. The Radiology of Emergency Medicine, 4th ed. Philadelphia, PA: Lippincott Williams and Wilkins, 2000.)

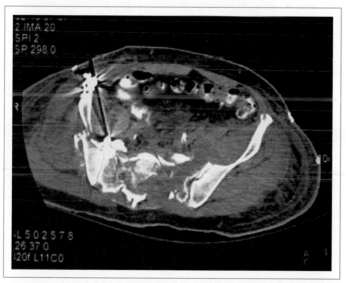

FIGURE 118.4: CT scan reconstruction of a typical vertical shear injury. (From Bucholz RW, Heckman JD, Court-Brown CM, et al. Rockwood and Green's Fractures in Adults, 7th ed. Philadelphia: Lippincott Williams & Wilkins, 2010.)

Angiography
- Allows for real-time imaging of vascular structures and injuries
- Therapeutic interventions are possible through direct embolization with wire coils, polystyrene spheres, and hemostatic sponges
- Requires a fully staffed angiography suite and experienced interventional radiologist

TABLE 118.7: Pelvic angiography/embolization

IV contrast	Yes, for evaluation of vascular injury
PO contrast	No
Amount of radiation	60 mSv

Classic Images

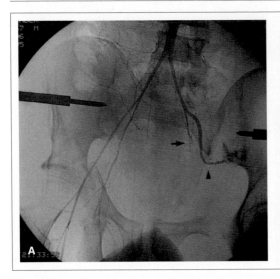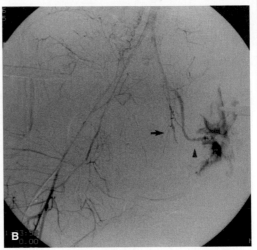

FIGURE 118.5: 29-year-old man run over by a backhoe had a large left groin hematoma and underwent external fixation of his pelvic ring disruption. The patient remained hemodynamically unstable, with falling serial hematocrit values. Note widening of the left sacroiliac joint, displaced left obturator ring fracture, diastasis of the pubic symphysis and a right acetabular fracture (**A**). Early (**A**) And late (**B**) arterial phase of nonselective pelvic arteriogram performed via right common femoral artery access shows multiple occlusions of the proximal branches of the left internal iliac artery (arrow), probably secondary to transection, and complete disruption of the left external iliac artery with frank extravasation of contrast (arrowhead). An occlusion balloon was introduced and inflated in the distal aorta, at its bifurcation, to decrease bleeding prior to surgical repair. (Reprinted with permission from Trauma Radiology Companion, Stern EJ ed. Philadelphia, PA: Lippincott Williams & Wilkins, 1997.)

Basic Management
- Follow ATLS algorithm
- Avoid excessive movement of the pelvis
- Suggest FAST examination to identify other bleeding sources, especially in a hemodynamically unstable patient; of note, uroperitoneum may be confused with hemoperitoneum on FAST examination
- Early emergent orthopedic surgery consultation
- Angiography and arterial embolization in cases of hemodynamic instability
- Avoid urinary catheter insertion in patients with possible urethral injury: vaginal bleeding, palpation of fracture edge on pelvic examination, high-riding or boggy prostate, scrotal hematoma, and/or blood at the urethral meatus
- Achieve adequate pain control with opioid analgesics

Summary

TABLE 118.8: Advantages and disadvantages of imaging modalities in Malgaigne fracture

Imaging modalities	Advantages	Disadvantages
AP pelvis x-ray	Low cost Less time-consuming Bedside availability	Less detailed images for displacement and ligamentous injury
CT scan	Detailed images of ligamentous injuries and posterior bony injuries	Availability outside the emergency department Time-consuming
Angiography	Potentially diagnostic and therapeutic for pelvic hemorrhages	Time-consuming Requires fully functioning angiography suite

119

Hip Fractures

Stacey L. Poznanski and James E. Svenson

Background

Hip fractures are the most common type of lower extremity fracture in the elderly and can lead to significant morbidity and mortality. For this population, as many as a quarter of hip fractures can precipitate death within 1 year and nearly half result in an inability to return to independent living. Most occur as a result of minor trauma, such as a fall from standing height, however fractures can occur in the absence of significant trauma in elderly patients, as well as those with significant osteoporosis, metastatic disease, and chronic steroid use. In young adults, hip fractures usually result from high-velocity injuries, such as motor vehicle collisions or falls from a significant height. Hip fractures are uncommon in children, but can be devastating if the growth plate or tenuous blood supply is disrupted.

TABLE 119.1: Classic history and physical

Hip fractures	Mechanism	Examination
Femoral head	75% due to motor vehicle crashes in younger patients; almost always associated with hip dislocation	Pain with palpation and rotation Lateral thigh contusion Deformity is rare without associated dislocation
Femoral neck	In the elderly, minor, direct trauma (fall) or indirect trauma (twisting with foot planted) Occurs only rarely in younger patients, almost always with high-energy mechanism	*Nondisplaced* fractures have minor groin, medial thigh, or knee pain, and exacerbated with active or passive ROM *Displaced* fractures usually present with severe pain, leg shortening, and external rotation
Intertrochanteric	Usually direct trauma (fall) or transmission of force along long axis of femur; muscles attached to each trochanter further displace fragments	Tenderness, swelling, ecchymosis, with significant leg shortening and external rotation (from traction by iliopsoas) Usually cannot walk
Trochanteric	*Greater:* avulsion in adolescent athletes or elderly who fall directly onto greater trochanter *Lesser:* forceful contraction of iliopsoas in young athletes	Able to walk No shortening, rotation, or limited ROM *Greater:* tenderness over the greater trochanter, worse with abduction *Lesser:* pain worse in flexion and rotation
Subtrochanteric	High-energy trauma, usually in younger patients	Pain and swelling in hip and upper thigh Deformity if displaced

ROM, range of motion.

TABLE 119.2: Potentially helpful laboratory tests

Complete blood count—Serial hemoglobin and hematocrit
Coagulation studies—May indicate need for FFP or vitamin K in a patient with coagulopathy
Blood type and cross

FFP, fresh frozen plasma.

Pelvis X-ray

- With suspected hip injuries, obtain the anteroposterior (AP) view of the pelvis and dedicated AP and lateral plain films of the hip
- Although the AP view will detect most fractures and dislocations, the cross-table lateral view and frog-leg views are better for evaluation of femoral neck and intertrochanteric fractures
- For evaluation of the lesser trochanter, obtain an AP view with the leg in supported external rotation
- Examine x-rays for alterations in the normal trabecular pattern, defects in the cortex, and shortening or angulation of the femoral neck

- Shenton's line extends from the inferior border of the femoral neck to the inferior border of the pubic ramus on the AP view—interruption suggests an abnormally positioned femoral head, such as in subtle cases of femoral neck and head fractures

 TABLE 119.3: Pelvis/hip x-ray: hip fracture

IV contrast	No
PO contrast	No
Amount of radiation	0.7 mSv per view

Femoral Head Fracture

- Uncommon
- Classification:
  - Type I: single fragment—usually caused by sheer forces, such as during dislocation
  - Type II: comminuted—usually caused by direct trauma
- May not be evident on plain radiographs; patients with persistent pain and negative radiographs may require MRI or CT imaging to further evaluate for occult fracture

Femoral Neck Fracture

- Typically occurs in the elderly, osteoporotic patients, with a female-to-male ratio of 4:1
- Very serious injury that may result in long-term disability because of loss of blood supply to the femoral head
- Garden classification used to describe the various femoral neck fractures

Intertrochanteric Fracture

- Most common type of hip fracture; represents almost half of proximal femur fractures
- Similar to femoral neck fractures, these are usually seen in elderly female patients (3:1)
- Unlike femoral neck fractures, the vascular supply to the cancellous bone here is ample; there may be significant blood loss (up to 3 units) due to injury of the well-vascularized cancellous bone; for the same reason, avascular necrosis and nonunion are uncommon complications
- *Stable*: a single fracture line transects the cortex between the two trochanters; no displacement, so may require MRI/CT to diagnose
- *Unstable*: comminuted with associated displacement between the shaft and neck; this is more common

Trochanteric Fracture

- If displacement of a greater trochanteric fracture is greater than 1 cm, there may be associated significant tearing of soft tissue and ligaments
- Lesser trochanter fractures are uncommon in adults and should prompt search for pathologic bone and/or metastatic disease (see image below)
- *Lesser trochanter Ludloff sign*: the patient is unable to lift the affected extremity in a sitting position

Classic Images

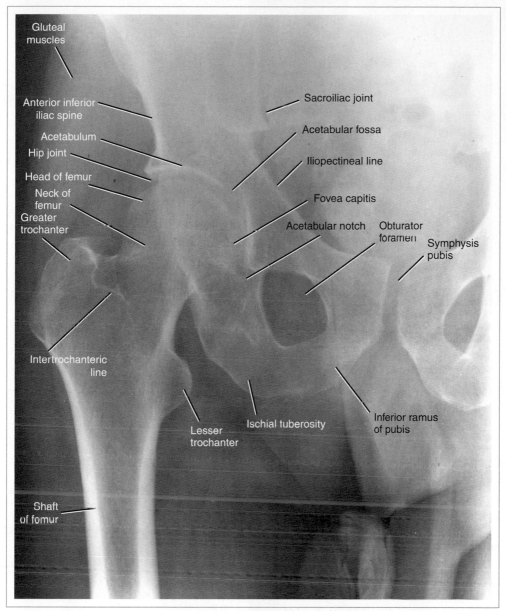

FIGURE 119.1: Anteroposterior radiograph of the normal hip joint. Note that the inferior margin of the neck of the femur should form a continuous curve with the upper margin of the obturator foramen (Shenton's line). (From Snell RS. Clinical Anatomy by Regions, 8th ed. Philadelphia, PA: Lippincott Williams & Wilkins, 2008.)

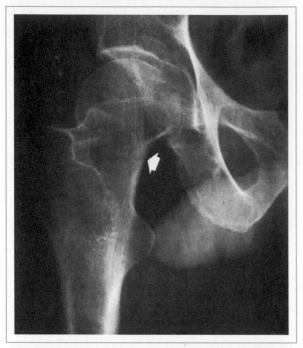

FIGURE 119.2: Type I femoral neck fracture. (From Bucholz RW and Heckman JD. Rockwood and Green's Fractures in Adults, 5th ed. Philadelphia, PA: Lippincott Williams & Wilkins, 2001.)

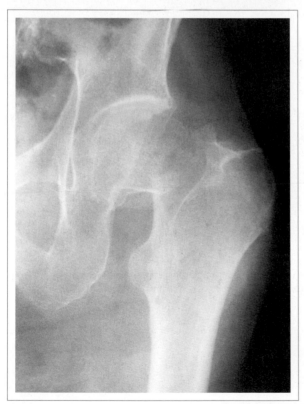

FIGURE 119.3: Type III femoral neck fracture. (From Bucholz RW and Heckman JD. Rockwood and Green's Fractures in Adults, 5th ed. Philadelphia, PA: Lippincott Williams & Wilkins, 2001.)

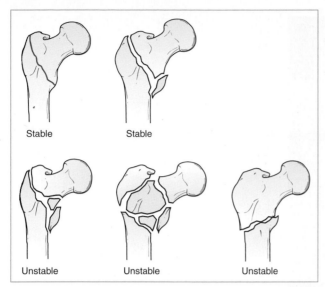

FIGURE 119.4: The Evans classification of intertrochanteric fractures. In stable fracture patterns, the posteromedial cortex remains intact or has minimal comminution, making it possible to obtain and maintain a reduction. Unstable fracture patterns, conversely, are characterized by greater comminution of the posteromedial cortex. The reverse obliquity pattern is inherently unstable because of the tendency for medial displacement of the femoral shaft. (From Bucholz RW, Heckman JD, Court Brown C, et al., eds. Rockwood and Green's Fractures in Adults, 6th ed. Philadelphia, PA: Lippincott Williams & Wilkins, 2006.)

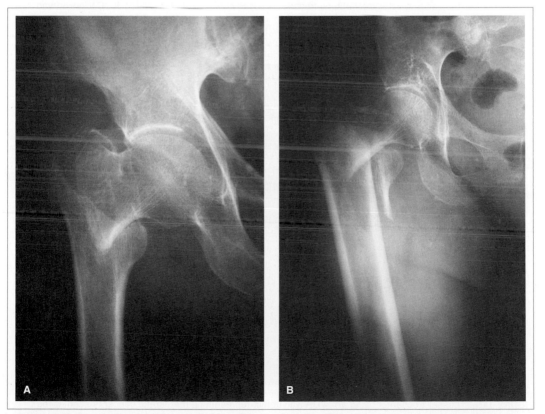

FIGURE 119.5: A: Stable intertrochanteric fracture characterized by an intact posteromedial cortex. **B:** An unstable intertrochanteric fracture characterized by disruption of the posteromedial cortex. (From Koval KJ and Zuckerman JD. Atlas of Orthopaedic Surgery: A Multimedia Reference. Philadelphia, PA: Lippincott Williams & Wilkins, 2004.)

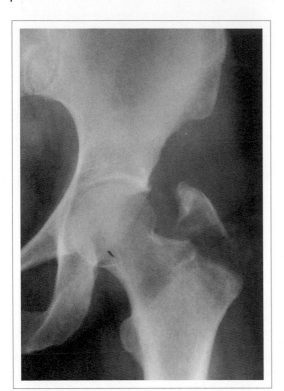

FIGURE 119.6: Displaced greater trochanteric fracture. (From Bucholz RW and Heckman JD. Rockwood and Green's Fractures in Adults, 5th ed. Philadelphia, PA: Lippincott Williams & Wilkins, 2001.)

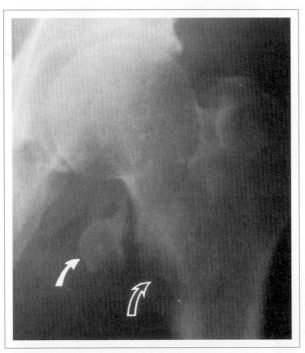

FIGURE 119.7: Lesser trochanter (*solid arrow*). A lytic defect representing metastatic cancer is seen at the femur attachment site (*open arrow*). (From Eisenberg RL. An Atlas of Differential Diagnosis, 4th ed. Philadelphia, PA: Lippincott Williams & Wilkins, 2003.)

CT Scan

- Detects most occult fractures, but may miss nondisplaced fractures that run parallel to the axial plane

 TABLE 119.4: CT scan: hip fracture

IV contrast	No
PO contrast	No
Amount of radiation	6 mSv

Classic Image

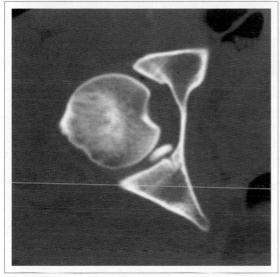

FIGURE 119.8: CT scan demonstrating a fragment of bone interposed between the femoral head and the posterior articular surface that requires removal. (From Bucholz RW and Heckman JD. Rockwood and Green's Fractures in Adults, 5th ed. Philadelphia, PA: Lippincott Williams & Wilkins, 2001.)

MRI

- Occult fractures are present in 2–10% of patients with trauma, hip pain, and negative initial radiographs
- Obtain MRI when plain films are equivocal and occult fracture is suspected; MRI is the diagnostic study of choice in this setting, with sensitivity and specificity close to 100%
- Provides complete anatomic characterization of the fracture and eliminates the need for repeated imaging or supplemental studies

 TABLE 119.5: MRI: hip fracture

IV contrast	No
PO contrast	No
Amount of radiation	None

Classic Images

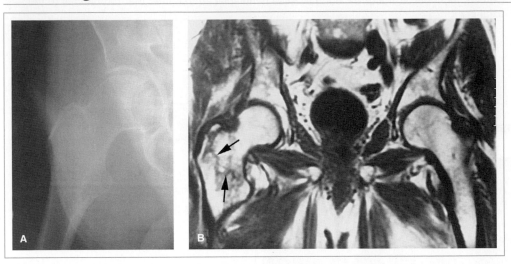

FIGURE 119.9: Posttraumatic hip pain: limited MRI scan. A: AP hip. Observe that the plain film is normal. B: T1-weighted MRI, coronal pelvis. Note the spider-like, low-signal intensity pattern and surrounding bone marrow edema within the intertrochanteric region of the right femur (arrows) These findings are consistent with an occult fracture of the proximal femur. (Courtesy of Steven R. Nokes, Little Rock, AR.) (From Yochum TR and Rowe LJ. Yochum and Rowe's Essentials of Skeletal Radiology, 3rd ed. Philadelphia, PA: Lippincott Williams & Wilkins, 2004.)

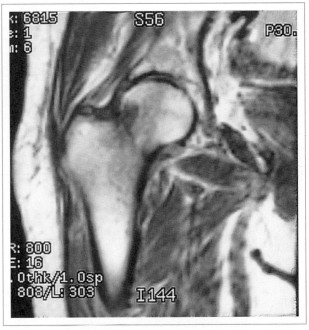

FIGURE 119.10: Magnetic resonance image shows a nondisplaced, right femoral neck fracture. (From Koval KJ and Zuckerman JD. Atlas of Orthopaedic Surgery: A Multimedia Reference. Philadelphia, PA: Lippincott Williams & Wilkins, 2004.)

Basic Management
- Achieve adequate pain control with opioid analgesics
- Emergent orthopedic consultation; prognosis varies by anatomic location and time to definitive management
- Femoral head fracture:
  - Single, small superior dome fragments of femoral head fractures may require operative removal or arthroplasty
  - Most comminuted femoral head fractures, however, will develop AVN if treated conservatively without arthroplasty
- Femoral neck fracture:
  - Ten to thirty percent of nondisplaced femoral neck fractures will become displaced if not operatively managed
  - Forty percent of untreated, displaced femoral neck fractures will develop AVN in 48 hours, while 100% will develop AVN in 1 week
- Intertrochanteric fracture:
  - The large amount of cancellous bone and good blood supply of the intertrochanteric region allows it to heal well if reduction and fixation are properly performed
- Trochanteric fracture:
  - Trochanteric fractures may be treated nonoperatively, especially if nondisplaced
  - Displacement of >1 cm for a greater trochanteric fragment or >2 cm for a lesser trochanteric fragment may require operative fixation

Summary

TABLE 119.6: Advantages and disadvantages of imaging modalities in hip fractures

Imaging modalities	Advantages	Disadvantages
Pelvis x-ray	Low cost Minimal radiation Bedside availability Less time-consuming	May miss nondisplaced fractures
CT scan	More availability than MRI	Radiation exposure May miss nondisplaced fractures
MRI	Gold standard Sensitivity and specificity nears 100%	Body habitus, metal implants, or claustrophobia may limit use Costly Time-consuming

120 Hip Dislocations

D. Paul Turley and Christian C. Zuver

Background

Given the intrinsic stability of the hip joint, dislocation of the hip joint requires significant force. The most common mechanism is blunt trauma, including motor vehicle collisions and motorcycle collisions. Falls, especially in those over 65 years old, are another significant mechanism. Ninety percent of hip dislocations are posterior dislocations.

Given the significant force required to dislocate a native hip, it is not surprising that the majority of patients have additional associated injuries. Causes of long-term disability include sciatic nerve injury (which may occur in 10–15% of posterior hip dislocations), post-traumatic arthritis, recurrent dislocation, and avascular necrosis.

TABLE 120.1: Classic history and physical

Significant blunt trauma, e.g., motorcycle and motor vehicle collisions
Posterior dislocation—hip flexed, adducted, internally rotated, greater trochanter unusually prominent
Anterior dislocation—hip abducted, slight flexion, externally rotated
Extremity usually shortened, although physical findings may be masked in setting of concomitant femoral shaft fracture
Significant pain with range of motion of hip, and possibly numbness and paresthesias
Sensory symptoms along the sciatic or femoral nerve distributions

TABLE 120.2: Potentially helpful laboratory tests

CBC: Serial hemoglobin and hematocrit
Coagulation studies: May indicate need for FFP or vitamin K in a patient with coagulopathy
Blood type and cross

FFP, fresh frozen plasma.

Pelvis and Hip X-ray

- Obtain anteroposterior (AP) view of the pelvis and lateral view of the affected hip
- Adequate AP pelvis should demonstrate the proximal one third of the femur and the entire pelvis
- Posterior hip dislocation
  - The head of the femur should appear smaller than the femoral head on the contralateral side
  - Because of internal rotation, the lesser trochanter should not be visible on the AP view; it should be directly behind the shaft of the femur and will be superimposed
- Anterior hip dislocation
  - The head of the femur should appear larger than the femoral head on the contralateral side
  - Because of external rotation, the lesser trochanter should be prominent and appear in profile
- Disruption of Shenton's line, a smooth curved line drawn along the superior border of the obturator foramen and the medical aspect of the femoral metaphysis, warrants consideration of hip dislocation, hip fracture, or a femoral neck fracture
- AP view of the proximal femur may be needed to completely evaluate for fracture
- Judet views (internal and external oblique views)
  - Centered on injured hip at 45 degrees
  - Useful in giving a more three-dimensional visualization of the dislocation
  - Useful in the setting of a prominent acetabular fracture
  - Helpful if CT scan is not available
  - Obturator oblique (internal oblique view)
    - Film taken parallel to the iliac wing
    - The posterior wall of the acetabulum, posterior segment of the obturator ring, and the pelvic brim are best visualized with this view
  - Iliac oblique (external oblique view)
    - Film taken perpendicular to the iliac wing
    - Posterior column and anterior wall is best visualized with this view

 TABLE 120.3: Pelvis/hip x-ray: hip dislocation

IV contrast	No
PO contrast	No
Amount of radiation	0.6 mSv per view

Classic Image

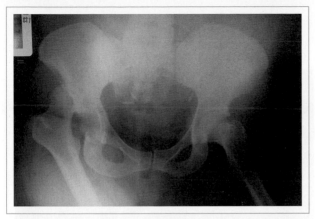

FIGURE 120.1: The trauma AP pelvis radiograph of this patient demonstrates a posterior dislocation of the right hip. Note the superior location of the femoral head and the internally rotated proximal femur. (From Bucholz RW and Heckman JD. Rockwood and Green's Fractures in Adults, 5th ed. Philadelphia, PA: Lippincott Williams & Wilkins, 2001.)

CT Scan
- Should be considered after successful closed reduction of the joint
- Allows better visualization of femoral head fractures
- It may be necessary to request multiple 3-mm cuts through the hips and sacroiliac joints when trauma scan reconstructions are performed

 TABLE 120.4: CT scan: hip dislocation

IV contrast	No
PO contrast	No
Amount of radiation	6 mSv

Classic Images

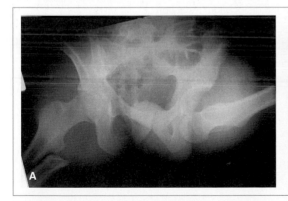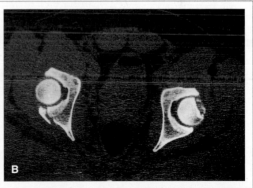

FIGURE 120.2: The anterior hip dislocation (**A**) was reduced successfully. The anterior femoral head impaction injuries were visualized on the CT scan (**B**) but not on the postreduction plain films. Note the impaction injury of the left femoral head and the contralateral posterior wall fracture. (From Bucholz RW and Heckman JD. Rockwood and Green's Fractures in Adults, 5th ed. Philadelphia, PA: Lippincott Williams & Wilkins, 2001.)

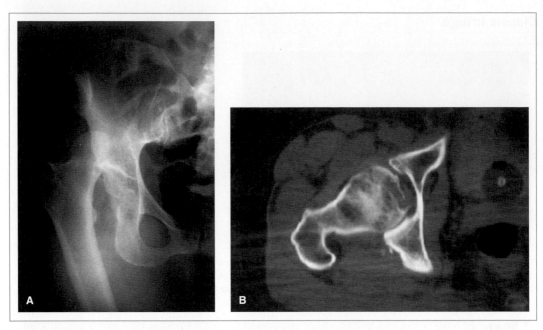

FIGURE 120.3: AP view of posterior hip dislocation with associated femoral head fracture (**A**). CT scan after reduction of the hip demonstrates an anatomic reduction of the fragment at the level of the fovea and a congruent joint (**B**). The injury was treated nonoperatively, and at 2 years the patient has no pain and no arthritis. (From Bucholz RW and Heckman JD. Rockwood and Green's Fractures in Adults, 5th ed. Philadelphia, PA: Lippincott Williams & Wilkins, 2001.)

MRI

- Limited role in the acute diagnosis of hip dislocation
- Useful for determining soft tissue entrapment or sciatic nerve damage that cannot be seen on CT scans or plain films
- May detect intra-articular fragments and femoral head fractures not otherwise seen

 TABLE 120.5: MRI: hip dislocation/reduction

IV contrast	No
PO contrast	No
Amount of radiation	None

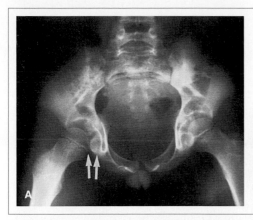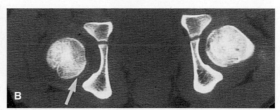

FIGURE 120.4: Radiographs taken following closed reduction of a right hip dislocation. **A:** The plain film demonstrates residual widening of the joint space (*arrows*). **B:** Widening is also apparent with MRI, as is entrapment of a portion of the posterior joint capsule. Under general anesthesia, further efforts at closed reduction were successful. (From Bucholz RW and Heckman JD. Rockwood and Green's Fractures in Adults, 5th ed. Philadelphia, PA: Lippincott Williams & Wilkins, 2001.)

Basic Management

- Follow advanced trauma life support (ATLS) algorithm as appropriate
- Achieve adequate pain control with opioid analgesics; moderate sedation is likely required for reduction
- Reduce hip dislocation as soon as possible, as earlier reduction leads to better results
- Primary contraindication to closed reduction is a femoral neck fracture
- Closed reduction of fracture-dislocations are not recommended for the emergency physician, and should prompt orthopedic consultation

Summary

TABLE 120.6: Advantages and disadvantages of imaging modalities in hip dislocation

Imaging modalities	Advantages	Disadvantages
AP pelvis x-ray	Low cost Bedside availability Less time–consuming	Poor visualization of femoral head and articular fragments
CT scan	Visualization of femoral head Can examine congruence of the acetabulum and femoral head Demonstrates intra-articular fragments	Radiation exposure
MRI	Can visualize entrapped soft tissue or sciatic nerve damage	Time-consuming No consensus on indications

Section Editor: Moira Davenport

121

Femur Shaft Fracture

Karen D. Serrano and Gregory S. Rebella

Background

Femoral shaft fractures are a common cause of morbidity in both the adult and pediatric populations. Femoral shaft fractures typically result from high-energy mechanisms such as motor vehicle crashes or falls from a significant height. Since these fractures often occur in the setting of multisystem trauma, they can be associated with potentially life-threatening cardiopulmonary and vascular complications. Femoral shaft fractures in children are more commonly isolated and may be due to falls from playground equipment or sporting injuries. In infants, these fractures are frequently associated with nonaccidental trauma. In all age groups, relatively low-energy accidents may result in pathologic fractures in bone weakened by osteopenia, bone cyst, or tumor.

TABLE 121.1: Classic history and physical

Significant pain and inability to bear weight
Swelling (tense thigh), tenderness, and deformity (shortening of leg)
Distal paresthesia, pain, and diminished pulses suggest arterial injury or compartment syndrome
History may be vague in infants: caregiver may report crying, fussiness, poor eating, and the infant may demonstrate decreased movement of the extremity

TABLE 121.2: Potentially helpful laboratory tests

CBC: Hemoglobin and hematocrit may be normal initially. Blood loss of up to 1–2 L into the thigh compartment is possible in adults
Coagulation studies: May indicate need for FFP or vitamin K in a patient with coagulopathy
Type and screen: To expedite transfusion and as part of preoperative work-up

CBC, complete blood count; FFP, fresh frozen plasma.

Femur X-ray

- Anteroposterior and lateral views are typically diagnostic
- Include ipsilateral hip and knee films (anteroposterior and lateral) because of high incidence of associated injury, particularly femoral neck and tibial shaft fractures
- Femoral shaft fractures should be described according to the fracture pattern (transverse, oblique, spiral, or comminuted), associated varus or valgus deformity, and degree of shortening of the leg
- Obtain skeletal survey and head CT to evaluate for nonaccidental trauma in all infants with femoral shaft fractures

 TABLE 121.3: Femur x-ray

IV contrast	No
PO contrast	No
Amount of Radiation	0.01 mSv per view

Classic Images

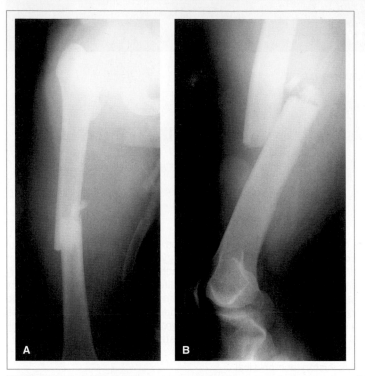

FIGURE 121.1: A 24-year-old man was ejected from a car during a motor vehicle collision, sustaining a grade IIIA open femur fracture (**A** and **B**). (From Bucholz RW and Heckman JD. Rockwood and Green's Fractures in Adults, 5th ed. Philadelphia, PA: Lippincott Williams & Wilkins, 2001.)

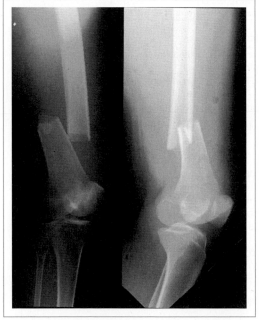

FIGURE 121.2: Type A distal femur fracture. (From Bucholz RW and Heckman JD. Rockwood and Green's Fractures in Adults, 5th ed. Philadelphia, PA: Lippincott Williams & Wilkins, 2001.)

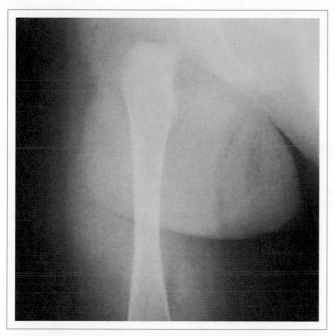

FIGURE 121.3: Hip films were obtained and were normal, but the full femur radiograph demonstrated a spiral femur fracture consistent with child abuse. (From Fleisher GR, Ludwig S, and Baskin MN. Atlas of Pediatric Emergency Medicine. Philadelphia, PA: Lippincott Williams & Wilkins, 2004.)

CT Scan
- Traumatic femoral shaft fractures do not usually require CT scan
- Due to high incidence of associated femoral neck and acetabular fractures, consider a noncontrast CT of the hip/pelvis as dictated by clinical suspicion

 TABLE 121.4: CT scan: hip fracture

IV contrast	No
PO contrast	No
Amount of radiation	6 mSv

Basic Management
- Follow advanced trauma life support (ATLS) algorithm as appropriate
- Early and aggressive fluid resuscitation and blood transfusion if indicated
- Achieve adequate pain control with opioid analgesics
- Immobilization and traction should be applied for comfort and stabilization
- Orthopedic consultation required for all femoral shaft fractures
- Frequent neurovascular assessments recommended to evaluate for femoral nerve and arterial injuries as well as to assess for compartment syndrome
- Child abuse specialist and social work consultations for infants with injury

Summary

TABLE 121.5: Advantages and disadvantages of imaging modalities in femoral shaft fracture

Imaging modalities	Advantages	Disadvantages
Radiographs	Low cost Minimal radiation Readily available Typically diagnostic	May miss subtle fracture
CT scan	Detects associated acetabular and femoral neck fractures	Greater cost Radiation exposure

122 Tibial Plateau and Tibial Spine Fractures

Marsha Tallman and Moira Davenport

Background

Tibial plateau fractures are increasingly common as the population ages. They account for 1% of all fractures overall, but 8% of fractures in the elderly.

The articular surface of the knee consists of medial and lateral tibial plateaus, which articulate with the medial and lateral tibial condyles, respectively. These two bony surfaces are separated by a bony ridge known as the tibial spine, or intercondylar eminence. The anterior cruciate ligament (ACL) and posterior cruciate ligament (PCL) both attach to the tibial spine. The medial tibial plateau is thicker and stronger and therefore not injured as frequently as the weaker, thinner lateral plateau. The lateral plateau is also injured more frequently as more traumatic events to the knee happen with valgus rather than varus stress.

Tibial spine fractures are more common in children and adolescents than in adults. In adults the ACL tears, whereas in younger patients the ligaments are stronger than the physeal plates and an avulsion fracture results. An adult with a tibial spine fracture frequently has an MCL tear or concomitant tibial plateau fracture.

TABLE 122.1: Classic history and physical—tibial plateau fracture

Direct trauma particularly twisting in hyperextension
Auto vs. pedestrian accident
Auto accident with knee striking dashboard
Fall from height
Hyperextension playing sports
Osteoporosis
Effusion
Difficulty bearing weight
Joint line tenderness
Ecchymosis
Associated ligamentous/meniscal injury possible
Popliteal artery injury possible
Peroneal nerve injury possible

Knee X-ray

- Obtain a standard anteroposterior (AP), lateral, or oblique film
- With minimally displaced vertical split fractures, the fracture line may sit in an oblique plane and may not be visible on AP or lateral radiograph
- Oblique projections should be added or carefully reviewed if clinical suspicion is high for this injury but not seen on standard projections
- Look for lipohemarthrosis, a fat/fluid level in the suprapatellar recess seen on the lateral view of the knee. The presence of fat from the bone marrow indicates an intra-articular fracture
- The medial tibial condoyle normally has greater trabecular density because it bears more weight; lateral plateau fracture should be suspected if there is greater trabecular density in this area on the AP view
- Definitive examination of range of motion and tests of laxity should be done only after radiographs have been reviewed
- Tunnel view radiographs provide an excellent view of the intercondylar eminence and any suspected tibial spine fracture
- Contralateral views may be useful to assure that adequate restoration of length and alignment of the leg is achieved during reduction

TABLE 122.2: X-ray: tibial plateau fracture

IV contrast	No
PO contrast	No
Amount of radiation	mSv

Classic Images

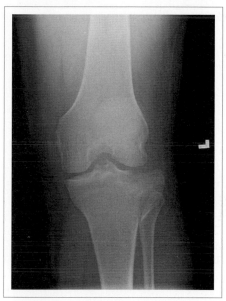

FIGURE 122.1: AP x-ray of the knee showing a lateral tibial plateau fracture. (*Courtesy of Richard H. Daffner MD, Allegheny General Hospital, Pittsburgh, PA.*)

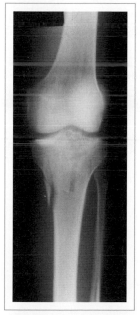

FIGURE 122.2: Comminuted fracture of the medial tibial plateau sustained by a motorcyclist with the knee in flexion. (From Bucholz RW and Heckman JD. Rockwood and Green's Fractures in Adults, 5th ed. Philadelphia, PA: Lippincott Williams & Wilkins, 2001.)

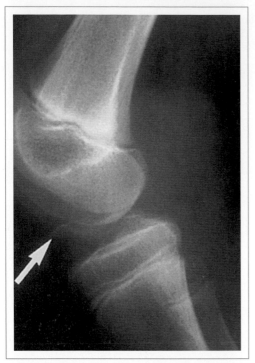

FIGURE 122.3: Avulsion fracture of the tibial spine in a 9-year-old girl. A significant hemarthrosis was present and was aspirated. (From Fleisher GR, Ludwig S, and Henretig FM. Textbook of Pediatric Emergency Medicine, 5th ed. Philadelphia, PA: Lippincott Williams & Wilkins, 2005.)

CT Scan

- CT scan may be necessary if radiographs do not show fracture but clinical suspicion is high
- CT scan can provide information regarding the fracture planes to determine the best surgical approach
- Image data can be reconstructed to show the sagittal and coronal planes
- Lipohemarthrosis, a fat-fluid level on lateral radiograph or CT scan, suggests intra-articular fracture

 TABLE 122.3: CT scan: tibial plateau fracture

IV contrast	No
PO contrast	No
Amount of radiation	mSv

Classic Images

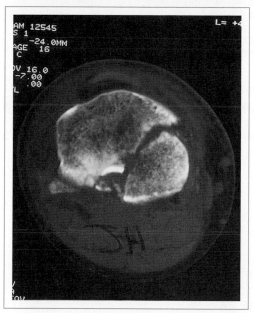

FIGURE 122.4: Lateral tibial plateau fracture, coronal view. (From Koval KJ and Zuckerman JD. Atlas of Orthopaedic Surgery: A Multimedial Reference. Philadelphia, PA: Lippincott Williams & Wilkins, 2004.)

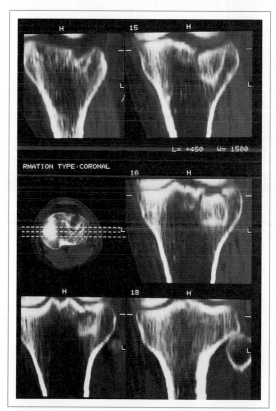

FIGURE 122.5: Lateral tibial plateau fracture, sagittal reconstructions. (From Koval KJ and Zuckerman JD. Atlas of Orthopaedic Surgery: A Multimedial Reference. Philadelphia, PA: Lippincott Williams & Wilkins, 2004.)

MRI

- MRI may be necessary if radiographs do not show fracture but clinical suspicion is high
- MRI can provide information regarding the fracture planes to determine the best surgical approach
- Image data can be reconstructed to show the sagittal and coronal planes
- MRI will also show concomitant ligamentous or meniscal injuries

 TABLE 122.4: MRI: tibial plateau fracture

IV contrast	No
PO contrast	No
Amount of radiation	None

Classic Images

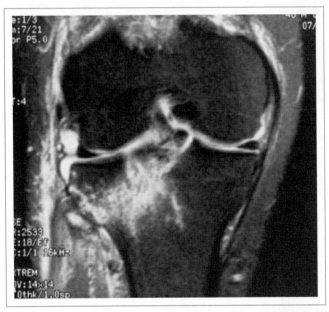

FIGURE 122.6: MRI scan showing a minimally displaced comminuted lateral tibial plateau fracture. The collateral and cruciate ligaments as well as the menisci are well visualized. (From Bucholz RW and Heckman JD. Rockwood and Green's Fractures in Adults, 5th ed. Philadelphia, PA: Lippincott Williams & Wilkins, 2001.)

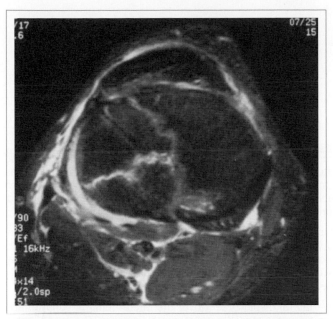

FIGURE 122.7: MRI scan showing a minimally displaced comminuted lateral tibial plateau fracture with stellate comminution of the articular surface. (From Bucholz RW and Heckman JD. Rockwood and Green's Fractures in Adults, 5th ed. Philadelphia, PA: Lippincott Williams & Wilkins, 2001.)

Basic Management
Tibial plateau fracture

- Carefully examine the skin surface for any punctures or lacerations
- Open fractures require immediate orthopedic evaluation
- Ice, compression, elevation
- Pain management
- Monitor for signs of compartment syndrome
- Immobilization in full extension and crutches
- Strict non-weight bearing is required for all fracture types
- Displaced, bicondylar, or comminuted fractures require orthopedic consultation as open reduction and internal fixation may be necessary
- Orthopedic follow-up is required for nonoperative cases
- Tibial spine fracture
- Non-weight bearing, immobilization in full extension, and orthopedic follow up

Summary

TABLE 122.5: Advantages and disadvantages of imaging modalities in tibial plateau and tibial spine fractures

Imaging modalities	Advantages	Disadvantages
X-ray	Low cost Rapid	Does not evaluate ligaments/menisci Limited information regarding fracture planes
CT scan	Soft tissues visualized Preoperative planning	Time-consuming Greater radiation exposure Not required emergently
MRI	Soft tissues clearly visualized Preoperative planning No radiation	Time-consuming Not required emergently

123

Acute Patellar Fracture and Dislocation

Michael Yeh and Moira Davenport

Background

The patella is a flat, triangular sesamoid bone that protects the knee joint from direct trauma and facilitates knee extension. The patella is embedded in the quadriceps tendon, which articulates with the trochlear groove of the femur and becomes the patellar ligament and inserts distally on the tibial tuberosity. Strong contraction of the quadriceps muscles against a flexed knee or landing on one's feet from a fall may produce forces sufficient to cause a fracture.

The knee joint capsule is also supported by the medial and lateral patellar retinacula, extensions of the vastus medialis, and vastus lateralis tendons. The retinacula attach proximally to the medial and lateral superior borders of the patella, and distally to the medial and lateral tibial condyles. Disruption of the retinacula associated with patellar fracture or dislocation results in inability to actively extend the knee.

Patellar dislocations usually involve lateral displacement over the lateral femoral condyle, and are almost always associated with a disrupted medial patellofemoral ligament. The medial patellofemoral ligament, which originates from the adductor tubercle of the femur and inserts on the proximal two thirds of the patella, provides most of the restraining force preventing lateral displacement of the patella. As the retinaculum and medial patellofemoral ligaments are disrupted, osteochondral fragments may be sheared off the articular surfaces of the medial patellar facet and lateral femoral condyles.

TABLE 123.1: Classic history and physical

Patella fracture
Direct trauma to the knee
Indirect mechanism involving forceful contraction of the quadriceps against a flexed
    knee (quadriceps avulsion fracture)
Localized tenderness, swelling, and knee effusion
Inability to ambulate or pain with weight bearing
Difficulty with knee extension

Patella dislocation
Noncontact mechanism of injury, classically occurring with external rotation of the tibia
    relative to the femur with the knee slightly flexed in valgus position; twisting of the
    knee and body while the leg is planted in a fixed position
Patients may report feeling a "pop" at the time of injury
Knee is generally held in a slightly flexed (20–30 degrees) position, with the patella
    visible and palpable laterally
Often patella has been reduced either spontaneously or by a prehospital care provider
Persistent subluxation can be detected by the apprehension test: the examiner pushes
    the medial aspect of the patella laterally with the knee in 20–30 degrees of flexion; a
    positive test occurs if the patient reports a sensation of dislocation and pain
Localized tenderness, swelling, and hemarthrosis of the knee
Inability to ambulate or pain with weight bearing
Difficulty with knee extension

X-ray

- Obtain anteroposterior (AP), lateral, and infrapatellar (sunrise or Merchant's) views
- The lateral view is useful for revealing the extent of separation between fragments
- The sunrise view may reveal osteochondral fractures
- Sunrise views may not be possible in patients with patellar dislocations because of the inability to flex the knee
- Direct blunt trauma often causes stellate or comminuted fractures
- Indirect trauma most often causes transverse fractures involving the central or distal third of the patella

- Vertical patellar fractures are less common and are usually caused by direct injury involving the lateral facet
- Contraction of the quadriceps muscle can pull a superior fracture fragment proximally, resulting in wide displacement requiring surgical repair
- Examine carefully for intra-articular fragments
- Bipartite or multipartite patellae are normal variants that appear as fractures; ossification centers of a bipartite patella are found at the upper outer areas of the bone, with smooth, continuous cortical borders and minimal distance between them
- Postreduction films are recommended after closed reduction of a dislocated patella to look for loose osteochondral avulsion fragments and confirm alignment of the patella in the trochlear groove

 TABLE 123.2: X-ray: patella fracture/dislocation

IV contrast	No
PO contrast	No
Amount of radiation	mSv per view

Classic Images

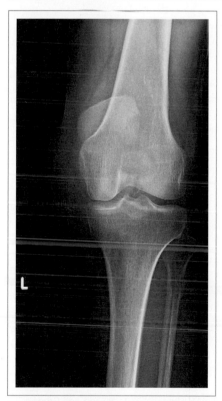

FIGURE 123.1: AP knee x-ray demonstrating patellar fracture (note the abnormality at the inferior pole). (*Courtesy of Richard H. Daffner, MD, Allegheny General Hospital, Pittsburgh, PA.*)

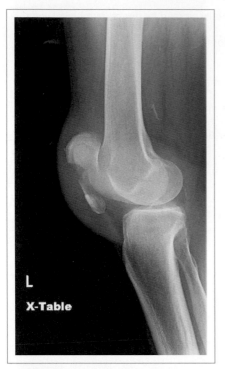

FIGURE 123.2: Cross-table lateral x-ray of the knee showing patella fracture with significant displacement of the inferior fragment. (*Courtesy of Richard H. Daffner, MD, Allegheny General Hospital, Pittsburgh, PA.*)

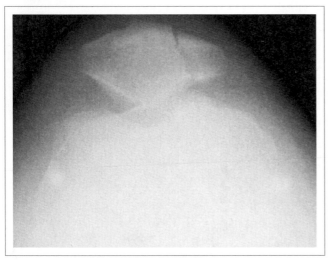

FIGURE 123.3: Sunrise view of a patella fracture. (From Bucholz RW and Heckman JD. Rockwood and Green's Fractures in Adults, 5th ed. Philadelphia, PA: Lippincott Williams & Wilkins, 2001.)

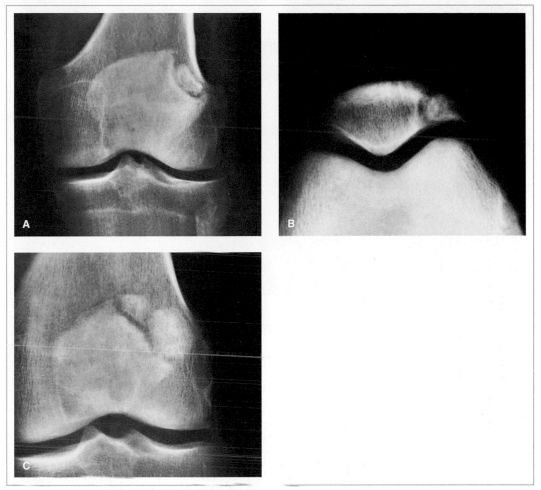

FIGURE 123.4: Bipartite patella. **A:** Anterior-posterior view **B:** Sunrise view **C:** Oblique view. (From Greenspan A. Orthopedic Imaging: A Practical Approach, 4th ed. Philadelphia, PA: Lippincott Williams & Wilkins, 2004.)

MRI

- MRI can evaluate soft tissue abnormalities that occur secondary to patellar dislocation
- MRI can be useful in determining whether joint laxity is present

 TABLE 123.3: MRI: patella fracture/dislocation

IV contrast	No
PO contrast	No
Amount of radiation	None

Classic Images

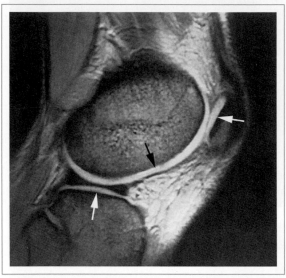

FIGURE 123.5: T2-weighted MRI, sagittal knee. Normal anatomy. (From Yochum TR and Rowe LJ. Yochum and Rowe's Essentials of Skeletal Radiology, 3rd ed. Philadelphia, PA: Lippincott Williams & Wilkins, 2004.)

Basic Management
Patellar Fracture
- Pain control
- Nondisplaced fractures with an intact extensor mechanism may be treated in the emergency department with a knee immobilizer or splint with the knee fully extended
- Protect the proximal fibula to limit peroneal nerve injury during splinting
- Elevation, ice, and compression as well as analgesics may help control pain and swelling; the patient should use crutches for ambulation, with no weight bearing on the affected knee
- Outpatient orthopedic surgery referral within 1 week
- Nondisplaced fractures with an intact extensor mechanism are usually treated with casting in full extension for 4–6 weeks as well as quadriceps muscles exercises
- Urgent orthopedic surgery consultation:
  - Surgical management of patellar fracture is generally indicated for patients with disruption of the extensor mechanism, intra-articular bone fragments, >2 mm displacement of the articular surface, or >3 mm diastasis between bone fragments

Patellar Dislocation
- Pain control
- Manual reduction
  - Place the patient supine with hips and the injured knee slightly flexed
  - Apply pressure to the lateral aspect of the patella, pushing medially, while the knee is slowly extended
- Obtain a postreduction x-ray
- Immobilize in extension for 3–6 weeks
- Crutches should be given for ambulation
- Rest, ice, elevation

Summary

TABLE 123.4: Advantages and disadvantages of imaging modalities in patella fracture/dislocation

Imaging modalities	Advantages	Disadvantages
X-ray	Immediate Little radiation	Unable to assess soft tissues Pain with manipulation to obtain all views
MRI	Able to evaluate soft tissues No radiation	Time-consuming Cost Availability

Background

A knee dislocation occurs when abnormal forces on the tibia and fibula result in complete loss of continuity with the femur. For this dislocation to occur, at least three of the four major knee ligaments (anterior cruciate (ACL), posterior cruciate (PCL), medial collateral (MCL), and lateral collateral (LCL)) must tear. The true incidence of knee dislocation is not known as reduction is often spontaneous and thus not often detected during the initial evaluation of multisystem trauma/obtunded patients. It is imperative that the emergency physician considers knee dislocation in the differential diagnosis as neurovascular deficits resulting from this injury can be devastating.

TABLE 124.1: Classic history and physical

Trauma, i.e., motor vehicle accident, severe crush injuries, or athletic activities
Obvious gross knee deformity
Unstable knee
Swelling/hemarthroses
Fullness in the popliteal fossa
Weak popliteal or dorsalis pedis and anterior tibialis pulses

TABLE 124.2: Types of dislocations—based on relative displacement of the tibia with respect to femur

Anterior	Hyperextension of the knee; most common type
Posterior	High velocity trauma to flexed knee (dashboard type injury); second most common type)
Medial	Varus force
Lateral	Valgus force
Rotational	Rotary force

TABLE 124.3: Potential complications

Popliteal artery injury–more common with posterior dislocations but also seen with anterior dislocations; associated with limb loss, especially if not revascularized within 6–8 hr
Peroneal nerve injury—foot drop
Compartment syndrome
Tibial nerve injury, ligamentous or meniscal injury

Knee X-ray

- Obtain three views—anteroposterior (AP), lateral, sunrise (patellar)
- X-rays are recommended prior to any ligamentous stressing during physical examination
- Fractures may be present (i.e., tibial plateau fractures)

 TABLE 124.4: X-ray: knee dislocation

IV contrast	No
PO contrast	No
Amount of radiation	mSv per view

Classic Images

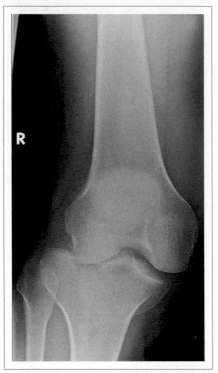

FIGURE 124.1: AP knee x-ray demonstrating lateral knee dislocation with lateral tibial plateau fracture. (*Courtesy of Richard H. Daffner, MD, Allegheny General Hospital, Pittsburgh, PA.*)

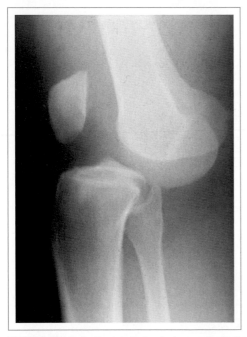

FIGURE 124.2: Lateral radiograph demonstrating an anterior knee dislocation with complete bicruciate ligament disruption. (From Bucholz RW and Heckman JD. Rockwood and Green's Fractures in Adults, 5th ed. Philadelphia, PA: Lippincott Williams & Wilkins, 2001.)

Knee MRI

- MRI is used to evaluate the disrupted ligaments after a knee dislocation

 TABLE 124.5: MRI: knee dislocation

IV contrast	No
PO contrast	No
Amount of radiation	None

Classic Images

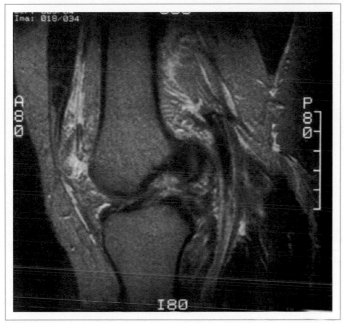

FIGURE 124.3: Anterior cruciate ligament and posterior cruciate ligament tears on MRI in a low-velocity knee dislocation. (From Bucholz RW and Heckman JD. Rockwood and Green's Fractures in Adults, 5th ed. Philadelphia, PA: Lippincott Williams & Wilkins, 2001.)

Lower Extremity Angiogram

- Remains the gold standard for vascular injury
- Risk of injury from direct arterial catheterization
- Extravasation of contrast is an indication of vascular disruption
- Time-consuming and special personnel required to perform

 TABLE 124.6: Angiogram: knee dislocation

IV contrast	Yes, to visualize the arterial vascular tree
PO contrast	No
Amount of radiation	4–5 mSv

Classic Images

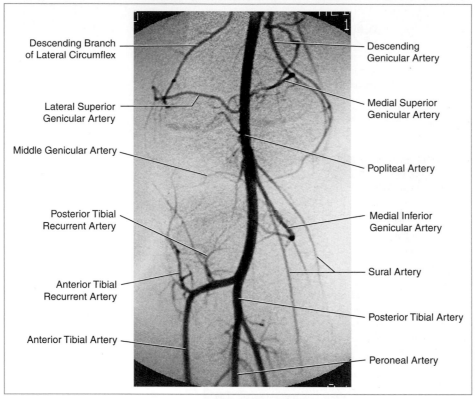

Descending Branch of Lateral Circumflex

Lateral Superior Genicular Artery

Middle Genicular Artery

Posterior Tibial Recurrent Artery

Anterior Tibial Recurrent Artery

Anterior Tibial Artery

Descending Genicular Artery

Medial Superior Genicular Artery

Popliteal Artery

Medial Inferior Genicular Artery

Sural Artery

Posterior Tibial Artery

Peroneal Artery

FIGURE 124.4: Anterior view of a popliteal angiogram showing the main branches. (From Uflacker R. Atlas of Vascular Anatomy: An Angiographic Approach, 2nd ed. Philadelphia, PA: Lippincott Williams & Wilkins, 1997.)

Basic Management

- Analgesia
- Immediate reduction
- Place the leg in a posterior splint (or a hinged knee brace fully locked) with 15–20 degree knee flexion
- Ankle brachial index (ABI) measurements
- Serial neurovascular examinations
- Angiography is recommended for patients with abnormal ABIs or neurovascular deficits
- Orthopedic surgery consultation
- Emergent vascular surgery consultation for any vascular deficit

Summary

TABLE 124.7: Advantages and disadvantages of imaging modalities in knee dislocation

Imaging modalities	Advantages	Disadvantages
X-ray	Low cost Rapid Study of choice	Pain with manipulation to obtain all views
MRI	Visualizes ligamentous injury Preoperative planning	Time-consuming Cost Availability
Angiogram	Gold standard for vascular injury	Arterial access Intravenous contrast Radiation Time-consuming Specialized personnel required

125

Ligamentous and Meniscal Injuries of the Knee

Ngozi Onyenekwu and Moira Davenport

Background

The joint capsule and the posterior and anterior cruciate ligaments help stabilize the knee against anterior and posterior displacement of the tibia on the femur. The medial and lateral menisci are crescent-shaped intra-articular fibrocartilaginous structures that function as shock absorbers while offering stabilization in all planes of motion. Externally, medial and lateral stabilization is provided by the collateral ligaments. The semimembranosus and pes anserinus tendons also contribute to medial stability. While the lateral collateral ligament is completely extracapsular, the medial collateral ligament has both a superficial extracapsular segment and a deep portion that is part of the joint capsule.

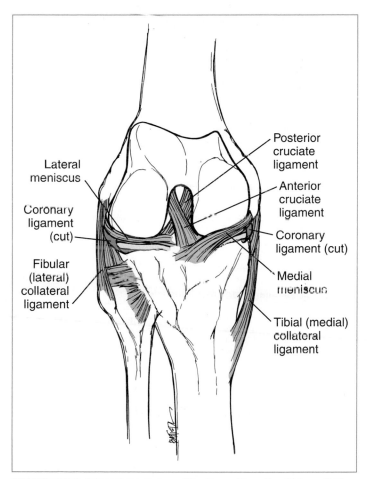

Lateral meniscus

Coronary ligament (cut)

Fibular (lateral) collateral ligament

Posterior cruciate ligament

Anterior cruciate ligament

Coronary ligament (cut)

Medial meniscus

Tibial (medial) collateral ligament

FIGURE 125.1: Internal structures of the knee. (From Hendrickson T. Massage for Orthopedic Conditions. Philadelphia, PA: Lippincott Williams & Wilkins, 2002.)

Anterior Cruciate Ligament Injury
- Most common ligamentous injury
- Lateral trauma to the knee can result in the terrible triad including injury to the anterior cruciate ligament (ACL), medial collateral ligament tear, and medial or lateral meniscus
- May be associated with knee dislocation and associated popliteal artery injury

Posterior Cruciate Ligament Injury
- Less common than ACL injury
- Ninety-five percent associated with other ligament injuries

Medial Collateral Ligament Injury
- Most common isolated knee ligament injury
- Most commonly associated with ACL tear
- Ninety-five percent associated with other ligament injuries

Lateral Collateral Ligament Injury

TABLE 125.1: Classic history and physical

ACL: High-speed, traumatic twisting movement, especially if accompanied by valgus stress
PCL: Injuries outside of sporting activities such as a fall striking the tibial tubercle, a direct posterior blow to flexed knee (dashboard injury), or severe varus or valgus load
MCL: Direct blow to lateral aspect of knee
LCL: Hyperextension with medial blow to knee
Associated with contact and noncontact sporting activities
Audible "pop" heard at time of injury
Sense of knee "giving out" or "locking"
Hemarthroses
ACL: Anterior drawer test—instability with anterior stress with knee in 90-degree flexion
ACL: Lachman's test—most sensitive; instability with anterior stress in 15- to 30-degree flexion
PCL: Posterior drawer test—instability with posterior stress in 90-degree flexion
MCL: Valgus (lateral) stress test—instability with valgus stress in 30-degree flexion and full extension
LCL: Varus (medial) stress test—instability with varus stress in 30-degree flexion and full extension

ACL, anterior cruciate ligament; LCL, lateral collateral ligament; MCL, medial collateral ligament; PCL, posterior cruciate ligament.

Medial/Lateral Meniscus Injury

TABLE 125.2: Classic history and physical—medial/lateral meniscus injury

Twisting maneuver on weight-bearing knee		
Joint line pain, swelling, and "clicking/locking" knee		
McMurray's test	Pain as the knee is brought from full flexion to 90-degree flexion and to full extension while the leg is externally rotated with compression over the medial join line and/or when the leg is internally rotated with compression over the lateral joint line	Medial joint line clunk is an indication of medial meniscus injury Lateral joint line clunk is an indication of lateral meniscus injury Pain without an appreciable clunk is not a true positive McMurray's test
Apley test	With the patient prone and the knee flexed to 90 degrees, pressure is applied to the heel while the tibia is rotated	Pain that resolves when the tibia is distracted from the femur while rotated is suspicious for meniscal tear

Knee X-ray
- X-rays should be performed in the acute setting, but are frequently unremarkable
- Obtain anteroposterior, lateral, and sunrise views
- Knee effusion may be seen on lateral x-ray
- A Segond fracture is an avulsion of the medial femoral condyle; when present it heightens the suspicion for an ACL tear

TABLE 125.3: X-ray: ligamentous and meniscal injuries

IV contrast	No
PO contrast	No
Amount of radiation	mSv per view

Classic Images

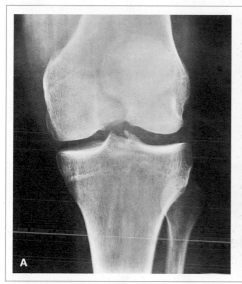
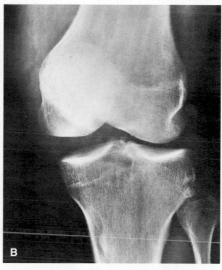

FIGURE 125.2: Tear of the medial collateral ligament. **A:** Anteroposterior radiograph of the knee shows the width of the medial and lateral joint compartments to be normal. **B:** The same projection obtained after application of valgus stress shows widening of the medial joint compartment, a finding consistent with the clinical diagnosis of tear of the medial collateral ligament. Note also the avulsion of the lateral tibial tubercle, which is occasionally associated with tear of the anterior cruciate ligament. (From Greenspan A. Orthopedic Imaging: A Practical Approach, 4th ed. Philadelphia, PA: Lippincott Williams & Wilkins, 2004.)

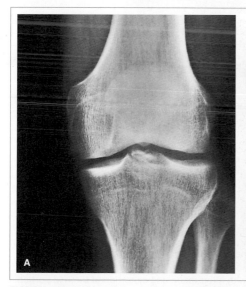
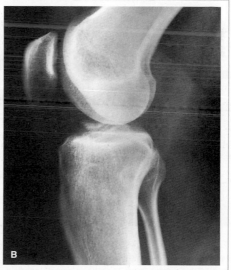

FIGURE 125.3: Tear of the anterior cruciate ligament. Anteroposterior (**A**) and lateral (**B**) films of the knee show avulsion of the tibial eminence, suggesting tear of the anterior cruciate ligament. The diagnosis was confirmed by arthroscopy. (From Greenspan A. Orthopedic Imaging: A Practical Approach, 4th ed. Philadelphia, PA: Lippincott Williams & Wilkins, 2004.)

MRI

- MRI is the gold standard for diagnosing ligamentous injuries
- This does not have to be performed in the emergency department setting
- The ACL originates on the lateral femoral condyle posteriorly and courses caudally in an anteroinferior direction to insert on the lateral portion of the intercondylar area of the tibia
- The posterior cruciate ligament (PCL) arises from the posterior surface of the intercondylar region of the tibia and attaches to the lateral surface of the medial femoral condyle, having an inverted hockey stick appearance; the PCL maintains a low signal intensity throughout and is broader and thicker than the ACL
- The menisci on T1-weighted images appear as diffusely low signal intensity structures; linear intermediate signal can represent a tear

 TABLE 125.4: MRI: ligamentous and meniscal injuries

IV contrast	No
PO contrast	No
Amount of radiation	None

Classic Images

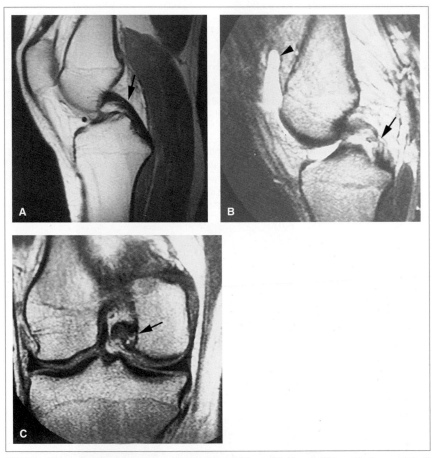

FIGURE 125.4: A: Normal anatomy: T1-weighted MRI, sagittal knee. The posterior cruciate ligament (PCL) is identified in virtually every examination of the knee and is seen in its entirety on this single slice (*arrow*). **B:** PCL tear: T2-weighted MRI, sagittal knee. Increased signal intensity with interruption and distortion of the mid portion of the PCL (*arrow*). Note the posterior subluxation of the tibia (posterior, drawer sign). In addition, there is a large hyperintense suprapatellar effusion (*arrowhead*). **C:** PCL tear: T2-weighted MRI, coronal knee. Heterogenous signal intensity of the slightly enlarged PCL (*arrow*), consistent with a tear. (From Yochum TR and Rowe LJ. Yochum and Rowe's Essentials of Skeletal Radiology, 3rd ed. Philadelphia, PA: Lippincott Williams & Wilkins, 2004.)

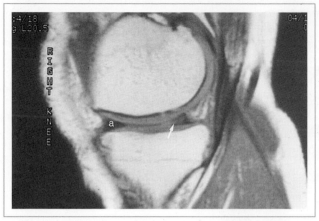

FIGURE 125.5: Sagittal T1-weighted spin-echo image of a medial meniscus depicts the normal anterior (A) horn as a diffusely low signal intensity triangular structure. The posterior horn contains linear intermediate signal extending to the inferior articular surface representing a tear (*arrow*). (From Koopman WJ and Moreland LW. Arthritis and Allied Conditions: A Textbook of Rheumatology, 15th ed. Philadelphia, PA: Lippincott Williams & Wilkins, 2005.)

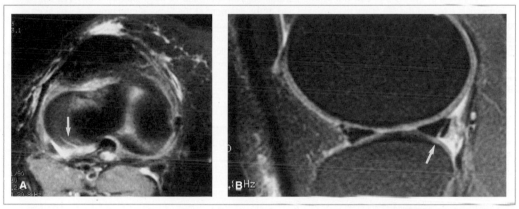

FIGURE 125.6: Tear of the lateral meniscus. **A:** An axial fast-spin-echo MRI shows a tear of the posterior horn of the lateral meniscus (*arrow*). **B:** A sagittal MRI confirms the presence of a tear (*arrow*). (From Greenspan A. Orthopedic Imaging: A Practical Approach, 4th ed. Philadelphia, PA: Lippincott Williams & Wilkins, 2004.)

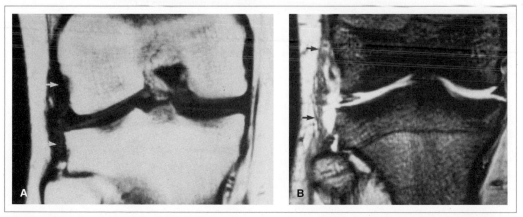

FIGURE 125.7: Tear of the lateral collateral ligament (*arrows*) can be seen on (**A**) T1-weighted and (**B**) T2-weighted coronal images. (From Greenspan A. Orthopedic Imaging: A Practical Approach, 4th ed. Philadelphia, PA: Lippincott Williams & Wilkins, 2004.)

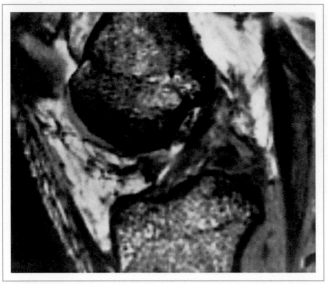

FIGURE 125.8: Tear of the anterior cruciate ligament (ACL). Sagittal spin-echo T2-weighted MRI (SE; TR 2000/TE 80 msec) shows a tear of the ACL. Only the proximal part of the ligament at the femoral attachment is well seen. The distal half shows lack of normal low signal intensity caused by swelling and edema. Arthroscopic examination demonstrated an acute tear of the ACL at its insertion to the tibia. (From Greenspan A. Orthopedic Imaging: A Practical Approach, 4th ed. Philadelphia, PA: Lippincott Williams & Wilkins, 2004.)

Treatment

- Analgesia
- Ice, elevation, rest
- Patients with suspected ligamentous or meniscal injuries may be discharged with the affected knee in a hinged knee brace (fully unlocked) and allowed to weight bear as tolerated
- Crutches may be needed
- Outpatient orthopedic surgery referral to facilitate MRI and physical therapy

Summary

TABLE 125.5: Advantages and disadvantages of imaging modalities in ligamentous and meniscal injuries of the knee

Imaging modalities	Advantages	Disadvantages
X-ray	Low cost Low radiation Rapid	Often unremarkable Pain with manipulation to obtain all views
MRI	Soft tissues clearly visualized Preoperative planning	Time-consuming Costly Availability Not required emergently

126

Lateral, Bimalleolar, and Trimalleolar Fractures

Ryan O'Neill and Brian Popko

Background

Lateral malleolar fractures result from ankle inversion and present similarly to the classic ankle sprain. Inversion injuries with a significant amount of force can result in fractures of both the lateral and medial malleoli. These injuries typically disrupt the surrounding ligamentous structures as well as the bony architecture. Approximately 20% of bimalleolar fractures are intra-articular. Because of the amount of force required to produce this injury, the incidence is lower than that of lateral malleolar fractures but the prognosis is significantly worse. Nonunion is reported in approximately 10% of bimalleolar fractures treated by closed reduction. Approximately 20% of intra-articular talar and tibial injuries will not heal properly with closed reduction. A trimalleolar fracture is a fracture of both the lateral and medial malleolus as well as the posterior malleolus, which is the distal posterior aspect of the tibia.

TABLE 126.1: Classic history and physical

Lateral malleolar fracture
Ankle inversion with or without "pop" sensation
Lateral malleolar tenderness
Tenderness over the anterior talofibular ligament
Ankle effusion
Lateral ankle ecchymosis
Difficulty ambulating

Bimalleolar fracture
Ankle inversion or eversion
Tenderness at medial and lateral malleolus
Tibia and fibula deformities
Ecchymosis common
Ankle effusion common
Ankle instability common
Inability to bear weight/ambulate
Neurovascular status rarely abnormal

Trimalleolar fracture
Talar inversion and posterior displacement injury
Tibia and fibula deformities and tenderness, joint
    dislocation may be present
Ankle unstable
Inability to bear weight/ambulate

Ankle X-ray

- Obtain anteroposterior (AP), lateral, and mortise views of the ankle
- Dedicated views of the tibia/fibula may also be helpful
- The Weber classification is used to describe fibula fractures:
  - Weber A: fracture distal to the ankle mortise; typically horizontal avulsion fractures; usually stable
  - Weber B: fracture at the level of the ankle mortise; may be stable or unstable depending on ligamentous injury and/or associated fractures to medial malleolus
  - Weber C: fracture proximal to the ankle mortise; usually unstable

 TABLE 126.2: X-ray: ankle fractures

IV contrast	No
PO contrast	No
Amount of radiation	mSv per view

Classic Images

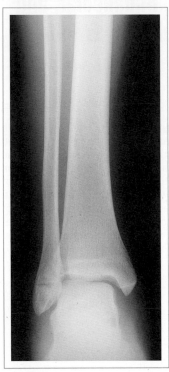

FIGURE 126.1: Anteroposterior radiograph of an isolated type A fibula fracture. (From Koval KJ and Zuckerman JD. Atlas of Orthopaedic Surgery: A Multimedia Reference. Philadelphia, PA: Lippincott Williams & Wilkins, 2004.)

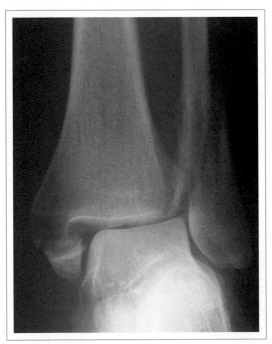

FIGURE 126.2: Type B ankle fracture in which the fibula fracture begins anteriorly at the level of the distal tibiofibular syndesmosis. (From Bucholz RW and Heckman JD. Rockwood and Green's Fractures in Adults, 5th ed. Philadelphia, PA: Lippincott Williams & Wilkins, 2001.)

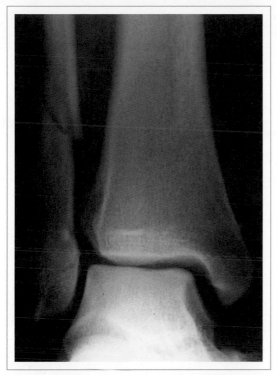

FIGURE 126.3: A mortise radiograph of a type C injury. The fibula fracture is completely above the distal syndesmotic ligament complex. (From Bucholz RW and Heckman JD. Rockwood and Green's Fractures in Adults, 5th ed. Philadelphia, PA: Lippincott Williams & Wilkins, 2001.)

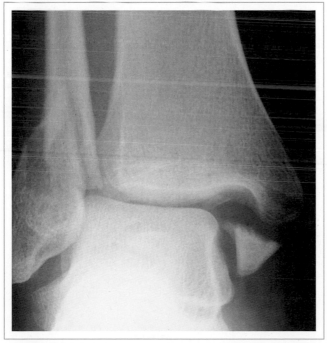

FIGURE 126.4: An anteroposterior radiograph of a bimalleolar fracture. (From Bucholz RW and Heckman JD. Rockwood and Green's Fractures in Adults, 5th ed. Philadelphia, PA: Lippincott Williams & Wilkins, 2001.)

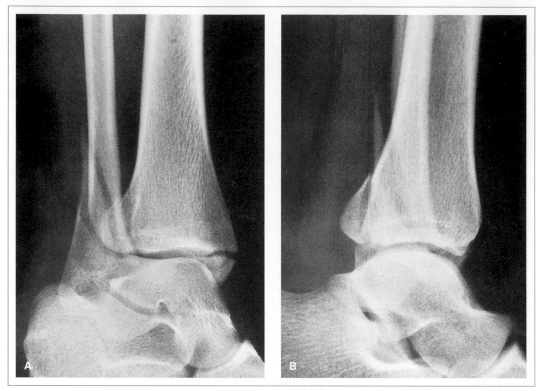

FIGURE 126.5: Trimalleolar fracture. Oblique (**A**) and lateral (**B**) radiographs of the ankle show a trimalleolar fracture affecting both malleoli and the posterior lip of the distal tibia. The latter feature is better seen on the lateral view. (From Greenspan A. Orthopedic Imaging: A Practical Approach, 4th ed. Philadelphia, PA: Lippincott Williams & Wilkins, 2004.)

Ankle CT Scan

- CT scan can further delineate fracture fragments and intra-articular involvement
- Useful in operative planning

 TABLE 126.3: CT scan: ankle fractures

IV contrast	No
PO contrast	No
Amount of radiation	mSv

Classic Image

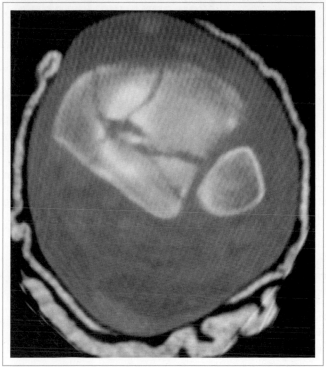

FIGURE 126.6: Transverse CT scan at the level of the tibial plafond type-C demonstrating an ankle fracture that is intermediate between a rotational injury and an axial loading injury. The medial malleolus fracture is vertical, and the fibular fracture is transverse, characteristic of a supination-adduction pattern. There is a large posterior malleolar component. The CT scan shows substantial intra-articular involvement, more characteristic of an axial loading tibial plafond fracture. (From Bucholz RW and Heckman JD. Rockwood and Green's Fractures in Adults, 5th ed. Philadelphia, PA: Lippincott Williams & Wilkins, 2001.)

Basic Management
- Analgesia
- Ice, elevation
- Lateral malleolar/fibular fracture
  - Weber A: air-stirrup splint, crutches (as needed), and outpatient orthopedic surgery referral
  - Weber B and C: orthopedic surgery consultation, posterior short leg splint with a sugar tong component; non-weight bearing and crutches
- Bimalleolar and Trimalleolar Fractures
  - Orthopedic surgery consultation, closed reduction with temporary placement of a posterior short leg splint with sugar tong component
  - Operative management is the preferred treatment

Summary

Table 126.4 Advantages and disadvantages of x-ray in malleolar fractures

Imaging Modalities	Advantages	Disadvantages
X-ray	Low cost Rapid Study of choice	Pain with manipulation to obtain all views
CT Scan	Soft tissue visualized Preoperative planning	Time consuming Greater radiation exposure Not required emergently

127

Maisonneuve Fracture

Ryan O'Neill and Brian Popko

Background

Common ankle sprains result from ankle inversion, and injuries to the lateral ligamentous complex are seen. However, the medial ligamentous structure (the deltoid ligament) is significantly stronger than its lateral counterparts and thus requires more force to produce injury. Such forces are seen with eversion of the ankle. Forces are transmitted across the interosseous membrane with residual energy resulting in a proximal fibular fracture. A true Maisonneuve fracture is an isolated proximal fibula fracture (commonly at the junction of the proximal and middle thirds of the shaft) while a Dupuytren's fracture is a Maisonneuve fracture with disruption of the ankle syndesmosis and medial collateral ligament.

TABLE 127.1: Classic history and physical

Eversion-type injury of the ankle
Tenderness at medial malleolus, syndesmosis, and proximal fibula
Ecchymosis
Ankle effusion
Potential ankle instability
Potential superficial, deep, or common peroneal nerve injuries
Potential anterior tibial artery injury

X-ray

- Obtain anteroposterior (AP)/lateral tibia and fibula; AP, lateral, and sunrise views of the knee; and AP, lateral, and mortise views of the ankle
- Widening of the tibiofibular syndesmosis without a fracture of the fibula is suggestive of a proximal fibula fracture
- There may be associated medial malleolus avulsion fracture or posterior malleolar fracture

 TABLE 127.2: Maisonneuve fracture

IV contrast	No
PO contrast	No
Amount of radiation	mSv per view

Classic Images

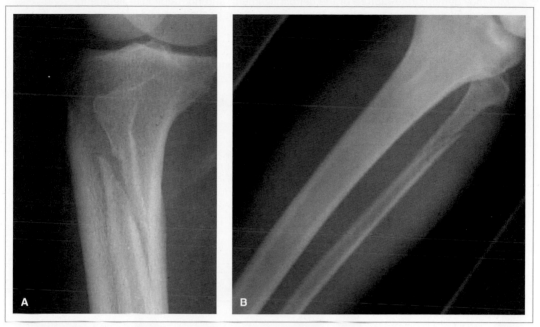

FIGURE 127.1: The AP (**A**) and lateral (**B**) tibia/fibula x-rays show a spiral fracture of the proximal fibula. (*X-rays courtesy of Richard H. Daffner, MD, Allegheny General Hospital, Pittsburgh, PA.*)

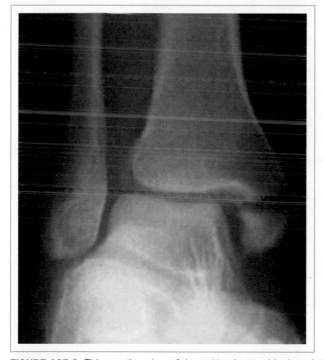

FIGURE 127.2: This mortise view of the ankle shows widening of the medial clear space, loss of the distal tibia-fibula overlap, and a medial malleolar fracture. This pattern is suggestive of a proximal fibula fracture. (*X-rays courtesy of Richard H. Daffner, MD, Allegheny General Hospital, Pittsburgh, PA.*)

MRI

- MRI may demonstrate rupture of the deltoid ligament, anterior talofibular ligament, calcaneofibular ligament, posterior talofibular ligament or syndesmotic ligaments
- There may be rupture of the interosseous membrane

 TABLE 127.3: MRI: Maisonneuve fracture

IV contrast	No
PO contrast	No
Amount of radiation	None

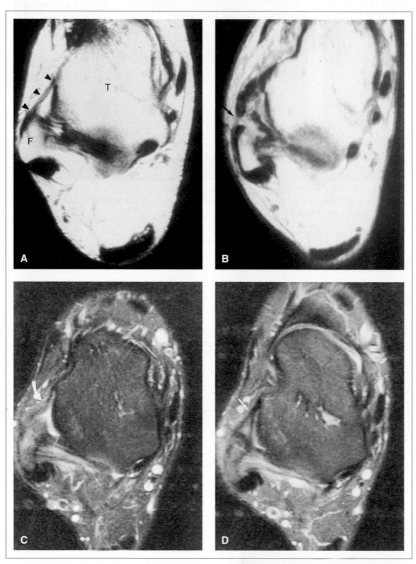

FIGURE 127.3: Magnetic resonance images of ligamentous integrity. **A:** Transverse T1-weighted spin-echo image of the ankle depicts the intact anterior talofibular ligament as a continuous low-signal intensity band (*arrowheads*). T, talus; F, fibula. **B:** Disrupted anterior talofibular ligament (*black arrow*) in another ankle appears thickened and discontinuous. **C:** Transverse fat-suppressed T2-weighted fast spin-echo imaging of another ankle in plantar flexion results in oblique sectioning and apparent discontinuity of the anterior talofibular ligament (*curved white arrow*). **D:** Repeat examination of the same ankle in dorsiflexion delineates an intact anterior talofibular ligament (*straight white arrow*). (From Koopman WJ and Moreland LW. Arthritis and Allied Conditions: A Textbook of Rheumatology, 15th ed. Philadelphia, PA: Lippincott Williams & Wilkins, 2005.)

Basic Management
- Analgesia
- Orthopedic surgery consultation
- Carefully attempt to reduce fracture if significantly displaced
- If the fracture is stable, the patient may be placed in a posterior leg splint (to the level of the mid quadriceps) and discharged with urgent outpatient orthopedic surgery referral
- Care should be taken to appropriately pad the proximal fibula when splinting to avoid damage to the peroneal nerve
- Rest, ice, elevation
- Strict non-weight bearing

Summary

TABLE 127.4: Advantages and disadvantages of imaging modalities in Maisonneuve fracture

Imaging modalities	Advantages	Disadvantages
X-ray	Immediate Low radiation	Unable to assess soft tissues Pain with manipulation to obtain views
MRI	Able to evaluate soft tissues No radiation	Time-consuming Costly Availability

128 Ankle Fracture and Dislocation

Joshua Ort and Mara Aloi

Background

The ankle joint is a modified saddle joint comprising the articulation of the talus with the mortise formed by the distal tibia and fibula. Dislocation of this joint is common and is frequently associated with concurrent fracture. Dislocations are described according to the direction of displacement of the talus in relation to the tibia, that is, posterior, anterior, medial, lateral, superior, or any combination thereof. Rapid assessment and reduction are necessary in these injuries to prevent neurovascular compromise.

TABLE 128.1: Complications of ankle fracture

Arterial injury (anterior tibial, posterior tibial, peroneal)
Entrapment of tendon(s) or fracture fragments
Osteochondral fractures of talar dome
Cartilaginous injury
Compartment syndrome (rare)
Decreased range of motion
Nonunion or malunion of fracture
Avascular necrosis of the talus
Synostosis

TABLE 128.2: Overview of fracture types

Posterior dislocation	Results from strong force applied to the posterior tibia in a posterior to anterior direction, usually when the foot is plantar flexed
	Associated with rupture of tibiofibular ligaments and/or malleolar fractures
	Foot will be held in plantar flexion and appear shortened
Anterior dislocation	Results from force causing posterior displacement of tibia on a fixed foot or forcible dorsiflexion of the foot
	Most commonly caused by deceleration injuries such as injuries such as motor vehicle collisions (MVCs)
	Associated with fracture of the anterior lip of the tibia and/or malleolar fractures
	Foot will be held in dorsiflexion and appear lengthened
Lateral/medial dislocations	Results from forced inversion or eversion of the foot, such as in contact sports
	Associated with malleolar and distal fibular fractures and deltoid ligament rupture
	Foot will be displaced laterally or medially with opposite skin tautness
Superior dislocation	Results from substantial axial force, such as landing on the feet after a fall from a significant height
	Associated with talar dome fracture and/or fracture of the tibial plafond
	Must evaluate for concomitant spinal injury
	Leg may appear shortened

X-ray

- Anteroposterior (AP), lateral, and mortise views of the ankle are required
- AP, lateral, and oblique views of the foot may be helpful
- AP and lateral views of the tibia/fibula may be helpful
- Look at the relationship of the talus to the distal tibia and fibula
- Look for symmetry/asymmetry on AP view of the mortise

 TABLE 128.3: X-ray: ankle fracture/dislocation

IV contrast	No
PO contrast	No
Amount of radiation	mSv per view

Classic Images

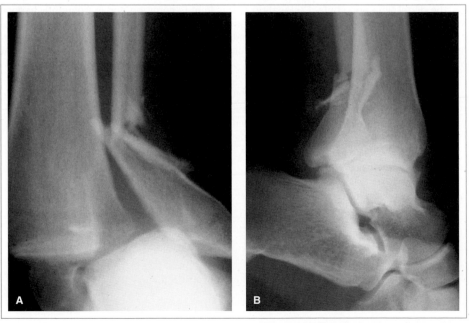

FIGURE 128.1: Fracture dislocation of the ankle. AP (**A**) and lateral (**B**) radiographs reveal lateral dislocation of the talus and comminuted fibular fracture. (From Bucholz RW and Heckman JD. Rockwood and Green's Fractures in Adults, 5th ed. Philadelphia, PA: Lippincott Williams & Wilkins, 2001.)

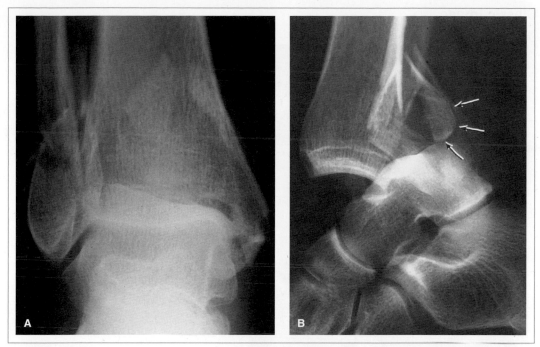

FIGURE 128.2: AP (**A**) and lateral (**B**) radiographs demonstrate a posterior fracture dislocation of the ankle. The arrows on the lateral radiograph indicate a posterior malleolar fracture. (From Buoholz RW and Heckman JD, Rockwood and Green's Fractures in Adults, 5th ed. Philadelphia, PA: Lippincott Williams & Wilkins, 2001.)

Ankle CT Scan
- CT is used to image complex fractures, especcially around joints because the area can be reconstructed in multiple planes
- Superior to x-ray in imaging small fracture fragments
- Not the test of choice since it may delay time to reduction
- Only to be considered at the request of the orthopedist in the absence of neurovascular compromise

 TABLE 128.4: CT: ankle fracture/dislocation

IV contrast	No
PO contrast	No
Amount of radiation	mSv

Classic Image

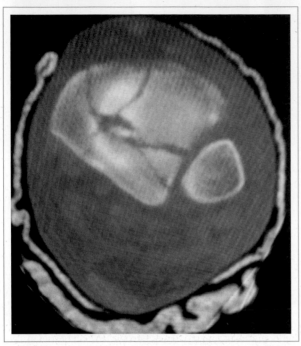

FIGURE 128.3: Transverse CT scan at the level of the tibial plafond shows substantial intra-articular involvement. (From Bucholz RW and Heckman JD. Rockwood and Green's Fractures in Adults, 5th ed. Philadelphia, PA: Lippincott Williams & Wilkins, 2001.)

Basic Management

- Evaluate for concomitant injuries in setting of trauma
- Neurovascular assessment must occur immediately as well as an assessment of tendon function
- Obtain prereduction radiographs if neurovascularly intact
- Emergent reduction of the dislocation in the setting of neurovascular compromise, for example, absent pulses, foot appears dusky
- Orthopedic consultation
  - Open dislocations
  - Superior dislocations
  - Neurovascular compromise
  - Inability to reduce dislocation after two to three attempts
- Pain control
- For open fractures apply wet, sterile dressing with gauze roll wrapping, administer antibiotics, and confirm tetanus immunization status
- Obtain postreduction radiographs and reassess and document postreduction neurovascular status
- Apply long-leg posterior splint with sugar tong component and provide crutches
- Arrange for orthopedic follow-up within 48–72 hours

Summary

TABLE 128.5: Advantages and disadvantages of imaging modalities in ankle fracture/dislocation

Imaging modalities	Advantages	Disadvantages
X-ray	Low cost Rapid Study of choice	Pain with manipulation to obtain all views
CT scan	Visualize complex fractures and small fracture fragments Preoperative planning	Radiation exposure Delayed time to reduction

129

Talus Fractures

Chuck Feronti

Background

The talus plays a major role in the complex motion of the foot and ankle, including dorsiflexion and plantar flexion (ankle) as well as inversion and eversion (subtalar joint). Tarsal fractures are uncommon as a whole. The talus is the only bone in the lower extremity with no muscular attachments. Accessory ossicles are found in 30% of the population and are often mistaken for fractures. Fortunately, neurovascular injuries are rarely associated with talar fractures as the posterior tibial nerve and artery are relatively protected by the flexor hallucis longus tendon. Fractures may involve the head, neck body, or posterior process of the talus with the neck being the most vulnerable site. Hawkins introduced a classification of talar neck fractures based on the blood supply and prognosis regarding healing, osteonecrosis, and need for operative repair.

TABLE 129.1: Classic history and physical

The patient may recall a "pop" sound or sensation at the time of injury
High-energy (falls and motor vehicle crashes) mechanisms involve hyperdorsiflexion of the foot or axial load through the talus
Low-energy (sports) mechanisms result in inversion or eversion of the subtalar joint; symptoms similar to traditional ankle sprains
Deformity, dorsal swelling and tenderness, ecchymosis, joint effusion of ankle
Ankle pain typically localizes at the syndesmosis rather than at the lateral malleolus/anterior talar fibular ligament
Normal inversion and eversion of the subtalar joint is at least 25 degrees in both directions. Ankle motion is often maintained; however, subtalar motion is often limited
Pain with flexion of the great toe should heighten suspicion for a posterior process fracture as the flexor hallucis longus tendon runs between the two tubercles of the posterior processes

X-ray

- Obtain anteroposterior, lateral, and 45 degree internal oblique views of the foot and anteroposterior, lateral, and mortise views of the ankle
- Overlapping structures make radiographs difficult to interpret and fractures are often minimally displaced
- Accessory ossicles have smooth, well-corticated edges compared to the jagged edge of fractures
- Talar alignment is best assessed on the anterior and oblique foot views
- The talar neck and subtalar joints are best evaluated on the mortise and the lateral ankle views
- The location of the fracture line relative to the lateral process of the talus (on a lateral foot x-ray) can differentiate fractures of the talar body from the talar neck injuries
- Fractures extending into or posterior to the lateral process are talar body fractures; injuries anterior to the lateral process are talar neck fractures
- Talar head fractures often involve the navicular and the talonavicular joint
- Lateral process fractures may be missed acutely and this injury should be considered in patients with ankle pain >3 months after presumed ankle sprain

 TABLE 129.2: X-ray: talus fracture

IV contrast	No
PO contrast	No
Amount of radiation	mSv per view

Classic Images

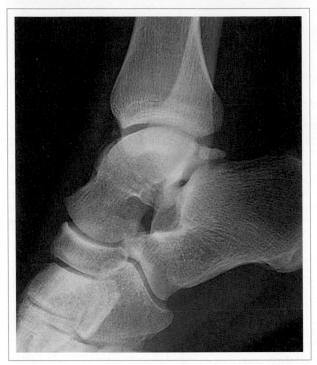

FIGURE 129.1: Lateral ankle x-ray showing talar fracture. (*Courtesy of Richard H. Daffner, MD, Allegheny General Hospital, Pittsburgh, PA.*)

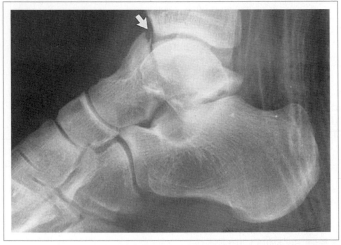

FIGURE 129.2: Vertical fracture line extending through the neck of the talus. (From Yochum TR and Rowe LJ. Yochum and Rowe's Essentials of Skeletal Radiology, 3rd ed. Philadelphia, PA: Lippincott Williams & Wilkins, 2004.)

CT Scan
- Overlapping structures make radiographs difficult to interpret and fractures are often minimally displaced; in these cases, CT scan will help to delineate injury

TABLE 129.3: CT scan: talus fracture

IV contrast	No
PO contrast	No
Amount of radiation	mSv

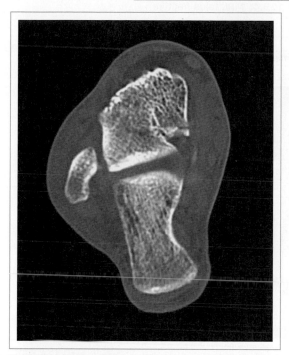

FIGURE 129.3: Axial CT image of a talus fracture. (*Courtesy of Richard H. Daffner, MD, Allegheny General Hospital, Pittsburgh, PA.*)

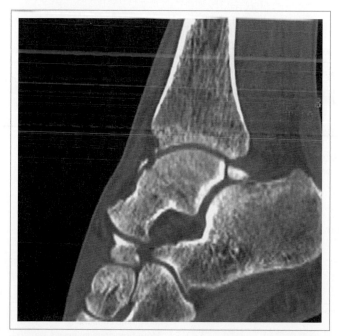

FIGURE 129.4: Sagittal CT image of a talus fracture. (*Courtesy of Richard H. Daffner, MD, Allegheny General Hospital, Pittsburgh, PA.*)

MRI

- Overlapping structures make radiographs difficult to interpret and fractures are often minimally displaced; in these cases, MRI will help to delineate injury
- MRI may also be used to evaluate for bone healing in patients with subacute or chronic pain

 TABLE 129.4: MRI: talus fracture

IV contrast	No
PO contrast	No
Amount of radiation	None

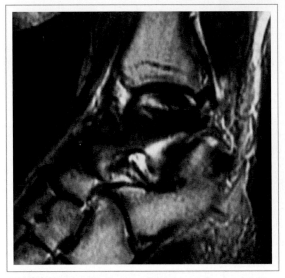

FIGURE 129.5: MRI of a type II talar neck fracture at 6 months. Note darker signal in talar body indicative of osteonecrosis. (From Bucholz RW and Heckman JD. Rockwood and Green's Fractures in Adults, 5th ed. Philadelphia, PA: Lippincott Williams & Wilkins, 2001.)

Basic Management

- Analgesia
- Assess and document the neurovascular status of the foot and ankle
- Reduce fractures causing neurovascular compromise
  - Flex the knee and plantar flex the foot to relax the gastrocnemius and soleus muscles; apply longitudinal traction and plantar flexion to the midfoot while stabilizing the hindfoot
- Orthopedic consultation
  - Displaced talar fractures
  - Open fractures
  - Fractures requiring reduction
- Minor talar fractures may be treated nonoperatively with a posterior leg splint with a sugar tong component and subsequent conversion to cast
- Strict non-weight bearing and outpatient orthopedic surgery referral in nonoperative cases

Summary

TABLE 129.5: Advantages and disadvantages of imaging modalities in talus fracture

Imaging modalities	Advantages	Disadvantages
X-ray	Readily available Low radiation Inexpensive	Pain due to manipulation to obtain all views Difficult to delineate because of overlapping structures
CT scan	Further delineates fracture for preoperative planning	Higher radiation More time-consuming
MRI	Gold standard Further delineates fracture for preoperative planning	More time-consuming

130

Calcaneus Fractures

Nathan Hemmer

Background

Calcaneal fractures are the most common tarsal bone fracture. The typical mechanism is axial loading, with falls from height landing onto the heels or a motor vehicle collision (MVC) with foot compression onto floorboards. There is a high rate of concomitant injuries including fractures of the contralateral leg (20%), spinal compression fractures (10%), and bilateral calcaneal fractures (9%). Compartment syndrome is relatively common (10–50%) and should be suspected with pain out of proportion to injury, tense swelling, weakness with toe flexion, or pain with passive dorsiflexion of the toes.

TABLE 130.1: Classic history and physical

Fall from height onto heels or motor vehicle collision
Pain/swelling over the heel
Unable to weight bear
Ecchymosis
Fracture blisters

Foot X-ray

- Emergency department (ED) physicians carefully reviewing films have very good accuracy (98%) in diagnosing calcaneal fractures without the aid of Bohler's angle or critical angle of Gissane
- Although imperfect (especially in severe compression) Bohler's angle (normal ~20–40 degrees) is useful in demonstrating fractures
- Bohler's angle is formed at the intersection of a line connecting the posterior tuberosity of the calcaneus and the apex of the posterior facet of the calcaneus and a line between the apex of the posterior facet and the apex of the anterior process of the calcaneus
- The critical angle of Gissane (normal 100–145 degrees) is not useful in diagnosing fractures. It is formed by two cortical struts that form an angle inferior to the lateral process of the talus. The first strut extends along the lateral border of the posterior facet and the second extends anterior to the beak of the calcaneus
- Intra-articular fractures have a poor prognosis in 25% of cases, whereas extra articular fractures have a good prognosis in 75% of cases
- The Harris view and Broden's view are additional x-rays used for visualizing the subtalar joint

 TABLE 130.2: Foot x-ray: calcaneus fracture

IV contrast	No
PO contrast	No
Amount of radiation	mSv per view

Classic Images

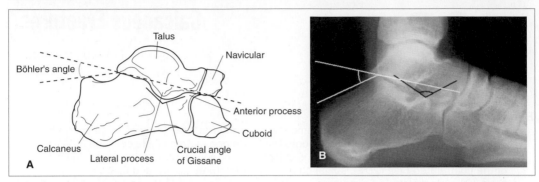

FIGURE 130.1: A: Schematic lateral anatomy of the calcaneus with surrounding structures. Note the angle of Bohler and the crucial angle of Gissane. **B:** Standing lateral radiograph of the same structures with the angles of Bohler and Gissane depicted. (From Bucholz RW and Heckman JD. Rockwood and Green's Fractures in Adults, 5th ed. Philadelphia, PA: Lippincott Williams & Wilkins, 2001.)

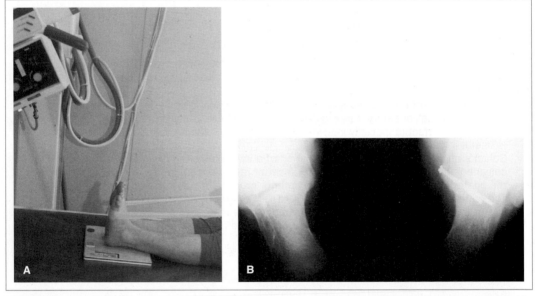

FIGURE 130.2: A: Photograph of the radiographic technique for obtaining the Harris or calcaneal radiographic view. Maximum dorsiflexion of the ankle is attempted to obtain an optimal view. **B:** Calcaneal views of bilateral calcanei. Normal is on the left; intra-articular fixation of sustentaculum fracture is on the right. (From Bucholz RW and Heckman JD. Rockwood and Green's Fractures in Adults, 5th ed. Philadelphia, PA: Lippincott Williams & Wilkins, 2001.)

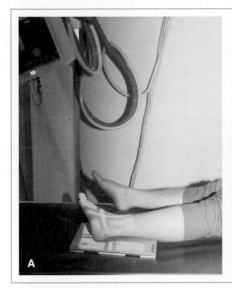
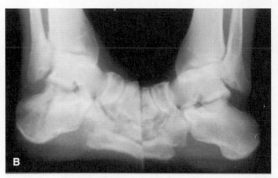

FIGURE 130.3: A: Photograph of the technique to obtain Broden's view for a direct view of the posterior facet of the subtalar joint. **B:** Corresponding radiograph of bilateral Broden's views depicting normal and pathologic anatomy of the calcaneus and the subtalar joint. (From Bucholz RW and Heckman JD. Rockwood and Green's Fractures in Adults, 5th ed. Philadelphia, PA: Lippincott Williams & Wilkins, 2001.)

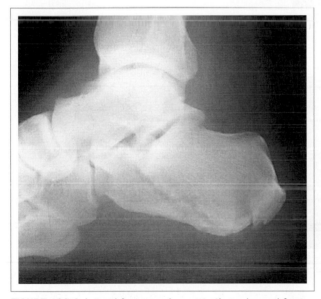

FIGURE 130.4: Lateral foot x-ray demonstrating calcaneal fracture. (*Courtesy of Richard H. Daffner, MD, Allegheny General Hospital, Pittsburgh, PA.*)

Calcaneal CT Scan

- If clinical suspicion is high and x-rays show no fracture, order a CT scan
- An ankle CT scan may be useful for any calcaneal fracture to further define fracture lines

 TABLE 130.3: CT scan: calcaneus fracture

IV contrast	No
PO contrast	No
Amount of radiation	mSv

Classic Images

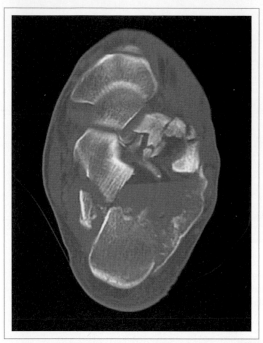

FIGURE 130.5: Axial CT image showing calcaneal fracture with lipohemarthrosis. (*Courtesy of Richard H. Daffner, MD, Allegheny General Hospital, Pittsburgh, PA.*)

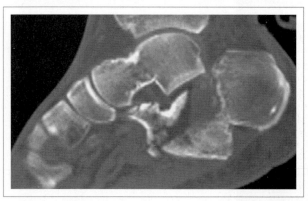

FIGURE 130.6: Sagittal CT image showing calcaneal fracture. (*Courtesy of Richard H. Daffner, Allegheny General Hospital, Pittsburgh, PA.*)

Basic Management
- Evaluate for concomitant injuries in setting of trauma
- Look for associated injuries, including, contralateral calcaneus, tibial plateau, lumbar spine
- Evaluate for compartment syndrome and open/tented fractures
- Evaluate for neurovascular deficits
- Pain management
- Apply ice, elevation, and a bulky dressing (posterior splint with sugar tong component)
- Strictly non-weight bearing
- Orthopedic consultation:
  - Compartment syndrome
  - Intra-articular and displaced calcaneal fractures
  - Expectant management

- Fasciotomy should be performed if compartment pressures are elevated (>30 mm Hg or within 10–30 mm Hg of diastolic blood pressure)
■ Disposition of the patient depends upon associated injuries and type of fracture

Summary

TABLE 130.4: Advantages and disadvantages of imaging modalities in calcaneus fractures

Imaging modalities	Advantages	Disadvantages
X-ray	Low cost Rapid Study of choice Imaging of small fracture fragments	Pain with manipulation to obtain all views Radiation exposure
CT scan	Preoperative planning Higher sensitivity	Higher cost Higher radiation exposure

131

Lisfranc Injury

Adarsh Srivastava and Moira Davenport

Background

Jacques Lisfranc, a French physician and field surgeon in Napoleon's army, was the first person to describe the anatomy of the Lisfranc joint as well as associated injuries.

The Lisfranc joint is made up of the articulations of the bases of the first three metatarsals with their respective cuneiforms as well as the fourth and fifth metatarsals with the cuboid. The complex bony and ligamentous anatomy of this joint allow supination and pronation of the forefoot. The Lisfranc ligament holds the metatarsal bases in place, maintaining the arch of the foot and anchoring the metatarsals to the rest of the body. Lisfranc fracture-dislocation is rare, occurring in less than 1% of all fractures and having an incidence of approximately 1 per 55,000 persons per year. These fractures are often overlooked because of the difficulty in assessing radiographs. Misdiagnosis has been reported to occur in approximately 20% of all cases.

TABLE 131.1: Classic history and physical

Axial load to a plantar flexed foot (e.g., stepping off a curb, high-velocity injury after high-speed motor vehicle crash)
Midfoot swelling
Midfoot pain
Tenderness to palpation over the tarsometatarsal area
Pain with passive pronation of the forefoot
Difficulty ambulating
Plantar ecchymosis

TABLE 131.2: Lisfranc fracture-dislocation patterns

Homolateral injury (all four metatarsals are displaced laterally)
Isolated dislocation (the first metatarsal is dislocated medially)
Divergent pattern (the first metatarsal is displaced medially and the second to fifth metatarsals move laterally
Associated injuries: metatarsophalangeal (MTP) joint dislocation, cuboid fractures, cuneiform fractures, and navicular fractures

Foot X-ray

- Obtain anteroposterior, lateral, and oblique views of the foot
- Weight bearing and non-weight bearing views should be performed
- The anteroposterior view demonstrates widening of the space between the first and second metatarsal heads when a Lisfranc disruption is present; gross displacement of more than 2 mm or a fleck sign (presence of a bony fragment) clearly indicates the need for operative stabilization
- Fracture of the second metatarsal base is virtually pathognomic of occult tarsometatarsal joint disruption
- The contour between the second metatarsal and the middle cuneiform is normally smooth
- The medial cortex of the fourth metatarsal should line up with the medial cortex of the cuboid in the oblique view
- Fractures of the cuboid, cuneiforms, navicular or metatarsal shafts are suggestive of disarticulation of the tarsometatarsal joint
- Weight bearing films may demonstrate Lisfranc joint subluxation as the bones separate when force is applied
- Comparison radiographs of the contralateral foot may be helpful in detecting subtle injuries
- Foot x-ray series may appear normal in up to 50% of patients with Lisfranc injuries, even when the injury is significant

 TABLE 131.3: Foot x-ray: Lisfranc injury

IV contrast	No
PO contrast	No
Amount of radiation	mSv per view

Classic Images

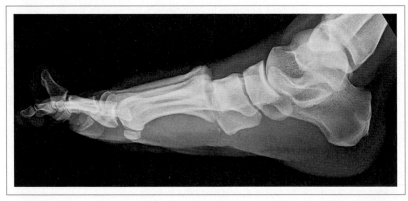

FIGURE 131.1: Lateral x-ray of the foot showing Lisfranc injury. (*Courtesy of Richard H. Daffner, MD, Allegheny General Hospital, Pittsburgh, PA.*)

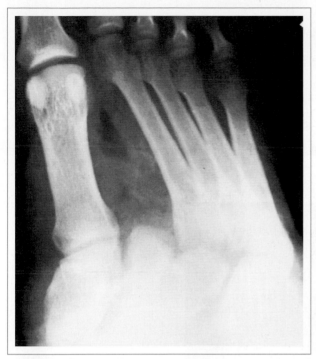

FIGURE 131.2: Lisfranc injury. Gross lateral displacement of the second through fifth metatarsals. (From Eisenberg RL. An Atlas of Differential Diagnosis, 4th ed. Philadelphia, PA: Lippincott Wllllams & Wilkins, 2003.)

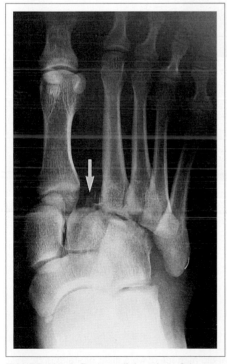

FIGURE 131.3: Fracture-dislocation of the tarsometatarsal joint (Lisfranc injury). The second through fifth metatarsals are dislocated laterally, with widening of the first to second intermetatarsal space. A small avulsed bone fragment from the medial base of the second metatarsal at the site of ligamentous insertion is visible (*arrow*). (From Yochum TR and Rowe LJ. Yochum and Rowe's Essentials of Skeletal Radiology, 3rd ed. Philadelphia, PA: Lippincott Williams & Wilkins, 2004.)

Foot CT Scan

- Foot CT scan series may appear normal in up to 50% of patients with Lisfranc injuries, even when the injury is significant
- CT scan or MRI can be obtained if the index of suspicion is high for Lisfranc injury despite normal radiographs

 TABLE 131.4: Foot CT scan: Lisfranc injury

IV contrast	No
PO contrast	No
Amount of radiation	mSv

Classic Images

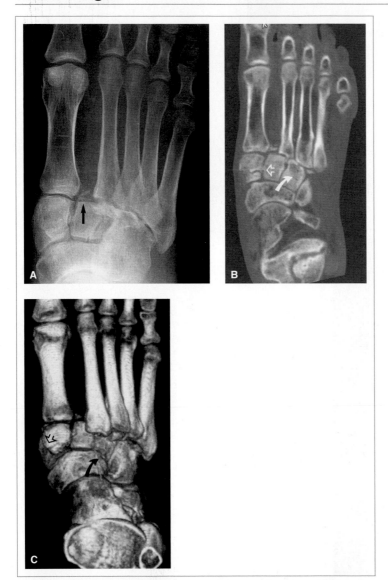

FIGURE 131.4: CT scan of a Lisfranc fracture-dislocation. A 54-year-old man fell down a flight of stairs and injured his left foot. Dorsoplantar radiograph (**A**) shows typical appearance of divergent Lisfranc fracture-dislocation. A small fractured fragment from the base of the second metatarsal is well seen (*arrow*). CT reformatted image in axial (transverse) plane (**B**) and three-dimensional CT (**C**) demonstrate an unsuspected fracture of the medial (*open arrow*) and lateral (*curved arrow*) cuneiform bones. (From Greenspan A. Orthopedic Imaging: A Practical Approach, 4th ed. Philadelphia, PA: Lippincott Williams & Wilkins, 2004.)

Treatment

- Analgesia
- Assess and document a neurovascular examination: a critical branch of the dorsalis pedis artery dives between the first and second metatarsals to form the plantar arch
- Manipulation of the foot should be kept to a minimum to prevent further displacement
- Emergent orthopedic consultation
- Immobilize foot in a posterior leg splint with a sugar tong component
- Strict non-weight bearing, rest, and elevation

Summary

TABLE 131.5: Advantages and disadvantages of imaging modalities in Lisfranc injury

Imaging modalities	Advantages	Disadvantages
X-ray	Fast Low radiation	Difficult to interpret May miss injury Pain from manipulation to obtain all views
CT scan	Better delineation of fracture soft tissue injuries Operative planning	Radiation

132   Jones and Pseudo-Jones Fractures

Adarsh Srivastava and Moira Davenport

Background

The base of the fifth metatarsal is commonly injured during inversion of the foot, particularly when the foot is in plantar flexion. A tuberosity avulsion fracture (pseudo-Jones) is the most common fracture of the midfoot. Two possible mechanisms of injury have been postulated: forceful contraction of the peroneus brevis and contracture of the lateral band of the plantar fascia. Current studies suggest that both play a role in this injury. A Jones fracture is a transverse fracture of the proximal diaphysis, occurring at least 15 mm distal to the proximal end of the fifth metatarsal. The tuberosity is not involved in this injury. Multiple mechanisms of injury are possible, including vertical or mediolateral forces exerted on the base of the fifth metatarsal while the heel is raised and the foot is plantar flexed and significant adduction force applied to the forefoot while the ankle is in plantar flexion. These injuries are frequently overlooked because forcible inversion injury usually causes more noticeable symptoms in the ankle.

TABLE 132.1: Classic history and physical

Inversion injury of the foot
Tenderness along the fifth metatarsal
Edema
Ecchymosis
Ankle effusion rare
Anterior talofibular ligament tenderness rare
Ankle and subtalar motion preserved
Able to ambulate

Foot X-ray

- Obtain anteroposterior (AP), lateral, and oblique views of the foot
- AP, lateral, and mortise views of the ankle should be performed if high suspicion for fracture and foot series shows no abnormality
- Pseudo-Jones fractures are an avulsion fracture of the tuberosity at the base of the fifth metatarsal proximal to the articulation between the bases of the fourth and fifth metatarsals
- Tuberosity fractures do not extend into the joint between the fourth and fifth metatarsals
- Pseudo-Jones fractures exit at the cuboid-fifth metatarsal articulation
- Jones fractures occur at least 15 mm distal to the proximal end of the metatarsal
- Jones fractures cross to the medial side of the metatarsal and exit the intermetatarsal facet

 TABLE 132.2: Foot x-ray: pseudo-Jones and Jones fracture

IV contrast	No
PO contrast	No
Amount of radiation	mSv per view

Classic Images

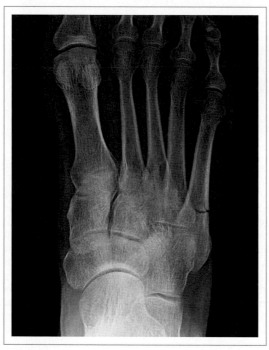

FIGURE 132.1: AP foot x-ray showing Jones fracture. (*Courtesy of Richard H. Daffner, MD, Allegheny General Hospital, Pittsburgh, PA.*)

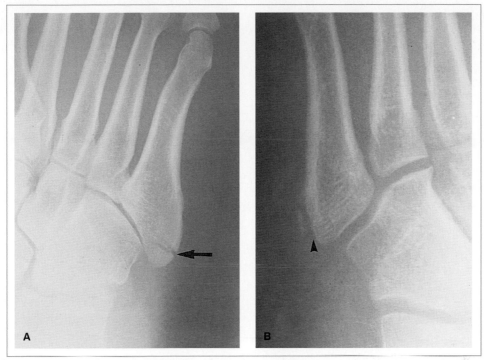

FIGURE 132.2: A: Pseudo-Jones fracture. The transverse orientation of the fracture line of the base of the fifth metatarsal (*arrow*) is demonstrated. **B:** Normal variation. The apophysis for the base of the fifth metatarsal is separated by a longitudinally oriented lucent cleft (*arrowhead*). With skeletal maturation, this radiolucent cleft will eventually ossify and become united to the base of the fifth metatarsal. (From Yochum TR and Rowe LJ. Yochum and Rowe's Essentials of Skeletal Radiology, 3rd ed. Philadelphia, PA: Lippincott Williams & Wilkins, 2004.)

Basic Management
- Pain control
- The treatments of Jones and pseudo-Jones fractures differ based on the variation in blood supply to different areas of the metatarsal

   Pseudo-Jones
   - The tuberosity has a good blood supply and therefore these fractures can heal with the patient bearing weight on the foot
   - Apply a hard-soled shoe
   - Outpatient orthopedic surgery referral

   Jones
   - The diaphysis has a relatively poor blood supply and a higher rate of malunion or nonunion. Internal fixation is often required
   - Immobilization in a posterior splint
   - Strict non-weight bearing
   - Close outpatient orthopedic surgery referral (3–5 days)
   - Immobilization for up to 6 months may be required for complete healing
   - Immediate fixation may be advisable in the competitive athlete

Summary

TABLE 132.3: Advantages and disadvantages of x-ray in Jones/pseudo-Jones fractures

Advantages	Disadvantages
Low cost	Pain with manipulation to obtain all views
Rapid	
Study of choice	

Index

Note: Page numbers followed by f and t indicates figure and table respectively.